W9-DJH-753

Walter Hruby (ed.)

Digital (R)Evolution in Radiology

Bridging the Future of Health Care

Second, revised and enlarged edition

SpringerWienNewYork

Univ.-Prof. Dr. Walter Hruby
Chairman, Department of Radiology, Danube Hospital, Vienna, Austria

Printed in Austria
SpringerWienNewYork is a part of
Springer Science + Business Media
springeronline.com

Typesetting: Scientific Publishing Services (P) Ltd., Madras
Printing: Druckerei Theiss GmbH, 9431 St. Stefan, Austria

Cover photo: Michael Mysik

Printed on acid-free and chlorine-free bleached paper
SPIN: 10981337

With numerous (partly coloured) Figures

Library of Congress Control Number: 2005927418

ISBN-10 3-211-20815-1 SpringerWienNewYork
ISBN-13 978-3-211-20815-1 SpringerWienNewYork
ISBN 3-211-83410-9 1st edition SpringerWienNewYork

Preface of the second edition

Since the first edition of "Digital (r)evolution in radiology" in 2001 several half-time cycles in the information- and computertechnology have passed with the well known implications on the fast ageing of these technologies. But while technological issues in Digital Radiology for the users, planners and decision makers become less important, while questions of practice and routine work as well as the wise application of information technology in health care become burning. It are these questions to which this book will provide solid answers. Due to the large and positive response the first edition of this book has received worldwide the publisher invited me to work on a second edition–a task which I gladly accepted.

In contrary to the first edition this revised and enlarged issue broadens and deepens the scope of digital radiology within a networked healthcare environment with its only one constant parameter: the continuous change. E-health has become a worldwide matter of importance and its challenges must be met if radiology has to survive. This includes not only new concepts of digital radiology concerning workflow, but also of cost-effectiveness matters. Furthermore the implementation and use of teleradiology and telemedicine raises new questions to the medical profession.

More than ever before we have to face medical responsibility within an always tighter legal environment and an increasing spread of health care. Interface and integration management of medical systems as well as migration from one system to the other is equally important as new advances in radiological modalities.

This book claims high demands on dealing with these issues, which are grouped into following categories:

1. Basics of Digital Radiology
2. Planning Digital Radiology
3. Applications and Methods
4. Economical and investment issues
5. Ethical implications

It is primarily the perspective of the planner and the user from which these issues are dealt with. So the practical approach is favoured versus a pure theoretical or technical approach. This concept has proven to be very successful for the first edition, so it will be kept for this revised and enlarged edition as well.

Innovations in information technology are shown to improve the quality of health care in particular facing an ever more increasing generation of medical data of various sources from within and outside radiology. While the public opinion very much overestimates the costs of radiology and information technology in health care, the focus must be set to communicate the improvements of the quality in health care which has direct effects on patients. This book informs and guides the reader through this rapid changing issue of the application of information technology in healthcare.

Vienna, June 2005 *W. Hruby*

Preface of the first edition

Three decades have passed since my first personal experiences, influences and contacts with computer applications in the field of medicine. These experiences were influenced by diverse presentations, publications and seminars concerning various applications of information technology as early as in 1970 (Univac International Executive Centre, Rome). The first clinical proposals and discussions during the first "World Congress of Intensive Care Medicine" (London 1974) strongly impressed me, since they demonstrated that the future of medicine would be changed rapidly by the use of computer technology.

In 1975, when I started my radiology residency, my clinical and academic interests were focused on two major topics: (i) interventional radiology and the clinical responsibility of the radiologist for the patient and (ii) the improvement of radiological services for both the clinician and the patient through the use of digital technology. These two topics, firstly interventional radiology and, secondly, computer technology along with all digital techniques developed in respect to examinations and modalities have been the basis for my "personal evolution" of medicine, especially of digital radiology.

In the late 1970s, my interests were focused on how digital modalities such as computertomography, digital subtraction angiography and the first clinical use of Hospital Information Systems (HIS) and Radiology Information Systems (RIS) were the initial changes in the way radiological examinations were performed. More and more clinical indications for radiological examinations and interventional procedures forced radiologists to use adequate technology to communicate online i.e. to electronically exchange examinations and reports and to be virtually available not only near the modalities but in the entire hospital.

In the early 1980s, with the first PACS-Conference (Ronald Arenson, AJ. Duerinckx, Samuel Dwyer III, H.K. Huang, Gerald Qu. Maguire jun. and M.P. Zeleznik), and the establishment of the CAR (Computer Assisted Radiology) by Prof. H.U. Lemke, I was pleased to know, that the basic technical research work in telematic technology was shifted to user-driven and user-orientated developments.

In 1988 when all chairmen had been appointed and designated to build the Danube Hospital in the Sociomedical Care Center East in Vienna, I strongly supported the decision made to design, develop and implement a filmless digital radiology department in a digital hospital. The aims, goals and objectives of 1988 have remained the same until today: to improve the quality of patient care, to overcome inherent problems of film-based systems, to improve the efficiency of patient data management, of image acquisition, image distribution, archiving, teaching, research, quality assurance, communication, and to create synergistic effects for an efficient and sufficient healthcare network. Additionally, to generate online communication and consequently integrate dose reduction, decreasing hospitalization time, speeding up the therapeutic reaction time by speeding up the report turn around time. In summary, to improve radiological services.

From the vision in 1988 to implementation in 1991 and since the opening of the hospital in 1992 until now (September 2000) 450,000 patients have been admitted to the hospital and 3,500,000 outpatients have been treated. 1,170,000 patients have undergone radiological examinations and procedures in this filmless radiology department. Since then, many publications, presentations, workshops and many visitors demonstrated that we went beyond all segments and limitations with dynamic progress to develop the system into an integrated health care enterprise.

Many people have contributed to the digital (r)evolution in radiology, and it is a great honor as an editor that most of them contributed to this book. In addition, all the other experts in this field who were not able to contribute for various reasons have influenced and guided our approach in many common conferences and personal discussions and visits. Our philosophy of improving the patient-orientated medical care from an ethical and sociomedical-legal, but also from an "electronic" point of view have been profoundly influenced by all these events and personal contacts and friendships.

The authors who are outstanding in their clinical and scientific work in digital radiology will share with you their knowledge and their expertise in the chapters following. Therefore this book consists of profound information provided by these outstanding radiologists and scientists. You will learn a variety of individual and different steps to transmit and handle the knowledge of information technology, digital radiography, hospital information systems, radiological information systems, digital archiving, teleconsultation, virtual reality, the integrated health care enterprise, the benefits of the World Wide Web and so on.

This book will address a wider audience than only radiologists or physicists, but also hospital administrators, health care consultants, insurance companies, and state and city administrators. Altogether the target audience consists of all readers reflecting on current trends and future aspects of digital radiology.

In accordance with our Hippocratic oath of improving health care with low risk at reasonable costs this book should be a little help fur further steps and implementations.

Vienna, September 2000 *W. Hruby*

Acknowledgments

I wish to express my sincere gratitude to all my staff for the encouragement to pursue this project. I would also like to express my deep gratitude to Mr. Dr. H. Mosser and Mr. Dipl.Ing. A. Maltsidis and all my staff members for their organizational skills and their enthusiasm, since their initial editing provided the framework for the entire book. I also want to acknowledge the superb editing and extraordinary patience of Mr. Petri-Wieder, Mrs. Dr. Kienast and Mrs. Mag. Eichhorn of Springer-Verlag. I want to offer special thanks to all authors who spontaneously accepted to contribute to this book and delivered their chapters professionally, well-prepared and on time.

It is a pleasure to express my long-standing gratitude to the Administration of the City of Vienna, the Mayor of Vienna Mr. Dr. M. Häupl, the former Mayor of Vienna Mr. Dr. H. Zilk, former Health councillor Prof. Dr. A. Stacher, city councillor and vice Mayor Mr. Dr. Sepp Rieder and Mrs. Prim. Dr. E. Pittermann MD and Mrs. Dr. R. Brauner, health councillor, and the former hospital administration of Vienna Mr. Prof. Eugen Hauke and Mr. Dr. L. Kaspar and Chairman of the KAV Mr. Dr. W. Marhold and Mr. DI J. Kastl and Mrs. S. Herbeck and for all the encouragement and support from Mr. Prim.Univ.-Prof. Dr. K. H. Tragl and Mr. AR W. Reinagl, the former Board of Chairman at the Danube Hospital, Chairman of the board Mr. Prim. Dr. Christian Sebesta, Technical Director Mr. DI M. Führer, Chair of the Nursing Department Mrs. J. Stich, Chairman of the Administration Mr. OAR G. Rudy and Members of the Administration Mrs. H. Schuh, Mrs. Ing. Kanzian, Mrs. D. Föda, Mrs. S. Kocher and Mrs. S. Schober.

I would like to take this opportunity to extend my thanks to the secretary of the department, Mrs. Wimmer and Mrs. Hudetz.

Above all I would like to express my love and sincere thanks to my children Stephan, Lukas, Lisa, Laura and my wife, Elke, for their understanding and support and their way of dealing with my busy clinical, scientific, administrative and congress schedule.

Contents

Contributors

Appel W., M.D., Kaiser Franz Josef Hospital, Kundratstrasse 3, 1100 Vienna, Austria

Backfrieder W., Ph.D., Department of Biomedical Engineering and Physics, University of Vienna, Austria, Vienna University Hospital, Währinger Gürtel 18-20, 1090 Vienna, Austria

Baldauf-Sobez W., M.D., Vice President, Siemens Health Services GmbH & Co. KG, Henkestrasse 127, 91052 Erlangen, Germany

Bale R., M.D., Interdisciplinary Stereotactic Interventions and Planning Laboratory Innsbruck (SIP-Laboratory), Medical University Innsbruck, Department of Radiology I, Anichstrasse 35, 6020 Innsbruck, Austria

Bautz W., M.D., Prof., Department of Radiology, Friedrich-Alexander-University Erlangen-Nürnberg, Maximiliansplatz 1, 91054 Erlangen, Germany

Bocionek S., Ph.D., General Manager, PACS Division, Siemens Health Services GmbH & Co. KG, Henkestrasse 127, 91052 Erlangen, Germany

Bulirsch R., Ph.D., Department of Mathematics (SCB), University of Technology, 80290 Munich, Germany

Clarke L. C., Ph.D., Cancer Imaging Program, National Cancer Institute, 6130 Execitive Blvd. MSC 7412, Bethesda, MD 20892-7412, USA

Dapra D., Department of Nuclear Medicine and Endocrinology, PET Centre, LKH Klagenfurt, St. Veiterstrasse 47, 9020 Klagenfurt, Austria

Diemling M., Department of Nuclear Medicine, PET Centre, Vienna University Hospital, Währinger Gürtel 18-20, 1090 Vienna, Austria

Edmunds D., M.D., M.P.H., Department of Radiology, Brigham and Women's Hospital, 75 Francis Street, Boston, MA 02115, USA

Engel A., M.D., Prof., Orthopaedic Department at the Socio-Medical Care Centre East/Danube Hospital, Langobardenstrasse 122, 1220 Vienna, Austria

Fellner F. A., M.D., Univ.-Doz., Central Radiology Institute, General Hospital (AKH), Krankenhausstrasse 9, 4021 Linz, Austria

Geiger B., Siemens Corporate Research Princeton Inc., 755 College Road, East Princeton, NJ 08540-6632, USA

Gell G., Ph.D., Institute for Medical Informatics, Statistics and Documentation, Engelgasse 13, 8010 Graz, Austria

Grosinger H., Mag., EDP-Management and Operation Management Centre, PM-CC, Viehmarktgasse 4, 1030 Vienna, Austria

Hanel R., M.D., Department of Radiology, Vienna University Hospital, Währinger Gürtel 18-20, 1090 Vienna, Austria

Hermann K.-P., Department of Radiology, Friedrich-Alexander-University Erlangen-Nürnberg, Maximiliansplatz 1, 91054 Erlangen, Germany

Hermann S., Ph.D., Univ.-Doz., Ministry of Traffic, Innovation and Technology, Radetzkystrasse 2, 1030 Vienna, Austria

Hruby W., M.D., Prof., Chairman of the Radiology Department at the Socio-Medical Care Centre East/Danube Hospital, Langobardenstrasse 122, 1220 Vienna, Austria

Hurley G. D., M.D., F.R.C.R., F.F.R.R.C.S.I., Consultant Radiologist, The Adelaide & Meath Hospitals Inc., The National Children's Hospital, Tallaght, Dublin 24, Ireland

Imhof H., M.D., Prof., Department of Radiology, Vienna University Hospital, Währinger Gürtel 18-20, 1090 Vienna, Austria

Kettenbach J., M.D., Prof., Department of Radiology, Vienna University Hospital, Währinger Gürtel 18-20, 1090 Vienna, Austria

Khorasani R., M.D., Department of Radiology, Brigham and Women's Hospital, 75 Francis Street, Boston, MA 02115, USA

Krampla W., M.D., Radiology Department at the Socio-Medical Care Centre East/Danube Hospital, Langobardenstrasse 122, 1220 Vienna, Austria

Kristen K.-H., M.D., Orthopaedic Department at the Socio-Medical Care Centre East/Danube Hospital, Langobardenstrasse 122, 1220 Vienna, Austria

Kumpan W., M.D., Univ.-Doz., Kaiser Franz Josef Hospital, Kundratstrasse 3, 1100 Vienna, Austria

Lind P., M.D., Univ.-Doz., Department of Nuclear Medicine and Endocrinology, PET Centre, LKH Klagenfurt, St. Veiterstrasse 47, 9020 Klagenfurt, Austria

Lindbichler F., M.D., Division of Digital Information and Image Processing, Department of Radiology, University Hospital Graz, Auenbruggerplatz 34, 8036 Graz, Austria

Lorang T., Ph.D., Department of Medical Computer Science, University of Vienna, Austria

Maltsidis A., DI, System Administrator at the Radiology Department, Siemens AG Austria, MED SHS, Erdberger Lände 26, 1031 Vienna, Austria

Mayrhofer R., M.D., Radiology Department at the Socio-Medical Care Centre East/Danube Hospital, Langobardenstrasse 122, 1220 Vienna, Austria

McInerney D. P., M.D., F.R.C.P.I., F.R.C.R., F.F.R.R.C.S.I., Consultant Radiologist, The Adelaide & Meath Hospitals Inc., The National Children's Hospital, Tallaght, Dublin 24, Ireland

Mohadjer D., M.D., Division of Digital Information and Image Processing, Department of Radiology, University Hospital Graz, Auenbruggerplatz 34, 8036 Graz, Austria

Mühlbauer M., M.D., Prof., Chairman, Department of Neurosurgery at the Socio-Medical Care Centre East/ Danube Hospital, Langobardenstrasse 122, 1220 Vienna, Austria

Nedden D. zur, M.D., Prof., Department of Radiology II, University Hospital, Anichstrasse 35, 6020 Innsbruck, Austria

Nyúl L. G., M.D., Division of Digital Information and Image Processing, Department of Radiology, University Hospital Graz, Auenbruggerplatz 34, 8036 Graz, Austria

Palagy K., Department of Applied Informatics, Josef Attila University Szeged, Arpad, 6720 Szeged K., Hungary

Pärtan G., M.D., Radiology Department at the Socio-Medical Care Centre East/Danube Hospital, Langobardenstrasse 122, 1220 Vienna, Austria

Peer S., M.D., Department of Radiology, University Hospital Innsbruck, Anichstrasse 35, 6020 Innsbruck, Austria

Pfisterer W., M.D., Department of Neurosurgery at the Socio-Medical Care Centre East/Danube Hospital, Langobardenstrasse 122, 1220 Vienna, Austria

Piraino D., M.D., Department of Radiology, 9500 Euclid Avenue, Cleveland, OH 44120, USA

Plihal A., DI, EDP-Management and Operation Management Centre, PM-CC, Viehmarktgasse 4, 1030 Vienna, Austria

Primo R., Siemens Health Services GmbH & Co. KG, Henkestrasse 127, 91052 Erlangen, Germany

Recheis W., M.D., Department of Radiology II, University Hospital, Anichstrasse 35, 6020 Innsbruck, Austria

Reiff K. J., Ing., Siemens AG Deutschland, Department Med. AXDM 2, 31301 Forchheim, Germany

Reinagl W., Chairman of Administration, Reg. Rat, Socio-Medical Care Centre East/Danube Hospital, Langobardenstrasse 122, 1220 Vienna, Austria

Reinhardt E. R., Ph.D., Prof., Siemens Medical Solution, Henkestrasse 127, 91052 Erlangen, Germany

Reiter U., Clinical Department for General Radiological Diagnosis, University Hospital for Radiology, Auenbruggerplatz 9, 8036 Graz, Austria

Rienmüller R., M.D., Prof., Clinical Department for General Radiological Diagnosis, University Hospital for Radiology, Auenbruggerplatz 9, 8036 Graz, Austria

Ros P., M.D., M.P.D., Department of Radiology, Brigham and Women's Hospital, 75 Francis Street, Boston, MA 02115, USA

Rueger W., Ph.D., Siemens Medical Systems, 186 Wood Avenue South, Iselin, NJ 08830, USA

Schäfer K., Ph.D., Institute of Human Biology, University of Vienna, Althanstrasse 14, 1090 Vienna, Austria

Schultz-Wendtland R., M.D., Prof., Radiological Institute, Friedrich-Alexander-University Erlangen-Nürnberg, Gynaecological Radiology, Maximiliansplatz 1, 91054 Erlangen, Germany

Seidler H., Ph.D., Prof., Institute of Human Biology, University of Vienna, Althanstrasse 14, 1090 Vienna, Austria

Sorantin E., M.D., Prof., Division of Digital Information and Image Processing, Department of Radiology, University Hospital Graz, Auenbruggerplatz 34, 8036 Graz, Austria

Staab E. V., M.D., Prof., Wake Forest University, 1834 Wake Forest Road, Winston-Salem, NC 27106, USA

Vannier M. W., M.D., Prof., Department of Radiology, University of Chicago, MC 2026, 5841 South Maryland Avenue, Chicago, IL 60637-1470, USA

Viethen U., Group Vice President, Siemens AG, Medical Solutions Health Services, Image Management Systems, Henkestrasse 127, 91052 Erlangen, Germany

Weber G., Ph.D., Institute of Human Biology, University of Vienna, Althanstrasse 14, 1090 Vienna, Austria

Weibel P., Prof., Chairman of the Centre for Art and Media Technology Karlsruhe, Lorenzstrasse 19, 76135 Karlsruhe, Germany

Weseloh D., Siemens AG, Medical Solutions Health Services, Image Management Systems, Henkestrasse 127, 91052 Erlangen, Germany

Wieser W. I., Ing., Siemens AG Austria, Medical Techniques, Erdberger Lände 26, 1031 Vienna, Austria

Ybinger T., M.D., Kaiser Franz Josef Hospital, Kundratstrasse 3, 1100 Vienna, Austria

Zetie C. A., M.A., Forrester Research Inc., 400 Technology Square, Cambridge, MA 02139, USA

Outlook

If everyone concerned commits to a given task to a sufficient degree then the technical progress and innovations that have happened in medicine will offer fantastic opportunities for health systems. Quality improvement and standards will benefit, and organisational and economic aspects will be improved through greater effectiveness. Available resources may be put to better use in serving patients. In the future holistic thinking will have to be applied as a guiding principle to a much greater extent than it has been so far. This is true for the whole of the person that is the patient, a biological-psychological-social entity. It is also true for the whole range of participants in the system, who will have to cooperate more closely in spite of greater technical specialisation. An effective health policy can be put into practice only when a joint effort is being made. The sentence that prefaced the constitution of the World Health Organization in 1946 should be our guiding principle:

"Health is a state of complete physical, mental and social wellbeing and not merely the absence of disease or infirmity."

To achieve this, structural developments will take place that regulate a patient's entry into the healthcare system and that regulate clearly the competencies for the process that ensues. Digitally networked data – patients' histories, laboratory results, or images obtained by investigations using imaging techniques – enable immediate access at any point in the system and optimise the process for inpatients as well as outpatients, shortens waiting times, avoids duplicate diagnoses, and thus achieves better results from a business perspective too. Clearly allocated competencies enable centralised management of the main processes, "curing" and "caring," which are being performed at the point in the medical system where they are required, and which therefore result in greater productivity.

For individual diseases, management pathways – developed by competency groups consisting of technical specialists and universally accepted – are available as guidance and for orientation. The Österreichische Gesellschaft für Radiologie (Austrian Radiology Society) developed its technical guidelines in 2000 and made these available to all colleagues running their own practices. In this way it is possible to apply exactly those methods that achieve objectives and avoid over-treatment as well as under-treatment. Decisions are made on the basis of medical knowledge and not, as has so often been the case in the past, on the basis of financial constraints. Ethical and humanitarian interests can be reconciled with business interests and are not mutually exclusive. An example for the kind of synergies that result from a considered, comprehensive use of modern information technology is the health network Donaustadt, where interdisciplinary cooperation overcame the problems at the interface of hospital, doctors with their own practices, social services, and care services by structuring and networking processes.

The opportunities offered by biotechnologies and the increasing insights at a molecular level open up methods and options for the future that will have a fundamental impact on our healthcare systems – prevention, care, treatment, and aftercare. Bioinformatics will enable us to produce a genetic map for every individual with his or her individual risk genes; the correlation of genotype and phenotype enables us to sketch an individual's risk profile; and medical informatics will enable us to plan customised and hence optimal treatment for cure and care. Altogether, molecular information enables optimised medical processes, but these have to be put into place where they are of immediate benefit to the patient: in early diagnosis of diseases. This means that what is at stake is not only confirming a disease but actually preventing it by enabling treatment at a stage where cure is possible. The objective is lifelong health care in the sense of total patient management: from the very beginning of life through ensuring quality of life at an advanced age and finally to a dignified death – support and company in all dimensions of life. As Greek philosopher Plato said in 400 AD, in a timeless sentiment: "One should not attempt to cure the eyes without the head and not the head without the body and not the body without the soul ... a part cannot recover if the whole is not sound."

Basics of digital radiology

All human beings are born free and equal in dignity and rights.They are endowed with reason and conscience and should act towards one another in a spirit of brotherhood[1]
Universal Declaration of Human Rights (1948), article 1

"Are the new technologies robbing us of our human dignity?" About the new "sciences" within medicine

S. Hermann

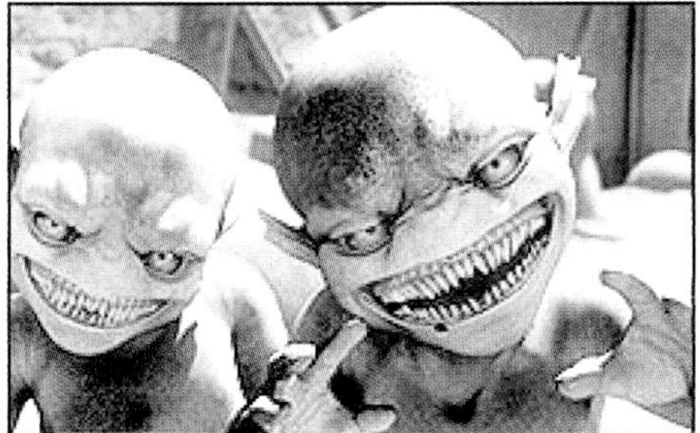

Fig. 1. Photo: Dreamworks, UIP

"In 1972, the ARPANET was presented at the International Conference on Computers and Communications. The computer network, which had been developed by the Advanced Research Project Agency (which is part of the US Ministry of Defense), formed the basis for the development of the internet. In the past 30 years the internet has grown, especially since 1992, when the www (world wide web) was introduced. Today, computer networks and telecommunications technologies (fixed line networks, mobile telephony, satellite telephony) form the technological heart of our modern information society."[2]

When I was a child, a millimetre was really tiny

When I was at university I was fascinated by the idea of "micro". Today's state of the art unit is the "nano". Nanotechnology has given us chips the size of molecules. An Intel transistor is three atoms thick[3] Keyboards are being replaced by microphones. Computers work with speech recognition. Personal computers are integrated into textiles, miniaturised and ever more powerful.

This new generation will hit the market in 2005. One computer will contain more than 400 million transistors. The processor speed will be 10 gigahertz. (One of today's Pentium 4 machines works with 1.5 GHz and has only 42 million transistors.) My former maths teacher would be turning in his grave. The mass of information that we don't understand but still have to work with is increasing. Our knowledge grows constantly, thanks to interdisciplinary thinking. My total amount of knowledge should double every seven years. But all the time I am all too aware of my total absence of knowledge. Is that a paradox? "Neuronomy" as the science of improving the brain and neural systems would not have bothered my grandfather, but I am worried by the situation. I don't know how to react, and I am writing this article. My workplace is changing at ever shorter intervals. Times are becoming difficult, and will be even more so for those who will follow in our footsteps.

In 1960 architect Le Corbusier demanded

Le Corbusier demanded that functional cities, residential areas, working and service areas (offices), etc should be planned separately. This idea has proved to be something of a red herring, but it has been put into practice in many cities and buildings. Now we are battling with the consequences that this planning concept has inflicted on us.

Every day, 170 000 people leave their rural settlements. Tokyo's population will be growing to 29 million by 2015. It is hard to imagine that in Asia, people live, sleep, cook, work, raise children, and are ill and infirm, all on 8 square metres. I cannot imagine that this will not affect society. Today, the

[1] http://www.lyriksite.de/courage/mrechte2.htm

[2] http://www.forschung-und-lehre.de/archiv/04-01/index.html

[3] http://www.spiegel.de/wissenschaft/mensch/0,1518,grossbild-78100-107329,00.html

world has 700 bill. motor vehicles. In 25 years, this number will have doubled. Green spaces in cities will make way for car parks. Telecommunications and the internet are functioning increasingly better in the desert of the conurbations. We are sealing up the Earth's surface with concrete. Can the outcome possibly be a good one?

Now we are learning once again from the so-called grown city

This city has remained interesting because it combines a whole range of functions. Smart technologies have helped correct planning mistakes. Cities have changed massively over the past 20 years. Just think of automatic traffic counting and surveillance, "intelligent" sweeping devices, the possibilities of wireless communications, sensory hydrants, electronic postmen, traffic-dependent street crossings, self-cleaning facades on buildings, online shops, and the networks that support each professional activity and life age. Almost half of the people will have to make do with 2 Euros per day, and industrialised countries will be faced with the new possibilities opened up by broadband communication. So is there any cause for envy in all this? Being part of it all, with 3D, holograms, in the virtual grid, will confront us with difficult decisions. Some will find their working time is too short, others that they have too much time. In the new, global world, your "friend" will be forever watching you from behind your back. Even if you are sitting down for afternoon tea or coffee and cakes, your cheque card and mobile phone will dominate the scene. Wide strata of the population who are impoverished in terms of information, so to speak, are turning into complete democratised consumer morons through shrill telecommunications. Political parties are degenerating into pawns on the chess board of the world. Life has increasingly fewer play areas. Human dignity is being put through the mincer of an omnipotent communications machine.

Much has started to evolve in the past few years

After a phase of being technology disciples and then thinking it through, we are now in a phase of balance. We live in a fast succession of innovations. Innovations that used to be plain revolutionary in the past now take place without public discussion and exclude the wide majority. Intelligent technologies produce vast amounts of data rubbish. The many positive contents seem to have gone missing. The entire scenario can be kept in check only through an even greater use of technology.

Medical doctors and molecular biologists are not only battling with the complexity of the matter but also with premature hopes and initial setbacks. Work is being done on deciphering genes and their respective functions. Molecular medicine, gene technology, stem cells, and genome are the new buzz words. Doctors are confronted with increasingly informed patients, who have obtained their information from the internet and who contact one another through interest groups. The step from a paper file to electronic data capture has been taken. Everyone has signed up to electronic work processes. Intelligent technologies revolutionise traditional work processes.

Strategic information networks are the backbone of the military[4]

Whereas only an oligarchy consisting of government officials, military personnel, and scientists was privy to the ARPAnet, the NSF (National Science Foundation) network has resulted almost in a democratisation process. In the US military it is not the shareholder value that dictates the organisation's business policy, but only the total result that its staff achieve.[5,6] Research institutions at universities and in the business sector are increasingly learning to use networks.

We are rethinking

Conventional analogue data – such as patients' files, radiograph, and print media – are being substituted by their digital equivalents – databases, digital images, and the internet. Processing and reproduction of information assumes a global dimension. The for-

[4]**Note**: The internet was developed some 20 years ago as the follow-up network to the ARPAnet. ARPA is an acronym for Advanced Research Projects Agency and is the predecessor of today's DARPA, the Defense Advanced Research Projects Agency, a military research and secret service of the United States. The ARPAnet was therefore a network entirely for research purposes. One of the main objectives from a military perspective was the creation of a network that links computers worldwide and that sustains operations even when parts of it have been put out of action, for example, as the result of a bomb attack by enemies.

[5]http://www.fas.org/spp/military/program/imint/warfighter.htm

[6]US Army's PEO C3S Knowledge Center, Program Executive Office, Command, Control and Communications Systems - PEO C3S Mission Statement ppt – 2000

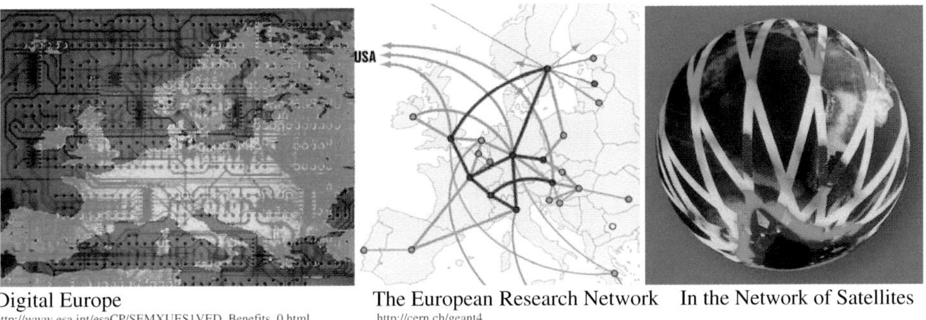

Fig. 2. Digital Europe............The European Research Network........In the Network of Satellites

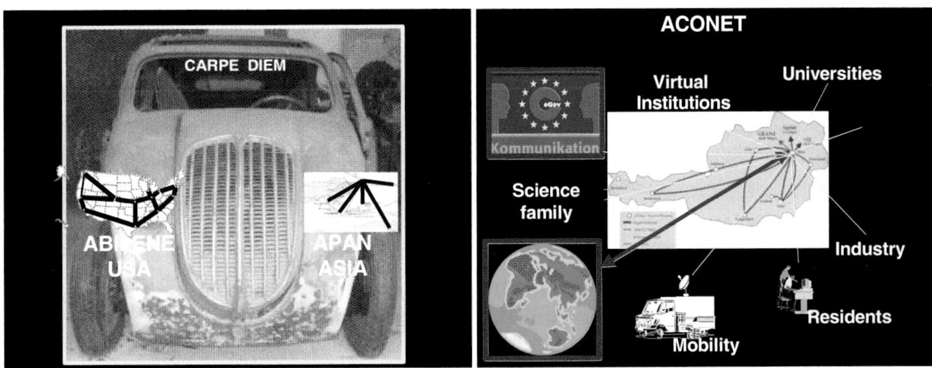

Fig. 3. Half a century ago, Austria produced a car, the Steyr-Daimler Puch[8]. On the basis of the Steyr type 70, built in collaboration with Porsche in 1940, in 1946 a car was built with a spec of 3250 ccm 87 PS V-8 engine[9]. The automotive industry in some ways anticipated today's developments in global broadband communication

mation of networks and collaborative ventures is resulting in new, interdisciplinary forms of healthcare provision in medicine. These range from internet contacts for free trade with no-longer-needed medical equipment in all disciplines[7]. In future, interdisciplinary teams will be working together to effect the quickest and most efficient care in hospitals. The development of networking technologies in general and the internet in particular opens up new possibilities for handling personal and professional transactions. Global networking in real time, through broadband communications networks such as GEANT, ABILENE, or ARPAN are changing the workplace.

E-Gov[10], e-commerce, and e-business applications are starting to accommodate the aforementioned conditions. In Austria, the remotest workplace in any research institution can be reached in real time immediately via ACONET[11]. Traditional routine actions are being speeded up. Screens visualise contents, with few words making up the text. Accompanying publications and worthwhile reading matter are offered as printable/portable document files. A new generation of information providers is arising[12]. Making contents visual is assuming an ever greater role. The values in our lives are shifting. Fairness is assuming a new position of importance. The fine balance between self confidence and sense of duty is being found in forms of active collaboration that have to be newly learnt. Intelligent technologies are creating active tolerance. This has not existed so

[7]http://www.medizin-equipement.de

[8]http://www.csse.monash.edu.au/~lloyd/4/Steyr/

[9]http://www.zuckerfabrik24.de/steyrpuch/steyr2000_1.htm

[10]http://www.gksoft.com/govt/en/

[11]http://www.aco.net/tn.html

[12]http://yokoya.aist-nara.ac.jp/research/storage/hayato-y/html/

far. Will this tolerance also affect the patient and care personnel?

The possibilities inherent in speedy data transfer are transforming the Earth into a global village

The "global village" described by Marshall McLuhan is becoming experienced reality[13]. *"There's an earthquake and no matter where we live, we all get the message. And today's teenager, the future villager, who feels especially at home with our new gadgets – the telephone, the television – will bring our tribe even closer together".*

Academic sciences are working mainly in an interdisciplinary fashion. Medicine has not been at the forefront for a long time, although highly interested and open-minded service providers are assuming importance. In 2010 we will not be carrying our computers within us just yet, but close. Computers are becoming invisible. Images are projected directly on to our retinas from our spectacles or contact lenses. The exploratory journeys into the fourth and fifth dimensions will be the next great step for science. Three-dimensional calculations, such as 4D CAD[14], will be changing entire professional groups.

Digital networks are inexorably transforming the structure of sciences. We are under pressure because we cannot control the flows of information any more. Opponents of globalisation, animal protection groups, and third-world activists exchange electronic data at great speed. Researchers are predicting "social network wars". Globalisation means a new beginning for some and the last phase of colonisation for others. Never before have so many people had such multiple access to power. The networked world is confronting us with gigantic tasks. Our children will not become more intelligent if we buy them a PC, laptop, or sophisticated mobile phone. But their idea of the world will be totally different from ours, however[16]. The crucial element that will really matter is well trained teachers. But who will train these teachers – surely not Alcatel or IBM? We deal

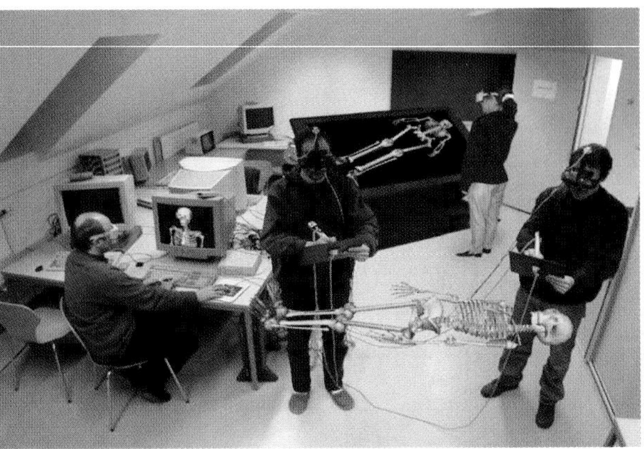

Fig. 4. VR Vis 2004 – Non-medics are playing with medicine. The VRVis Research Center for Virtual Reality and Visualization is a joint venture in Research & Development for virtual reality and visualisation, undertaken by five academic institutes and renowned Austrian companies. VRVis bridges the gap between scientific research and commercial development and supplies the necessary transfer of knowledge between the academic community and industry[15]

with information in our normal lives by default, and no one has fully grasped that we have a lot to learn about this. New jobs in hospitals are created by lifelong learning. This knowledge reaches us through networks that deal with knowledge and information.

Data protection and copyright are breaking the network of central elements guaranteeing order

People are voicing their desire for greater safety from bugging devices, protection from pirate copying, and continuous data transfer. Professor Manuel Castells from the University of California at Berkeley[17] thinks that people were forced from a rural lifestyle into the time discipline of machines and urbanisation. New forms of goverment had to be fought for. The situation in our information society is similar. Austria is not last in the queue. The country's young people are living in a transnational global society.

In addition to the existing internet, scientists use intensified active research networks such as GEANT[18], ABILENE, and APAN[19]. These networks are adapted to globalisation. They are 100–1000 times faster than the internet and are used for data

[13]http://archives.cbc.ca/IDC-1-69-342-1814/life_society/mcluhan/clip2

[14]http://www.stanford.edu/~fischer/ am 10.7.02

[15]http://www.vrvis.at/center/index.html

[16]As a 5-year-old I stood in the stream with my dad. We built waterwheels and dams. Our imagination had no limits.

[17]http://globetrotter.berkeley.edu/people/Castells/castells-con4.html am 1.7.02

[18]http://wwwasd.web.cern.ch/wwwasd/geant4/geant4.html

[19]http://abilene.internet2.edu/

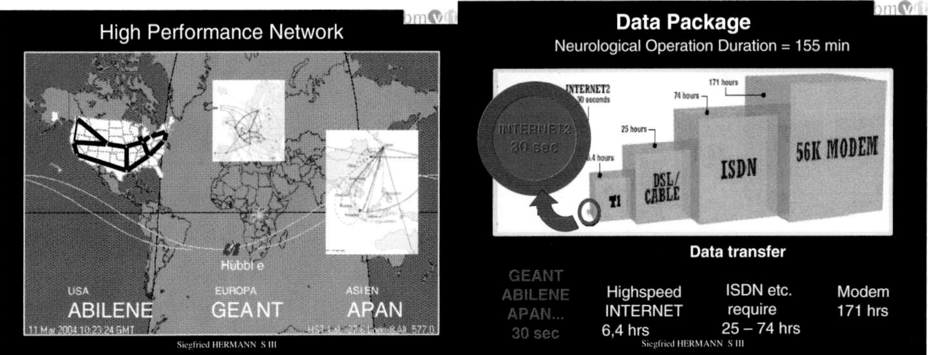

Fig. 5. Existing networks are resulting in a speedy interdisciplinary exchange of ideas in real time

transfer in real time. The former live broadcast of an surgical procedure does not raise an eyebrow among the new specialists. Different scientific disciplines can now witness events as well as participate in them. Participation of active partners has increased. They can be present and if required participate in the medical proceedings, seemingly virtually. Potential audiences are always welcome but do not have a dominant role. It is important that people have a common goal and that problems are resolved by continual dialogue.

The new networks are adapted to globalisation. If in future we deal with intelligent, socially interactive machines[20] the world will change even more drastically. "Real" socialism has failed because it did not turn the industrial revolution into reality. Capitalism will fail too because, although it has realised industrialisation, it cannot control the sorcerer's apprentice. Even the mightiest will forever be shackled by a residual powerlessness to the residual power of the powerless.

In order to bring the networks back down to a human level

The "Berliner Zukunftssalon" [Berlin Salon for the Future] has been founded by salonière Bettina Pohle,[21] who directs the show perfectly. Elegantly dressed, she welcomes her guests, introducing those to one another of whom she finds that they might enjoy a chat. Networking in evening attire. All is as it should be, but some things a subtly different. The idea is traditional, but the concept is new. Tomorrow's managers are on the guest list. Topics of conversation include topics from society, politics, and economics that have a future dimension: virtual illusion, media in the knowledge society, knowledge revolution, art on the web, the courage to stand up for one's beliefs. Those on the guest list are people who are passionately interested in life.

Communication technologies are today's giant growth markets

Voice dial, GPRS (general packet radio service[22]), SMS (short message service[23]), WAP (wireless application protocol[24]) or UMTS (universal mobile telecommunication system[25]), analytical applications[26] are synonymous with high-speed data interchange. These high-tech standards in speech and data transmission are approached through huge amounts of development work, which can be too easily forgotten. Modern economies could not perform without telecommunications. Only those who have greater knowledge,

[20]*http://www.uk.research.att.com/augmentedvehicles/,* http://www.astrosurf.com/lombry/philo-sciences-paradigme-comp.htm

[21]http://www.berliner-zukunftssalon.de/ und http://www.welt.de/daten/2001/01/31/0131b01219350.htx

[22]Data transmission technology that is based on parcelled data transfer within the traditional mobile telephony network.

[23]Short messaging service. SMSenables transmission of short messages of up to 160 lines [Don't you mean „Zeichen, ie „characters"?]

[24]This standard protocol emables direct access to the internet from the mobile handset.

[25]Mobile telephony standard that is supposed to provide higher bandwidths and thereby enable data transfer rates of up to 2MB

[26]Software programs that enable the user to analyse historical transaction data and changed parameters and study their effects on the business by simulating them.

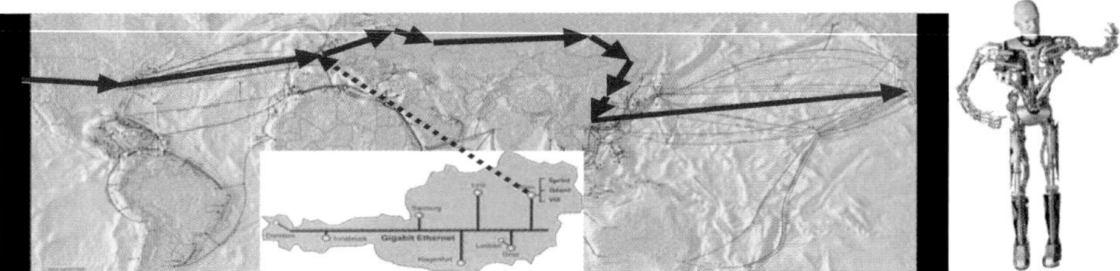

Fig. 6. Existing broadband networks, such as the "GLORIAD" network (GLObal RIng for ADvanced application technologies[27]), will promote such information sharing and exchange. The internet, riddled with viruses and advertising, will not be needed any longer. There will, however, be other harmful elements

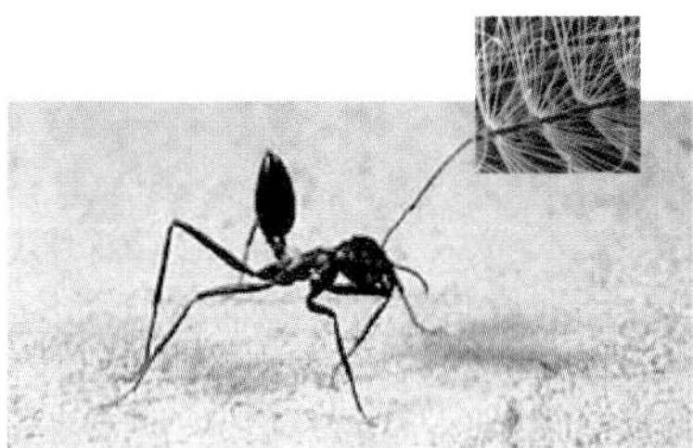

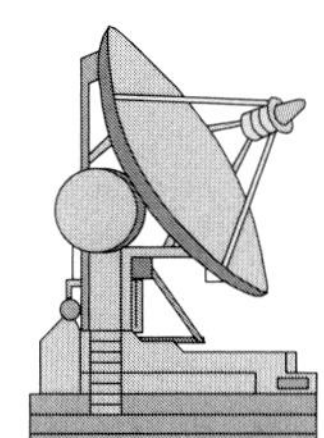

Fig. 7

creativity, and innovation can achieve growth and employment. New ideas are born at the interface of disciplines. Telecommunications has set the course for the future through technologies and innovative products that point the way. Innovation at high speed is changing many industries fundamentally.

Maybe we are not on the right path if we wait until we know everything

In the new internet, broadband internet, many things are defined anew. Everyone seems to benefit in a new culture of independence. People learn together and look beyond their own horizons. Computers are unbeatable in calculating, storing, and searching data, to the point where humans cannot compete any more. Human beings, however, are irreplaceable when it comes to assessing and recognising forms and shapes. Within five years, surgeons will perform rare procedures at the console. The patient, accompanied by a robot, is in a different location to the surgeon. The hospital has a broadband link to a smart surgery and care unit. The teams of doctors and care staff could not ever be replaced with technology. The only advantage is that in this way, many hospitals can benefit from a surgeon with special experience. Learning, however, is only possible from one's own experiences.

We thus have no choice but think about the cooperation of humans and machines. Robots can do the handiwork while humans do the thinking and lifelong learning. Computer manufacturers think that life can be planned. Everyday life is managed by intelligent technologies. In future, even intelligence will be created artificially, so that in a foreseeable space of time we will be dealing with intelligent, socially interactive machines[28]. And what will happen when energy resources break down?

Human beings do the thinking, but machines do the directing

Robots guided by chip technology will be handling the scalpel in the operating theatre. Almost anything is possible. Conventional analogue data, such as patient data and images, can be accessed anywhere in the hospital. People who live and work with this technology will be the colleagues recruited in the future.

Nature remains the model

We are now keen to learn more intensively from and invest more research into the natural scenarios that surround us. A desert ant, for example, has an extremely complex orienteering system, which uses the magnetic force field of the Earth. The ant perceives the world from a totally different perspective. Its sensors show up our clunky space telescopes. Evolution has provided the solutions for so many problems of telecommunications for such a small creature. We can only hope to answer arising questions with added value if we use global data networks.

New ideas are born out of adaptive thinking

The differences between human skin and the walls of a house will seem to disappear. The layers of the wall will consist of smart materials. The brickwork will

[27]http://www.gloriad.org/gloriad/index.html

[28]http://www.uk.research.att.com/augmentedvehicles/, http://www.astrosurf.com/lombry/philo-sciences-paradigme-comp.htm

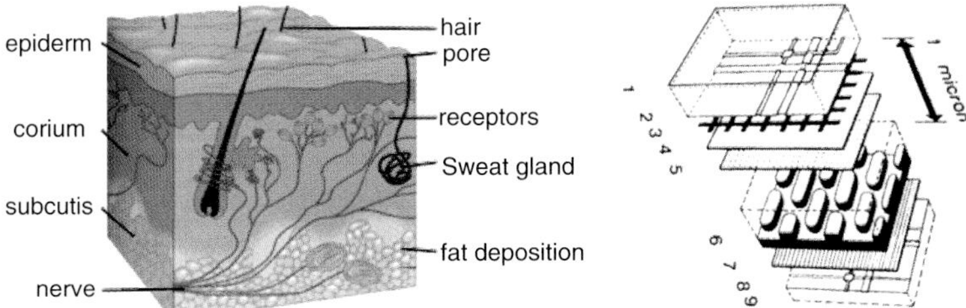

Fig. 8. Human skin and building façades will have similar structures. 1. Silicaweather skin and deposition substrate weather skin and deposition substrat – 2. Sensor and control logic layer – external – 3. Photo electric grid – 4. Thermal sheet radiator/selective absorber – 5. Electro reflective deposition – 6. Micro pore gas flow layers – 7. Electro-reflective deposition – 8. Sensor and control logic layer – 9. internal layer

have external foils for diverse sensors on the plaster surface. Photoelectrical foils measure the thermic properties with electrostatic sensors. Internal sensors and control systems are in all places where they are needed.

The Jet Propulsion Laboratory[29] in Pasadena, USA, has produced the lightest solid substance in the world, AEROGEL. The material, is a sponge made from silicium, consists of 99.8% air and has a density of only 3 mg/cm^3. Future roof tiles will not be made from clay but from silicium cells, walls not from brick but from glass. All this will be substituted by the new building material AEROGEL. The facades will be "lifted" or exchanged. This material is equally interesting in a medical context.

In 2020 we will be working with systems that think like humans and behave like them too. Everything is constantly shrinking in size and getting faster – "micro" and "nano" are the key technologies of the coming century. Man will be a clumsy Gulliver in the realm of the techno-dwarves. This is scary as well as fascinating. We do not even have the most basic answers to how the brain works or understand all its multiple achievements. Computers "think" in a programmed fashion. They are neither creative nor guided by their feelings. At the moment, computers are socially illiterate. Their brain distinguishes between hardware and software, but they know nothing about the language of human neural cells. Even the visual chip for blind people is only in the early stages of its development. The everyday, seemingly effortless, achievements of the human brain have not been explored – what a relief! Vigilance is called for, however, the moment when it will be possible to manufacture electrochemically stable, highly integrated chips, with thousands or even millions of contact sites[30].

Everything will change. Decentralised organisations will find homes in period buildings and reform with new, flat organisational structures. Satellite working centres will increase in number. Satellite working centres (tele-offices) that are situated in easily accessible suburban locations of large cities or rural areas will provide an infrastructure to outsource

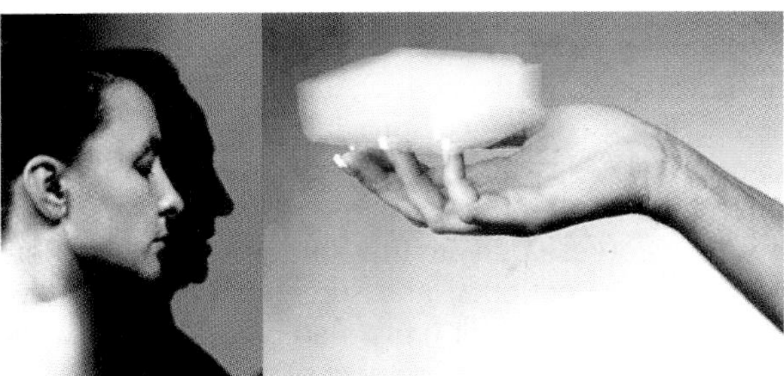

Fig. 9. Ageing with dignity does not happen only through facelifts[31]. The new building substance AEROGEL is akin to a facelift for buildings. Any application and correction requires searching discussion

[29]http://stardust.jpl.nasa.gov/tech/aerogel.html

[30]http://www.biochem.mpg.de/mnphys/publications/96fro-kopp/abstract.html am 28.5.02: Peter Fromherz; Die Technik auf dem Weg zur Seele. Forschungen an der Schnittstelle Gehirn/Computer [Technology on its way to the soul. research into the interface between brain and computer]. Rowohlt Hamburg, 1996

[31]http://www.metka.at/altersv.html ; Dr. Wolfgang Metka; „Das Altern mit AEROGEL hinauszuzögern wird den „test of time" benötigen. Die Komponenten für die Verträglichkeit sind sorgfältig zu prüfen" [Only time can tell whether ageing can be delayed with AEROGEL. The components will have to be tested carefully for their acceptability and possible side effects] Credit: AEROGEL-NASA/JPL)

certain administrative activities of private or public-sector companies. The aim of this outsourcing will be to avoid the high office rents in city centres and the parking problems as well as, from a town planning perspective, to reduce the number of private cars in city centres. Everything will be calculated. Are humans cost-effective?

Almost everything will be possible. Conventional analogue data such as sickness notes, radiographs, and print media will be replaced by the respective digital equivalents – databases, digital images, and the internet. Processing and reproducing information will assume a global dimension. The formation of networks and collaborations will result in specialty-transcending forms of healthcare provision in medicine.

Thanks to an implanted hearing aid, the cochlear implant,[32], (CI) deaf people will be able to access and appreciate the world of sound, music, and speech/language. In patients of profound deafness, the sensory cells will be replaced by a technological implant.

Hi-tech eyewear such as the critical data viewer[33] will be used to expand the field of vision. Contents in the forms of text will be reflected directly in front of the eye, as a quasi-overlay. Our world is three-dimensional. Books and screens represent the world in a two-dimensional fashion. Distorted areas (which cannot be outlined or sketched) can be represented, such as biomolecules or cancer cells. Autostereoscopic liquid crystal display monitors[34] provide a new window into reality. To clarify the real situation even better, computer generated 3D images are created. Images from all sectors of research are thus understood better. Car mechanics, geneticists, and surgeons can gain new insights. This has never happened before in this way. Our senses for research are becoming more acute.

In 1966 I saw the film "The Phantastic Journey" with my eyes and ears wide open. I saw Raquel Welch plough through the aorta of an ageing professor in a microvehicle. Fact is now catching up with fiction. New prototypes are going to be launched in the coming decades: nanoparticles, agglomerations of particles the size of a few to several hundred atoms or molecules. These will transport DNA fragments into human cells. Viruses will be attacked and genetic defects repaired. The microchips that we use today are veritable giants compared with those that will rule the nanocosm. Much is as yet unexplained and opens up new research questions – for example, how can we propel the health-bringing particles circulating round the human body? We can imagine that biocompatible neural implantates will help improve the memory function of the brain. Connections will be made between the human brain and computer networks. A person's entire memory of a lifetime might be kept "alive" on a data storage device in the future. The vision: the contents of each single brain will be scanned and thus preserved. Thank God I am living today. But in future, everything will be new, and different. Can this be reconciled with human dignity as we understand it now? Computers are neither creative nor are they ruled by feelings. At the moment they are socially illiterate. Are they going to remain that way, and what will happen when Pandora's box is opened?

Wireless technology is supported by ever smaller devices

People will carry them in their pockets like pens or pen-knives. Communication will be strictly wireless[37]. We cooperate in a diversity of life's areas. Images and data will be captured via speech recognition. We work, without having been trained for it,

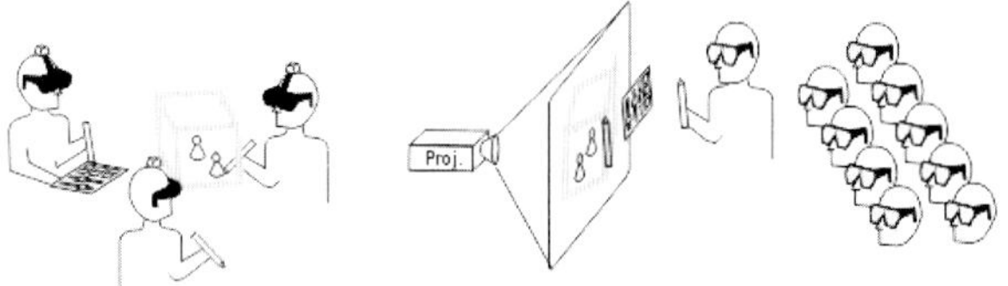

Fig. 10. The next techologies[35] .... In a Viennese coffee house[36] (Franz Hubmann)

[32]http://www.gschwaninger.de/ohrenseite/download.html (25 Jahre CI in Wien [25 years of cochlear implantation in Vienna])

[33]http://www.microopticalcorp.com/products.html

[34]http://www.visureal.de/3d_medizin.htm

[35]http://www.vrvis.at/br1/vrss/index.html

[36]copyright Franz Hubmann, Wien

[37]http://www-5.ibm.com/ch/franklin/images/atapuercas_gross.jpg

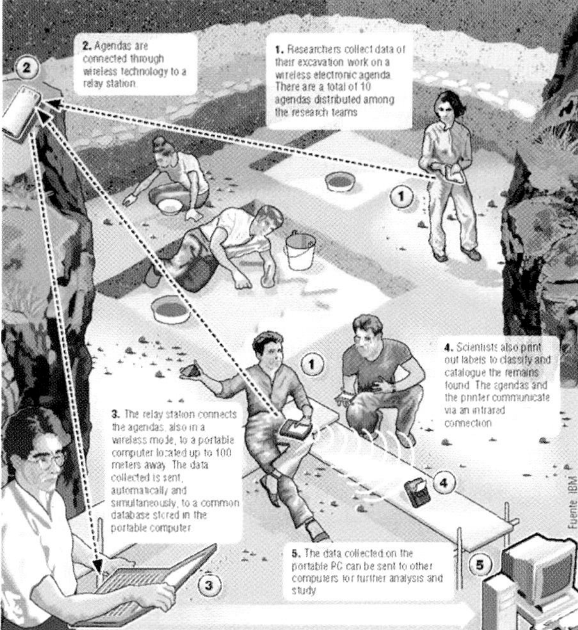

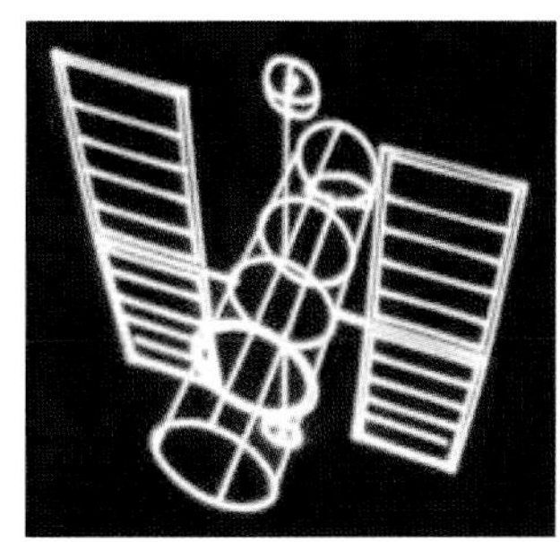

Fig. 11. "Archaeology" as an area where new technologies will be used Chip technology puts us in a position to do many things[38] and yet is small enough to be placed on the tip of a finger. Even the Hubble space probe offers new insights if focused towards the Earth

in so-called real time. Learning and problem solving will take place at once. This will be achieved by virtual group work. Complicated and large paper volumes with instructions for users will become surplus to requirement. The computer shows where foci for disease are located and where treatment has to be initiated. My grandparents could have never done their work in such a way. Today's world of employment is already home to the children of the former „amusement arcade generation."

Digital cameras the size of credit cards are already available[39]. Critical data viewers in combination with with intelligent clothing, can project virtual sitemaps from inside the patient at every section directly in front of the eye of the beholder.

Tomorrow's textiles are more than just en expression of fashion

People's clothing in future should do more than just keep them warm. It is, after all, only the human being that embodies the elastic, ever changing interface. "Invisible" personal assistants[40] will be woven into the fabrics[41]. The clothing (smart shirt[42]) will measure the inner and outer temperature of the fabric and

[38]http://www-5.ibm.com/ch/pressroom/images/technologien/chip_kiwistraw.jpg

[39]http://www.uni-weimar.de/~burger1/umts_lin.htm, http://www.exilim.jp/ **Note:** Exilim is 11.3 mm thin, 88 mm wide, und 55 mm high, and it weighs 86 g without charger and storage disk. The expanded model Exilim EX-M1 integrates additionally an MP3-Player, Movie-Player, and a voice recording function. The 1/2.7" CCD has a resolution of 1.31 million pixels in total or an image format of 1280×960.

[40]http://www.techexchange.com/education.html

[41]Spring fashions from companies Infineon and Levis, 2003: The intelligent waistcoat incorporates an MP3-Player, mobile telephone, and remote control. The garment is fully wired anmd always in receiving mode. Each device has its own separate pocket and plug and can be operated centrally via remote control. Headphones and a microphone are in the collar. Levis brought 320 items on to the market in its spring collection. This is a computer you can wear, with 40 MB and a Pentium 3 processor. It weighs about 900 g and has sensory, signal processing, and communications components – for example, to search data. Recommended retail price: 2328 Mark. http://www.wearabl.e-electronics.de/photos/highres/Thermo.jpg See: W.D. Hartmann, K. Steilmann, A. Ullsperger; High-Tech-fashion, Heimdall-Verlag ISBN: 3-9807087-4-8

[42]http://www.cc.gatech.edu/fce/house/proposals/final-preproposal.doc

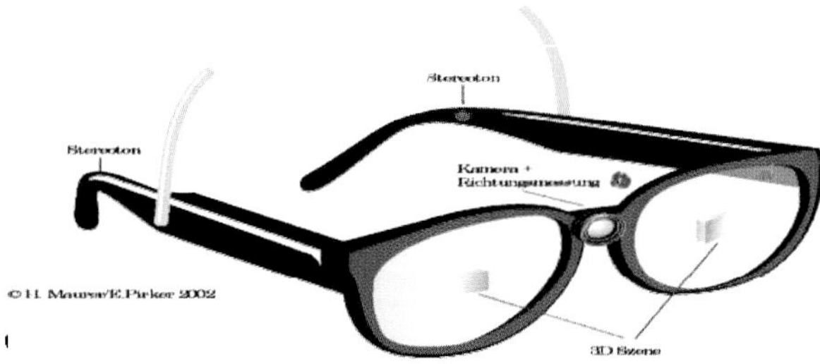

Fig. 12. C.H.Maurer, E.Pirker; "stereo" critical data viewer–Universität Graz, 2002

control the wearer's heartbeat. Innumerable tiny sensors will be being wove in, same as wires for telephone aerials, A body area network[43] and its wireless links will monitor body variables, such as blood pressure, heartbeat, temperature, etc, around the clock. It will transmit signals from body implants, visual and hearing aids. Blind people may regain a certain amount of their sight through implants. This is within the realm of the possible in pathologies where the photoreceptors in the human retina have deteriorated or the eye's macula has degenerated through accident or disease.[44] Ultra-thin materials will protect against UV radiation. Body tolerability will always be the prime consideration. People's attention to their own natural body signals will be sharpened; if problems occur they will attend the relevant specialist immediately.[45]

On cool summer days it is difficult to decide what to do with one's shirt sleeves: rolling them down because it is too cold one minute, rolling them up because the sun has appeared, and then rolling them down again when a cloud materialises. An Italian clothes manufacturer has found a solution: a shirt that rolls up the sleeves automatically when it gets hot. And even better: the shirt does not have to be ironed.[46] Thin vibration layers have also been worked into the fabric.[47] The accidental vibrations this layer causes apparently results in a new body consciousness and feelings of wellbeing, totally unnoticed by others.

Smart textiles will become an integral part of people's intricately intertwined worlds, consisting of work and life.[48] The individual experiences, on his or her laptop and with the critical data viewer – in connection with smart clothing – the globalisation of the planet (which still amounts to nothing much when we look at the universe around it).

Medics and material scientists are collaborating to find solutions for problems –

For example, in the area of implants. Medical experts know about problems with tolerability. Science experts know about alternative materials. Both sides contribute their technical knowledge, identify problems and set objectives, and work on solving the problems together. It takes guts to leave one's own research ivory tower and share one's knowledge with others. The so-called decoding of the human genome marked the start of the biotechnological era.

We see progress in gene technology and nano technologies is accelerating exponentially. The dawning biotechnological age and its ideologies have the potential to change society substantially; the nuclear age will appear a veritable dwarf in comparison. The capacities of personal computers are increasing exponentially too. Thinking computers will be approaching reality in the coming decades. So-called intelligent fabrics, "smart clothes", will have chips woven in. The will be planned as a recycleable textile – they can be washed and recharged by the professionals. In case their wearer has an accident, they will call for help via a global positioning system after 30 seconds. They will function as a compass to find directions. The increase "water-

[43]http://www.phmon.de/deutsch/kommunikation.html

[44]http://www.victorianweb.org/cpace/prosthesis/stein/vision.html - Note: „creation and implementation of fully implantable lenses, which actually replace (or in some cases merely enhance) the old, dysfunctional lenses. The lenses are very small (as seen compared to a penny) and are put into the eye by a clever surgical procedure. Take, for example, a patient with cataracts. This means that there has been a clouding of the lenses (Cataract is a Greek word meaning "white water falling." Early Greeks thought the blurred vision of a cataract was like looking through a waterfall). A small opening is made in the sac which holds the eye's diseased natural lens . A chemical is injected into the opening which dissolves the lens and the remains are vacuumed out. A special "folding lens" is put into a needle like tube, and is injected into the now emptied sac. Within a short amount of time, vision is restored to the patient, and vision is rendered almost perfect (glasses may be necessary for reading)." http://www.acm.org/cacm/newstrack/2002/points_of_light.html

[45]http://www.gtwm.gatech.edu/, http://www.e-ssist.fraunhofer.de/technologien/index.html, http://www.sensatex.com/

[46]http://www.expeditionzone.com/start_hi.cfm?story=2984&business=&club=&member

[47]Lycra T 400, Du Pont de Nemours, Dr. Alexandra Fede

[48]http://www.sensatex.com/smartshirt/index.html

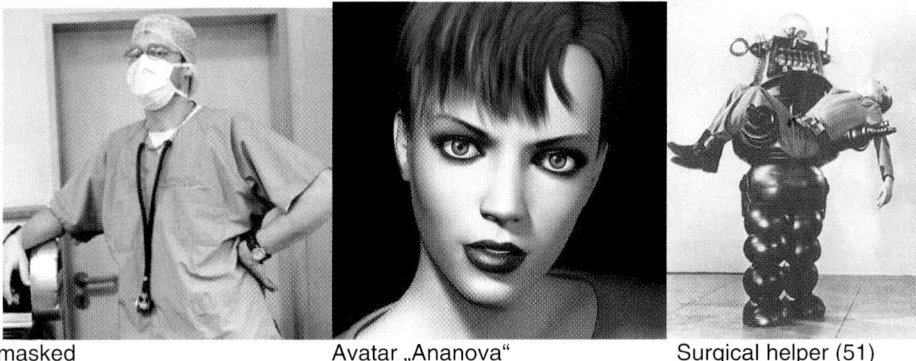

Fig. 13. Masked ... avatar "Ananova" .... surgical helper[51]

friendliness" and therefore bind the components of human sweat. Their modified fibre surfaces can serve as a skin-friendly repository for pharmaceuticals. Harmful UV rays will be stopped from penetrating by the fibres.

The future microcomputers will accompany humans every step of the way

They are woven into people's clothing or implanted into the people themselves. Even smaller neuro-implants with a learning capability will be able to listen into the human nervous system and communicate with it. A circuit diagram will be transferred lithographically on to a chip, which means that smaller, structral details will be visible only when the wavelength of the light used for the lithography process is short. New solutions for problems will be found by using electronic structural elements based on biomolecules.[49] These are an integral part of nanotechnology.

In Hinduism, avatars are reborn beings that descend to earth. In the early 1980s, the term was used for the first time for the human artefacts in computer simulation games.The British Press Association presented the green-eyed, green-haired Ananova, the first new-look, virtual newsreader on the internet[50], and a new face is part of this: the presenter was styled to the last detail.

Avatars move in worlds that were especially created for them, in which social activities happen as much they do in the physical world. Today, the most well-known virtual personalities are Lara Croft, the star of the computer game Tomb Raider, and Kyoko Date, who became an idol for young people and a popstar in Japan. In the computer age, avatars are novel identities. After entry into the virtual world an avatar could provide advice for acute situations and emergencies on the screen of the Socio-Medical Center East (SMZO), City of Vienna, Austria. A virtual moderator should also be able to show emotion. Ananova was therefore designed with 36 facial muscles. She can roll her eyes, raise her eyebrows, and move the corners of her mouth – but all this is still rather unsubtle. "Human warmth comes from body language and eye contact," says Jonathan Jowitt, "and that is difficult for an animated person,"

And this is what plans for hospital buildings look like:

The former hospital typologies, such as large blocks with many wings or or pavilion-style buildings, are being changed depending on the network. Where it makes sense, large offices and cell offices will be built. Smart, hi-tech groups of rooms will complete the intelligent building design. Mirror projects will be started.[52] The Mirror Project, University of Arizona, enables participants to simulate meetings around a (virtual) conference table. Participants are in different locations. Virtual communication will be introduced into administration buildings. The term "virtual" is being used to point out in networks and particularly on the internet that something does not have a physical, but only a simulated existence ("virtual rooms"). The first prototypes are being developed for

[49] http://www.infobiogen.fr/services/deambulum/english/ http://home.a-city.de/claudia.borchard-tuch/

[50] http://www.mmjp.or.jp/amlang.atc/worldnow/00/apr/20-ananova-big.gif

[51] http://www.genmed.org.uk/images/robodoc/robby.jpg

[52] http://www.3sat.de/3sat.php2/http://www.3sat.de/nano/cstwecke/06262

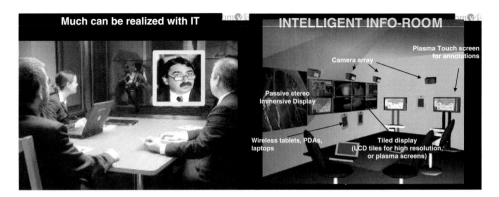

Fig. 14

future interiors, such as surgical groups in operating theatres intensive care wards, storage, and specialised research sectors[53].

In the surgical tract a group of rooms will be available where chip-guided robots guide the scalpel. The advantage is obvious: the so-called robodocs are always on top form, at any time of day or night. They merely need regular, thorough servicing and never take holidays. They do not have family problems. For years, the size of a surgeon's hand has determined the surgical technique and therefore the size of the sutures. Now the master surgeon will sit at a console. His manual movements will be transferred by a computer on to the mechanical surgical tools. The new mechanical hands have endoscopes the size of fingers. These will do the inspecting, gripping, palpating, clamping, and cutting via a screen (in future critical data viewer, contact lens). The tools will be placed inside the patient. The computer will compensate for the tremors of the human hand. A sort of "automatic transmission" will minimise the centimetre movement of the human hand. Reduction will enable the tools to cover only one-third of the distance. Computer are unbeatable in calculating, storing, and searching data. Human beings cannot compete any more.

If human beings do the thinking, is it actually the machines that do the directing? Within five years, a surgeon will be able to perform uncommon procedures at the console. The patient, together with a robot, will be in another hospital. What will be needed for this: the hospital's network link; the specialised, intelligent robot, and an additional surgeon in case of any emergencies. The advantage is obvious: many hospitals benefit from one surgeon with special expertise and experience.

Fig. 15. Young people are learning to handle virtual reality machines. Tomorrow she will be placed at the robodoc[54]

The new hospital buildings will be built for a mobile society

This society will consist of people who start walking in the hospital department every morning. A person's location will be situated in an every-changing in-between. One example of this has already been realised in a concept, but not in a hospital.

The brave new world of the dvg Hannover Datenverarbeitungsgesellschaft mbH (Hanover Data Processing Company Ltd) (Heinle-Wischer & Part-

[53] http://www.psu.edu/dept/cs/projects/farming.html

[54] http://uk.dk.com/static/cs/uk/11/clipart/future/image_future010.html

ner) is an innovative office landscape covered by 15 000 square metres of glass.[55] Office work has adopted a new structure. Each partner in a cluster shares in the overall workload and stays within his or her area of expertise. The result is a service that has not been possible thus far. Each partner in a cluster can handle new business acquisitions. He or she uses the advantages of the group. The many small and large organisational units are given interesting activities, and synergies form. The services on offer are delivered more rapidly. The risk is spread evenly (different countries, disciplines, languages...). Personnel and infrastructures are used more efficiently. Specialisation is enhanced – the service improves. New experiences benefit the company's image. Communication between cluster partner and client is immediate. Finances are managed better. An image of togetherness is being cultivated and people appear together. Joint ventures are formed, etc.

The real inhabitants of buildings will be the nomadic managers and employees who walk from project to project, rather than go to the office every morning. The real workplace is a constantly changing in-between. The new workplaces will be created in ever increasing numbers by the new tasks in everyday life. No school has prepared the workers for this. Since the nomadic worker can declare any place in the world his or her office, designers and architects have relinquished their responsibilities. Most of them limit their input to the design and proportions of the outer hull of the building. Furniture firms determine the floorplans. Maybe architects have declared professional bankruptcy altogether. Information specialists are creating networks, and the virtual shadow of the nomad worker travels within these networks.

In the geriatric centre Favoriten of Vienna's association of healthcare facilities (KAV)[56], designed by Anton Schweighofer,[57] the central corridor has been transformed into a residential street. The rooms have windows that can be opened and look out into this street. Residents decide for themselves whether they want to participate in the social interaction or rather close the window and remain by themselves, undisturbed. The medicine cluster might be seen as the structure of the future.

Tomorrow's buildings will be kinetic[58]

The breathe, the move and consist of components that can be exchanged/swapped. Centres of excellence, technologies, innovation centres, iDTV technologies[59], multimedia labs, science centres, science portals, AplusB, competencies, impulse centres, start-ups, technology parks, think-tanks, value-added services[60] are clearing houses, corporate universities, corporate information technology[61], data warehousing, digital networks, dot.coms, GRID and clusters ... are fashionable terms that are of no particular meaning to architects. They plan for old dressed as new. Many hospital buildings are originally industrial and administrative buildings that were badly planned, shabby, and short-lived. The pressure to re-think comes from intensive application of telecomms and development of new building materials.

It's a remarkable fact that the buildings inhabited by the Austrian Empire were continually newly adapted; this was possible only because they had enough space and air. Today we do not plan in such a generous way. Jobs should be secure but also attractive. The objective is to maintain pole position in the global race for innovation. Only those who have more knowledge, creativity, and innovative thought can achieve growth and create jobs. The smart infrastructure of buildings is integral to this. Planning a regional hospital appropriately as a competency centre (cluster) takes more than creating a gimmicky facade to the building.

Back to everyday life

Faced with increasingly complex technological systems, the shorter lifespan of top-of-the-range technology products, and costs rising exponentially,

[55]http://www.heinlewischerpartner.de/projekte/dvg_hannover/index.html

[56]http://www.wienkav.at/kav/gzs/

[57]http://info.tuwien.ac.at/histu/pers/11608.html

[58]http://destech.mit.edu/akilian/projectpages/tower.html

[59]Interactive, digital television – a rival for the internet.

[60]for example, banking or travel bookings via mobile phone. The SIM application toolkit helps improve the user-friendliness of new services by some margin. Users of mobile telephones can navigate quickly and simply in (additional) menu functions and can reach the desired application via mouse click – users thus will not have to remember user dialogues and instructions.

[61]Development of functional business applications for global use

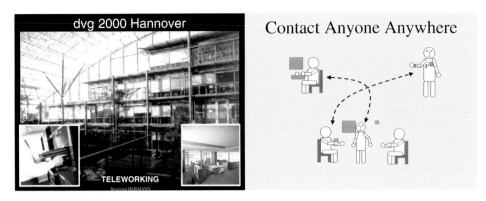

Fig. 16. Desk sharing – 1350 work places, 1850 employees – the work processes are task-oriented

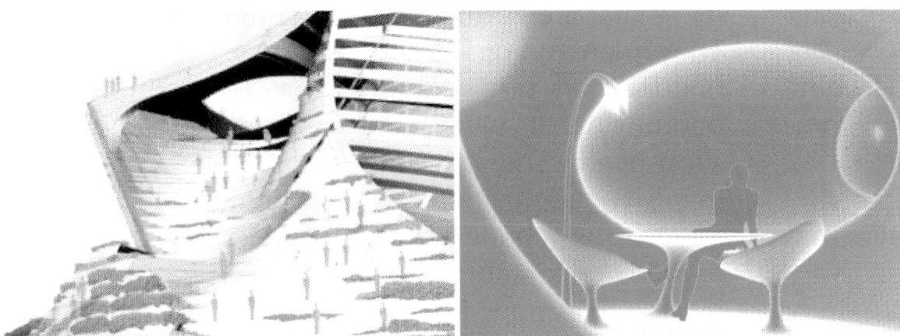

Fig. 17. A possible future: Buildings that turn towards and move with the sun – architectural structures and furniture could be made from genetically modified plants[62]

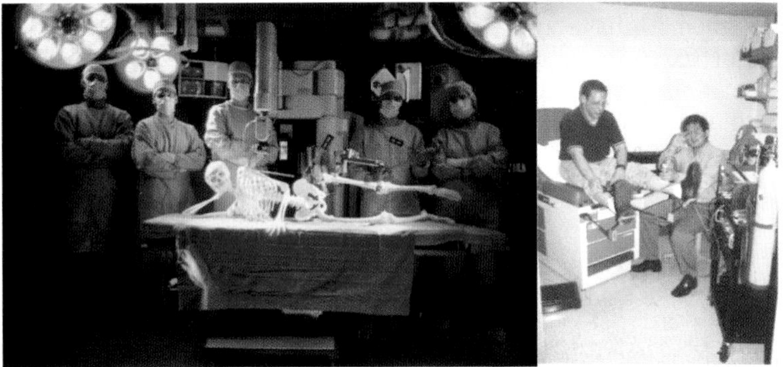

Fig. 18. How do RoboDoc hip replacement surgeons, Pittsburgh, USA,[63] go together with health care in windowless rooms?[64]

companies are having to form alliances. This creates access to complementary know-how, and risks can be shared.

Everything will be accessible from anywhere (via the internet) – for example, telemedicine guides, 2004[65]. In the United States, a total service exists that encompasses everything, including housekeepers and babysitters. The current thinking is that in the future, people can work in whatever they desire and whenever suits them. Everyobody will be able to make independent decisions about their work.

[62] http://www.beyond-design.de/

[63] http://www.georgesteinmetz.com/images/science/robodoc.jpg

[64] http://www.mgh.harvard.edu/depts/neuroimaging/gollublab/photo%20gallery.html

[65] http://www.telemedizinfuehrer.de/

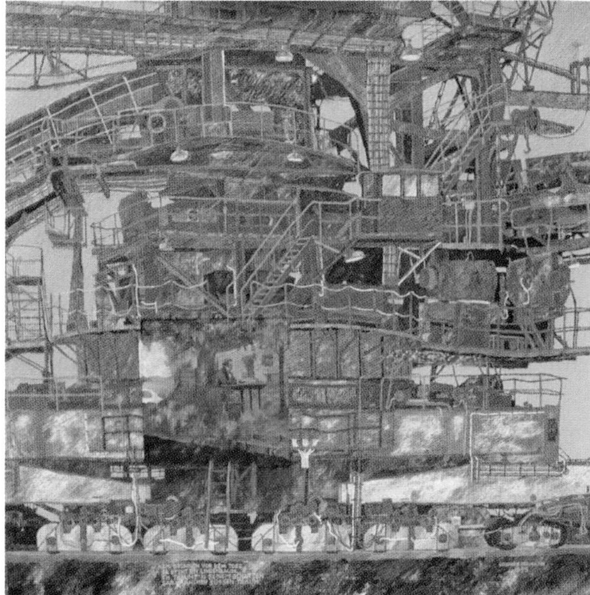

Fig. 19. Here's the solution to the problem: coal digger in the former German Democratic Republic (Siegfried Herrmann 1991 (Oil, 180 cm/180 cm)

Everyone will take on more responsibilities and

Modern, automated buildings	Modern workplaces
• Securing physical comfort through appropriate regulations	• Securing ergonomically designed workstations
• The possibilities of using rooms flexibly	• Abolishing desolate workplaces
• Centralised and decentralised governance	• Flat organisational structures
• Intelligent linking of systems from dierent companies	• Time management and capture systems that enable documentation of actual workload
• Communications, etc	• Worldwide (broadband) internet, etc

assume decision making powers. Flat hierarchies in decentralised businesses will open the doors for new tasks. Useful and useless "items" will determine our actions to an extent that we have not anticipated. To date, it is certain that:

- We are evolving from a manufacturing society to knowledge and service society
- Different cultures interpret the same trends in different ways
- Whatever happens HERE does not mean the same the world over

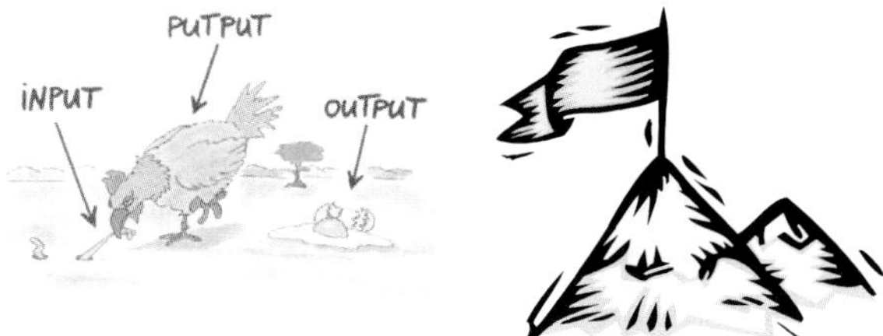

Fig. 20. In a world of biocomputers, buidling sandcastles is difficult

- To understand the world we will need not only natural sciences, engineering, and social sciences, but also the arts and philosophy.
- Completely new independent disciplines will arise in medicine, which will be impossible to integrate into the existing disciplines.

The demands are similar everywhere. The main issues are

The two aims are:

Making workplaces human and maintaining and continuously improving IT infrastructures. This has always been always a tightrope walk between investment and technical compromise. Service level management[66] can create new ways of thinking. Standardisation may be important for technologies, software, applications, and processes. In each scenario, the individual situation will have to be considered and assessed. This will necessitate new forms of learning and teaching, which our universities will carry on developing. Lifelong learning is the order of the day.

Human beings must remain the measure of all things. The pioneering phase is coming to the end

The link between work clothing and technology began when people started carrying equipment around. The invention of the computer has made this into an intelligent companion.

The near future might look like this:

1. **Free international exchange of information will be possible via GRIDs and CLUSTERs**
2. **As communication via networks will be increasing, language and spoken communication will change**
3. **We will talk increasingly in "images." Imaging techniques are of benefit.**

[66]This is a platform that supervises the dependencies of working processes, develops them further, and implements them.

4. **Our culture, politics, society, the environment, and relations between nation states will be affected directly.**
5. **The individual will have not only rights but also obligations – even if it is not modern to talk about these.**
6. **Making money or even profits out of education will have lost its stigma.**
7. **The main issue will be that in global competition, the brightest minds should remain most successful.**
8. **Every transaction will be based on clear financial interests. Unfortunately good samaritans will be no more.**
9. **The consequences of these processes will not be limited to the healthcare system. They will be interdisciplinary. Today's adolescents will find these entirely normal.**

Marketable products will be competing at an ever-faster speed. Everything is becoming speedier and smaller. "Micro" and "nano" will be the key technologies of the coming years. The high speed at which innovation happens will result in changes and losses in many industries. In 2020 we might be working with systems that think like humans and even behave like them too. I am finding this scary but also fascinating. All of us, young and old, will have to learn to cope with the information society. Not everyone will find this easy.

Basics of computer technology and digital imaging

W. Krampla

Radiology Department, Danube Hospital, Vienna, Austria

To understand what happens to a digital X-ray image, we will accompany such an image on some of its steps. First, the examination is performed on the modality in the way already familiar from systems based on conventional X-ray films; there are no discernible differences here for the patient, or, with very few exceptions, in respect to exposure technique. The sole exception, and only to a limited extent, is the use of phosphor storage plates as a digital equivalent to the conventional survey X-ray. In order to exploit the technical possibilities provided by this modality, the person performing the examination must attend to certain details when generating the examination; this is the subject of another section. When an examination has been concluded, the images produced are not printed out on a laser printer or any other similar output unit, but are sent to a workstation. To make the details more comprehensible, I would first like to clarify.

The nature of a digital image

With this in mind, we will first look at the composition of an analog image. Consider a painting. With each single brush-stroke, paint is applied in a way that cannot subsequently be precisely replicated (Fig. 1). No individual brush-stroke is exactly like any other; not even the artist can reproduce it. Thus, each painting is unique, and in its uniqueness can never be perfectly replicated, not even by the artist her/himself. Any reproduction necessarily involves deviations from the original. It is just as impossible to take a painting apart and then re-assemble it. We come a step closer if we consider a mosaic. Each element in the image is localized to a defined place (Fig. 2). Assuming that this is a mosaic for which identical tesserae (=image elements) are available, and that these are arranged in a reproducible way in a matrix, it is possible to produce a copy that is indistinguishable from the original. Each tessera is uniquely defined within such an image by its position and its color (or its gray-value). Thus, without knowing the original, it is still possible to produce the image from information about the color of the tesserae and their position in a grid system. All digital X-ray images are quite similar to "mosaics," where the image is uniquely defined by individual reproducible elements. Every image on a computer monitor is made up of a precisely defined number of points. These "tesserae" are called **pixels**. Each pixel can be displayed only at a precisely defined location on the monitor, since it is assigned a value on the *x*- and *y*-axes. In addition, its gray-value or color level is uniquely defined. The number of image points in both dimensions is called the **matrix**. **Image depth** refers to the number of possible colors or gray tones. It follows from what we have said up to here that a digital X-ray image can be displayed at all locations where the information about its composition is available. We can already see one of the important advantages of such a system: any image can be transmitted or reproduced in its original quality simply by transmitting the information about its composition; it is not the image itself that must be communicated, but only the information about its composition.

The effect of the matrix and image depth on the image

Every image point has a homogeneous color or a single gray-value. Details within the individual pixel cannot be displayed. To yield the highest possible resolution, the size of the individual points must be small. At the same time, this means that in order to make very small details visible, there must be as many points as possible per cm (or any other unit of distance). **Spatial resolution** is a function of the number of pixels per cm; the total number of pixels depends on the size of the image. If the number of pixels per image is predetermined, resolution is

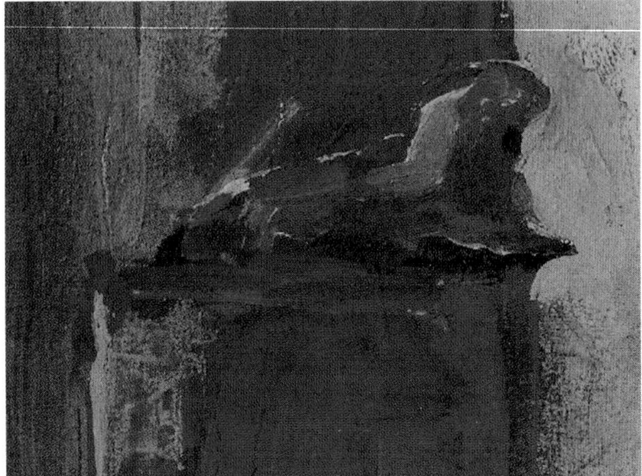

Fig. 1

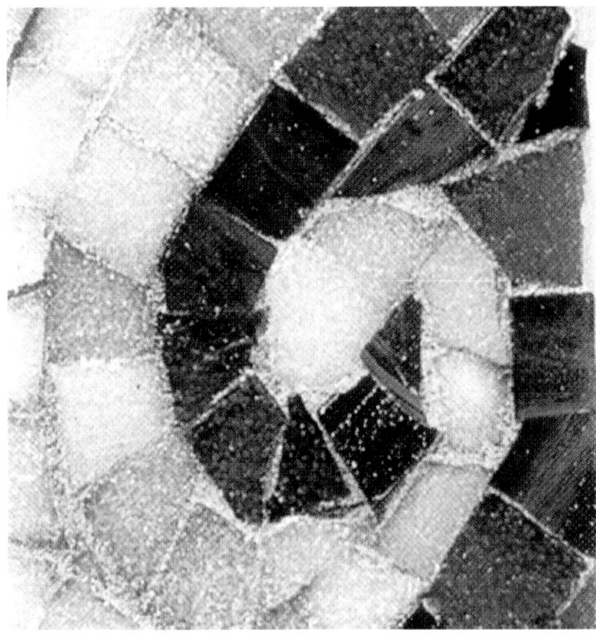

Fig. 2

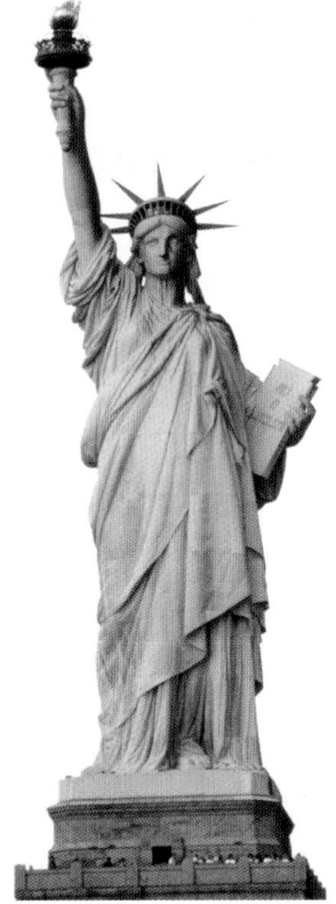

Fig. 3

diminished as image size increases. On the other hand, image size is automatically predetermined if the number and size of the pixels are predetermined. To double the resolution, both the number of pixels per row and the number of rows must be doubled. Thus, the number of pixels is increased by a factor of 4 (Figs. 3 and 4). All slice image examinations must also take the third dimension into account; in addition to the *x*- and *y*-axes, the value along the *z*-axis must also be determined. In these examinations, one speaks not of an image point, but of a volume element, or **voxel**. The number of voxels is the product of the number of elements along the *x*-axis (or image rows) multiplied by the number of elements along the *y*-axis (or image columns) and the number of elements along the *z*-axis (usually the same as the number of slices). In many examinations, the dimensions in the three planes are not the same, resulting in box-shaped voxels; it is also possible, though, to have cubical voxels, where the edge-length is the same in all directions. Regardless of the shape of the voxel, when spatial resolution is to be doubled, the amount of data required is raised to the third power (and thus by a factor of 8). It is easy to see that requirements for the visibility of details result in rapidly increasing demands on the memory and speed of the computer system. Naturally, image depth, already discussed above, also has a significant effect on the need for memory; this, however, stands in a linear relation to the volume of available data. In the simplest case, an image point can have only one of two values: black or white. To put it "digitally," this case can be encoded with one **bit** (a bit is the smallest unit of digital information and can have a value of either 0 or 1). Two bits are needed to encode 3 or (at most) 4 gray-values. With 8 bits, 256 values can be encoded. Eight

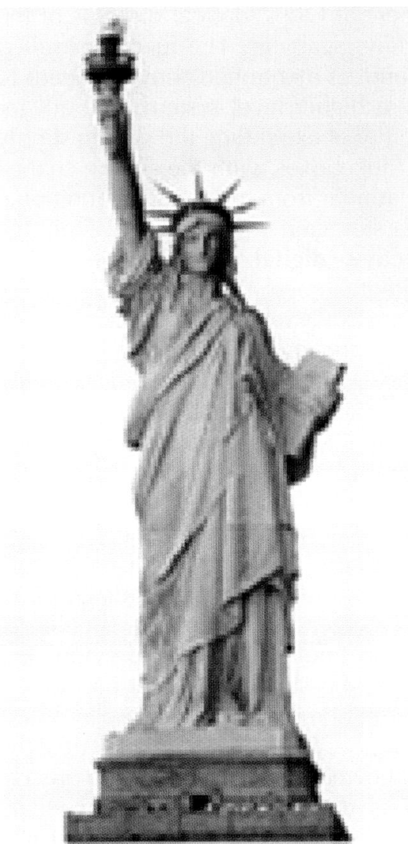

Fig. 4

bits correspond to 1 **byte**, which is the unit for digital storage capacity. Since significantly larger amounts of data are involved in digital imaging, multiple quantities of byte are usually indicated, furnished with the prefixes "kilo" for 10^3, "mega" for 10^6, "giga" for 10^9, and "tera" for 10^{12}. (Note the peculiarity that the prefix "kilo" does not stand for exactly 1000, as it is used otherwise, but for 2^{10}, thus 1024.)

Regarding memory, multi-slice CT became the most challenging modality. In 1990 an average CT examination consisted of far less than 100 images. The matrix was usually 256 × 256 pixel. Up-to-date CT scanners produce images in a 512 × 512 matrix. It comes quite easily to more than 1000 images in a modern multi-slice CT scan. After multiplanar reconstruction there can be 2000 images or more. The necessary memory has increased by a factor of almost 100 in 15 years for the same type of examination. As computer technology has advanced in a similar way, today's computers can keep up with the required speed but digital imaging still challenges high end products.

Organization of data-transfer between modalities and workstations

In addition to the image data themselves, information of a technical or organizational nature is also translated in an appendix to each image. This "attached image description" includes information about the patient, examination modality, etc., and information identifying the image. While this information is indispensable to the flow of the procedure, it is usually processed by the image processing system so that the user is completely unaware of it. This information is significant for the application, not for the user, and will be disregarded in the remainder of this chapter. In the following, when we speak about the transmission of images and examinations, we should be aware that we invariably mean the transmission of information about the composition of the image; at no time is there any actual exchange or transport of material objects. When an examination is concluded, the images are sent to a workstation. In technical terms, the information is copied from the modality's storage to the storage facility of the workstation. The condition between the modality and the site of diagnosis can be either a point-to-point connection or a connection to a network. The data can be transmitted via a (co-axial) cable, a fiber optic cable, or, to a certain extent, in wireless fashion, for example, via an infrared interface. It depends on the circumstances which type of connection is the most appropriate; the most important factors are the amount of data and the transmission speed. Technically, the data are divided into smaller packages furnished with the sender and destination address and instructions for the receiving workstation about the composition of the image information. All this is invisible to the user. After a brief time, the user has access to the information at the destination. After the completeness of the image material on the diagnostic console has been confirmed, the examination can be deleted from the examination modality. This procedure can be done manually, or an automated process can be implemented. The examination is available on the workstation itself for further use.

Archive-levels and logistics

Typically, the radiologist performs the diagnosis there. The data volume for images is large (each image corresponds to several hundred kilobytes, up to 8 megabytes); at the same time, the memory on the workstation is limited. In practice, this has resulted in an archive architecture providing for a short-term storage memory and a long-term storage memory.

The long-term memory can also be divided into one part for mid-term storage and the part for definitive storage of the data. Currently, a magnetic-based medium makes sense for the short-term storage. This is typically a magnetic hard-disk of the type familiar in all computers. The capacity is of a magnitude ranging from 40-200 gigabytes. All examinations needed here at the moment for diagnosis are stored on the **local hard-disk**. The previous examinations and comparison images, as required, are also stored locally. The image viewing stations in the clinical departments are comparable in capacity. These devices are not only used for diagnosis, but also enable the viewing of examinations together with the diagnosis that has already been made. Usually, the current examinations are available of those patients who are in the department at present. For practical purposes, thus, a storage medium is needed that enables rapid call-up of the images in the working memory, and that can at the same time be updated at any time and for which no usage costs arise. The workstation's hard-disk meets these criteria in an ideal way. A magnetic hard-disk is also most appropriate as interim storage for examinations that are very likely to be accessed again, namely, all the examinations from the most recent days or weeks and the previous examinations required for diagnosis. Given that such examinations will be accessed from many different points, a central location within the network is required. The size of this storage place is a good ten orders of magnitude larger than that of the local hard-disk. Extreme flexibility is required at this location as well, since the likelihood that an examination will be accessed again diminishes drastically after the passage of just a few weeks. This means that the mid-term memory must also be erasable and if at all possible should not require the use of any materials. The situation with regard to long-time memory is completely different. The emphasis here is on safe, permanent archiving. The storage medium must be unmodifiable and unerasable. Naturally, this will involve the consumption of a storage medium, which should be inexpensive and offer much storage room; the terabye range is desirable. Reading speed, on the other hand, is of only secondary importance. **Optical disks** have worked well for this up to now. Currently DVDs are a reasonable medium to store high quantities of digital information. Both optical discs and DVDs are administered in automatic disc changers. They are administered in automatic disk-changers (**jukeboxes**). They are controlled via a higher-level archiving system, which sees to it that new examinations are burned onto an optical disk or that previous examinations are read back from such a disk. The capacity of normal commercial OD's (optical disks) is of the magnitude of a few gigabytes. The jukebox itself is "unintelligent," and, as mentioned above, it needs to be controlled by a higher-level system. The advantage is the possibility of expanding the system simply by adding further jukeboxes, with the simple change in configuration familiar from installing an additional hard-disk or other storage medium in a PC. From the financial perspective, **digital optical tapes** would also be an excellent storage medium for permanent archiving. Their great advantage is an otherwise unattainable storage capacity at an unparalleled low price per megabyte. Their reading speed is lower, though, than that of a jukebox with OD's; this is attributable chiefly to the much slower access time, since the tape must first be wound to the right place. In practice, if the control of the archive is set up in such a way that previous examinations can be preloaded before diagnosis, this is not a disadvantage, especially since it is vanishingly rare that diagnosis of an unscheduled emergency examination should depend exclusively on information from previous images. Unfortunately, this storage medium has not yet made the step from the research laboratory into day-to-day routine practice. This chapter will not treat the remaining path followed by the image, as the process for the dataflow is described precisely elsewhere. What is of essential importance is the fact that it is not a real image in the physical sense that is transmitted, but only information about the image's composition. Forwarding the information from one point to another is always simply a matter of copying – without any decrease in quality. If this transmission of information involves transfer of the image to another location (as is the case, of course, for transmission between the examination modality and the workstation, or for forwarding from the workstation to the long-term archive), the "original" can be deleted after this transfer has been accomplished. (Do not forget, of course, that there can be neither an "original" nor a "copy"; only the identical information can be available simultaneously at different locations.) What is significant in this connection is that an examination can be deleted only when it is available at least at one other location. This makes it desirable for the system to recognize whether saving on the associated workstation has been concluded before it is deleted by the modality to make memory space available. This is true as well for the workstation's storage in its interaction with the central archive.

The described availability of images at different locations at the same time is also the key to scientific databases. As all images can be accessed from every workstation and the criteria for image retrieval can be determined to your personal requirements, all examinations that meet certain criteria can be accessed in no time at all. All that has to be done is to enter the required information into a digital query-form. The patient directory (this is the highest level of the data storage system) will then find all examinations that meet the specific requirements and will present a list with all matches to the user. For example: at the radiology department a large clinical trial was performed in which all 75-year olds of particular districts of Vienna were asked to participate. (The main aim of the study was to identify prognostic criteria to predict Alzheimers disease.) All participants underwent an MRI examination of the brain. All these MRI studies have been reviewed several times for other purposes. The information is stored in the central archieve as in any other examination. There is no need to have a dedicated section for scientific purposes. A query with the criteria "MRI AND brain AND age 75" will bring the required information. Within seconds such a list is created. The retrieval time of the actual study depends on the level of storage ranging from seconds (if still in the short term archive) to several minutes (if in the long term archive). No conventional system will make it as easy to access studies that meet a combination of criteria.

Data compression

It will usually make sense to reduce the size of the large data volumes that are involved. This step is most important before saving on the final storage medium. Absolutely nothing stands in the way of reversible, loss-less **data compression** using appropriate algorithms. The compression factor here, however, is not much higher than 2. (Nevertheless, this still means halving the volume of data to be archived without any loss of quality.) Compression procedures that are not completely reversible enable data compression of the order of a power of ten; this involves some loss of quality when the image is reconstructed, however. This is often hardly noticeable, but at least from a legal perspective it raises questions that must be considered individually for each user in each case, and must ultimately be answered according to the situation in the given country. This is true as well when data are reduced by archiving only those images selected by the physician. This type of data reduction also involves the additional effort required for selection.

We should not forget that archive media has become considerably bigger and cheaper. In 1992 storage capacity on optical discs(OD) cost about 7 (Euro-)cent per Mbyte. At that time a typical OD could hold app. 800MB. Today a standard DVD has at least 5 times this capacity and costs something like 0.05 cent/MB. As reading and writing speeds of digital archive media have been increased tremendously since the 1990s, it has to be discussed if there is a need for data reduction after all.

Generally, as much work as possible should be automated. The physician should be able to concentrate on his or her medical activity, rather than becoming a slave to the digital system.

Digital radiology: more than a PACS

The technical assistants, too, should be able to concentrate on the examination. A good digital X-ray system should see to it itself that the correct images are at the right place at the right time. Digitial radiology is concerned not only with the generation, archiving, and de-archiving of images, but encompasses all the steps, from entering a request to returning a diagnosis with the images; it is concerned as well with teaching and research, with the logistical, legal, and technical aspects of procuring outside opinions, and more. Such a system must be able to do much more than a PACS in the classical (by now nearly the historical) sense. The patient's master data and the specific data from the patient's location (referring ward...) must be available, as must the statement of the problem with clinical information, previous diagnoses, etc. Furthermore, such a system should provide statistical and searching functions, and be usable for billing. Of course, it is possible to integrate all these functions into a PACS, thus upgrading it as a digital radiology system. In most cases, however, this is not practical, since systems administering these data and providing these functions are typically already in place in a hospital. Data administration is usually performed in a hospital information system in conjunction with a radiology information system. Redundant administration represents additional effort and expense, in terms of work and costs, without providing any simultaneous benefits. The exchange of information between these two systems in both directions is vital, though. Experience has shown that it is very difficult in practice to connect different systems that are not adjusted to each other in any way. This fact has not escaped the engineers either (who are equally aware of the necessity for system integration). While great improvements have been made in recent years, resulting in a good rapport, further improvement in shared standards is necessary to make the integration of different systems unproblematic. A "plug-and-play" system from different manufacturers is still far in the future. Promising approaches have resulted from the widespread use of the **DICOM standard** in imaging. In contrast, no international standard for alphanumeric systems (HIS and RIS) is foreseeable.

Useful technical terms in digital radiology

The term "workstation" has already been used several times above. We turn to this component in the following. Under "**workstation**," we understand in general a computer in a computer network connected to a central processor with which it exchanges data. The important components are the **motherboard**, which includes the **main processor** at the "heart" of the computer with the **working memory**; the local **hard-disk**; the **graphics card**; the keyboard and mouse as control elements; and, of course, one or usually more monitors. Most calculation operations take place in the main processor. The speed of the workstation depends to a great extent on the main processor's performance. An important parameter in this connection at a range of up to several thousand MHz is the **clock frequency** (at a range of several hundred MHz). The higher this value, the more calculation operations are performed per second, and the faster this component works. Only those data that are loaded at the moment in the working memory (RAM) can be processed directly. Thus, if images are to be displayed, they must be loaded simultaneously with the **application** (by which we understand the computer program being used) and parts of the **operating system**. The operating system is essential for every function of a computer, since the computer cannot perform even the smallest functions or understand any computer program. For practical reasons, it must be possible to load extensive examinations together with any comparison examinations simultaneously into the working memory. If we consider that an MRT examination frequently consists of some hundreds of individual images, a working memory of 1Gbyte or more makes sense for the matrix and image depth currently used. Of course, amounts of data even larger than this can be transferred to external **virtual memory**, although this slows speed considerably and in day-to-day operation is acceptable only in individual cases.

The graphics card and the monitors are responsible for displaying images. The most important parameters here are the possible **resolution** and the **refresh rate**; the diagonal measurement (as a measurement of size) and brightness of the monitor are also important. Resolution must be high enough to be able to display the pixels in the images. The refresh rate indicates how many images can be displayed per second. Although the human eye cannot resolve many more than 25 images per second, image frequencies of less than approximately 70 per second seem quite unpleasant, since the image is not steady, and the monitor flickers. Values of 72 frames/s (=72 Hz) are acceptable, but higher values are preferable, with values in excess 100 Hz providing no practical advantages. The term "**bandwidth**" is also used in this connection; it indicates how many image points per second can be displayed (the necessary bandwidth results from the number of image points and the refresh rate). Usually, images with lower resolution can be displayed more often than when the displayable matrix is used to its full extent. In addition to these values, the brightness and contrast of the display are also significant to the quality of viewing. The brighter the room in which diagnosis is performed, the brighter the monitor must be. Contrast, however, must not be neglected either. In this connection, image sharpness should also be considered. Images displayed on tube monitors tend not to be in focus in all segments when the devices are operated at brightness and contrast settings at the limit of the device's specific capabilities. Today, there are commercially available devices with sufficiently good display characteristics that satisfy high requirements without raising any doubts as to their durability. For our specialized purposes (namely, diagnosis of radiological examinations), a good gray-value display is of far greater importance than the capacity for color display. The color monitors available today are still inferior to high-quality black-and-white monitors in their gray-value display. Recently TFT-screens have reached a spatial and contrast resolution that makes them an alternative to cathode-ray-tube based conventional monitors. With TFT-screens the problem of inappropriate low refresh-rates does not exist. Because of the different principles at work in TFT monitors, they do not have the problem of unfocused display at the edges.

We have already seen some of the requirements for the hard-disk as local short-term storage. In addition to an appropriate capacity, **access speed** and the **data transfer rate** should be as fast as possible. Access speed is a parameter usually indicated in ms; it provides information about the speed with which certain contents of the hard-disk can be accessed. This value should be as low as possible. The data transfer rate gives the maximum transmittable data mass per second. This is dependent on several factors that affect transfer from the hard-disk to the working memory or the memory of the graphics card. As in almost any chain, the weakest link is the decisive one. Because there are so many factors, a practical test is especially appropriate here. We must not forget that the prerequisites in daily operation are different than those for a display model in a showroom, which is usually already equipped with test images. Opening and manipulating images in laboratory conditions lets the workstation make its capabilities available for the function required at that moment. In daily operation, though, the workstation is often communicating with the central archive, receiving previous examinations and other new examinations, performing database reconciliations, and performing many other activities simultaneously "in the background," which puts demands on the system components and reduces actual working speed. Most of these functions cannot be controlled in respect to time, but are demanded from the workstation at any time. The possible system times are adequate for all these activities, but even today high-end products are required. If a device cannot perform several functions in parallel, but is set up for sequential processing, too many unaccomplished tasks will pile up, thus making clinical use in routine operation impossible.

The digital radiology in the digital hospital of the future

S. Bocionek, W. Baldauf-Sobez, and R. Primo

Siemens Medical Solutions, Erlangen, Germany

Introduction

Digital Hospitals can be seen as a goal-oriented vision of how to improve healthcare delivery and operations by means of modern *Medical and Information Technology*. The driving forces behind the vision are the business needs of healthcare delivery organizations, in particular better quality of care and improvement of their economic situation (revenue, market share, expense growth, cash balance). These needs can be fulfilled through business re-engineering based on *people* (new roles) and *processes*, supported by leading-edge *products* (innovative technology), together forming new *solutions* like the *Digital Hospital*.

A systematic construction principle leads to more sophisticated workflow management to support teamwork, as well as desktop integration for ergonomic roles-based workplaces. The basis is a clear platform strategy for software applications spanning both, *Medical and Information Technology*.

Based on the advantages of the platform-based system construction approach, it is possible to demonstrate the additional capabilities of such a *Digital Hospital* concept in terms of *value adding services* that help maximize the utilization of the technology investment. Examples of such services include hosting all software applications in a supplier's data center (ASP concept), (information) technology outsourcing in the hospital through the technology partner, but also non-technology services like combined business office, accounts receivables collection or supply chain management.

We will use the example of the *Digital Radiology* to explain in more detail the technology infrastructure and its ability to provide improved workplace ergonomics and teamwork automation throughout the whole *Digital Hospital*.

Digital Hospitals: The idea

The idea of *Digital Hospital* is not brand new. Earlier articles describe a vision of the *Hospital of the Future* [1, 2]. The *Hospital of the Future* focused almost entirely on leading edge technology and its capabilities, while the *Digital Hospital* is a much more goal-oriented process re-engineering approach. This approach looks at how to improve healthcare delivery and operations by means of modern *Medical and Information Technology*. The reasoning behind the *Digital Hospital* is that technology should be seen as the enabler rather than the driver of this vision. (Interestingly, the term *Digital Hospital* has already be used in the first filmless hospital project in Vienna, see [3]).

Hospital workflow

A key objective of the *Digital Hospital* is to use technology for increasing quality and productivity in healthcare. Central to this objective is the support of teamwork through modern workflow management tools [4], add parantheses. The prerequisite for tool support in healthcare teamwork is the understanding of healthcare processes and their optimization as the first step. The introduction of software applications with embedded workflow capabilities (like Soarian, see [5]) is the second step.

Hospital processes can be modeled as depicted in Fig. 1. The standard workflow starts with an *administrative cycle* where patients are scheduled, then admitted in an ADT system, and finally discharged. This cycle ends when their claim is generated.

The next cycle after admission is the the *clinical cycle*, where a physician order entry system (POE) may be used to enable doctors to give their orders online (the positive results of POE are quantified in Ahmad A. et al. [6]). During the clinical cycle, everything happening to the patient must be documented. Procedure codes are sent back to the administrative cycle that allows the billing system to produce the claim.

During the *clinical cycle*, the physician first gathers information by sending the patient into the

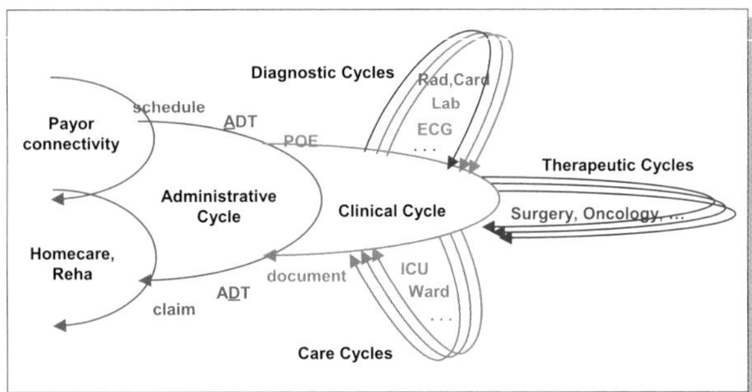

Fig. 1. Process model of hospital operations

diagnostic cycles, and then decides on the best treatment. At this point, the patient enters the *therapeutic cycle*. Therapy can range from simple medication administration to surgery, or to complex combined treatments like radiation and chemotherapy for a cancer patient.

After treatment (or during the process of treatment) the patient remains in the *care cycle*, which may include days in intensive care, or in the ward only.

Currently, the "pain points" in hospital workflow are the various and highly disconnected process cycles.

- Example 1: Patients are registered more than once, in more than one place. Result: Patient data resides in multiple databases, leading to inconsistent data sets and, hence, to inconsistent documentation and claims.
- Example 2: Doctors don't have access to the patient chart in real time, or sometimes not at all, at the moment they have to give an order. Result: Medication errors that could have been avoided (7000 deaths in the USA annually caused by medication errors only, 90000 deaths due to so-called adverse events; see Institute of Medicine [7]).
- Example 3: The different care providers in a hospital work in quite an uncoordinated way. Result: A diabetic patient is scheduled for a radiology exam at 11:30 a.m. When he returns to his bed at 12:30 p.m. his meal is cold or being taken away. The person bringing the food was not aware of the exam and not informed to delay meal delivery.

The above examples of "pain points" provide us with a straight-forward understanding of the term 'hospital workflow;'

The flow of patients, information and resources in a coordinated way.

Process re-engineering goals for a *Digital Hospital*

Re-engineering of the hospital workflow is, therefore, the systematic change of all processes toward measurable goals. These goals are very similar to those described for the optimization of task flows in the *diagnostic cycle* of radiology (see [8]), but on the level of a complete hospital. They include:

1. Cycle time goals – shorter length of stay, length of a diagnostic cycle (from the order to the reception of the result), or average duration of tasks like bed turnaround time.
2. Punctuality goals – the percentage of radiology exams performed at the time they were scheduled, or surgical operations started at the hour they were planned.
3. Quality goals – reduced error rates (medication, transcription, others), or reduced number of follow-up treatment needs (like re-stenosis removals).
4. Financial goals – lower cost per surgical procedure, reduced IT spending per adjusted patient day, fewer A/R recovery days, increased market share.
5. (Customer) Satisfaction goals, which include all constituents – patients, physicians, nurses, administrative personnel.

A massive introduction of leading-edge innovations in medical devices, information and communication technology, software workflow solutions, and infrastructure management (security, energy, light) to form the *Digital Hospital* is the logical next step to maximize the results of re-engineering efforts.

Quality management needs in the *Digital Hospital*

Improving quality is a major reason for all re-engineering efforts. As one example, let us look at the quality management in the *Digital Radiology* that plays a major role in many disease management workflows.

Disease management outcome is based on assessing whether a specific treatment is likely to have a positive effect on the quality of life. This attention to total quality is in its infancy, as health care faces a true "quality revolution." In the following paragraphs, we will look into quality issues in a digital radiology department.

Examples of the quality revolution can be found in almost every industry. William Edwards Deming (1900–1993; see [9]) was an American statistician and quality control expert. He used statistics to examine industrial production processes for flaws and believed that improving product quality depended on increased management–labor cooperation and innovative design and production processes.

Industries utilize quality management techniques to improve outcomes and lower costs. The "re-engineering" of business practices is routine. Long a laggard in adopting management practices; the health care industry must develop its own tools to achieve similar gains in quality improvement if it wishes to control its own destiny.

It is clear that "digitization" will have direct implications for the quality and outcome of radiology services. Many variables with a direct impact on quality (e.g. quality of display device, imaging modality, and radiology processes) are under direct control of radiologists and can be managed by resources inside the radiology department.

Many other variables, however, are located beyond the departmental boundaries (e.g. quality of enterprise patient scheduling and registration, information technology and communication networks and access, or training of nurses and physician's using Enterprise PACS viewers). That means, the complete enterprise must be involved. A structured quality approach using methods like Continuous Quality Improvement (CQI; see Crosby [10]) and ISO 9000 accreditation (see ISO WebSites [11]) will be required.

Implementing quality management systems such as CQI and securing the results of CQI with ISO 9000 are long and tedious processes. CQI (and ISO 9000) require a strong commitment from top management in the enterprise. Failing to allocate the required resources and commitment from the top of the organization will result in disappointments during implementation. It is therefore good practice to set modest, credible, and reachable QA targets.

The "Plan – Do – Check – Act" cycle can then start. "Act" means that changes are documented and consolidated, and staff is trained on the new procedure. The organization is now ready for the next improvement cycle.

Technology needs of a *Digital Hospital*

Based on the process and quality goals for a *Digital Hospital* one can list the requirements for the technology to be applied.

1. Ease of use: Technology is for people and requires their acceptance. Therefore, all user interaction with technology has to be made easy, and as short as possible. This includes the need for desktop integration.
2. Smart behavior: The software applications have to interact *smartly* with the user, exploiting anticipation (predict what the user needs), feedback (propose better alternatives), and automation (do what is known) concepts.
3. Application support of teamwork: Teamwork support has to maximize *push technology*, to forward information or requests automatically to the person(s) responsible for the next step(s) in the workflow chain.
4. Consistent technology behavior: Independent from the tools and applications technology has to act or re-act consistently, from simple user login to complex surgery team coordination.
5. Connectivity of all applications: Connectivity within the *Digital Hospital* is needed to allow for accessing ALL information anywhere, anytime.
6. Scalability: Technology solutions have to work with the same performance in environments of any size, from small hospitals to complex university facilities.
7. Safety: The technology, in particular the workflow support parts of the applications, have to work in a way that excludes any risk for patients and hospital personnel.
8. Consolidation: Consolidation of technology is needed to simplify today's complex configurations (networks, computers, storage, applications).
9. Cost efficiency: Cost efficiency is partly a construction principle (e.g. decide on scalable computers) for the *Digital Hospital*, partly a design goal, but ultimately an outcome (like reduced IT expenses per adjusted patient day).

Digital Hospitals: The technology approach

To understand our technology approach for the *Digital Hospital* it is first necessary to explain the distinction between *solution integration* and *solution construction*.

Solution integrators take products and integrate them as much as possible following established standards (in healthcare HL7, DICOM, often aligned with the IHE interoperability model as described in [12]). Examples of successful companies in healthcare providing solution integration are Accenture,

Cap Gemini Ernest & Young, and also IBM Global Services. Such companies typically cannot influence the R&D (research and development) of the products they integrate. As a consequence, they mainly address the technology needs 5 – 9 as described above, but have no real means to fulfill the requirements 1 – 4.

Fulfilling the technology needs 1 – 4 is the difference between technology and solution. A *solution* is an answer to a problem (see [13]), in terms of applying technology to solve the re-engineering goals of a *Digital Hospital* as stated above. To give these answers and provide solutions for all needs of the *Digital Hospital*, one needs a systematic bottom up engineering approach that we call *system construction*.

System construction: The basis for the *Digital Hospital*

The construction of the system *Digital Hospital* is based on four technology layers of increasing complexity. Each lower layer is consistently used in the next higher layer. Technology components are embedded in technology platforms. Technology platforms are the basis for products. Workflow-oriented combinations of products are forming solutions, of increasingly higher complexity up to the level of a *Digital Hospital*.

Technology *components*: This layer starts with off-the-shelf components like operating system, database, network protocol, UI toolkit, etc. It just needs a determination of what to use, but then it must be used consistently (e.g. the decision to use the Windows or the Linux operating system).

Based on off-the-shelf components, higher-level basic application modules must be purchased or developed. They include security components (like PKI based authentication and authorization), session management components (like single sign-on, context sharing), data modeling and access tools (masterfile toolkit or CMF, enterprise master person index or EMPI, terminology server), one interface engine (to map HL7, DICOM, EDI transactions), one workflow management system (WfMS for process automation), one output management component, and others.

Technology *platforms*: The platform layer is key for the development of efficient products with consistent behavior, thus fulfilling in particular the technology requirements 1 – 5 described above, and also supporting fast and cost-efficient development by the vendor.

Why? Let us use the example of the three Siemens Medical Solutions software platforms:

- syngo (for all medical imaging applications; see syngo WebSites [14]).
- SIENET (the PACS for large-scale image data management, see [15]).
- Soarian (for complete administrative and clinical workflow, see [16]).

Users of Siemens products expect that all platforms work well together and show consistent 'behavior' (e.g. in terms of security and session management). Siemens engineers integrate all components like PKI, CMF, EMPI, WfMS as named above in exactly those three platforms. This ensures identical integration of the components and consistent behavior of all products: the perfect case of re-use in software development, and a unique differentiator for Siemens solutions.

Products: Products are typically developed on one platform, like the software of a CT scanner on syngo, a PACS archive on the SIENET data management platform, or a specific cardiology data management system on Soarian. Although the products utilize only one platform, they mostly need all components.

Solutions: The platform-based products can now be combined in a way that fulfills the re-engineering needs much better than systems integrators could ever provide. The resulting optimal desktop and workflow integration give the buzzword 'seamless integration' a clear meaning.

Desktop integration allows for the deployment of *workplaces* that combine the features of multiple products in an ergonomic way. For example, the integrated cardiology exam workplace (ICEW) is a workstation providing cardiology specific syngo image examination and post-processing functionality. This is combined with the Soarian based cardiology data management system – on one (multi-) screen setting, operated with one mouse and one keyboard, accessed by one single sign-on, sharing the patient context of studies in the SIENET archive with electronic medical records in the Soarian repository.

Workflow integration is achieved by modeling healthcare processes in a workflow editor, and making the models executable, i.e. let the Soarian workflow engine push tasks and results automatically to referring clinicians, to nurses or to the hospital pharmacy.

In the same way, integrated radiology, oncology, OR, ICU and other workplaces and workflows can be designed for the other clinical specialties. Ergonomics driven integration is key for the acceptance of physicians to better utilize modern technology.

Combining workplaces (e.g. diagnostic and/or therapeutic devices) with workstations in a value-adding approach leads to digital departments, like the *Digital Radiology, Digital Oncology,* and so on.

Combining the digital departments with an enterprise wide workflow-oriented hospital information system finally forms the *Digital Hospital.*

Operational options for a *Digital Hospital*

Improving financial goals, in particular through the optimization of technology and the non-medical activities, is not really unique in a hospital environment and thus can be approached like typical operational excellence initiatives in other industries. The key idea to tackle such non-core activities is the *utilization of scale effects,* with regard to the technology infrastructure (networks, servers, desktops), and the utilization of personnel, in particular coping with the needs of highly specialized experts.

Outsourcing of technology is a service provided by companies that take over the responsibility to operate the technology in a hospital for costs lower than the hospital IT department could do. The cost advantage comes from scale effects across more than one customer, e.g. running software applications of various customers on the same computer mainframe, or deploying one expert in billing software for consulting or trouble shooting across many locations in a specific territory.

Outsourcing of business processes is another service where specialized companies provide back office services like payroll management, accounts receivables collection, or supply chain management. For example, one can typically realize cost savings up to 50% by outsourcing payroll services.

Hosting of software applications is a special type of technology outsourcing where the servers and mainframes are located at one central data center of the service provider, and the client workstations in hundreds of hospitals are connected through a data network. Hosting allows the provider to utilize the highest possible scale effect. A good example is the Siemens Health Services data center in Malvern, PA, where about 100 Siemens employees operate the software applications of more than 1000 customers 24 × 7. Those customers would need an accumulated equivalent of 10000 or more IT staff to provide the same service at the 1000 different sites locally.

Digital radiology for diagnostic workflow in the Digital Hospital

Diagnostic workflows in the *Digital Hospital* are happening at various places, where ever assessments of a patient's condition are needed. Examples are the laboratory (e.g. for blood tests), the ECG lab for stress tests and other examinations, as well as the units for diagnostic imaging mainly in Radiology and Cardiology. In this section we want to focus on workflow solutions inside a *Digital Radiology* (early references can be found in Hruby et al. [3]).

The workflow of a *Digital Radiology* is well described in the IHE model [12]. The main steps are (in this sequence):

- Patient registration (manually in the RIS, or transmitted from the HIS).
- Order placing (in the RIS, or transmitted from a referring physician order entry).
- Scheduling time, location, personnel, and device.
- Sending a DICOM work list entry with all patient, order and scheduling information to the modality; in parallel triggering pre-fetching of previous studies from the PACS archive to the reporting workstation; see [8]).
- Performing the examination on the modality, and sending the resulting images to the reporting workstation of the PACS.
- Performing the interpretation on the PACS workstation, writing the report in the RIS application.
- Sending results (report and selected images) back to the referring physician, and the study into the PACS archive.
- Sending a billing code (ICD-9, ICD-10, others) back to the HIS.

Additional steps, like pre-processing a radiography image on the QC workstation, post-processing of studies to generate 3D views, and the clinical demonstration can extend the workflow depending on the case.

Ease of use: Ease of use focuses on *ergonomic workplaces* (for doctors, radiographers, nurses, administrators), since those workplaces are the points of contacts for humans with technology.

Ease of use starts with ease of access: Modern biometric authentication devices (like the fingerprint mouse in Fig. 2) allow the doctor to login without *typing* passwords.

Combined with a central user administration like the Soarian Common Master File Toolkit (CMF), login is possible at any workstation in the network that has a biometric mouse connected.

Based on the CMF, an integrated desktop for the radiologist (like the Sienet Command Center) can even provide a *single sign-on* (e.g. the doctor performs one login, and is then authorized to use all

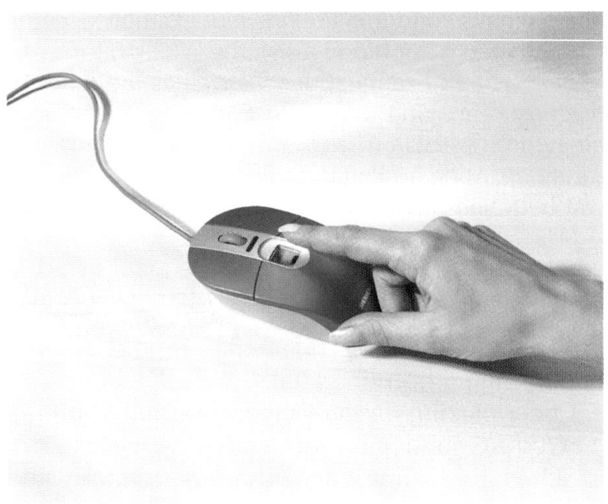

Fig. 2. Biometric mouse: The touch sensor in the middle of the mouse recognizes the fingerprint of an individual. (Photo: Siemens)

applications – PACS, RIS, EPR browser, speech recognition, word processing), as well as access to all databases connected (PACS archive, EPR repository, others). A global session manager (GSM) preserves the context of the patient data manipulated within the various applications.

'Smart behavior': The easy to use workplace becomes 'smart' if automated steps are incorporated that speed up the radiologists work. A good example is the *hanging protocols* in a PACS workstation. The radiologist hits the 'next study' button and the study is automatically arranged on the multi-monitor screen as pre-defined, simulating the layouts he was used to at the lightbox.

Further 'smart' interaction could be provided by the concept of *embedded analytics*, as first introduced in Soarian (see [16]). Such mechanisms are not yet part of RIS-PACS applications today, but can be envisioned within the next two – three years. The embedded analytics would enable the application to automatically and continuously monitor and measure key performance and quality parameters of the radiology workflow. Examples are automated reminders if a study is not completed and delivered to the referring physician within the targeted cycle time, or automated alerts if a report comes to different conclusions based on similar findings as a previous one.

Support of teamwork: Technology-enabled support of teamwork in Radiology is not a new approach. Since the inception of PACS in the early nineties, such concepts have been incorporated. A good example is pre-fetching and auto-routing (i.e. the automated transmission of images between archive and workstations at the earliest possible moment). Another good example for a *Digital Radiology* is the consequent utilization of speech recognition in the KFJ, Vienna (see [15]).

Additional progress – besides the automated image management – has been made in data access, order management and results distribution. Web-based portals (like the Dashboard from Siemens) allow access to all possible sources of clinical information. The portal unifies and personalizes the interaction with the specific browsers (like MagicWeb for images or Soarian Clinical Access for patient record data). Furthermore, Soarian Clinical Access includes mechanisms to actively notify the user that new information is available. Results notification is not only automated, but also 'smart' in the sense that it contains the notion of 'importance' (e.g. a doctor is informed of a critical new lab data of a patient immediately).

Connectivity and scalability of all applications: Connectivity is the pre-requisite for teamwork automation as discussed above. Key for 'economic' connectivity is the rigorous adherence to standards, like DICOM, HL7, EDI and others. Proprietary, maybe even point-to-point, connections within one vendor's product line prevent economics of scale, combination and migration toward other solutions, and result in increasing costs for maintenance.

Furthermore, the scalability of such solutions is often limited, thus leading to problems if the throughput in the *Digital Radiology* increases (more procedures to be performed, more doctors and nurses online, more studies and data in digital form, etc.).

Technology consolidation drives cost efficiency of investment and maintenance costs: Connectivity and scalability considerations 'naturally' lead to a consolidation of the technology used in the *Digital Radiology*. The goal is to limit the ever-growing hunger for hardware investment, the subsequent increase of the maintenance costs, and all other associated negative implications.

One first solution is the so-called *broker-less RIS-PACS integration*, as provided in the SIENET radiology command center. Broker-less RIS-PACS means that no integration engine (like a PACS broker) is needed inbetween RIS and PACS. The results are savings overall of about $100K, one less point of possible failure, and better ability to integrate RIS and PACS on one desktop with a single-sign on. Further quantified positive results have been reported from Bethesda Memorial Hospital in Florida [17].

An expensive investment in the *Digital Radiology* is the need for huge storage capacity, large RAID banks for online access, as well as big tape robots for long-term storage. The discussion whether 'cheap'

RAIDs will make tape libraries obsolete soon is ongoing; the author is not in a position to predict the outcome. Independent from the outcome is the concept of SAN / NAS (storage area networks, network archive systems). Both are a scalable approach to provide the 'technology service' archiving to a PACS without making a difference between the media (RAID, OD, CD, tape). From the PACS application point of view SAN / NAS stores all studies and allows for retrieval within acceptable response times.

The future: from Digital Hospitals to Digital Healthcare Environments

The healthcare process is not only limited to a (digital) hospital. In more general terms it includes all activities of a person related to his or her health status, from wellness and prevention activities, through acute care encounters, subsequent rehabilitation phases, until homecare and even assisted leaving becomes important. Utilizing modern technology for the entire span of health-related needs extends the idea of the *Digital Hospital* toward fully integrated *Digital Healthcare Environments.*

Support patient and family needs: One strategic goal of a *Digital Hospital,* in particular if it is fighting for market share as many such institutions do in the United States, is the support of whole families – for prevention, acute care, rehabilitation.

Prevention has much to do with information. Resources like healthcare information on public Web pages, personalized Web pages for patients and family, individual dietary programs for at-risk patients, and continuous support for individuals with chronic problems (disease management for diabetes, asthma or congestive heart problems) are in their infancy today but will soon be part of the service offering of many *Digital Hospitals.*

Supporting the family of a hospitalized patient by simple technology means is another target for the *Digital Hospital* of the future (esp. in rural areas). Installing a $50 WebCam on each patient bed would allow the patient to talk to relatives face to face, an important means to make the family feel more comfortable and maybe even help the patient recover faster.

Support business people: A specific variation of the WebCam approach described above is the integration of a 'business office' in every patient room. Certainly, the impact on the healing process needs to be discussed for any single case. However, for many business people – with simple problems like a broken leg – the access to video conferencing, email, and other business office tools can easily become the driver for them to decide which *Digital Hospital* to chose.

Support the mobile citizen: The *Digital Hospital* will become a service provider for the mobile society. Chronically ill patients can travel, but will be connected and monitored online throughout the whole trip. Persons having accidents and in need of a hospital abroad will give the doctors there an access code so that they can login to the patient's data (history, digital images, etc.) provided by the *Digital Hospital* where the patient has subscribed for this service.

Furthermore, by means of video conferencing, even doctors from the *Digital Hospital* can consult with the physicians in the other country, or even assist in complicated operations through tele-surgery support.

Connect to the community and the future responsibility of a Digital Hospital: Besides services for individuals and their families the *Digital Hospital* will also become an integral part of community life, thus forming the overall *Digital Healthcare Environment.* This is driven by both the desire of individuals to avoid healthcare encounters because they are generally considered as unpleasant, as well the need of the healthcare system to reduce healthcare encounters in order to limit healthcare expenditures.

The new role will include responsibilities for information and education, for children as well as for adults. It will include the objective to make healthcare /wellness activities a pleasant, interesting and convenient part of everybody's life, including prevention, rehabilitation, disease management and assisted living. Technology is the enabler for such a modern world but not the driver.

It will be interesting to see, how far today's multi-trillion dollar healthcare industry will step up to redefine all the interdependent healthcare processes so that information technology can be applied as a true enabler for providing better and more cost effective solutions to patients.

References

[1] Lundine S (1996) Hospital gambles at celebration. Orlando Business Journal, October 11th 1996

[2] Geisler E, Krabbendam K, Schuring R (2003) Technology, health care, and management in the Hospital of the Future. Quorum Books

[3] Hruby W, Mosser H, Urban M, Rüger W (1992) The Vienna SMZO-PACS-project: the totally digital hospital. Eur J Radiol 16 (1): 66–68

[4] Jablonski S, Bussler C (1996) Workflow mangement: modeling concepts, architecture and implementation. International Thomson Computer Press

[5] Haux R et al (2003) Soarian – Workflow management applied for health care. In Methods Inf Med 1 / 2003
[6] Ahmad A et al (2002) Key attributes of a successful physician order entry system implementation in a multi-hospital environment. JAMIA 9: 16–24
[7] Institute of Medicine (2000) To err is human. National Academy Press, Washington, DC
[8] Bocionek S (2000) PACS 2000+ from networks to workflow and beyond. In: Hruby W (ed) Digital (R)Evolution in Radiology. Springer, Vienna
[9] Denning WebSites: Yahoo's Management Science/ Deming section (http://dir.yahoo.com/Business_and_Economy/Management_Science/Deming_Dr_W_Edwards_1990_1993_/) has links to the principal Deming sites.
[10] Crosby P (1996) Quality is still free. McGraw Hill Professional Book Group, New York, NY
[11] ISO WebSites: http://www.iso.ch/ The home page of the ISO organization.
[12] IHE Technical Framework (1998) http://www.rsna.org/IHE/tf/
[13] Bocionek S (2001a) Editorial, electromedica 69, Nr. 1, 2001
[14] syngo WebSites: http://www.syngo.com/
[15] Kumpan W, Karnel F, Nics G. (1999) 18 Month Experience with an Integrated Radiology System: HIS-RIS-SPEECH-PACS, CARS '99: 524–528
[16] Bocionek S et al (2001b) Built for Success – The new clinical and financial IT solutions from Health Services. electromedica 69, Nr. 2, 2001
[17] Bethesda Case (2002) proof.esiemenshealthcare.com/content/talk/bethesda.htm

Planning digital radiology: practical approaches

Radiology information systems in the digital hospital

G. Gell

Institute for Medical Informatics, Statistics and Documentation, Graz, Austria

Hospital information systems and RIS/PACS

The Handbook of Medical Informatics [5] gives two definitions of a Hospital Information System:

The goal of an HIS is to use computers and communication equipment to collect, store, process, retrieve, and communicate patient care and administrative information for all hospital-affiliated activities and to satisfy the functional requirements of all authorized users.

or another definition:

An information system for the benefit of a hospital, in which data are coherently stored in a database, from where they are put at the disposal of authorized users at the place and at the time the data are required, in a format adapted to the specific needs of the user.

These definitions include radiology as being part of the hospital. From a logical point of view Radiological Information Systems (RIS) and PACS are therefore parts or subsystems of the hospital information system (HIS). For practical and historical reasons however RIS have been developed as stand alone systems because the functional demands of the departments of radiology could not (and very often still cannot) be implemented in the HIS, because the HIS were mostly adapted to the needs of the hospital administration.

Of course, radiology reports and images are parts of the patient record and must be integrated or at least interfaced to the HIS and the patient record. This chapter deals with the question of integrating RIS and PACS. The ideal solution would be an integration of HIS, RIS and PACS in such a way, that each user, a radiologist, a clinician, a nurse has access to all the patient data he/she needs to care for the patient in a seamless way, with only one user interface (for each group of users) for all types of data regardless of their origin.

There are two possibilities to approach this ideal solution (which is still far away), depending on whether the emphasis is given to integration or to functionality.

- One monolithic system. RIS and PACS are implemented within the HIS with the same software system and with the same data base. There is only one HIS that covers all clinical functions.
  - Advantages: high integration concerning workflow, data base and user interface.
  - Disadvantages: less functionality because a general system usually cannot offer the same specialized services as a dedicated RIS or PACS (see below).
- Specialized systems (RIS, PACS) that are linked to the HIS through (hopefully standardized) interfaces.
  - Advantages: the systems are fine-tuned to the needs of radiology with its high volume of reports, the need to manage enormous amounts of image data which must be integrated in the workflow and the specialized interfaces to modalities.
  - Disadvantages: interfaces provide weak integration, with differences in data structures, different user interfaces etc.

The definition of the HIS given above requires, that authorized users have access to the information they need for their tasks. Since these users are human beings, they need the information in a form they can understand and process, i.e. as natural language texts, as images etc. and not in the form of codes or numbers. There are however many goals, that need computer processing of stored data, to produce statistics, to make automatic decisions about branches in the workflow etc. This questions will be dealt with in the paragraph on documentation and evaluation.

In the next chapter we will give examples, so called scenarios, for the specific processes in a radiology department and for the functional requirements for a RIS. A general scenario for a complete RIS/PACS solution is given in Ref. [1].

RIS-scenarios/business processes

The main goal of a radiology department is to perform diagnostic procedures and establish, document and distribute diagnoses effectively and efficiently. Therefore there are some basic activities (processes) common to all or most radiologies.

- Scheduling
- Admission
- Examination
- Image interpretation/reporting
- Report transcription/report verification by radiologists
- Ancillary services (e.g. billing, documentation, statistics, quality control).

Functional building blocks of a RIS

Scheduling: the planning of requested radiological examinations for the patient for a certain time and date, taking into account the availability of resources like room, modality, radiologist, radiographer etc. Scheduling may trigger other processes like printed or electronic worklists for wards about the preparation of the patient, worklists for transport services, worklists for radiologists, anesthetists etc.

Admission: the identification of the patient upon his/her arrival in radiology, basic data entry, printing of labels, triggering prefetching of images, generating worklists for modalities etc.

Examination: the radiographer selects a patient from a worklist that was generated by the admission process, performs a procedure, where patient data are automatically sent to the modality to identify images (DICOM worklist), enters additional documentation about the procedure if data cannot be acquired directly from the modality (e.g. films, contrast media, exposure), confirms end of procedure etc. Note that there are some points like patient selection from a worklist, where the distribution of tasks between PACS and RIS is not clear – there are several options how to realise this either in the RIS or in the PACS.

Image interpretation/reporting: film reading is usually a PACS function but needs assistance from the RIS, because the radiologist needs information about previous exams, clinical data etc., which are supplied by the RIS/HIS. There are also several options for reporting (dictation):

- Traditional dictation on tape with later transcription
  - advantage: very convenient for radiologists
  - disadvantages: time gap between dictation and transcription, dissatisfaction of clinicians, waste of time of clinicians and radiologists by frustrating efforts to get results by telephone calls.
- Digital dictation where the voice is stored digitally and becomes available simultaneously and immediately to typists as well as to referring physicians.
  - advantage: convenient handling to radiologists, fast availability of preliminary (voice) results to clinicians, streamlined operation of transcription
  - disadvantages: still need of transcriptionists with delays, errors, overhead, need for proof reading etc.
- Automatic voice recognition where the computer translates the dictation into written text
  - advantage: in theory, this is the ideal solution, immediate availability of written reports
  - disadvantages: in practice most available systems transfer work from typists to radiologists and are as yet not as convenient to use as normal dictation
- Generation of reports by radiologists using text-processing, decision trees etc. Except for short reports in emergency situations these methods have not been adopted widely by radiologists.

Report transcription and verification: Typing of reports on the RIS (see above). Written reports must be verified by the dictating radiologist and sometimes authorized by a senior radiologist either by signing a printed report or by signing on a computer display after proper identification. Reports may be distributed as written and signed originals on paper, or distributed in electronic form.

Ancillary services: A full RIS provides a gamut of ancillary services to the department, to mention just a few:

- Billing: either transmit necessary information for billing to the HIS or the financial system of the hospital or print bills directly
- Administration of the film archive: keep track of the lending of films, request missing films etc.
- Workload analysis: documentation of workload, statistics of workload for resource planning (budget, personnel etc.)
- Scientific retrieval and case finding for scientific work.

Each of these processes has a complex structure and consists of several subprocesses. To better understand the requirements for a RIS we will describe some of them in detail.

Admission, the scenario

At some point in time, the patient arrives in the department of radiology. There are many different possibilities:

- the examination has been scheduled or
- the patient arrives unscheduled because
  - there is no scheduling policy for this examination
  - there is an emergency.
- the patient is already in the HIS/RIS because
  - he is an inpatient
  - he is an outpatient but has previous encounters, or
- the patient is not yet in the HIS/RIS.
- the patient arrives at a dedicated admission desk or
- the patient goes directly to the examination room.

Technically admission may mean: entering patient data on a keyboard, reading a bar code label or some other ID-device. If the RIS is linked to a HIS, the typing of a short patient ID (or the selection of the patient from a list of scheduled patients) may be sufficient, the rest of the data can be requested from the HIS. The correct identification of the patient, i.e. the matching with data, which are already in the system, may be a very complex process which may be error prone and time consuming. If the patient is an outpatient which comes for the first time, more data have to be acquired: first name, surname, birth name, birth date, address, employer, relatives, social security data, billing information (e.g. private insurer), medical information like type of requested examination, clinical problem etc.

As a result of admission, the patient is entered into a worklist for the requested examination, a new patient record may be created in the database with patient data, time stamps (e.g. time of admission) etc. are recorded, labels may be printed, the prefetching of images of previous examination may be started according to some algorithms etc.

Admission, modelling

The scenario describes in plain language the real activities in the real world and also what kind of support is wanted. It can easily be seen, that the scenario is still incomplete; we did for example not describe the details of the patient identification process, what happens, when the patient claims, that he already had a previous examination but was not found in the database: phonetic matching, check for a change of name because of marriage, different spellings of first names like Bob and Robert etc.

In order to implement a RIS, all these facets of the real-life activities must be described, preferably in a formal abstract model for workflow [6] and data.

To design a new RIS, the model must be abstract and flexible enough to include all the variations of the workflow in different departments. To implement a given RIS for a given department, the model must describe the workflow at hand and it must be checked, if the RIS is able to represent it adequately.

To illustrate the problems arising from inadequate modelling we will discuss a detail of the admission process with two scenarios. For both of them, we assume that the RIS is not coupled to the HIS and patients arrive with an examination request form with all the necessary data for the RIS.

a) The admission desk belongs to an examination area with scheduled examinations (e.g. MR). Patients arrive one at a time and the clerk at admission has time enough to enter all the data from the examination request form.
b) The admission is in an area with unscheduled examinations with high throughput (chest or skeletal X-rays), where patients come in clusters. To avoid long waiting times admission is organized differently. The clerk at the desks types only the ID-data and collects the examination request forms for later entry during off-peak hours or even at a different location, e.g. by administrative personnel.

If a RIS is designed under the assumption that scenario a) is the universal model for admission, then there will be a sequence of steps, where after the identification data all the data for this patient are requested and entered by a series of screen masks, which are displayed automatically and must be filled in properly. To apply such a system to scenario b) will result in disaster. The short admission will take too much time, because the clerk must skip over several screen-masks that will not be filled yet (he/she is lucky if the system does not insist on filling the entries) and the process of filling in the rest of the data later will again be hindered by a time consuming selection process to get the correct patient mask to complete the data. An optimised system for scenario b) will have two processes, a short mask for primary admission which produces a worklist for the second process of entering the remaining data.

This example illustrates the need for a precise description and modelling of processes and workflow and the need to run realistic benchmark tests with precise timing of crucial processes. System a) can correctly claim that it is in principle able to implement process b) – but the modelling is inadequate and practical operation would be far too slow to be acceptable.

Data protection

A RIS and a PACS contain data about patients which must be protected against unauthorized access, misuse, data loss, data corruption etc. There is a directive 95/46/EC of the European Union about data protection, which has been (or is going to be) transferred into the national legislature of the member states.

The protection against misuse by unauthorized access relies on three basic principles:

- Public policy and awareness: public opinion as well as the law must perceive unauthorized access to personal data, and in particular to sensitive data as a crime, as something that is not done by a normal citizen (even if no harm is intended) as one does not open and read a private letter for somebody else.
- Company policy and education: the hospital must have a consistent policy about data access and data protection and must educate the users about their duties in keeping patient data confidential and protected.
- Organisational an technical measures including restricting physical access to computers, separating local networks form the internet by so called firewalls, a backup policy to prevent loss and destruction of data and to ensure continuous availability of the system etc. Concerning data access, basic security mechanisms include:
  - User authentication. This is the identification of an individual user within the system, traditionally by typing a user ID and a password. More secure authentication is provided by ID-cards or biometric methods like fingerprints. In a modern system, the authentication of the individual user is a must. No group entries are permitted because the responsibility of the user for his actions in the system, for the accuracy of the data etc. must be guaranteed.
  - User authorisation. Authorisation defines a set of transaction rights for the authenticated user. These rights can be assigned to user groups or classes (or functions). The individually identified user belongs to a user class and inherits the transaction rights of this class: a billing clerk may only have access to administrative data necessary for his/her job, a junior radiologist may not have the right to finally approve a report etc.
  - Digital signature and encryption. Whenever there is a technical risk of unauthorized data access – e.g. when patient data are sent over wide area networks – data should be encrypted. If the department aims at film- and paperless operation, digital signatures should be used to establish and guarantee the integrity and the origin of stored data.

In addition to the national data protection laws CEN, the European standards organisation has issued and is working on European standards on data protection. If the acquisition of a new RIS is planned, the tender should ask for and the vendor should guarantee the compliance to national laws and European standards. CEN papers provide valuable input for risk analysis and data protection measures.

Documentation and evaluation

Documentation means the collection, classification and storage of information, to be able to use it later for specific purposes [4]. Historically, the first goals of what was to become a RIS were often documentation of diagnoses for scientific purposes [2,3]. However, documentation as a separate activity is difficult to sustain. In a modern RIS/PACS it is integrated in the workflow of a department in such a way, that documentation of activities and results is a mere byproduct of routine operation.

What are the most important purposes of documentation in radiology and in clinical medicine in general? The most important goal is, of course, patient care. Important, but secondary goals are quality control, documentation for legal purposes, evaluation of workload for planning, scientific evaluations, teaching files etc.

In a RIS data are collected in different forms and during different processes in the workflow. The form is usually determined by the primary purpose for which the data are collected. The radiologic report for example has the primary goal to document the state of the patient as perceived by the radiologist and to transmit this information to the clinician to serve as a basis for therapeutic decisions. Secondary goals are the documentation of procedures for legal purposes and for quality audits, scientific purposes etc. To serve the primary goal, the report is "processed" by humans, the radiologist must express his perception and diagnostic judgement and the clinician must understand the report. The most natural way for that is natural language, which allows the expression of any individual item that may be important.

On the other hand, in applications like workload statistics or scientific retrieval, we want automatic processing of the stored data by computer and therefore the data should be stored in a standardized way as codes or numbers. So, in the case of the radiologic report we face a certain dilemma because different purposes require different data formats. A RIS must be designed very carefully to be of maximum value in the use of the data.
The general rules are:

- Use standardized data then and only then, when they are an adequate model for the process (a standardized list of procedures is an adequate model for billing and, if coupled with other items, for workload statistics, but not for a full documentation of what happened – here free text additions, must be possible).
- If there are conflicting interests, the most important goal must decide the data format (a radiological report cannot be replaced by a set of diagnostic codes, because this would limit the communication between radiologists and clinicians in an unacceptable way).
- Collect data only once and, whenever possible, where they are generated.

We will study two applications, i.e. scientific evaluations and workload statistics in some detail:

- Scientific evaluations. Scientific work in radiology usually means a reinterpretation of images from a new point of view, under some hypothesis. This must be done by radiologists and the rôle of the computer is to provide the basic material, e.g. to select those patients, that may be relevant for the problem under study. The RIS merely serves as an index to the cases. This case retrieval can be accomplished with high sensitivity by a word search in natural language documents, admittedly at the cost of low specificity (or high recall with lower precision). With a careful selection of search words one can retrieve a high percentage of the interesting cases but will also get redundant reports that must be discarded by hand (as a simple example when looking for "carcinoma of the mamma" one might get a case, where the text reads "no carcinoma of the mamma has been found"). However, in reality, this is not a real problem and discarding redundant cases is a minor effort.
- Workload. The information collected in a RIS together with time stamps – i.e. the recording of the time when the patient is admitted, when the procedure begins and ends, when the report is dictated and when it is written and signed – provide a wealth of data for analysing, modelling, planning and optimising the operation of the department. However here again, data must not be used at face value and without analysis. As an example, in our RIS radiographers had to record the final discharge of the patient after a physician had checked the technical quality of the examination. A first evaluation registered very long times to discharge (seemingly indicating that physicians were lazy in checking the quality). The real cause was, that this discharge was not properly inserted into the workflow of radiographers, who would have to interrupt their work, to call up the screen mask for the discharge. So they decided to discharge patients en bloc at great intervals – in reality the patients had been sent away much sooner.

At the end of this chapter we come back to data protection. A RIS contains implicitly data about the personnel of the department. It would be possible to compute for example the individual workload for each employee, the percentage of repeated examinations for each radiographer, the number of performed procedures and the percentage of complications for each physician.

When introducing a RIS there must be a clear and transparent policy, which evaluations are allowed, who might order them etc. In our own RIS evaluations about individual employees are generally forbidden, with a few exceptions like planning the night shifts etc. Each physician may ask for his own data, for example to document the number and type of procedures he had performed.

Outlook

Logically, there should be one HIS covering all the functions of the RIS and the PACS. In reality however, separate subsystems will stay for some time to come. The most likely candidate to vanish soon is the stand alone RIS with interfaces to PACS and HIS.

Tendencies in the industry seem to indicate that the probably scenarios for the next years are either

- a PACS coupled to a HIS where the HIS also serves the radiology department or
- a PACS/RIS in one system coupled to a HIS for the rest of the hospital.

In all cases, integration of the systems will become stronger so that each user gets with his/her accustomed interface seamless access to all the data needed, regardless if they are stored in the HIS, the RIS or the PACS.

References

[1] Gell G (1994) PACS-2000. Radiologe 34: 286–290
[2] Gell G, Oser W, Schwarz G (1976) Experience with the AURA Free-text Documentation System. Radiology 119: 105–109
[3] Kricheff II, Korein J, Chase NE (1966) Computer processing of neuroradiological reports by variable-field-length format. Radiology 86: 1100–1106
[4] Leiner F, Gaus W, Haux R (1955) Medizinische Dokumentation. Schattauer, Stuttgart, p 5
[5] Van Bemmel JH, Musen MA (eds) (1997) Handbook of Medical Informatics. Springer, Heidelberg, p 346
[6] Wendler T (1999) From Image Management to Workflow Management. In: Lemke HU et al (eds) Computer assisted radiology and surgery. Elsevier, Amsterdam, pp 404–413

Radiology information system and picture archiving and communication system: interfacing and integration

D. Piraino

Department of Radiology, Cleveland, Ohio, USA

Introduction

In the past several years picture archiving communication systems (PACS) have become increasingly important to the practice of radiology, just as radiology information systems (RIS) several years ago became important to the practice of radiology. These systems now constitute the major infrastructure of electronic radiology practices. It has become increasingly apparent that these two systems need to communicate in a robust manner in order to optimize the operation of an electronic radiology department. In order for these systems to work together they must be interfaced or integrated throughout the radiology practice. The technology to do this integration has been developing rapidly over the last several years. This chapter will discuss the needs for interfacing RIS and PACS, the history of RIS and PACS interfacing, and future directions that RIS/PACS interfaces are taking.

Need for interfacing

RIS systems and PACS Systems have developed separately over several preceding years. Both of these systems have matured in their ability to provide full function services to electronic departments and referring physicians. In addition these systems have proven to be cost effective. There is an acute need for these systems to intercommunicate. First, for patients to be correctly identified you need patient identifiers, patient names, patient birth dates and other demographic information to be consistent within the RIS and PACS Systems [2]. Also all updates to patient identifying information needs to be communicated between the RIS and PACS. Radiographic interpretation in the form of a report needs to be associated with the proper images to provide both the images and reports electronically to referring providers and radiologists [26]. Change in exam information also needs to be communicated bi-directional between RIS and PACS Systems. Economic analysis of integrated PACS–RIS Systems has shown increased technologist productivity [29]. Integration of PACS and RIS Systems also allows easier image retrieval and management [21].

Modalities also need to communicate with the RIS for patient demographic information to insure correct patient information. Modalities should communicate exam information to RIS systems for exam completion and to communicate quantitative exam information such as measurements. Modalities should also communicate similar information exam and patient information as well as images to PACS systems.

With decreasing reimbursement there is an increased need for streamlining workflow within radiology departments. PACS and RIS Systems can contribute to improve efficiency only if they are able to communicate patient demographics, exam information and report information. In addition these systems also need to be able to access information within the wider hospital information system [14]. For example it is important for RIS and PACS systems to communicate in order to develop enterprise radiologists' work-to-do lists based on exam status, modality and anatomy.

Yesterday

In initial implementations of RIS and PACS Systems, these two systems may have been completely separated and not communicated at all (Fig. 1). These types of implementations typically consisted of modality specific PACS systems that were primarily confined to the radiology department. The interface between the two systems was human interface with either the radiologist or technologist providing this correlation between the two systems. The fact that

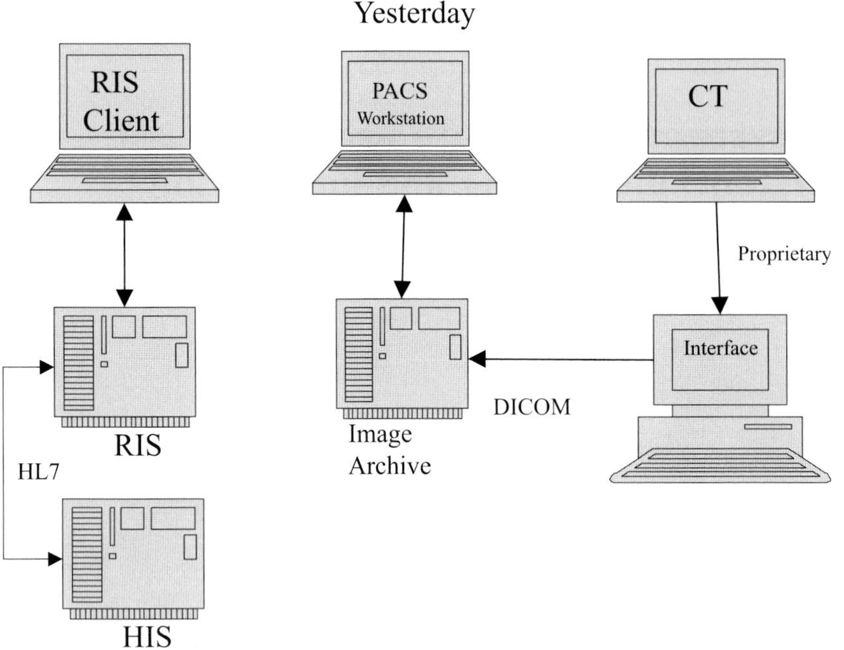

Fig. 1. Shows PACS and RIS systems of the passed where there was no interface between the two systems

the RIS and PACS Systems did not communicate eliminated the possibility of automatically pre-fetching images, distribution of reports and images electronically, and validation of patient demographic and exam information within the PACS archive [5]. These types of systems can function within a radiology department but lack the ability for enterprise image and report distribution and were unable to optimize workflow.

Today

Current state-of-the-art RIS and PACS interfaces can be seen in Fig. 2. Presently most RIS systems communicate text information using the Health Level 7 (HL7) standard. Most PACS systems communicate image information using the Digital Imaging and Communication in Medicine (DICOM) standard [7]. In order for the RIS and PACS Systems to communicate there needs to be an interface which translates HL7 messages to DICOM messages or a proprietary communication format [32].

Exam information is sent from the RIS System to the interface system which translates new exam information into PACS system with the correct patient demographic information and exam information. The exam information can be used by the PACS System for pre-fetching of previous images and can be used for demographic and exam comparison when new images are actually received by the PACS System. Non-matching exam or patient information can be corrected manually by a systems administrator. This type of interface allows development of consistent patient and exam information on the RIS System and the PACS System. It also allows pre-fetching of images based upon activity within the radiology department. These interfaces, however, allow only limited bi-directional communication between the RIS system and PACS system [30]. There is also no direct communication of demographic data to the modalities. Demographic information is usually input into modalities manually or through barcodes and similar mechanical devices. In addition this structure does not allow for workload redistribution, automated correction of demographic information and reports, but does allow enterprise-wide distribution of radiology images and reports. In this type of system the exam information may include reports that are then accessible from the PACS workstation along with the images [22].

RIS/PACS interfaces may be unidirectional with the RIS sending information to an interface broker on certain events. These events include patient registration, scheduling of examinations and report generation. This information is then typically stored in a temporary database by the interface broker. The interface broker then communicates using DICOM or proprietary application interfaces to the image archive and PACS system [30]. The information in the interface broker is available to the archive for a set

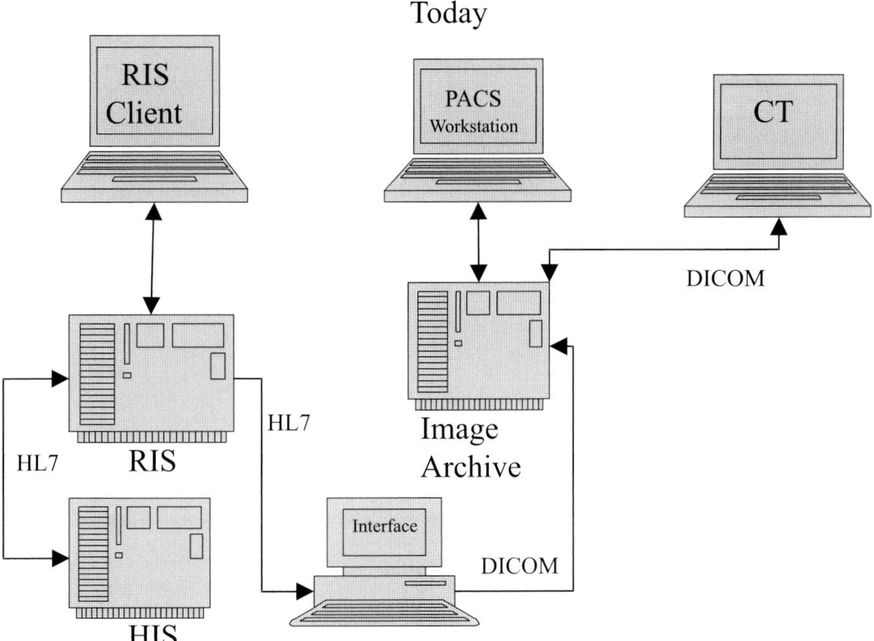

Fig. 2. Shows a typical PACS and RIS implementation of today with limited communication between the PACS and RIS. There may be a separate system used as a protocol converter between the PACS and RIS

period of time. In some implementations, the PACS system may query the RIS for certain pieces of information including reports [12].

Tomorrow

New generation PACS and RIS Systems are beginning to communicate directly without the need for an interface system (Fig. 3) [19]. Communication between the RIS system and PACS system can either be HL7, DICOM or both. In these interfaces the RIS and PACS systems may send information to each other on certain events [22]. For example, the RIS may send scheduled or complete exam information to the PACS System as the exams are scheduled or completed. The PACS system may send image information to the RIS System when images are received. ADT information may also be communicated bidirectionally to ensure correct ADT information on both the PACS system and RIS system.

The RIS may communicate exam and patient information directly with the modality using the DICOM Modality Work List standard [9]. Also the modality may communicate procedure information to both the RIS and PACS system using the DICOM perform procedure step [10]. This allows the modality to transfer exam information about a completed examination including number of images and technical perimeters to both systems.

In the near future the DICOM Structure Reporting will allow modalities to communicate additional information to both the PACS and RIS systems such as measurements, in addition to the images. Structured reporting will also allow communication of complex radiology reports between RIS and PACS systems using an accepted standard allowing easier and better communication of reports between systems.

At the workstation level the concept of context sharing will allow different systems to automatically display information simultaneously about the same patient or same exam. This allows a single workstation to be used for PACS image viewing, access to RIS information and access to hospital information. The concept of context sharing allows a user to have a single log-in to access multiple systems. The context may be related to a specific patient or a specific exam. With context sharing if you are viewing a specific image in the PACS viewer, the RIS client on the same workstation would then display information concerning the exam information associated with that image and the HIS System may display lab data pertaining to that patient.

Future

In the future the concept of a single workstation accessing multiple software components that may or

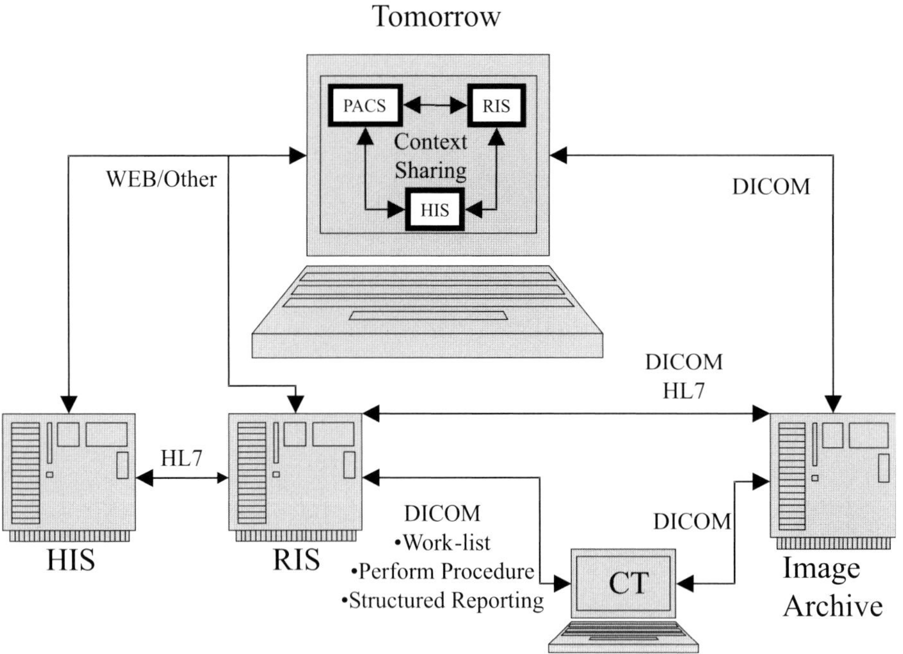

Fig. 3. Possible configuration of future systems with robust PACS, RIS, and modality communication. Workstation also allows for patient context sharing between RIS, PACS and HIS

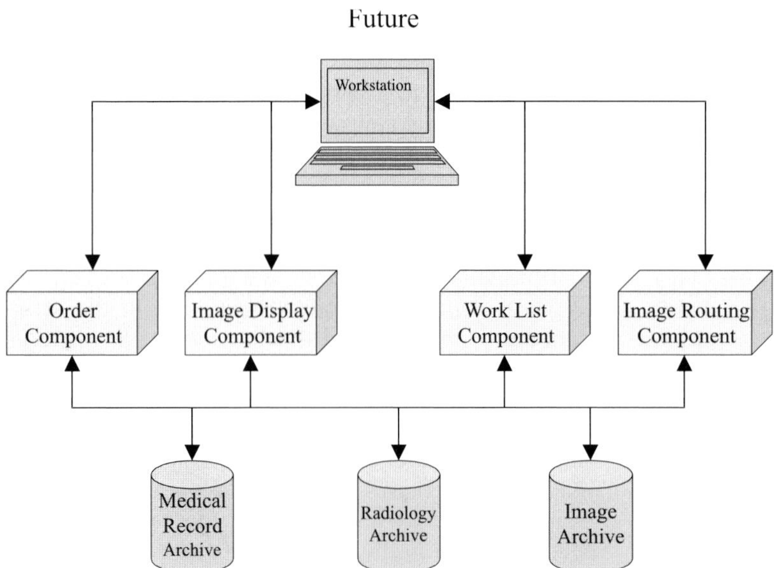

Fig. 4. Future possible configuration where the functions of PACS, RIS and HIS are distributed over several different distributed software components that could be supplied by various vendor

may not be provided by the same vendor appears to be a major direction of software development (Fig. 4). These separate components may access many different information and image archives to process appropriate information and display it for the specific user [20]. The software components will interact using object oriented technology and will work together to provide a more seamless display of all patient information including images, reports, laboratory data and patient visit information.

Interface standards

In the past many RIS/PACS interfaces used propriety commands to communicate information between systems. Proprietary interfaces cost both users and developers additional time and money, as many different interfaces need to be supported by a single system. The development of standards has made it possible for better communication between component systems.

The two major standards used in Healthcare are the Health Level 7 (HL7) standard used to communicate textual information and the DICOM standard used to communicate image and image related information. Both of these standards are in the process of evolving to more robust communication standards and are in the process of working to make the interactions of these standards better.

DICOM

DICOM is a standard developed by the American College of Radiology and the National Electrical Manufacturers Association (DICOM Home Page: http://www.nema.org/nema/medical/dicom/). DICOM stands for Digital Imaging and Communication in Medicine. DICOM has become the major standard for communication of medical images. The DICOM standard describes a uniform and well understood set of rules for communication of digital medical images [6]. DICOM uses standard communication protocols such has ethernet and TCP/IP for communication. During a DICOM communication, the communicating systems initially negotiate what services each system is capable of providing and establish which types of communications the two systems will be performing. Once the common types of services are negotiated a DICOM association is established. This association then can be used to perform several functions including query retrieving of images, sending of images and other services that the two systems have negotiated. DICOM has adopted an object-oriented approach. Things such as, reports, patients and images are called DICOM objects. Certain pieces of information in a DICOM message receive unique identifiers such as reports and images that are transmitted from one device to another medical device. DICOM uses these unique identifiers to identify information objects. The two fundamental components of DICOM are an information object and a service class. Service classes and information objects are combined to form the functional DICOM units, the Service Object Pair or SOP [13].

Present implementations of DICOM support transmissions of various image types from one device to another. For example, transmission of CT images from the CT scanner itself to a diagnostic workstation or an image archive. DICOM also support query retrieving of images from an image archive. Other portions of the DICOM standard which are presently being implemented include the modality work list and perform procedure step. These standards allow communication of patient demographic information and exam information from a RIS to a modality. They also allow modalities to communicate exam specific information back to the RIS or PACS system such as, the number of images and types of images.

The Structured Reporting Draft of the DICOM standard would allow transfer of observations from the image acquisition devices or image interpretation devices to an archive system or other workstations. This may allow transfer of numeric information such as, head and abdominal circumference measurements along with the related images. This standard also allows production of diagnostic reports that may include simple text or multimedia.

Health Level 7 standard

The Health Level 7 or HL7 standard is a set of standards primarily used to transmit text-based data between systems (HL7: Health Level 7: http:/hl7.org). HL7 has defined data messaging standards for the exchange of healthcare information. It has focused extensively on data formats for exchange of information within organizations. As such, HL7 has focused on text based messaging standards used to replicate data between systems.

HL7 subgroups are looking into object-oriented technology and the use of extensible markup language for translation of the current HL7 data. HL7 standards provide for many optional components and in the typical implementation requires additional programming effort for systems to intercommunicate. HL7 messages can be sent to other systems based upon certain trigger events in the sending system or the messages may be sent in response to a query. HL7 can be criticized for lack of an information model to standardize the semantics of the information being exchanged.

The visual integration subgroup within HL7 is working on a standard for transfer of contextual patient related information between the different systems at the client or server level. The patient context link standard provides for visual integration of independent healthcare applications at the point of use. This allows the user to be using several different independent systems but maintain the same patient or exam context when switching between the separate software systems. An example of this would be in switching from an image viewing application to an electronic medical record would allow access of the patient's record at the same time as viewing the images without having to re-enter the patient's demographic information into the second application.

Interface implementations

There are several methods of implementing DICOM and HL7 communication standards. The major focus in software development has been object-oriented technologies. The basic unit of software development becomes an object. An object hides the intricacies of implementation within the object and communicates with other objects or other components by passing specific reference information. Object technology allows for easier and more robust communication between objects and hides the programming intricacies within the object itself. Also objects allow for code reuse by the ability of objects to inherit functions from other objects.

In the interfacing area there are several object-oriented implementations of the HL7 and DICOM standards which are being developed. These include Common Object Request Broker Architecture (CORBA) Med, which uses the CORBA's standard to encapsulate interface standards as objects, Microsoft Healthcare Users Group which uses ActiveX and other Microsoft object technology to encapsulate interface information and the Andover Working Group sponsored by Hewlett-Packard which uses several different object technologies to encapsulate communication standards.

The HL7 Standards Committee and DICOM Committees are also considering the use of extensible mark up language (XML) to be used in data communication in future HL7 and DICOM standards. This would allow flexible communication of diverse information including images, video and text using these standards.

Implementation of HL7 and DICOM standards to provide seamless communication between RIS and PACS systems is in the works. The Radiological Society of North America (RSNA) has established a project called Integrating the Healthcare Enterprise (IHE). In association with Hospital Information Systems Management Society (HIMSS), RSNA is sponsoring a demonstration showing the potential of integrating different hospital systems. A technical committee has been developed to establish methods to be used in the demonstration for communication between various components of RIS, modalities and PACS systems. This implementation uses HL7 and DICOM standards to communicate information (IHE Year 1 documentation, RSNA: http://www.rsna.org/IHE/iheyr1/ihe_yr1docs.html).

The technical committee has established a group of functions and standard ways to communicate these based on a patient visit scenario. Table 1 shows the major actions that occur with a patient's visit at a radiology department that were identified for the first year or second of IHE (IHE year 2 scope, RSNA: http://www.rsna.org/IHE/ihe_yr2_techsum.pdf). At each level the IHE establishes standard communication between Actors which are defined functional system components. The standards based communication between Actors are defined for each step in the patient flow process. By following this suggested implementation different vendors should be able to communicate appropriate information at appropriate stages in the patient's visit. The purpose of IHE is to establish a group of standard interactions that if supported by different vendors, would allow more for seamless communication of information from HIS to RIS systems to modalities to PACS components.

CORBA MED

The Object Management Group (OMG) is a non-profit entity engaged in developing standards for system integration using object technology (Object Management Group: http://www.omg.org). CORBA has developed a standard of inter-operability of distributed object computing or components. This standard allows different software components to intercommunicate using a standard architecture, thereby allowing a more plug and play distributed software architecture. CORBA Med is a task force of OMG to establish interface specifications for distributive objects in the healthcare arena. These objects would include functions such as, patient identification, clinical observations, clinical image access and Lexicon query service. The focus of CORBA Med is on inter-operable services using the CORBA standard. In this context, the various distributed components could provide their services to multiple systems or other components in a distributed healthcare system. CORBA Med's focus is on inter-operable services rather than establishing standard message passing formats.

Standard based implementations

Several groups are working on standard implementations of HL7 and DICOM in order to provide a more plug and play functionality for various systems

Table 1. Integrating the Healthcare Enterprise: Table shows in outline form the follow of patient information that occurs when a patient has a procedure in the radiology department. The steps are shown at the highest level of the outline and the corresponding actors (information system components) that correspond to that process are shown and what standards are required for participation in the IHE demonstrations. Further steps and incorporation of non-radiology systems will occur in later years

1) Patient registration
   a) Actors
      i) ADT-Patient register – sends ADT information
      ii) Order placer – receives ADT information
      iii) Department system placer – receives ADT information
      iv) Master Patient Index placer – receives ADT information
   b) Standards
      i) HL7
2) Duplicate patient checking
   a) Master person index
3) Order procedure
   a) Actors
      i) Order placer – sends new order, receives new order and order status
      ii) Departmental system scheduler or order filler – receives order, sends order status, sends new order
   b) Standards
      i) HL7
4) Check appropriateness of order
5) Schedule procedure
   a) Actors
      i) Order filler/department system – sends procedure information
      ii) Image manager – receives procedure information
      iii) Relevant information manager – receives procedure information
   b) Standards
      i) HL7
   c) Assign protocol for procedure
6) Compile Relevant information for this procedure
7) Patient arrives
   a) Patient Update (Year 2)
8) Communicate procedure information
   a) Obtain patient and procedure information
      i) Actors
         (1) Department system/order filler – sends procedure information in response to worklist query
         (2) Modality – queries for worklist, receives procedure information, stores procedure information in image header
      ii) Standards
         (1) DICOM: Modality Worklist SOP Class
   b) Make any changes to procedure information
9) Communicate procedure step started
   a) Actors
      i) Modality – send start procedure
      ii) Perform procedure step manager – received start procedure, send start procedure
      iii) Image Manager – receive start procedure
      iv) Department system/order filler – receive start procedure
   b) Standards
      i) DICOM: Modality perform procedure step Management Service Class
10) Communicate procedure is in-progress
11) Communicate procedure is completed
   a) Actors
      i) Modality – send procedure complete information
      ii) Perform procedure step manager – receive procedure complete information, send procedure complete information
      iii) Image Manager – receive procedure complete information
      iv) Department system/order filler – receive procedure complete information

(*continued on next page*)

Table 1 (*continued*)

- b) Standards
  - i) DICOM: Modality perform procedure step Management Service Class
- 12) Communication of images
  - a) Images sent to workstation or archive
    - i) Actor
      - (1) Image Archive – receives images
      - (2) Modality – sends images
    - ii) Standard
      - (1) DICOM Storage SOP Class
  - b) Transfer of image ownership is requested
    - i) Actors
      - (1) Modality – sends storage commitment request
      - (2) Image management system – acknowledges request
    - ii) Standards
      - (1) DICOM Storage Commitment Push SOP Class
  - c) Softcopy Present State Storage (Year 2)
- 13) Communication of image status and information
  - a) Communication that images are available and validation of procedure information (Year 2)
  - b) Images accessible
    - i) Actors
      - (1) Image Archive – sends images
      - (2) Internal or External user – queries for images, receives images
    - ii) Standard
      - (1) DICOM Storage SOP Class
      - (2) DICOM Query study root FIND and MOVE SOP Class
      - (3) DICOM Query patient root FIND and MOVE SOP Class
  - c) Corrected procedure information communicated to image archive (Year 2)
  - d) Corrected procedure information communicated to other systems
- 14) Interpretation with appropriate associated information (Year 2)
  - a) Query/Retrieve and Storage of Images
  - b) Query/Retrieve and Storage of Softcopy Present State
  - c) Interpretation Step Started/Completed
  - d) Softcopy Present State and Image Storage
- 15) Report is generated
- 16) Report and images distributed to other systems (Year 2)
  - a) Draft report submission
  - b) To be decided
  - c) Final/Draft report submission
- 17) Provider review of report and images (Year 2)
  - a) Query/Retrieve of final/draft report
- 18) Patient follow-up

in using these standards. The two major groups working on these solutions are the Andover Working Group (AWG) and the ActiveX for Healthcare Committee.

The ActiveX for Healthcare (AHC) is a part of Microsoft Healthcare Users Group (AHC: http://www.healthcare.agilent.com/mpgawg/). This group's goal is to develop an ActiveX based implementation of HL7 messaging objects. They have released ActiveX for healthcare messaging components. They also have plans for certification of components and developing specifications for other areas in healthcare (AHC – Initiative Overview, Microsoft Healthcare Users Group, http://mshug.org/ahc/overview.asp).

The Andover Working Group is a vendor consortium sponsored by Hewlett Packard (Andover Working Group: http://www.healthcare.agilent.com/mpgawg/). This group is devoted to providing standard solutions using CORBA and ActiveX technology. The Andover Working Group is developing enterprise communicator software which encapsulates or wraps HL7 messages in object-oriented transport mechanisms either CORBA or ActiveX. The Andover Working Group's goal is to establish a specific and full featured implementation of standards such as, HL7 and DICOM which can be used for a plug and play type implementation of these communication standards.

Conclusion

The ability of RIS Systems and PACS Systems to communicate and to provide a more integrated environment for the radiology department of the future is progressing rapidly. As these interfaces become better, bi-directional and robust we will see additional functionality provided by the systems which will help provide better patient care, enterprise wide distribution of radiology information and enhance radiology workflow.

References

[1] ActiveX for Healthcare (AHC): http://www.healthcare.agilent.com/mpgawg/

[2] Adelhard K, Nissen-Meyer S, Pistitsch C, Fink U, Reiser M (1999) Functional requirements for a HIS–RIS–PACS-interface design, including integration of "old" modalities. Methods Inf Med 38 (1): 1–8

[3] AHC – Initiative Overview, Microsoft Healthcare Users Group, http://mshug.org/ahc/overview.asp

[4] Andover Working Group: http://www.healthcare.agilent.com/mpgawg/

[5] Bergstrom S, Karner G (1994) PACS–RIS interconnection: results of a feasibility study. Comput Methods Programs Biomed 43 (1–2): 65–69

[6] Bidggod WD, alSafadi Y, Tucker Y, Prior F, Hagan G, Mattison JE (1998) The role of DICOM in an evolving healthcare computing environment: the model is the message. J Digit Imaging 11 (1): 1–9

[7] Creighton C (1999) A literature review on communication between pictures archiving and communication systems and radiology information systems and/or hospital information systems. J Digit Imaging 12 (3): 138–143

[8] DICOM Home Page: http://www.nema.org/nema/medical/dicom/

[9] Garland HT, Cavanaugh BJ, Cecil R, Hayes BL, Lavoi S, Leontiev A, Veprauskas J (1999) Interfacing the radiology information system to the modality: an integrated approach. J Digit Imaging 12 (2 Suppl 1): 91–92

[10] Hayes B (1999) A new approach to RIS/DR interconnection. Radiol Manage 21 (2): 44–47

[11] HL7: Health Level 7: http://hl7.org.

[12] Honeyman JC (1999) Information systems integration in radiology. (1999) J Digit Imaging 12 (2 Suppl 1): 218–222

[13] Horii SC (1996) A Nontechnical introduction to DICOM, National Electronic Manufactures' Association. Digital Imaging and Communications in Medicine (DICOM). Rosslyn, Va:NEMA, PS 3.1–1996–3.13–1996

[14] Inamura K, Umeda T, Sukenobu Y, Matsuki T, Kondo H, Takeda H, Inoue M, Nakamura H, Kozuka T (1998) HIS/RIS contribution to image diagnosis and maximization of efficacy of PACS when coupled with HIS/RIS. Comput Methods Programs Biomed 57 (1–2): 41–49

[15] Inamura K et al (1997) Time and flow study results before and after installation of a hospital information system and radiology information system and before clinical use of a picture archiving and communication system. J Digit Imaging 10 (1): 1–9

[16] IHE Year 1 documentation, RNSA: http://www.rsna.org/IHE/iheyr1/ihe_yr1docs.html

[17] IHE year 2 scope, RSNA: http://www.rsna.org/IHE/ihe_yr2_techsum.pdf

[18] Jagannath VJ, Wreder K, Glicksman B, alSafadi Y (1998) Objects in healthcare – focus on standards, ACM Standards View

[19] Keayes RG, Grenier L (1997) Benefits of distributed HIS/RIS–PACS integration and a proposed architecture. J Digit Imaging 10 (3 Suppl 1): 89–94

[20] Kim JH, Lee DH, Choi JW, Cho HI, Kang HS, Yeon KM, Han MC (1998) Three-tiered integration of PACS and HIS toward next generation total hospital information system. Medinfo 9 Pt 2: 1086–1090

[21] Kondoh H, Washiashi T, Sasagaki M, Arisawa J, Nakamura H, Inamura K (1998) Development and evaluation of PC-based HIS–RIS–modality–PACS coupling: the results of evaluation of initial state with personal computer application. Comput Methods Programs Biomed 57 (1–2): 63–68

[22] Kotter E, Langer M (1998) Integrating HIS–RIS–PACS: the Freiberg experience. Eur Radiol 8 (9): 1707–1718

[23] Kotter E, Langer Ml (1998) Integrating HIS–RIS–PACS: the Freiburg experience. Eur Radiol 8 (9): 1707–1718. Review

[24] Kroger M, Nissen-Meyer S, Wetekam V, Reiser M (1999) [Economic effects of integrated RIS–PACS solution in the university environment]. Radiologe 39 (4): 260–268 (German)

[25] Martens FJ et al (1993) HI8PIN – a generic HIS/RIS–PACS interface based on clinical radiodiagnostic procedures. Eur J Radiol 17 (1): 38–42

[26] Mosser H, Urban M, Durr M, Ruger W, Hruby W (1992) Integration of radiology and hospital information systems (RIS,HIS) with PACS: requirements of the radiologist. Eur J Radiol 16 (1): 69–73

[27] Object Managemant Group (OMG): http://www.omg.org

[28] Offenmuller W (1997) Expectations and solutions for HIS/RIS/PACS dataflow and workflow. J Digit Imaging 10 (3 Suppl 1): 95–98

[29] Reiner BI, Siegel EL, Hooper FJ, Glasser D (1998) Effect of film-based versus filmless operation on the productivity of CT technologists. Radiology 207 (2): 481–485

[30] Shook KA, O'Neall D, Honea R (1998) Challenges in the integration of PACS and RIS databases. J Digit Imaging 11 (3 Suppl 1): 76–79

[31] Shook KA, O'Neall D, Honea R (1998) Challenges in the integration of PACS and RIS databases. J Digit Imaging 11 (3 Suppl 1): 75–79

[32] Takeda H, Matsumura Y, Kondo H, Inoue M, Kondo H, Taked I, Miyabe S (1995) System design and implementation of HIS, RIS, and PC-based PACS at the Osaka University Hospital. Medinfo 8 Pt 1: 430–433

Horizontal PACS deployment in an integrated system

D. Edmunds, R. Khorasani, and P. Ros

Department of Radiology, Brigham and Women's Hospital, Boston, MA, USA

Introduction

In today's society there exists a continual evolution and enhancement of technology in all realms of industry. This evolution has been becoming much more noticeable in recent years in the medical domain. Of particular significance has been the impact of digital evolution in radiology, in part due to radiology's heavy reliance upon imaging processes, techniques, and equipment. Of particular interest to radiology departments has been the concept of replacing analog (film-based) imaging with digital imaging. Such a system is broadly known as PACS, or Picture Archival and Communication System, a system that allows for the transmission, archiving, and display of images in an electronic environment. This electronic transformation has the potential to provide substantial benefit and improvement to imaging operations, particularly as they affect integrated delivery systems. This chapter will attempt to use the horizontal PACS implementation experience of two academic radiology departments, and their affiliated community facilities, in order to provide a useful guide to the successful horizontal deployment of PACS in such an integrated system.

Partners HealthCare System

Overview of Partners HealthCare System

Partners HealthCare System, Inc., established in March 1994, is the corporation overseeing the affiliation of Brigham and Women's Hospital and The Massachusetts General Hospital. This affiliation has resulted in the development of an integrated health care delivery system throughout the region that offers patients a continuum of coordinated, high-quality care. This system includes primary care physicians and specialists, community hospitals, the two founding academic medical centers and other health-related entities, all of whom are dedicated to delivering high quality, cost effective health care and, in conjunction with Harvard Medical School and Harvard University, participating in the research and teaching missions of Partners HealthCare System, Inc. In so doing, Partners is attempting to create a framework in which all aspects of the health care delivery system are coordinated between and among providers and facilities. The integrated system will also allow for the design of new approaches to medical management, as well as measures to document outcomes in order to improve care continuously.

For the radiology departments of the integrated Partners HealthCare System, this has translated into the exploration of management strategies and endeavors designed to enhance radiological services throughout the system. The most major of these endeavors, and perhaps the most important, has been the large-scale horizontal deployment of PACS throughout the system, which is composed of the two founding academic medical centers and its fifteen off-campus radiology sites. This radiological system is quite extensive in its provision of services: Partners Radiology performs well over 1,000,000 imaging procedures annually, and is comprised of approximately two hundred radiologists at these sites. Such a large expanse of service sets this integrated delivery system apart from any other in the area.

Radiology departments at both academic centers have been committed to achieving a successful deployment of PACS, and this commitment is evidenced by the formation of a Partners PACS Committee. The Partners PACS Committee has as its mission "...the development and integration of systems" for the capture, storage, transmission, display, and management of digital medical images within the local, metropolitan, and wide area networks of the institution and affiliates. The Partners PACS will use state-of-the-art componentry and systems to create a secure and seamless environment in which digital images and information can flow freely to appropriate destinations as needed, while ensuring the integrity and security of patient information at all times. The result will be a system that will deliver Partners HealthCare System radiological services effectively, and impact positively on patient care. The strategy includes the following steps: 1) define goals; 2) analyze existing Radiology/Informational System infrastructure; 3) create a project planning team for each Partners Institution; 4) create a strategic vision at each Partners affiliate; and 5) develop a tactical approach for a phased implementation plan. In order to fulfill the mission described above, the PACS Committee has approached the deployment of PACS by focusing on each component of this strategy.

PACS models

Through the implementation process outlined above, the two major academic radiology departments have been able to identify a particular philosophy by which they have arrived at their current strategic vision for PACS deployment, with each department utilizing PACS for primary interpretation and secondary display of images. The overall goal for the Partners HealthCare network is to have these two systems integrated in such a way as to enhance radiological services throughout the integrated network. The fundamentals of this philosophy will be outlined for each of the two academic centers. Then, the remainder of the chapter will focus on the implementation plans and methods that have been developed in order to achieve this, and the lessons learned to date in the implementation process.

The Radiology Department at Massachusetts General Hospital began their PACS development by enlisting the use of PACS primarily for the purpose of primary interpretation. In effect, this means that the digital infrastructure is composed in such a way as to allow for the interpretation and delivery of images and reports electronically throughout the Healthcare enterprise, which is composed of seventeen separate interpretation areas. The interpretive focus involves the primary radiological interpretation of digital images from within the network. The ultimate goal is to allow any physician from within the integrated system to easily access radiology images and reports, regardless of where they conducted within the Partners HealthCare enterprise [1].

A fully functional PACS infrastructure has also been developed at the other main academic medical center, Brigham and Women's Hospital. Here, the Department of Radiology has focused primarily on deploying a horizontal PACS integrated throughout the main academic center and its fifteen off-campus sites. This system is also organized in such a way as to concentrate on providing primary interpretation of digital images, and distribution of electronic data for secondary viewing. This particular PACS infrastructure has been implemented in response to the need to provide consultative patient care services to the fifteen off-campus sites that utilize radiological services within the network. It corresponds to the philosophy of this particular department, i.e. that there are in effect two primary goals for PACS: 1) to provide a superior information management system that is able to integrate image and non-image information, as well as provide a means for transferring images throughout an integrated system that is composed of nineteen different interpreting areas; 2) to provide an integrated network of off-campus, or community, sites who can utilise PACS consultative services through primary interpretation at the main campus.

Implementation strategies

Traditional PACS implementation

Most early PACS implementation efforts were initiated by large academic hospitals and academic departments, and by research laboratories of major imaging manufacturers, without the added involvedness of horizontal deployment throughout large integrated systems [2]. Consequently, the following three methods can be considered to be the original methods of PACS implementation that have been described previously in the digital imaging literature:

- Homegrown system – The radiology department creates a multidisciplinary team that uses their technical knowledge to develop system interfaces, and writes specific PACS software to fulfill the clinical need. It then selects the PACS components from various manufacturers.
- Two-team effort – A team is assembled with members both from outside and inside the hospital and radiology department, which acts to write detailed terms for the PACS for a particular clinical environment. A manufacturer is then contacted to implement the system.
- Turnkey approach – A manufacturer is contracted to develop the PACS in its entirety, and then installs it in the department [2].

Current PACS strategies

It can be surmised that a large integrated system must elaborate upon the main concepts employed by the above three implementation methods. The development of a horizontal PACS deployment plan for an integrated network of health care delivery involves many additional contributing factors, all of which necessitate the design of a systematic and organized approach. Consequently, the Partners HealthCare System has devised an implementation plan that takes into consideration the uniqueness of all of the individual sites and their respective health care delivery needs. This implementation plan has evolved into an approach characterized by a sense of commitment by all involved, and by a particular commitment by each academic center to drive this implementation process locally at each site.

With the benefits of a horizontally deployed Picture Archival and Communication System being of such a multitudinous scale, it follows that the challenges in the implementation process for PACS rollout are equally abundant. As with any technologically rooted adaptation, there are constant changes and advances that add to the complexity of successful integration. Through the experience of the Partners HealthCare System, it can be deduced that an important first step in the implementation process consists of carefully defining goals for the process of PACS deployment. It is then necessary to conduct a comprehensive assessment of the current environment in order to understand the existing operation. Once this is accomplished, it is essential that project planning teams be created for each institution. A fourth step involves the mutual creation of a strategic vision, which paves the way for the final and most important task: developing a tactical approach for a phased implementation plan.

A. Defining goals

Since integrated delivery systems can benefit from achieving many desirable goals from successful PACS deployment, one of the first involves defining the ultimate goals for the PACS deployment. These goals should include such things as improved workflow, improved productivity, enterprise integration, improved service, reduction of lost images, and finally, improved overall quality of care. Evidently, these are long-term goals, realizable through the ultimate success of the PACS deployment. However, it is important that a planning process be built around these long-term goals in order to arrive at clearly delineated short-term goals. Short-term goals of fundamental importance include: 1) arranging for the necessary resources, which may include the formation or restructuring of a PACS Committee, as well as a working team locally situated at each site, to deal with the substantial efforts required in such a large undertaking, and 2) the selection of an appropriate vendor. Once these goals are attained, the path is paved for an organized process of PACS implementation planning.

B. Analysis of existing radiology/informational system infrastructure

The Partners PACS Committee identified the need for each institution to conduct a thorough analysis of the current radiology and information technology environment throughout all of the sites within the integrated network. Some of the main features that were considered in this analysis include:

- the presence of physical space, as well as construction requirements, that will be needed for PACS deployment;
- the conformity of pre-existing systems to DICOM standards;
- radiology Information System (RIS) and Hospital Information System (HIS) integration;
- workflow processes, including such things as number of radiologists, the actual number of locations in use for each radiological service, and difference in hours and days when services are provided (i.e. the different nights and weekends of operation for the different locations).

Two of the most important of these features include the presence of DICOM compatible systems, and accurate non-image information in the form of adequate RIS/HIS integration. Evaluation of workflow processes also deserves particular attention in the analysis of the existing radiology environment.

DICOM, or Digital Imaging and Communications in Medicine, refers to one of the common standards in use today in the employment and integration of diverse information systems. It is described as an "object-oriented standard", defining information objects, services, and classes of devices to perform the exchange of information between imaging modalities [3]. Before the adoption of DICOM standards, it was common for each imaging or PACS vendor to have its own proprietary image format and communication protocol. This led to difficulty in the interfacing of equipment in the setting of a multivendor environment. The employment of DICOM compatible systems has enabled the sharing of data among systems, leading to the ability to successfully develop truly integrated systems. Consequently, DICOM compatibility is one of the most important requirements for information system infrastructure, especially when horizontally deploying PACS across a network.

It is also crucial for any picture archival and communication system to be able to access information from, and communicate with, the other information systems within the network. The two information systems of primary importance in this regard include the RIS and the HIS. Easy access to patient information is pertinent to maintaining the overall quality of patient care, and can therefore be considered a major contributing factor to any successful deployment of PACS. In many radiology departments, there exist anywhere from five or more different information systems relating to such aspects as patient information, scheduling, billing, reporting, teaching, research and imaging. In order to achieve adequate functionality in a horizontal PACS it is necessary to ensure integration between the requisite systems, and of utmost importance is the connectivity with the RIS and HIS databases. Linking with these databases will allow for the necessary non-image information to be transmitted throughout the network. The Partners HealthCare experience in PACS rollout unveiled the presence of many different systems within the planned PACS enterprise for Partners HealthCare. Although a difficult endeavor, integration is possible in such a system and brings with it many practicalities, one of which is a successful PACS operation.

An additional requirement necessitating close examination in an analysis of existing infrastructure concerns that of the workflow processes, i.e. those processes currently employed in each area of the network. Horizontal PACS deployment has the potential to provide extensive improvements and efficiencies in radiological workflow processes, especially as they relate to network efficiencies. But for the maximum benefit to be obtained, the workflow processes in existence before PACS implementation must be explored in detail. The primary purpose of such an exploration is to gain an understanding of, and appreciation for, the wide range of complexities that require inclusion in the PACS planning process. These include the workflow processes performed by all "users", both technologists, radiologists, and support staff, and involve identifying the specific tasks, matching these tasks to skill sets and resources, and coordinating this with the detailed processes involved in the daily flow of information and procedures. Quality of process depends on accurate and timely transfer of information pertaining to both patient demographics, i.e. non-imaging information, as well as imaging information. It is one of the goals for digital technology across an integrated system to adequately preserve and enhance information throughout the work processes, so as to maximize the full potential of system integration.

DICOM gateways facilitate communications across different vendors, but do not necessarily ensure that the data being entered into the acquisition device is validated with regards to the RIS. Problems may arise when the study and associated patient information are "pushed" into the PACS via a gateway, and include such problems as demographic errors, and incorrect image segmentation for routing to different workstations [4]. One of the academic radiology centers, the Brigham and Women's Hospital, has approached the challenge of connectivity of databases by developing a relay software program, known as a relay station. This software program was designed and built under an academic-industrial collaboration (Mitra, Canada) to address two common problems that exist for cross sectional imaging modality interfacing. These include: 1) reconciling the alphanumeric demographic discrepancies with the existing HIS and RIS prior to entry into the PACS; and 2) segmentation of the image dataset in order to route studies to the appropriate workstation [4]. The relay station deployed by this department is successful at prospectively eliminating these demographic errors, and effectively segmenting the images from the same study so that they can be seamlessly integrated into the technologists' current workflow. The functions are performed prospectively, so as to effectively eliminate retrospective maintenance of the PACS database, thus facilitating radiologists' and technologists' workflow in a subspecialty oriented practice environment. It has been found to be a low-cost and scalable solution, as opposed to dedicated PACS Quality Control workstations, thereby contributing to improved PACS interfacing [4].

C. Project planning teams

The creation of project planning teams at each Partners institution was identified as another essential element of the Partners HealthCare PACS Committee. This step involves the formation of planning teams whose responsibility includes a wide array of activities and tasks as they relate to PACS deployment at each particular institution across the system. These planning tasks can be further broken down into the following applications:

Acquisition

Acquisition tasks refer to such elements as: automated capture, query, and retrieval of all digital exams via DICOM; automated validation of ownership and exceptions handling; bi-directional modality interfaces with Radiology Information Systems and Hospital Information Systems; and DICOM conformance.

Modality coordination

For implementing coordination of film digitization across all modalities, including computed tomography, magnetic resonance imaging, computed radiography, ultrasound, nuclear medicine, mammography; implementation of modality gateways and protocol converters where necessary.

Storage

Hierarchical and distributed image storage management; DICOM storage class services; and long-term digital archives to replace film as the archive copy.

Display

Planning the installation of: soft-copy primary interpretation systems throughout radiology; clinical review stations where appropriate with specialized applications; World Wide Web based server and display for intra/internet access; and integration into the Partners HealthCare-wide electronic medical record.

Reporting

Exploration of: continuous speech recognition systems; capture of sub-selected images; composition of multimedia diagnostic reports (including audio annotation); access to full image data sets for interventionists and research; results coding; provider profiling; technology/outcomes assessment research; electronic teaching files.

Information systems

Planning of aspects related to: electronic order entry via intra/internet; utilization management; next generation Radiology Information Systems with multi-site capability; integration of PACS with Partners HealthCare System master patient index; integration of PACS with Hospital Information Systems and Radiology Information Systems; integration with Clinical Application System via API (Application Program Interface).

Network

Ensuring implementation of: support for very high-speed networks for primary interpretation where appropriate; seamless connectivity for local and wide area networks; real-time network for conferencing where needed; information system support for the local and wide-area user community; Integrated Service Digital Network (ISDN) and cable modem support where appropriate.

Teleradiology

Employing full integration of teleradiology systems and applications; World Wide Web-based teleradiology capability; support for commercial teleradiology ventures; and integration with Partners HealthCare System telemedicine effort.

Work flow

Developing a Work Flow Director position for management of data through the system; ensuring auto routing of image studies to appropriate station(s) after image capture and validation; and prefetching of previous relevant exams.

Systems integration

Implementing a support structure for any and all DICOM conformant componentry; developing of redundant systems architecture to assure no single point of failure; development of automated electronic monitoring; build secure systems that include password protection, data encryption, certificate authority, and digital watermarking; object oriented systems compatibility (Common Object Request Broker Architecture (CORBA), Active-X, JAVA); complete systems support with 24 hour, 7 day on-call and automated paging.

Compression

Responsible for ensuring compliance with evolving DICOM standards, and compliance with in-house standards for lossless compression.

Film printing

Employing filmless environment wherever possible.

Growth and marketing

Coordination of efforts towards potential growth areas, as well as PACS marketing issues.

D. Creation of a strategic vision

The fourth step defined by the Partners PACS Committee involves creation of a strategic vision by the institutions involved in the PACS deployment initiative. Building a long-term strategy not only allows for a higher level of planning processes to occur, but also ensures that all participants involved in the project are aligned with regard to interests and ultimate goals for PACS. This is a very important concept in the planning of such a large-scale deployment of digital imaging systems. Since there is the potential for many conflicting or differing ideas and opinions to arise throughout the network, the creation of one unifying and collaborative vision, on which the remaining planning process can be based, permits the construction of a solid foundation for the deployment strategy. This step was achieved in the Partners network through the actual formation of the PACS Committee, and continues to be realized through the everyday workings and accomplishments of the self-defined tasks of this committee.

E. Tactical approach for a phased implementation plan

The final element related to the PACS Planning Committee activities involves the use of a calculated approach for a phased implementation plan in the horizontal deployment of PACS in a large integrated network. Due to the complexities alluded to earlier in this chapter, a horizontal PACS deployment plan must be executed by a well-organized, well-constructed methodology. This entails corroboration of all personnel involved in the planning process, so as to arrive at a project plan that emphasizes an organized, step-wise fashion of deployment among all institutions, with the overall implementation and application being controlled locally. The leadership of this planning committee is a key resource, and one of the most important in this process. It is the leadership of the overall implementation plan that determines the extent of the "buy-in" ideology held by all users of the PACS. Employment of a phased plan with ample opportunity at each phase for input by any user within the network, as well as the necessary staff training, will result in a well-constructed and efficient horizontal PACS rollout.

Lessons learned

A. Resources needed

Since the start of the horizontal PACS deployment process, the Partners PACS Committee has been able to identify several key lessons in successfully deploying the Picture and Archive System throughout an integrated network. One of the lessons learned surrounds the importance of clear delineation of the resources necessary for the implementation process. Monetary resources are, in effect, the foundation for most networks that are implementing a horizontal PACS. Due to the complex nature inherent in a large integrated network composed of numerous diverse facilities, the monetary resources may sometimes end up being somewhat unspecified as a result of assumptions made by those involved in the planning process. Such assumptions may result in inopportune effects resulting in untimely delays in the planned schedule for phased deployment, no matter how well prepared the planning team may be with their strategic plan. A rule of thumb involving monetary delineation can be shown in the following calculation for an approximation of Total PACS Expenditure:

Total PACS Expenditure (US Dollars) = (Number of Workstations $\times$ 20–40,000) $\times$ (2–3).

However, this calculation is only applicable to individual facilities and institutions, as it only looks at workstations per facility. It can be, however, a starting point for those integrated enterprises wishing to estimate the PACS deployment resources required at the institutional level. Also of note is that it only approximates purchase-related costs; maintenance and future upgrade costs are not included in this calculation. Maintenance costs can be estimated at 8–10% of purchase price.

Another important resource necessitating consideration is that of personnel. The people who are working on the large, multifaceted project of a horizontal PACS deployment must be committed to exploration and innovation as they relate to systems integration. Consultants may be useful, as they may bring with them the expertise and knowledge that is required at a particular phase of the planning process. However, a limitation may be that these outside authorities do not possess sufficient understanding of the integrated network, and all of the unique intricacies involved in the extensive horizontal PACS deployment. For this reason, it is of utmost importance to construct a team, or workforce, who are already part of the participating enterprise, and therefore possess the technical and workflow knowledge of the system and its requirements therein. This team would also have, by way of its makeup, the necessary authority for decision-making and project management, so as to contribute to the progress and ultimate success of the PACS deployment plan.

B. Selection of vendor/product

In the selection of a vendor and product, it is essential that the appropriate functional requirements be met. One of the most important requirements includes choosing products that have appropriate functional capacity for PACS. This includes DICOM compatibility, as well as the capacity for RIS integration, which as discussed is essential to any PACS. Other functional requirements include such factors as ease and availability of supportability, integration into already existing information systems, and future direction of the product or vendor; i.e. are they likely to remain up-to-date with future developments and expansion. Price should not be a deciding factor to come into play when deciding on products, as the previously described aspects are probably the greatest determinants of overall PACS deployment success.

C. Training, support, and maintenance

Training, support and maintenance are all essential elements to successful PACS deployment operation. Without sufficient training, any informational technology initiative will not proceed in a timely manner. For a PACS, training has an even greater role, as most of the users within the system will be required to possess full user ability in a short period of time. Additionally, the support availability will need to be provided and maintained in such a way so as to supply all users with the necessary resources to address and repair any technical or procedural problems in a timely and comprehensive manner.

D. Installation

Project management in this realm has one of the greatest and most substantial tasks related to horizontal PACS deployment. As there exist so many sites and/or facilities involved in the PACS implementation, each of these will require a sectional representative(s) who is responsible for ownership of PACS installment at that particular site. This aspect of project planning and management is complicated by many extenuating factors, not the least of which include the actual construction and physical space requirements of implementation. The network foundation and server location are also important factors requiring special attention in horizontal deployment of PACS, as well as the creation of a "survival guide" approach by the PACS Committee, to provide essential assistance and instruction in times of crisis.

Conclusion

Additional applications and benefits

The deployment of a Picture Archival and Communications System carries with it several advantages other than the obvious ones relating to direct cost savings. Indirect savings also exist, in the form of improvements in efficiency, productivity, workflow, enterprise integration, and quality of care. In a PACS environment, images relevant to further medical decision-making are available to the referring physician more rapidly, and therefore may lead to improved patient care, and possibly such favorable outcomes as reductions in hospital stays, and decreased incidence of double-imaging. Likewise, an increase in overall workflow efficiency may occur as a result of just integrating the Radiology Information Systems and the Hospital Information Systems within the network [5].

Additionally, PACS has the potential to lead to enhancement of other undertakings, one of which is of considerable interest to academic centers. The research applications available in a PACS are of utmost usefulness and effectiveness. For instance, a Picture Archival and Communications System that is shared over a large horizontal network will be beneficial to the sharing of clinical information suitable for large studies and trials. A similar benefit arises in the potential for teaching applications, in which PACS may be utilized as a tool in the sharing and retrieval of clinical images useful for educational purposes. The internet has now been established as a vehicle for providing opportunities for the wide distribution of educational materials, such as teaching files [6]. Such a teaching file could be especially beneficial in the setting of a horizontal PACS shared among an integrated network, thereby increasing exposure to a variety of teaching files cases. Since a teaching file is both a tradition and a requirement in an accredited diagnostic radiology training program, many of the same resources can be committed to designing it for internet access, as well as for integration with digital images provided by PACS. One of the main academic centers, the Brigham and Women's Hospital Department of Radiology, has developed such a software system. It allows easy and rapid input of digital radiology images and text reports, at the time of interpretation, into an easily searchable electronic teaching file database using the internet and the World-Wide Web protocols, servers, and browsers [7]. The advantages of such a teaching system are numerous, and include such things as easier availability of images, communication among a wider audience, the opportunity for collaboration among different institutions, and a more rapid availability of information and images than with more traditional, film-based teaching tools [6]. This inexpensive and simple interactive software program for building a digital teaching file allows a rapid single-step process for building a teaching case at the time the study is interpreted by the radiologist [7]. The system has the potential to significantly improve the quality of radiology educational materials available to users, and to reduce expenses for generation, management, storage, and duplication of teaching materials in radiology departments.

Measuring the return on investment

This chapter has attempted to describe the processes involved in deploying a Picture Archival and Communications System in a large, integrated system. Due to the enormity of this particular topic, it is impossible to provide detailed information on all of the issues that are involved in such a deployment. Hence, this discussion has focused on those aspects relating to implementation methods, and some of the main issues and problems that exist therein. In concluding, it seems appropriate to include a final facet to this discussion; that concerning the return on investment.

The process of PACS deployment in an integrated network is not an overnight operation, and may take up to four, five, or more years for completion. However, the longer the amount of time to full implementation, the less chance for a substantial return on investment. And since implementation of PACS is a capital-intensive process, it involves the need to justify and clearly document returns on investment. To justify the large capital investment necessary for its deployment, PACS needs to cut costs associated with film handling, improve the efficiency of radiologists and non-radiologists personnel, and improve overall quality of care. Measuring the monetary return on investment is therefore very important, and involves the following two key aspects: 1) turning off film, and 2) subsequent reduced film-handling costs. Film-handling costs are two to three times the cost of film; thus, merely turning off film can attain a major gain in return on investment. This particular return on investment, however, is often very difficult to accomplish, due to the fact that others in the HealthCare System outside of radiology also require access to films and images. The Brigham and Women's Hospital Department of Radiology has dealt with this important issue by first turning off film in the Ultrasound department, an area where film is not commonly required by others in the HealthCare System. This allowed the department to begin measuring the reduction in film handling costs almost immediately in this particular area, and thus measuring return on investment.

Another element that this academic center has successfully achieved within their local PACS network is one that enables another substantial return on investment; it has successfully exported the PACS solution to the rest of the hospital, outside of radiology. In this way, the PACS solution can serve to cohesively bring the different pieces of this particular institution together. This methodology has consequently provided the institution with the expertise and ability to implement a completely compatible PACS in the other parts of the hospital-wide network.

Regardless of the cost aspect of return on investment, there are several others that deserve inclusion. Improvements in service, quality of care, and productivity are all substantial and realizable returns that can be accomplished through a horizontal PACS deployment. Some of the aspects contributing to such improvements in service and quality of care include the potential for improved timelines of reporting, improved image availability regardless of time or place, and reduction in lost images. Also deserving of mention is the subsequent capability of improving report generation tools with the co-implementation of a structured reporting system such as voice recognition, thus adding to the improvements generated by a PACS implementation across a large network. An important factor for a large enterprise to keep in mind throughout the implementation process is to systematically measure such details, and then use the results and the process as a learning opportunity to aid in improving their organization. In this way, a PACS deployment process can be beneficial in not only the obvious sphere of digital imaging efficiency, but additionally in many other areas, which are only now being explored in this new era in radiology, the era of continuing PACS evolution.

References

[1] Dreyer KJ, Mehta A, Sack D, Thrall J (1998) Filmless medical imaging: experiences of the Massachusetts General Hospital. J Digit Imaging 11 (4) (Suppl 2): 8–11

[2] Huang HK (1999) PACS: basic principles and applications. Wiley-Liss; pp 1–13, 389–456

[3] Honeyman J (1999) Information systems integration in radiology. J Digit Imaging 12 (2) (Suppl 1): 218–222

[4] Carrino J (2000) Modality interfacing: the impact of a relay station. (To be published as a supplement in the Journal of Digital Imaging in June 2000)

[5] Bick U, Lenzen H (1999) PACS: the silent revolution. Eur Radiol 9: 1152–1160

[6] Mammone GL, Holman BL, Greenes RA, Parker JA, Khorasani R (1995) Inside BrighamRAD: providing radiology teaching cases in the internet. RadioGraphics 15 (7): 1489–1498

[7] Khorasani R, Lester JM, Davis SD, Hanlon WB, Fener EF, Seltzer SE, Adams DF, Holman BL (1998) Web-based digital radiology teaching file: facilitating case input at time of interpretation. Am J Roentgenol 170 (5): 1165–1167

Hospital PACS as an agent of continuous change

D.P. McInerney and G.D. Hurley

The Adelaide & Meath Hospitals, incorp. The National Children's Hospital, Tallaght, Dublin, Ireland

Abstract

Following the transfer of three old hospitals to a 600 bed teaching hospital in Dublin a HIS/RIS/PACS solution was implemented which was filmless from the day of opening of the new hospital in 1998. We review the planning and commissioning arrangements and the experience over the ensuing years. PACS has been a great success and the decision to adopt it in one single episode has been justified. The subsequent development of the system and its effects on the radiology department, the hospital and on wider medical practice are described.

Introduction

Seventeen years of planning preceded the opening of the new hospital, with a catchment area of 330,000, in 1998. A specific PACS sub-committee was set up to administer the PACS programme. The project was run by an equipping and commissioning group consisting of radiologists, radiographers, medical physicists and clerical staff with representatives of hospital management, architects, project managers and equipment suppliers. We found the assistance of an experienced equipment procurement specialist invaluable [1]. Senior hospital staff were persuaded to support the PACS project on the basis of cost, staff and space savings enhanced environment and patient care, and better academic facilities. PACS objectives also included patient satisfaction, clinical needs, and market positioning. The contract was awarded to the supplier providing the financially most advantageous solution. The project was implemented in 'Big Bang' fashion in time for the hospital opening [11].

Configuration

The radiology department consists of 23 diagnostic rooms including separate paediatric radiology and emergency radiology areas (Fig. 1).

Twin radiographic rooms are served by two single plate CR readers One reader each is situated in the Fluoroscopy and Mammography areas. There are two readers for the two radiographic rooms in the Accident and Emergency Department. Three hard-copy dry laser cameras are networked on the system. These are used mainly for images of patients transferring to other hospitals, where teleradiology is not appropriate.

A CCD based film digitiser is used for digitising films on to the PACS. Scanning of previous images has diminished over time. The older C arm equipment in operating theatres etc., produces spot films which are digitised and transferred to PACS. Newer C arm equipment produces digital images which are transferred directly. Each of the main processing areas is provided with quality control (QC) workstation at which the radiographers review and prepare images for transfer to PACS. Since opening further upgrades have included an archive upgrade, ward block extension and out patient Ward Service, and a RAM upgrade for clients. There has also been an upgrade of RIS hardware and installation of new PACS viewing software.

There are ten servers in the PACS room catering for the different functional areas in the hospital and running DICOM viewing software and RIS. All DICOM viewing servers had 9GB (the highest capacity available in 1998) and were later replaced by servers with 72GB hard discs. This alleviated the problem of older images being auto deleted from the server before the patient had left the ward. A RAM upgrade has been carried out on each client PC to the max of 128MB. This makes for faster image viewing and is essential in order to run the newer software.

The disc storage space on the reporting workstations was unchanged at 8Gb which caused occasional trouble due to auto deletion when images accumulated.

The decision to base permanently a vendor PACS engineer on site for support has been fully justified.

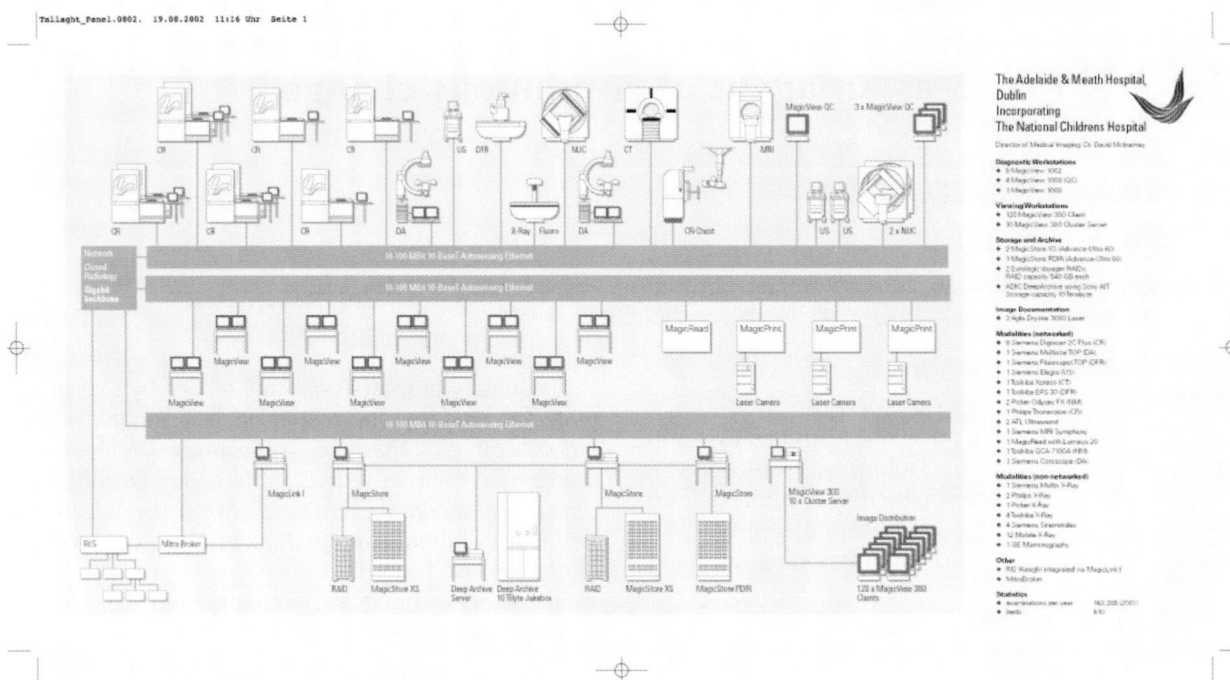

Fig. 1

The down time of the PACS over 5 years has been virtually zero. A cheaper alternative is on-line service from the vendors. Larger departments may be able to afford the permanent presence of a vendor technician or real time on-line supervision but smaller departments need a local solution.

Managing the information network is vital. While a good working relationship with the hospital IT department is necessary, it is important that the RIS/PACS environment is controlled and managed from within the Radiology Department as the staff are familiar with managing radiology services.

HIS/RIS issues

Before transfer a common RIS was established in the base hospitals and the professional staff harmonised activities across the hospitals. Discussions between suppliers led to an integrated HIS/RIS/PACS solution using a broker for RIS/PACs and an integration engine for HIS/RIS.

DICOM issues

We have installed DICOM worklists where possible. Some older equipment does not have DICOM worklist capacity including some gamma cameras and a fluoroscopy room. DICOM issues arose in connecting the equipment of different manufacturers to the PACS and underlines the necessity for clear cut contractual commitments regarding DICOM issues.

An early modification sought was a DICOM worklist for all modalities in order to speed up the workflow through CT and ultrasound areas and to avoid double entry of data with potential errors and inconsistencies.

Outside digital image data can be troublesome if the format is unsatisfactory for putting into PACS. In addition, inputting outside images breaches software security protocols and this is an ongoing issue. Computer network security is now becoming recognised as a critical component. Technology is available to provide strong defence against attacks on network and network computer systems in radiology. Vigilant supervision and management of users and systems is important [7].

Image archive, short and long term

Short-term storage is provided by two 96 Gigabyte redundant arrays of inexpensive discs (RAID). This arrangement offers resilience in that, if one RAID breaks down, activity can be switched to the other. In l998 there was 180 Gigabytes of RAID space which held 3 weeks images plus older pre fetched images. Since then capacity has been increased to 1.26 Terabyte. Now 10 weeks images are available on RAID despite the introduction of MR and extra clinics. Image retrieval times of 1–2 seconds from the RAID are maintained. We propose to implement RAID for all images.

For long term storage, there is a robot-operated archive with image retrieval time of 2 to 20 minutes depending on system traffic which varies with the time of day. The estimated total storage in 1998 was four and a half to five years images with all data on tape. Total tape storage has been increased to 60 Terabytes. The speed of technical advance in memory capacity may mean that we can indefinitely store the images in an uncompressed form.

Daily backup tapes are produced and are stored on site. We originally used digital linear tape but have upgraded to advanced intelligent tape (Sony) which has an embedded microchip to enhance performance. There is duplication of all images for added security. It can now process 100 read requests at any one time, thus reducing the queuing time for clinic manual pre-fetching which is a major improvement. We are changing from batch pre-fetching to serial pre-fetching with HIS/RIS connectivity. Compression is not used at any stage. Radiologists are reluctant to do primary reading on compressed images both for professional and medico-legal reasons.

Transmission

Images from different source modalities are transferred to specific reporting workstations but are also available for retrieval from the general archive and thus can be reported on any workstation. Images for teaching, research and conferences are transferred to a separate file. The tutorial room workstation is connected to a beamer allowing the display of images on a large screen for case conferences. Open access to the archive is restricted to prevent excessive network traffic and to optimise performance.

The hospital is wired with a separate PACS network which is a dedicated active network with Gigabit backbone. Transmission of images throughout the hospital is by a separate cable network supporting l20 PCs with 17 inch monitors, 1024 by 768 matrices and 64 megabytes of RAM on which images and reports are available to the referring doctors. These 120 image viewing stations are grouped by medical speciality into logical clusters. RIS reports are also available on these viewing stations. We have replaced ward and OPD monitors with LCD monitors as they have higher luminance and low reflectivity for reviewing on the wards where viewing conditions are very bright. Low level lighting should be provided in viewing areas. We have subsequently installed high resolution monitors in all theatres and some outpatient clinics. High spec monitors similar to those in radiology reporting were then installed in the vascular theatre and in orthopaedic outpatients.

In order to transmit images and reports more widely to the surrounding area, we are planning to instal a web server and software, with order communications also. Web access provides images to any PC anywhere in the network or over the internet and fulfils the requirements for most consultation rooms. However it limits the physician to one low to medium resolution monitor and is not as fast or efficient as a workstation. It does however solve the problem with pre fetching which can be done directly by the client. At present, we cannot anticipate all patient movements within the hospital for adequate pre fetching. With web based technology, clinicians have ready access to any image anytime, from any site. A radiologist can cover multiple sites from a single location. We are planning web viewing on the wards to replace the current DICOM viewing software, thereby utilising better the PC's already in situ on the hospital network and also enabling the possibility of remote viewing of images in radiologist's homes, clinics, and other locations.

Image transfer to the National Neurological Centre for urgent neurological cases is available via ISDN. Image transfer to the radiologists' home is possible.

An additional ward block and an Out patient clinic have been opened and have been directly wired for PACS.

Workflow

For a successful implementation, major changes in working habits must be accepted and dedicated training must be set up. Every person's work pattern will change and the most difficult operation is to accept these changes at the individual level. Natural leaders within the staff should be encouraged. Staff must be involved in workflow redesign During this time of change, the pressure of routine work should be diminished and the staff should have some free time from routine tasks to facilitate planning and implementation. Workflow optimisation is well recognised in the industrial engineering literature. Imaging department productivity has being studied in a similar manner and a significant increase in radiographer productivity has been shown to follow workflow improvement [17].

PACS can be used as a tool to re engineer workflow not only in radiology but also throughout the hospital and this is one of its greatest advantages [19]. Processes need to be completely reengineered to get the full advantages of PACS. Workflow alterations have been more easily set up through the RIS than the PACS in our hospital [6]. Software alterations are easier to achieve for the RIS than the PACS.

Patient details, code and referral source are downloaded from HIS to RIS. PACS reads this information from the RIS through a special broker interface. Paper multipart request forms are still used. These contain important clinical information, are signed by medical practitioners and are thus an important element of the justification process statutorily required before carrying out a radiological examination. While the patient is passing through the department, radiography staff involved in a particular examination may enter comments on the request form which may be helpful to the reporting radiologist. We found that digitally scanning the request forms into the system was too slow.

When patients arrive for their scheduled examination they are checked in and the examination room worklist is updated. For conventional x-ray examinations the worklist is displayed on the CR reader. For the other modalities, the worklist is displayed on the console screen using a DICOM "Get Worklist". CR examinations are optimised by the radiographer at the QC station. The image folder is then auto-routed to the designated reporting workstation and to the requesting location (A&E, Ward etc.). Simultaneous storage on the RAID also takes place. Image printing can also take place at this time if necessary. Examinations acquired on direct digital modalities are routed directly to the designated reporting workstations.

When examinations are completed the radiographers place the request forms in boxes located in the central reporting area and classified by source. Thus it is clear at a glance to the reporting radiologists what work requires to be done. It also provides a fail-safe to prevent an examination being forgotten and images going unreported. Examinations may be dealt with by a specific radiologist who takes the request forms. Reporting is via portable dictating machines. This allows report dictation at any point in the department at any time. It is convenient for radiologists who may perform special examinations throughout the department during the day, to keep on their person the request forms and to report on them as they go along. Voice recognition technology is commencing with a pilot project for urgent A & E work.

After typing and verification, reports are then available throughout the hospital. Each radiologist can avail of a personalised icon based reporting package. CT and MRI images can be viewed in stack or tile mode. The RIS reports are also available on the viewing stations.

These workstations are currently distributed in one centralised reporting room. This facilitates case discussion, teaching and consultation. The reporting workstation will also auto query the RAID for other images belonging to that patient, whether reported or not. Reports are downloaded automatically and instantaneously from the RIS to the reporting workstation. The radiologist dictates the report and signs off the image folder. The image folder is then stored on the RAID and archive.

The workstations were initially located in the consultant radiologist's offices. After a trial these were centralised into a single central area where consultants and trainee staff now report together, enhancing teaching opportunities.

Enhancement of radiologist viewing is achieved by darkening the reporting room to almost complete darkness, rendering the room quiet with carpet and soft coverings, restricting access to reporting areas and a programme of planned QA and maintenance of VDU's to maximise human perception factors [25].

The radiologists have after a short interval found soft copy reporting preferable to hard copy particularly in multi image examinations[18]. Soft copy reading is as reliable as hard copy interpretation [12]. Adaption of workflow process includes having a standard hanging protocol for radiographic images so that radiologists see them in the same structure and sequence at all times.

In moving from film to PACS many file clerk functions must be carried out by the radiologists such as, selecting previous images for comparison, arranging images for viewing, pulling previous reports and clearing images from the work station.

Acceptance by junior medical staff is high as they no longer have to search for x-rays in the department and wards.

Training

To prepare for the arrival of PACS, staff should visit working PACS departments. A workstation should be installed in the department so that staff can see how it operates. The implementation group will identify natural leaders among the staff and also diehard opponents. It will train clinical colleagues, and identify leaders and opponents similarly. Different staff categories should be invited to targeted teaching sessions, taking account of users day to day time constraints. PACS conferencing should be demonstrated. This is such an improvement on film conferences that both clinical radiology and teaching staff will be won over.

Two radiographers were trained as specialist PACS system managers by the PACS vendors. The people best suited to become PACS managers are senior and experienced Radiographers. Working together with IT staff they constitute a more effective working group than IT staff alone. They have played a pivotal role in the training of staff within the department and throughout the hospital. In turn they have trained several other radiographers to act as "super users" providing backup for holidays, illness, etc. A reporting workstation was commissioned early for training radiologists. The PACS system managers ran training courses for clinical and nursing staff and instruction handbooks were distributed. On site system monitoring is done by PACS administrators.

The help desk should be overstaffed in the first two weeks after implementation. Small follow up group sessions should be provided in the first two weeks. PACS training should be incorporated in the induction programme of all junior doctors arriving at the hospital. There were difficulties in training staff, and in particular non-attendance of key members of clinical staff at training sessions. An emergency line availability of support staff for on the spot training in the early stages of PACS proved very helpful. A lot depended on whether doctors were ready to devote sufficient time to formal training in handling computers.

Discussion

Preparing the ground for a PACS installation by meticulous communication and dialogue with clinical colleagues is essential.

The proposal should specify the advantages and disadvantages of the proposed and present systems and stress the level of training required to be able to operate the new system successfully [1,2,3,5,8,9,20] It must be preceded by a number of presentations and site visits. The long-term technical advantages of PACS in the integration with technological developments in the wider area of HIS should be stressed [8]. An assessment of time taken from patient examination to completion of report showed a 150% reduction compared with the pre PACS situation in our departments. [3,5,21,22]. Soft copy reporting is a major change in their fundamental work for Radiologists and adequate training is essential [20,21,22] The more softcopy reporting one does, the easier it gets. In our experience, radiologists who perform softcopy and hardcopy reporting in different locations find that softcopy reporting is easier and preferable and they make the adjustment with ease.

The filmless department is a major component of the drive to reduce the time to deliver structured information to clinicians. Until the advent of PACS, the radiology report generally reached the clinician before the images. With PACS the radiology images now reach the clinician immediately and the report follows later. Radiologists must close this gap and ensure that the report accompanies the image. PACS offers the possibility of delivering radiology in real time [10]. Voice recognition and structured reports are very helpful in this [13]. Added value in Radiology occurs when a report is delivered to the clinician. We plan to use speech recognition systems to type reports in real time so that a digital report is available for transmission simultaneously with the image. This will place extra time pressures on radiologists. It will be implemented first for emergency and urgent examinations Our future plans are to integrate the hospital system to drive an electronic patient record. This requires management of image, text, and voice information integrated into advanced communication technology.

In the future we will have desktop integration of the radiologist workstation. Instead of having to sign into one system for the RIS and HIS and another system for the PACS, all systems will be accessible on a single work station. A study can then be located on RIS and simultaneously opened on PACS, with reporting via voice recognition effectively integrated on one workstation. This will facilitate real time reporting.

New PACS software will intelligently anticipate the workflow patterns of clerical, technical radiologists and clinical staff and will anticipate their needs so as to continually diminish the amount of repetitive and routine tasks [19]. Increased productivity in radiologist reporting of CT with PACS compared to conventional film boxes has been reported [16].

Automatic structuring of radiology reports will be a second information revolution in Radiology [13]. If radiology reporting is systematised as has been done with the Birad structure of mammography reporting, it can both assist in real time reporting and it can use automated reasoning e.g. diagnostic suggestions for unusual cases, automatic index and retrieval of online teaching files or peer reviewed literature relevant to specific cases.

PACS is a hybrid between Radiology and IT each totally dependent on the other. The facility requires on-going management involving the Imaging Dept, outside contractors and the IT Dept. Though it is more difficult to install a PACS system piecemeal in an existing old hospital, this may be necessary where financial and other constraints obviate a "big bang" approach.

Big bang implementation of PACS is better. In an incremental process there are problems associated with the use of dual systems and consequent increased workload. Conversion of archives and databases to new systems is complex and infrastructure upgrades are usually needed. New hospitals which are now preparing to go filmless are starting from a technical base which has widespread digital imaging, one or more mini-PACS situations within the x-ray department and a variety of digital facilities of variable degrees of modernity. A mini PACS could be created by linking several digital modalities with workstations, but this does not realise the major benefits of PACS. It is necessary to move into a uniform modern PACS to reap the full benefits in cost reduction, improved productivity and quality. Moving to new technology raises a new set of problems even when it is an updated version of the original vendors PACS. These issues include workstations, data base and media migration, archives, compression, RIS interfaces, new DICOM services, worklists.

The vision is to integrate the Healthcare Enterprise [4]. This involves bringing together radiologists, clinicians, administration, and commercial representatives for framework sharing to integrate workflow and IT processes in radiology. This closes the loop between HIS, RIS, PACS, diagnostic workstations, radiologists, and the patient to create seamless flow.

Conclusion

PACS has become the prime agent of continuous change in the radiology department through its effects on workflow.

PACS optimises the handling of the multiple images produced by multislice CT and MRI scanners and is far more efficient than film based systems.

The workload of the department has increased from 85,000 Examinations per annum pre PACS to 120,000 on the year of opening (1998) to 165,000 examinations annually in 2003. This has been achieved with a 20% increase in clerical staff, a 25% increase in radiographic staff and a 15% increase in radiology staff. The reject rate in radiography decreases when PACS is instituted [26]. All examinations are now presented for reporting whereas in the pre PACS department up to 20% of examinations were not returned from the wards in time for a report to be of value. The report turnaround time has greatly improved [24]. 99% of all radiological studies are reported compared with a reporting rate of 82% before PACS despite a dramatic increase in workload. The new system has reduced the time from issuing a request to availability of the x-ray report by a factor of 3.

Freeing up of space formerly used for film storage and filing is a major benefit. A large percentage of the floor area of any traditional Radiology department is given over to these functions. As most x-ray departments are situated in the centre of the hospital. this real estate is extremely valuable [14].

PACS has changed relationships with our clinicians. Since they can see images anywhere in the hospital they no longer need to meet face to face to review cases. Phone consultations have become common with the radiologist and clinician viewing the same image on different monitors in the hospital. If the department cannot report images quickly the clinicians will read the images themselves and form their own view. PACS-based multidisciplinary radiology conferences are now the most popular in the hospital. Physician acceptance is good. The most difficult group to satisfy has been the orthopaedic surgeons and they have been given dual high performance monitors. In addition software solutions to their requirement for long cassettes to measure scoliosis and limb length have been installed. Patient stay time is decreased and this benefit is magnified in the busiest short-stay stay departments such as A & E.

Our experience of implementation of PACS since 1998 confirms the central significance of change management, planning, and comprehensive training. A "big-bang" installation is better than piecemeal. Going into PACS is an irrevocable step which requires continuous assessment and support with ongoing investment and quality control. The planning groups that set up the original system should remain in existence for this purpose.

PACS is in a state of rapid evolution with increasing integration and fusion of RIS and PACS and with improvements in both hardware and software. This will lead to multimedia reporting and communication in the future.

References

[1] Allison DJ, Faulkner JJ, Glass HI, Mosley J & Reynolds RA (1994) "PACS" at the Hammersmith – the implementation of a clinically orientated system. Proceedings of the Twelfth International Congress of the European Federation for Medical Informatics

[2] Barneveld Binkhuysen FH (1992) Required functionality of PACS from clinical point of view. Int J Biomed Comput 30: 187–191

[3] Bick U, Lenzen H (1999) PACS: The silent revolution Eur Radiol 9: 1152–1160

[4] Bryan RN (2002) The digital revolution in radiology. President's Address, Scientific Program 21
[5] Bryan S, Weatherburn D, Watkins J, Roddie Mc Keen J, Muris N, Buxton MJ (1997) Radiology report times: impact of picture archiving and communication systems. AJR 170: 1153–1159
[6] Carty AT, O'Dowd B (2003) Preparing for a digital department/hospital. Published abstract ECR 2003, Scientific Program, 27
[7] Eng J (2001) Computer network security for the radiology enterprise. Radiology 220: 303–309
[8] Fiedler V (1997) Do HIS, RIS and PACS increase the efficiency of interdisciplinary teamwork? In: Lemke HU, Vannier MW, Inamura K (eds) Computer-assisted radiology and surgery. Elsevier, Amsterdam, pp 504–510
[9] Foord KD (1999) PACS Workstation respecification: display, data flow, system integration, and environmental issues, derived from analysis of the Conquest Hospital pre-DICOM PACS experience. Eur Radiol 9: 1161–1169
[10] Guiney M, McInerney D, Hurley GD (1999/2000) Mammography Hospital Health Care Europe D1: 17–19
[11] Hurley GD, McInerney DP (2001) Going filmless in a new hospital setting. In: Hruby W (ed) Digital revolution in radiology. Springer, Wien New York, pp 65–72
[12] Kundel HL, Polansky M, Dalinka MK, Choplin RH, Gefter WB, Kneelend JB, Miller WT (Sr) Miller WT (Jr) (2001) Reliability of soft-copy versus hard-copy interpretation of emergency department radiographs. AJR177: 525–528
[13] Langlotz CP (2002) Automatic structuring of radiology reports, harbinger of a second information revolution in radiology. Radiology 224: 5–7
[14] O'Dowd B, McInerney D (2000) The Tallaght PACS. Radiography Ireland 4 (2): 1–3
[15] Peters PE, Dykstra DE, Wiesmann W, Schluchtermann J, Adam D (1992) Cost comparison between storage-phosphor computed radiography and conventional film-screen radiography in intensive care medicine. Radiology 32: 536–540
[16] Reiner BI, Siegel EL, Hooper FJ, Pomerantz S, Dahlke A, Ralllis D (2001) Radiologists' productivity in the interpretation of CT scans. AJR 176: 861–864
[17] Reiner BI, Siegel EL (2002) Technologists' productivity when using PACS: comparison of film based versus filmless radiography. AJR 179: 33–37
[18] Rogers LF (1999) PACS: new age radiology. AJR 173: 1159
[19] Siegel E, Reiner B (2002) Workflow redesign: the key to success when using PACS. AJR 178: 563–566
[20] Strickland NH, Allison DJ (1995) Default display arrangements of images on PACS monitors. Br J Radiol 68: 252–260
[21] Strickland NH (1996) Review article: some cost-benefit considerations for PACS: A radiological perspective Br J Radiol 69: 1089–1098
[22] Strickland NH, Martin NJ, Allison DJ (1997) A study of the effects of PACS on working practices and patient care after one year's totally filmless operation of a hospital-wide PACS: the Hammersmith experience (Abstract). Radiology 205: 401
[23] Strickland NH, Shadboldt C, Byneveldt M, Williamson R, Allison DJ (1997) Efficiency of reading plain radiography images: soft copy reading on PACS monitors compared with hardcopy conventional film. (Abstract) Radiology 205: 401–402
[24] Twair A, Torregiani W, Ramesh N, Hogan B (1999) The first complete PACS Radiology Department in Ireland: "Is it more efficient?" Ir J Med Sc 168(2): 138 (Abstract)
[25] Wang J, Langer S (1997) A brief review of human perception factors in digital displays for picture archiving and communications systems. J Dig Imag 10 (4): 158–168
[26] Weatherburn GC, Bryan S, West M (1999) A comparison of image reject rates when using film, hardcopy computed radiography and soft copy images on picture archiving and communication system (PACS) workstations. Br J Radiol 72: 653–660

Large PACS projects

S. Peer

Department of Radiology, Innsbruck University Hospital, Innsbruck, Austria

Introduction

Since the installation of the first prototype PACS in the late 1980s large scale PACS projects have always received special attention by the scientific community. Pioneers in the field such as the Vienna SMZO [5], the Hammersmith Hospital [14], the Baltimore Veterans affairs Hospital [12] or the Hokkaido University Hospital in Japan [6] have catalyzed the technical and logistical development of PACS components in close collaboration with the industry. When the first edition of this book was written in the year 2000 a substantial part of this chapter was devoted to basic technical features of large PACS installations and to experience with workflow aspects gained in the aforementioned installations. It is only three years since then, but oh what a change we have experienced in almost every aspect related with PACS from network infrastructure to workstation design and workflow integration. Much of this development came along with the progress of important initiatives such as the Integrating the Healthcare Enterprise (IHE) initiative technical framework initiated by the RSNA as well as the Healthcare Information Systems Society (HIMSS). The following paragraphs will consequently focus on new insights on basic PACS aspects gained during this period of change and draw the readers attention to new trends and probable future directions of PACS development.

Image acquisition

State of the art digital imaging systems are a prerequisite for a successful digital workflow and in a way the ongoing development of digital imaging systems was one of the main triggers for evolution of PACS. While digital radiography was still in an early state of development when the first edition of this book was published, meanwhile a digital alternative exists for practically every aspect of radiologic imaging including direct digital radiography, mammography or dedicated dental systems. As far as integration of these modalities into a PACS environment is concerned a lot of what has been said in the first edition of this book is still valid and some of the most important aspects will be discussed hereafter.

Data volume

Digital images require storage capacity in the PACS archive and the design and maintenance of this archive depends strongly on the amount of data that have to be handled. With further development of digital modalities, this task has become more and more demanding as far as storage capacity, network speed and routing concepts are concerned. A digital image normally comprises 0.5 to 8 MB/image, the exact size depending on the modality. Traditionally a typical CR study with an ap and lateral exposure comprised some 5 MB, for newer high resolution CR plates and digital detectors however this rose to more than double the traditional size. A similar development has been noted with the integration of MSCT (multi slice computer tomography), which suddenly has boosted the volume of daily data production into previously unknown heights due to the application of sophisticated examination protocols with scanning in different phases of contrast administration and a trend to thinner and thus more slices [15]. With the Innsbruck University Hospital PACS serving as a representative example we will show how an originally well planned and successfully operating digital archive had to be changed to adjust to these new demands.

When the Innsbruck PACS after more than one year of continuous development was fully operational at the end of 1998 some 90GB of losslessly compressed data were acquired per month. At this time five CR units, a digital chest stand, two helical CTs, two MRIs, four fluoroscopy systems, three ultrasound scanners and an x-ray film scanner were integrated in the radiology PACS. With exchange of the two CTs (adding one four row MSCT and one sixteen row MSCT), addition of a digital mammography (GE Senograph) and a skeletal DR system (Philips Digital Diagnost) the data volume rose rather abruptly to almost 200GB per month. With this development the original design of an online RAID archive with some 50GB of capacity and longtime storage of data on CDROM jukeboxes (each with 500 media, giving a total of approximately 1 TB of archive capacity) was no longer sufficient. Consequently the archive was completely remodeled: The size of the RAID was increased to more than 400GB to handle the daily load of new image data. Additionally a large online disk pool was designed with an array of 16 servers plus attached 100GB disks to achieve an online storage capacity of almost 2 TB, which allows for quick online access to relevant patient studies of the past six to eight months. This decision was not only demanded by the increasing data volume but also a reaction on the spread of PACS to wards and outpatient clinics. To make the best use out of PACS for the clinician quick accessibility of data is a must and therefore imaging data need to be online for the whole inpatient stay, which could not be achieved with the original short term archive configuration.

A second step to a new archive concept concerned long term storage: The original design with archival on CDROM jukeboxes proved to be troublesome and personal demanding in operation. When many read operations had to be performed on a jukebox, while new CDROM's had to be burnt, the burning process was often interrupted and in one case a CDROM was even corrupted, which resulted in irreversible loss of data. An attempt to improve this situation with introduction of a whole cluster of jukeboxes (finally nine jukeboxes were added) failed to definitely improve this situation. Finally the whole long term archive was outsourced to a tape archive at an offsite privately run computer enterprise (connected via a 622Mbit/s metropolitan area network). This turned out to be a definite improvement in many aspects: With integration of IBM's ADSM software (advanced distributed storage management) it is a very versatile archive concept, which implies high flexibility for the future use of new archive media. All studies are kept in double copies, to guarantee data access without loss of patient related information for a minimum of ten years, which is enforced by government law. Security in general is kept on a high level with operation in underground bunkers with efficient fire prevention, uninterrupted power supplies, etc., which may not as easily be obtained within a hospital setting.

Networks for PACS

The data network is one of the key features in a successful PACS, as transfer of patient demographics form HIS to RIS and PACS, as well as of images from modalities to archives and workstations, has to be quick and reliable. Even in a small PACS installation the network will rather quickly become very complex and the physical properties of the network need to be robust and at the same time networking protocols and software have to be easy to handle for network technicians. In this respect the development of the Innsbruck PACS again shows how things may change quite unexpectedly. When the installation was planned in 1996 the only networking technology fulfilling the specifications stated before was ATM (advanced transfer management) at 155Mbit/s. At that time it was a very promising technology – probably the standard for all future data and telecommunication networks – allowing for construction of a switched network, where all attached components have the full bandwidth of 155Mbit/s (as opposed to 100Mbit FDDI networks, where the bandwidth has to be shared among the attached stations). In daily routine maintaining the ATM network proved to be rather complicated, because of a very sophisticated and complex service layer, and despite a promising future it stayed a rather expensive network option. Slowly a new, cheap, easy to use alternative appeared on the market: Fast Ethernet. With evolution from 100Mbit/s Ethernet to Gigabit Ethernet and a future development to 10Gbit Ethernet, this technology fulfills all requirements of network speed. At the same time it proved much easier in network configuration and maintenance. Thus the complete PACS network at the Innsbruck University hospital installation is slowly replaced by Fast Ethernet connections, and our experience shows, that transfer rates and image loading times for attached workstations are not inferior to ATM.

Display workstations

The display workstation is the workhorse of radiologists and clinicians in a digital hospital and has to handle all the tasks known from conventional film reading procedures [1a]. Display of newly acquired and historical images in a logical way suited for comparison of pathologic findings, display of patient demographics and clinical information, sufficient spatial resolution and luminance are some of the features, that have to be fulfilled by the workstation and its software. With more sophisticated integration of PACS with HIS and RIS and the addition of speech recognition software or CAD (computer aided diagnosis) the key position of the workstation in the radiology workflow has become even more important for a functioning daily clinical routine, and a variety of new aspects have to be considered.

One important feature of the display workstation is its monitors ability to display medical images in sufficient resolution and brightness. While in the early PACS installations options for workstation monitors were limited (mainly relying on high luminance grayscale cathode monitors), meanwhile there are various options of monitors suited for different viewing purposes. As far as gray scale monitors are concerned, we may meanwhile choose from a spectrum of 1K to 5K resolution high luminance cathode monitors, and with high resolution LCD monitors as a possible alternative, the choice for the optimum workstation specification has become even more difficult to decide. For a radiology enterprise changing to digital radiography and PACS several questions concerning workstation monitors arise:

- Which matrix size is suited best for softcopy reporting of radiology studies (keeping in mind that specifications may be different, depending on the type of images to be viewed – i.e. sonograms, CT-images, X-rays, etc.)?
- Do I need high resolution cathode monitors or may I go for an LCD alternative, without a compromise in image display?
- How many monitors should combine to a single workstation (again depending on the reporting purpose)?

Besides this the monitor problem is twofold, as not only clinical demands have to be concerned, but due to the high cost of the higher matrix displays economic factors play an important role and this is especially true for large scale PACS installations. In fact the price for a medical grade dual monitor display system can cost from \$1,500 to \$30,000. Compared to this a consumer grade 19-inch color LCD monitor may be purchased at only about \$2,500. The price for the video card further adds to this expense with \$2,500 to \$12,000 for a medical grade compared to about \$160 for a consumer grade video card.

Several recent studies have been reported in the literature, which tried to tackle the above mentioned questions. In a recent study by Hirschorn et al LCD and CRT monitors were compared regarding their suitability for reporting of CT exams [4]. Their rationale for this comparison was the inherent difference in the pixel data of CT or MRI images and radiographs. While the native resolution for the single CT and MRI image is about 0.25 megapixels (MP), a conventional radiograph has a resolution of about 5 MP. From a technical point of view a consumer grade LCD color monitor operating at up to 2 MP may thus be able to display CT and MRI images in sufficient quality. The results of the before mentioned study nicely support this presumption, by showing no difference in the accuracy of CT readings on 1024 × 768 pixel CRT monitors and color LCD monitors with the same matrix size. In a similar setting Pärtan and coworkers did not find any significant differences for the reading of cerebral CT images, when comparing a 1600 × 1280 pixel CRT with a 1280 × 1024 pixel color LCD monitor workstation [7]. In a study by Reiner et al a similar trend is even reported for soft copy viewing of computed radiographs [11].

The problem of monitor matrix requirements for different viewing purposes has been addressed by different workgroups. Our own experience with comparison of 1K and 2K CRT displays in a phantom experiment showed only small and probably insignificant differences in the correct detection ratio for small low contrast objects [8] and are in good accordance with the results of other research groups testing the same types of monitors for the detection of pulmonary nodules [3].

The number of monitors needed in a workstation for different reporting purposes has been subject to debate since the beginning of PACS. In the early installations workstations were regarded as a substitute for the film changer or alternator used in film based departments and many radiologists and PACS companies tried to copy the film based environment when changing to soft copy reporting. Thus a larger number of monitors (three or four monitors in a single workstation) were for example considered more effective for reading of MRI or CT studies with multiple sequences, but meanwhile there has been a paradigm shift among radiologists using PACS for a period of time [2]. With the evolution of workstation software radiologists change their reporting habits, with preferential viewing of cross sectional studies in stack mode instead of the tile mode known from traditional hard copy reporting. Comparative displays often rely on the presentation of two studies on one monitor each, and the maximum number of studies displayed on one monitor is decreasing with ongoing use of the workstation, with four on one probably being most effective in relation to image size for comparative CT or MRI studies.

All these findings are experienced in large PACS installations in a similar way and have great implications for planing of a PACS. With fewer monitors and a modular concept providing high resolution displays for certain applications only and a change from high cost medical grade to low cost consumer grade products PACS gets easier affordable for smaller budgets. Nevertheless we want to point the reader on certain threats or alternative considerations: Longevity and constancy of technical equipment is to be considered and may be a vote for the products derived from a dedicated medical technology company. Legal issues may demand certain constancy testing protocols, which are easier achieved with a monitor and/or video card, that comes together with a software package derived from a medical supplier. With new software applications or a higher end integration of information systems (HIS-RIS-PACS integration, inclusion of digital dictation systems) an extra monitor for the display of other than image related data may be necessary to improve radiology workflow.

PACS workflow and system integration

Ever since the onset of PACS, workflow aspects and integration of information systems have been the key issues for a successful operational installation. The use of PACS and other IT technologies can reduce the inefficiencies known from conventional film based radiology departments. These inefficiencies mainly relate to the use of film, which is a somewhat tricky media as far as workflow is concerned. Film images may only be in one place at a time, which implies a need for sequential working of radiologists and clinicians. Especially for the emergency setting, this may result in unacceptable delays in patient management. At many departments – and the same was true for the Innsbruck University Hospital – films of emergency patients were consequently viewed first by the traumatologist or emergency physician, and were reported by a radiologist only some time later, however only a certain amount of radiographs reached the reporting radiologist, due to the well known loss rates in film based departments. The threat of an overlooked coexisting finding, which is not of traumatic nature is straight forward.

While PACS is a suitable tool to cope with these general insufficiencies of film based radiology, many benefits which may be gained by a PACS installation are not straight forward and a redesign of departmental workflow is to be performed in order to fully exploit the potential of digital radiology [13]. In this regard PACS has to be viewed in the larger context of a digital hospital with interaction of PACS with RIS, HIS or departmental information systems, as many benefits can only be gained with sophisticated integration of these systems [9]. What we aim for when introducing information technology into radiology is improvement of patient care, which may be achieved at a local level in the radiology department, but strong links and interactions with clinical departments exist. So when planning a PACS installation the first step to success will be a critical evaluation of the current "non electronic" workflow, to see which steps in a work process have to be covered by the electronic system. From a radiology point of view, we always have to keep in mind that we are a service provider for clinicians and therefore clinical matters have to be included in this consideration. As an example for the importance of this aspects of PACS planning we may use a study performed at the Innsbruck University Hospital and the Potsdam Regional Hospital in Germany combining the workflow aspects included in the provision of urgent and scheduled chest X-rays and CT-exams for ICU patients in a PACS based and film based environment [10]. According to the analysis performed, there is a comparable basic workflow structure in conventional and digital departments, however marked differences in the execution of different workflow steps exist. With the use of a PACS for example radiology no longer has to physically provide image access to ICU physicians for clinical image consultation or conferences, as images are generally available from the archive via a simple worklist entry at the ICU viewing station. Changes in the working habits of ICU physicians were noted after transition to PACS. Every clinical round at the ward for example starts at the viewing workstation with consultation of the recent patient images. Consultation of radiologists were substantially reduced due to unlimited availability of images for the ICU, and when necessary were often reduced to a kind of teleconference between the ICU physician and the radiologist viewing the same imaging study at the workstation in their local department. With simultaneous availability of imaging information for clinicians and radiologists, the times for clinical decision and/or radiology report generation have been reduced dramatically. In general a trend to more frequent use of radiology services is noted, due to better and quicker access to image based information.

Despite these beneficial workflow changes, the study at Innsbruck University Hospital also revealed problems related with poor system integration, which are similarly addressed in the aforementioned study by Eliott Siegel et al. Several analogue process steps in the interdepartmental workflow of radiology and intensive care, such as ordering of radiology exams via telephone calls, manual entry of patient and exam data in the RIS after handwritten filling of order forms at the ICU, among others were noted. These "media breaks" in the otherwise digital workflow were mainly due to the use of an old HIS, which allows only for electronic transfer of basic patient demographics, but not for a higher level integration. This is one reason, why meanwhile the HIS is completely redesigned, with a future possibility for direct ordering into the RIS from a dedicated HIS software mask, direct access to radiology reports in the HIS with a possibility to directly view selected X-ray or CT-images in a HIS based image viewer, etc. So what we learnt from this is: you may never get to a high and clinically satisfying level of integration, if one of your electronic systems, that are to be interfaced, is not able to speak the same language as the others. Or in other words: Germans, Austrians and Swiss speak German, but due to differences in their local dialects, they may still not understand each other in daily conversation except on a very basic level. This leads us back to what has been said in the introduction of this article: interfacing relies on compatibility, and in this regard medical software and electronics are far from "plug and play" despite important initiatives such as the IHE or HIMSS. DICOM and DICOM are not alike and DICOM (or HL7) compatibility does not necessarily imply good system integration in terms of workflow improvement.

Besides this, simply transferring the working habits of a film based department into digital work-steps will not automatically result in an efficient electronic workflow. Digital technology enables the user to perform various tasks in a way not possible with conventional workflow. Let me just mention a very simple example: with soft copy reporting we always have the option to view a CT data set in different window/level settings (lung, bone, soft tissue), we may even manipulate images with additional edge enhancing filters or view them in interactive 3D mode with perpendicular image planes. Consultation of historical images for reporting will improve report quality [16] and is possible at any time, given a good prefetching algorithm in your PACS. The use of speech recognition software will strongly enhance report turnaround times [Antiles 2003], which is even more important if clinicians gain unlimited access to radiological images.

Conclusion

To implement and run a large scale PACS is a highly sophisticated task. Careful planning of the installation with respect to the interdepartmental workflow and the required performance is crucial – always keeping in mind, that these requirements may change, once the system is operational and users got to know its benefits. Many technically demanding components are included in such a system, which ask for a high level of in house expertise among radiologists, radiographers and technical staff. To get the clinicians into your boat early is important to find out, which relations to workflow on the wards and outpatient clinics exist and which clinical requirements are to be met by the PACS. The transfer of a conventional department to a digital environment requires a substantial amount of change at almost every level of workflow and involves every staff member. This change may also impose fear on people (fear to loose ones job, fear to work with digital technology, fear to get a higher workload or worse working conditions) and this implies an often neglected need for intensive information and training of staff from the planning phase to the operational PACS. Key to success is to involve every staff member from the beginning and to make sure that digital technology is not a goal for its own sake, but a set of tools to perform our foremost aim – to give our patients the best care we can – in a more efficient, more rewarding and hopefully relaxed and stress free way.

References

[1a] Antiles S, Couris J, Schweitzer A (2000) Projects planning, training, measurement and Sustainment. Radiol Manage 22(1): 18–31

[1] Arenson RL, Chakraborty DP, Seshadri SB, et al (1990) The digital image workstation. Radiology 176:303–315

[2] Bennett WF, Vaswani KK, Mendiola JA, Spigos DG (2003) PACS monitors: an evolution of radiologists's viewing techniques. J Digit Imaging 15 [Suppl 1]: 171–174

[3] Graf B, Simon U, Eickmeyer F, Fiedler V (2000) 1K versus 2K monitor. A clinical alternative free response receiver operating characteristic study of observer performance using pulmonary nodules. Am J Roentgenol 174: 1067–1074

[4] Hirschorn DS, Dreyer KJ, Schultz T (2003) Are consumer grade flat panel monitors comparable with medical grade CRT monitors for primary diagnosis of abdominopelvic CT exams? J Digit Imaging 16 [Suppl 1]: 31–32

[5] Hruby W, Moser H, Urban M, et al (1992) The Vienna SMZO PACS project: the totally digital hospital. Eur J Radiol 16: 66–68

[6] Irie G, Miyasaka K, Miyamoto K, et al (1990) PACS experience at the University of Hokkaido medical school. Pro SPIE 1234: 26–32

[7] Pärtan G, Mayerhofer R, Urban M, Wassipaul M, Pichler L, Hruby W (2003) Diagnostic performance of liquid crystal and cathode ray tube monitors in brain computed tomography. Eur Radiol 13: 2397–2401

[8] Peer S, Giacomuzzi SM, Peer R, Gassner E, Steingruber E, Jaschke W (2003) Resolution requirements for monitor viewing of digital flat panel detector radiographs: a contrast detail analysis. Eur Radiol 13: 413–417

[9] Peer S, Vogl R, Peer R, et al (1999) Sophisticated HIS, RIS, PACS integration in a large scale traumatology PACS. J Digit Imaging 12: 99–102
[10] Peer S, Sander H. Marsolek I, et al (2003) Radiography for intensive care: Participatory process analysis in a PACS equipped and film/screen environment. J Digit Imaging (in print)
[11] Reiner B, Siegel E, Brower S, Moffitt R (2003) Clinical comparison of CRT and LCD monitors in the evaluation of non-displaced fractures. J Digit Imaging 16 [Suppl 1]: 76–77
[12] Siegel EL (1994) PACS at the Baltimore Veterans Affaires Medical Center – planning implementation strategies and preliminary experience. Proceedings of the Korean Society of PACS, pp 1–8
[13] Siegel E, Reiner B (2002) Workflow redesign: the key to success when using PACS. AJR 178: 563–566
[14] Strickland NH (1996) Some cost benefit considerations for PACS: a radiological perspective. Br J Radiol 69: 1089–1098
[15] Tamm EP, Thompson S, Venable SL, McEnery K (2002) Impact of multislice CT on PACS resources. J Digit Imaging 15 [Suppl 1]: 96–101
[16] Völk M, Strotzer M, Lenhart M, et al (2000) Analysis of the availability and completeness of previous radiological examinations related to plain films. Acta Radiologica 41: 106–110

A view to the past of the future – Digital (r)evolution at the Danube hospital

W. Hruby[1] and A. Maltsidis[2]

[1]Chairman of the Radiology Department, Danube Hospital, Vienna, Austria
[2]Senior Consultant, Siemens AG Austria, MED SYS, Vienna, Austria

Introduction

Clinical experiences in digital radiology including intra- and interhospital communication have been documented in literature since the late 80ies. The world's first strictly-digital radiology system was planed in 1988 and implemented in 1992 in the Danube Hospital at the Socio Medical Care Center East of the city of Vienna (SMZO). The objectives of this project were firstly to overcome inherent problems of film-based systems, e.g. the loss of films, as well as to improve the efficiency and speed of patient data management, image acquisition, image distribution, archiving and reporting. The implementation of an integrated digital radiology system was expected to improve the quality of research and patient care and to support administrative tasks in connection with radiology and hospital information management systems (RIS, HIS), thus improving the efficiency not only of the radiology department but of the whole hospital.

The scope of this article is to give an overview of a decade's experience in digital radiology and of the various aspects that have to be considered when implementing it. This experience has proven us that digital radiology is an excellent working clinical tool for improving health care, since it allows the functional integration of physically separated systems, centralized archiving and image display, rapid access to images from multiple locations and effective image communication.

History – review

The hospital

The Danube Hospital (Fig. 1) is the youngest newly build hospital in the city of Vienna and features a complete power spectrum of two internal medicine departments, departments for dermatology, general surgery, traumatology, neurology, neurosurgery, orthopedic surgery, pediatry, child surgery, otorhinolaryngology, nuclear medicine, radio-oncology, urology, psychiatry and outpatient clinics for all faculties. The Danube Hospital is part of the Socio Medical Care Center East of the city of Vienna (SMZO), which covers, besides the hospital, a geriatric nursing home with 405 beds, a geriatric daily care center, a nursing school, as well as 500 personnel dwellings, and is considered as the authority center for medical and social supply in the eastern part of Vienna (Fig. 2).

Planning of the Danube hospital began in 1979. After a two-year planning interruption, building was initiated in 1985. The first implementation phase, featuring 573 systemized beds, went into clinical operation on the 27th April 1992. A clearer insight to the dimensions and the growing workload of the hospital is given in Tables 1 & 2 and is comparable with the growing workload and requirements to the department of radiology.

The radiology department – History-review

Planning for the radiology department started in 1988. The decision to implement it in strictly digital manner was made primarily considering the qualitative advantage for the patient. A further objective was the improvement of departmental and hospital-wide efficiency through the automated dispatch of image and examination report data. The potentials of teleconsulting were a strategic target pursued on from the beginning (e.g. for consultations between radiologists and referring physicians in cases with abnormal findings). The economic factor was of course also a key issue for the financial providers of the city of Vienna, and as was proven later the costs of digital radiology were, despite its substantial

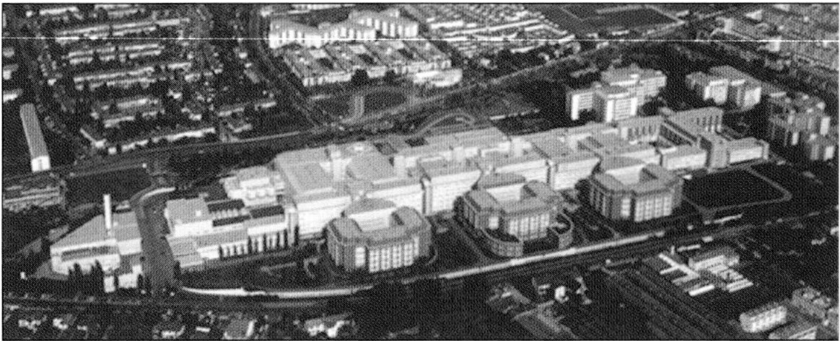

Fig. 1. Socio Medical Care Center East (SMZO) – Danube Hospital

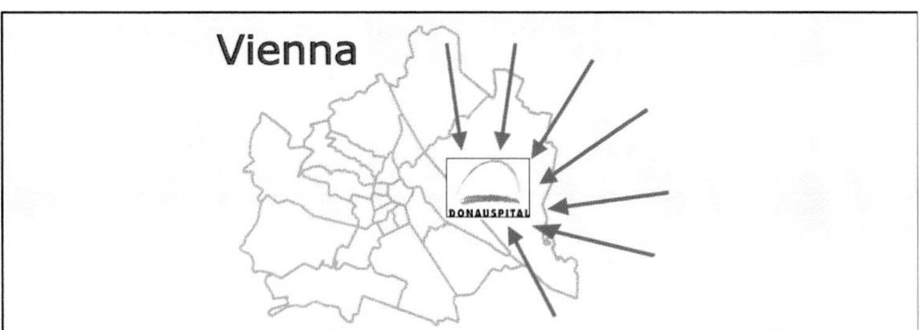

Fig. 2. Service Area of the Socio Medical Care Center East (SMZO)

Table 1. General hospital facts

Metropolitan area	1,800,000
Service area	250,000
Average number of systemized beds	933
Number of beds in the geriatric nursing home	405
Personnel	2,781

Table 2. Annual hospital facts

	1997	2000	2003
In-patient frequency	44,473	50,182	50,498
Out-patient frequency	129,317	137,834	132,874
Hospitalization days	323,411	340,120	341,883
Short term stays	8,174	10,634	10,390
Average length of stay (days)	7.27	6.78	6.78
Average utilization of beds	81.9%	84.9%	85.6%
Number of births	1,823	1,858	1,934
Number of deaths	845	894	914

qualitative advantages, not higher than those of conventional radiology.

After termination of the medical and radiological specifications the project became subject of a competitive bidding. From a technical point of view, two main problems/challenges arose in the context of digital radiography, namely the challenge for image data transmission and storage and the challenge of interfacing all subsystems and modalities. From a medical point of view the main challenge was that reporting workstations and their software should be able to handle at least all tasks known from conventional film reading procedures. The main hardware prerequisites were sufficient spatial resolution and luminance intensity. The workflow (software) prerequisites were e.g. display of present and previous examinations in a way suited for comparison, display of patient demographics and clinical information etc.

The installation began in the summer of 1991. Following the implementation phase, a half year test run was started as phantom operation, the purpose of which was to optimize the newly applied technology for practice and to check the EDP supported local organizations and communications for system consistency. A further goal of the test operation was the determination of parameters for quality control and quality assurance, and thus the exact documentation of exposure doses in the context of digital radiography compared with film-screen radiography. These data were analyzed and documented under economic and ecological criteria as well as regarding the legal radiation protection. The successful termination of this simulation was the prerequisite for a successful introduction into daily clinical practice. A technical review of all major implementations in the radiology department during the last years is shown in Table 3.

Today's standard

Today's technology

We have achieved to be a filmless radiology department within a filmless hospital. Today's status is the result of the constant adaptations to the changing needs within the hospital and the change in technology regarding imaging modalities and computer technology. The principle of the network and the archive configuration remained unchanged since the first planning period. New imaging devices have been added during the years or have been replaced by new ones.

Digital network

The implemented digital network is equipped with two types of connections, which are used depending on the requirements of the connected workplaces. The first and faster one is the FDDI-connection,

Table 3. Technical review of all major implementations in the radiology department

1988	Vision – Decision		
1989/90	**Planning**		
1991	**Implementation:**		
	Workstations:	Sun Sparc	Monitors: Simomed
	Archive:	Sun Sparc 2; 35 GB RAID	
	Jukeboxes:	NKK, media 680 MB WORM	
	Network:	Ethernet FDDI	(5 GB/day expected)
	RIS:	Simedos	
	Modalities:	2 CT, 2 Digiscans, Digital Chest, 3 Angiography units, Coronary-Angiography unit	
09/1991	**Preopening phase**		
04/1992	**Start of Clinical Operation**		
1994	**Archive Upgrade:**		
	Jukeboxes:	media 1.7GB WORM	
1995	**MRT – Radiation Thearapy:**		
	Networking, Neuronavigation		
1995	**Upgrade ISA – MagicStore:**		
	Network:	complete upgrade to fiber optics	
	Archive:	Sun UltraSparc ; 90 GB RAID	
1997	**Upgrade Sun UltraSparc 2:**		
	Workstations:	Sun UltraSparc 2	
1998	**Prepared for the year 2000:**		
	Archive:	MagicStore; 100 GB RAID	
	Jukeboxes:	media 4.8 GB WORM	
	Network:	Fast Ethernet FDDI (15 GB/day expected)	
	RIS:	MagicSAS, PC based, support of autorouting and prefetching	
	strictly-digital radiology in the **trauma center** with Digiscans and reporting WS, DICOM standard in ultrasound examinations		
1999	**Upgrade MagicStore & Modalities:**		
	Archive:	Sun UltraSparc 2	
	Modalities:	Angiostar Plus, Polytron TOP (DS) Iconos, Fluorospot TOP (DF)	
	3D:	3D Virtuoso	
2000	**No Y2K related problems**		
2000	New Technologies: Ampex Long Term Archive; 7,6 TB capacity on tape cartridges Thorax FD, Polydoros Lx50 Lite (Flat Panel Detector, CR) Exposure Dose, automated documentation embedded in the RIS		
2003	**Opening of the new "Mamma Vital" center**		
2004	**Preparations for the next decade of digital radiology** competitive bidding for the next ten years of all-inclusive digital radiology		

which was realized according to a combined ring-star-architecture and operates on fiber optics with a data transmission rate of 100 Mbit/s. FDDI is used for workplaces with high requirements on transmission rate, e.g. modalities, reporting workstations, heavily used viewing workstations. All other workplaces, e.g. radiology information system (RIS) workstations, less used viewing workstations etc. are integrated through a ETHERNET-connection, which operates on common copper wire with a transmission rate of 10 Mbit/s.

Digital archive

The digital archive (Fig. 3) serves both the Picture Archiving and Communication System (PACS) and the Radiology Information System (RIS) and is the electronic correspondent of a conventional film archive including the radiological reports. The unique master over the digital archive is the so called Patient Directory (PDIR) database. Following the PDIR-database in hierarchy are three Information Management Systems (IMS). The IMS form modules, which consist of an IMS database-workstation, a Redundant Array of Independent Disks (RAID) and up to two jukeboxes with Magneto Optical Disks (MOD). IMS modules can be added freely to the system and this modular structure allows a extension and adaptation of the archive to the increasing requirements of a radiology department.

In the PDIR patient demographics, clinical information and radiological reports are stored according to a relational database model (SYBASE database). In this relational database, data are organized in tables, which are named PATIENT, STUDY, EXAMINATION, REPORT in accordance with the typical workflow in a radiology department. The PDIR is used commonly from the PACS and the RIS and contains only the reference to the respective digital images of every examination.

The actual storage of radiological images is managed and organized by the IMS-modules. The most recent images (especially not reported ones) are stored in the RAID. Older and reported images are compressed (at a loss-free compression rate of 2.5) and stored on MODs – in a Write Once Read Many (WORM) manner –, which are arranged in jukeboxes. Finally, all images including those, which are too old to be kept online on a disc jukebox, are additionally saved in the Long Term Archive.

This distributed database structure guarantees short response times, since if a query is performed at e.g. a reporting workstation then the superordinate PDIR determines first the exact localization of the pictures within the IMS, then the images are located by the IMS and sent to the workstation (Fig. 4).

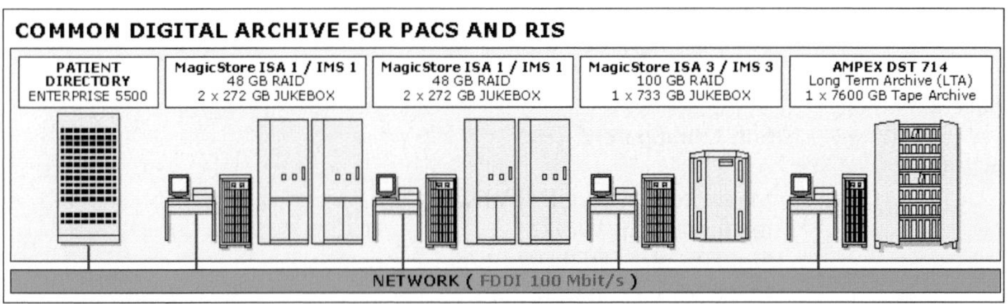

Fig. 3. Digital archive in the radiology department

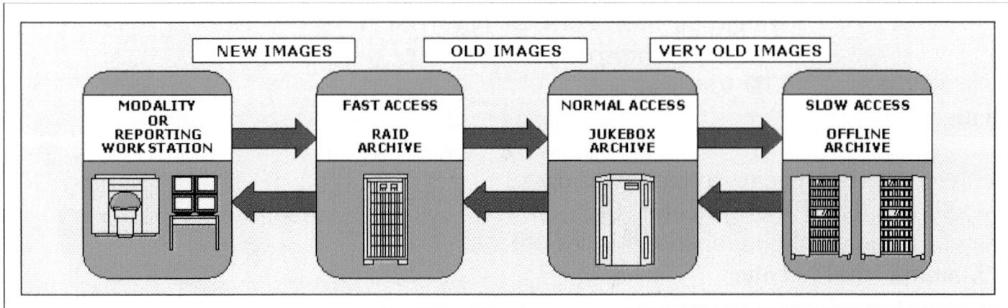

Fig. 4. Data-flow of radiological images – Storage hierarchy

The functions of the digital archive can be summarized as follows:

- handle the entire data-flow of the RIS.
- receive examination folders from modalities and reporting workstations.
- save examination folders on fast error-tolerant RAIDs.
- compress examination folders at a loss-free compression rate of approx. 2.5.
- save examination folders on optical disks.
- control the functionality of the jukeboxes.
- organize archived examination folders in a database.
- handle query requests from reporting workstations.
- send examination folders to reporting and viewing workstations.

Modalities and workstations

The extent and complexity of the hospital-wide digital network, as well as the digital modalities and workstations in use are shown in the Figs. 5–7 and in Table 4.

Radiology department

In the main radiology department (Fig. 5) RIS terminals (PCs) are installed in the reception, adjacent to all modalities, adjacent to all reporting workstations and in the transcription office, allowing a complete documentation of the radiological workflow. Since RIS functionality is based on status-dependent worklists, it seems for the users as if the patient record makes its own way through the department. In the reception, RIS terminals are used for patient admission. The terminals at the modalities are used for exam documentation. These near reporting workstations are used both for worklist control and for reporting and verification of written reports, and those in the transcription office are used - during normal working hours – for the transcription of reports dictated on tape.

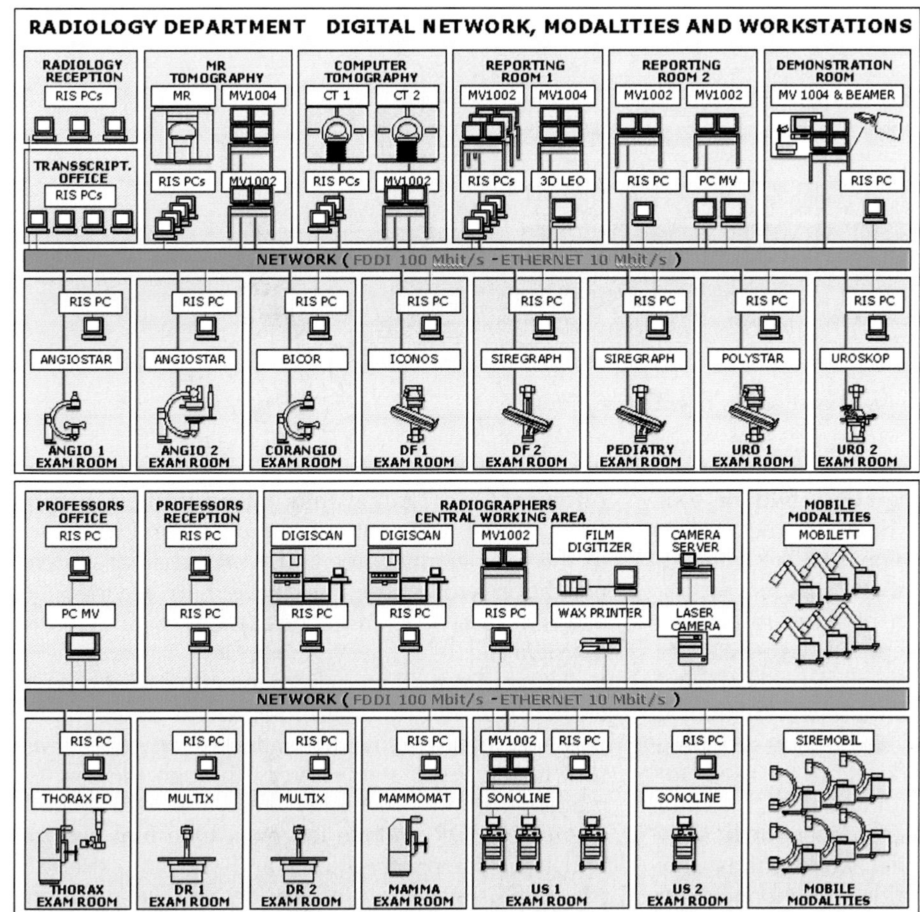

Fig. 5. Digital network, modalities and workstations in the radiology department

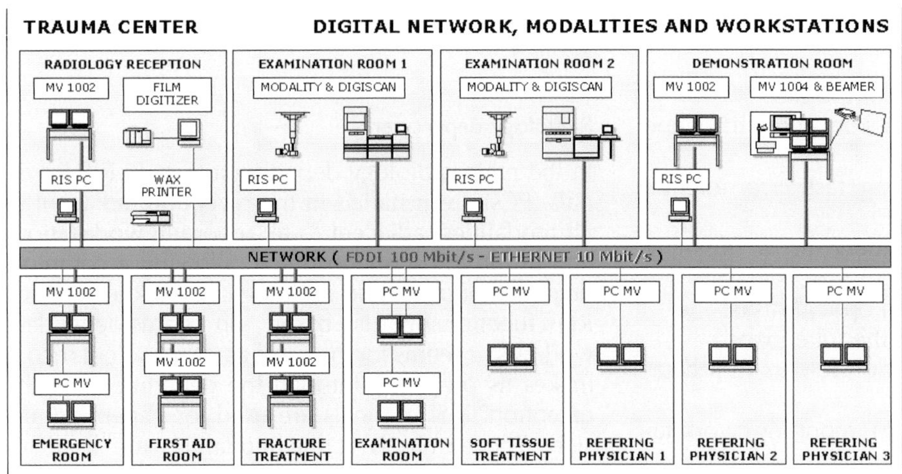

Fig. 6. Digital network, modalities and workstations in the trauma center

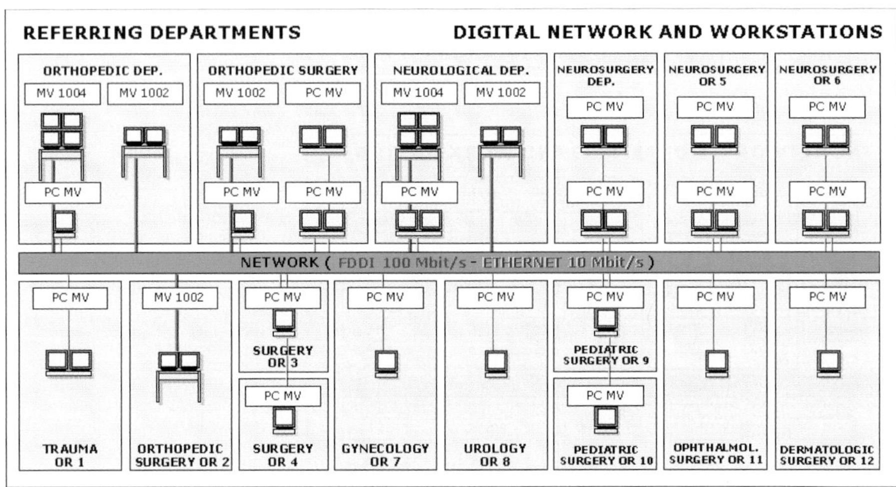

Fig. 7. Digital network and viewing workstations in referring departments

Reporting workstations in the radiology department are equipped with either one, two or four monochrome landscape size monitors, depending on the needs of the examination type assigned to them. All are integrated to the PACS via a fast FDDI-connection. Images from different modalities are auto-routed to specific reporting workstations but are also available for retrieval from the digital archive and can be reported on any workstation in the radiology department. In the main reporting room, one four-monitor workstation is used for skeletal examinations and three dual monitor workstations are used for other conventional x-ray examinations. Several additional workstations in a second reporting room provide redundancy for cases of technical problems or high workload and are also used by radiographers for quality control (i.e. review and preparation of images for reporting). Additional workstations are placed in the CT exam room, in the MRI room, in the ultrasound room and in the radiographers' central working area. A demonstration workstation, connected to a video beamer, is used for case conferences with referring physicians.

Images from all modalities are either sent directly to the PACS (e.g. CT, MRI, ultrasound, angiography, coronary angiography, digital fluoroscopy etc.) or are sent to the PACS semi-directly through the two CR readers installed centrally near the radiographic rooms (e.g. DR, mobile DR etc.). One film digitizer and two film printers (laser and wax) are used for importing images from outside the hospital and printing images for designated out-patients, respectively.

Table 4. Technical summary of the integrated hardware in the radiology department

Diagnostic Workstations	
6	MagicView 1004
22	MagicView 1002
17	MagicView 300
1	Leonardo AX Workstation
1	3D Virtuoso
Viewing Workstations	
48	MagicView 50
Storage and Archive	
1	PDIR Enterprise 5500
3	MagicStore RAID (2 with 48GB each, 1 with 100GB)
4	Jukebox (272GB each, 1.7GB WORM media)
1	Jukebox (733GB, 4.8GB WORM media)
1	Ampex DST 714 Long Term Archive (7,600 GB, 100 GB tape media)
Image Documentation	
1	Camera server with Sterling LP400
2	MagicRead
2	Sterling Solid Ink Jet 400 (Post Script Level 2)
Modalities (networked)	
Siemens Somatom Plus 4 Power (CT)	
Siemens Somatom AR.T (CT)	
Siemens Magnetom Impact Expert (MR)	
Siemens Angiostar Plus, Polytron TOP (DS)	
Siemens Angiostar, Polytron 1000VR (DS)	
Siemens Sonoline Elegra (US)	
Kretz-Technik VoluSon 530D (US)	
2 Siemens Siregraph D1, Fluorospot H (DF)	
Siemens Iconos, Fluorospot TOP (DF)	
Siemens Thorax FD, Polydoros Lx50 Lite (Flat Panel Detector, CR)	
2 Siemens Digiscan 2 (CR)	
Siemens Digiscan 2C Plus (CR)	
Siemens Digiscan 2H Plus (CR)	
Siemens Polystar, Fluorospot H (DF)	
Siemens Uroskop D3, Fluorospot H (DF)	
Siemens Bicore (DS)	
Other	
48	SIENET MagicSAS RIS PC's
Interface to HIS of City of Vienna	

Trauma center

The trauma center can be considered as a high-speed micrography of the radiology department including its referring departments (Fig. 6). The radiology sub-department in the trauma center is equipped with two DR modalities and two CR readers and is completely integrated in the PACS and the RIS of the main radiology department. This allows for image, report and workflow communication between main radiology and its sub-department, as well as workload dispatch in cases of emergency.

As in the main department a quality control workstation is used for the review and preparation of images. A demonstration room workstation, including a video beamer, is used here also for case conferences. A film digitizer and a wax printers are used for importing and exporting images from and to "non-digital" radiologists. As for referring departments, all referring exam rooms are equipped with viewing workstations depending on their needs.

Referring departments

All referring departments directly related to and relying on radiological examinations (Fig. 7) are equipped with viewing workstations. These are either standard (reporting quality) workstations, as in the radiology department, equipped with one, two or four high resolution monitors, or PC-based viewing

Table 5. Used storage capacity of the digital archive

	Number of exams	Number of images	Capacity in MB
CR	90,935	146,659	1,428,278
CT	92,181	4,952,116	2,504,190
DF	5,042	88,273	198,677
DR	773,311	1,438,704	7,928,518
DS	23,356	196,022	267,975
MG	886	1,691	43,259
MR	45,714	4,154,115	738,547
OT	22,757	49,955	64,302
PT	6	621	20
RG	2,536	6,391	23,292
RT	19,574	50,926	9,235
SC	9,563	28,762	92,677
US	43,458	405,158	332,389
XA	2,789	38,404	49,129
Other	271	4,690	9,943
TOTAL	1,132,379	11,562,487	13,690,431

workstations with one or two standard PC monitors. The number and quality of workstations, as well as the number and quality of the respective monitors installed, depends on the actual needs of the departments as experienced after many years of clinical practice with digital radiology.

Growing along increasing needs

The average data-volume per study is constantly increasing as there is a clear tendency towards higher resolution images, thinner slices in cross-section imaging in general and additional sequences in MRI-imaging. The amount of digitally archived images in the last years consumes a storage capacity of over 13.6 million Megabytes.

The increasing number of patients per year and increasing number of examinations per patient also contribute towards a highly increased number of new images each month (Table 6).

All this was foreseeable when the network and the central archive were set up. The technology concerning the network itself was already available at this stage and did not have to be altered. The need for increasing archive capacity was also clearly foreseeable but has not been available at the time of the implementation. Right from the beginning it was perfectly clear, that the system had to grow with the clinical needs. For this reason the complete system was designed in a modular concept, allowing to exchange and replace components that are out of date without any significant changes to the structure. Unforeseeable changes in the future such as new imaging techniques must not be a significant problem for a newly built digital radiology system either. This is another essential reason for a flexible system that is

Table 6. Number of examinations and patients during the last 4 years – Continuous growth

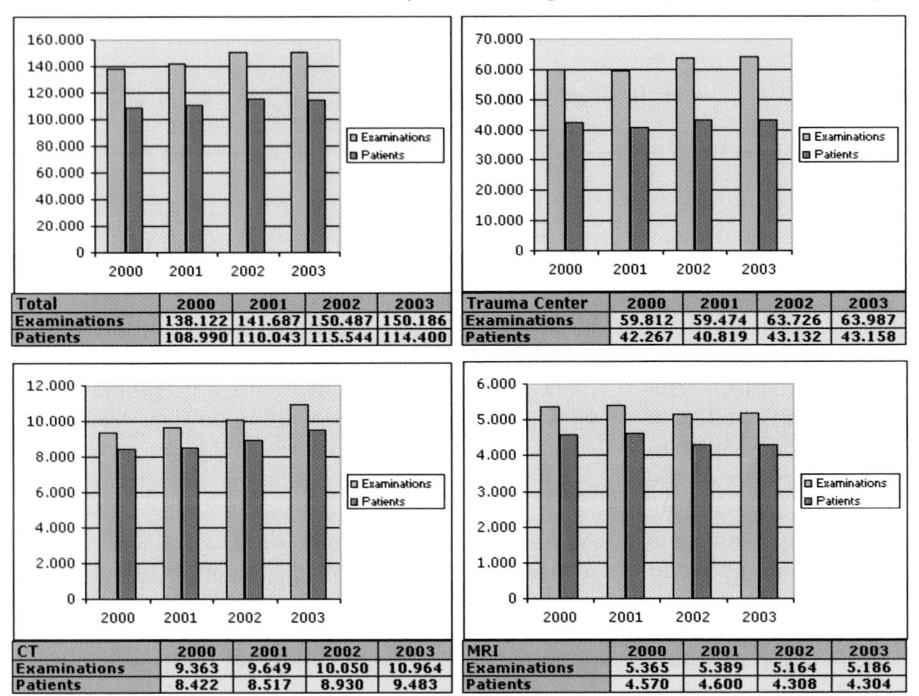

Total	2000	2001	2002	2003
Examinations	138.122	141.687	150.487	150.186
Patients	108.990	110.043	115.544	114.400

Trauma Center	2000	2001	2002	2003
Examinations	59.812	59.474	63.726	63.987
Patients	42.267	40.819	43.132	43.158

CT	2000	2001	2002	2003
Examinations	9.363	9.649	10.050	10.964
Patients	8.422	8.517	8.930	9.483

MRI	2000	2001	2002	2003
Examinations	5.365	5.389	5.164	5.186
Patients	4.570	4.600	4.308	4.304

open for future demands. The rapid development in computer technology made it possible, to switch from especially designed hardware to commercially available workstations in 1997. This was one of the major steps to improve cost-efficiency. During the first decade, the archive costs have dropped significantly as the price for long-term digital archive media have dropped tremendously.

Radiology Information System (RIS)

The development of a Radiology Information System (RIS) that serves as the master of the imaging part of the digital radiology system was one of the major steps in the improvement of time-efficacy, because a feasible automatization of the workflow depends on the integration of the sub-systems.

The newly integrated RIS introduces a new-generation of administration systems; it is a comprehensive, easy-to-use system, modeling the optimal work flow within the radiology department together with the PACS. The client-server architecture with Windows-user interface, the common data base from RIS and PACS allow for the following advantages:

- Integrated database, i.e. no interface between RIS and PACS. No special implementation work during software updates necessary.
- Guarantee of data consistency (e.g. when modifying patient data).
- Common data backup for all PACS and RIS components.
- Less work for system administrator due to the use of a common database.
- Controlling of prefetch and autoroute mechanism via PACS. Automatically images relevant for reporting will be loaded from the archive and sent to the reporting workstation.

The functionality of the RIS corresponds to the entire administrative workflow at the radiology department and that includes:

- **Communication:** Exam requests are interfaced from the HIS. Verified reports are interfaced back to the HIS, including billing information.
- **Scheduling:** Exam requests are planned for a certain date, time and modality, considering availability of resources.
- **Examination:** Documentation of performed examination and additional data, such as used contrast media, exposure dose, complications etc.
- **Reporting:** Assistance to the reporting radiologist by providing information not easily available in the PACS (e.g. clinical data, exam request form). Facilitation of report transcription and verification.
- **Analysis:** Management of cases for scientific work, statistical analysis and documentation.

Workflow – example of an examination

Before examination

The exam request is booked electronically at the HIS terminals (Fig. 8) at a referring department and con-

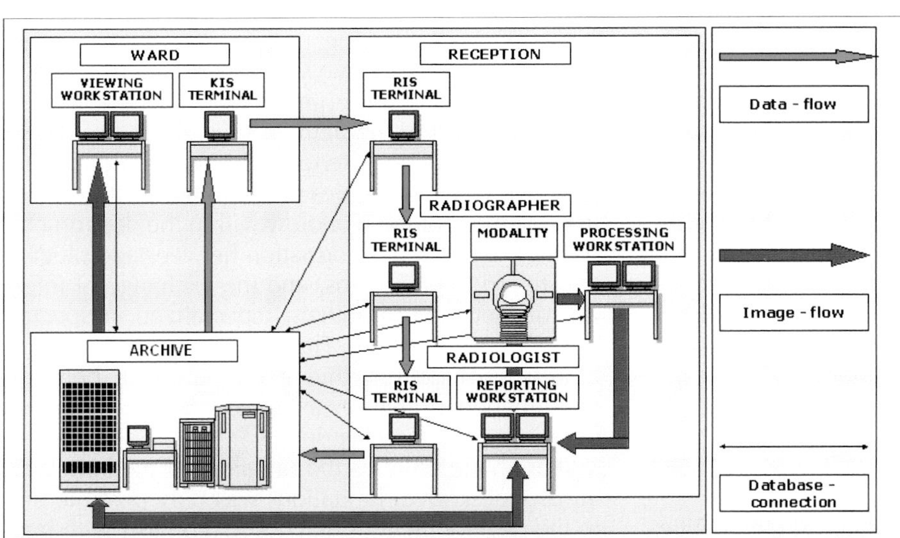

Fig. 8. Workflow and dataflow diagram of an examination

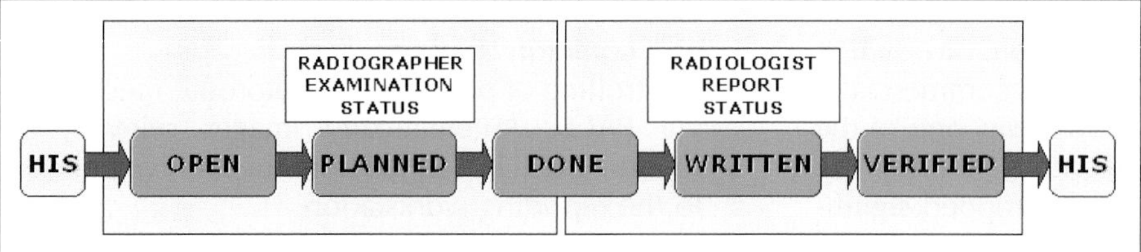

Fig. 9. Status diagram of an examination and report in the RIS

sists of the obligatory patient demographics, preferred date and time of the exam and examination type. The exam request is then transferred automatically, via an proprietary interface, to the common database for RIS and PACS (PDIR). Triggered by this input the PDIR allocates all relevant previous images according to specified rules and initiates pre-fetching and autorouting. Thus, where possible, exam requests are booked one day before the examination as this facilitates overnight pre-fetching and autorouting. At this point, radiographers or clerical staff schedule and specify the "open" examination (Fig. 9) at a RIS-terminal and depending on the scheduled modality the exam request appears on the respective RIS-worklist, having the examination status "planned". For conventional x-ray modalities, the same worklist is also displayed on the CR reader's console. For modalities supporting "DICOM worklist", the worklist is displayed on the modality's console. The common database for RIS and PACS guarantees for data consistency between these worklists.

During examination

When the patient arrives for the scheduled exam he/she is checked in at the reception and the examination room worklist is updated. The patient is then examined according to the information entered in the exam request. During and after examination, information, such as number of CT slices, X-ray dose, involved staff etc., is recorded in the RIS and is available for statistical analysis and documentation. Additionally, while the patient is passing through the department, the involved staff may enter comments on the electronic request form, which may be helpful to the reporting radiologist. The examination is then signed by the radiographer and disappears from the "planned" RIS-worklist, now having the status "done".

After examination

Images acquired from conventional x-ray modalities are routed to a designated quality control workstation, are optimized by a radiographer and are then auto-routed to a specified reporting workstation. Images acquired from direct digital modalities (CT, MR, US) are auto-routed directly to a reporting workstation. All relevant patient and exam information, as well as all previous images are naturally also accessible at this workstation. To the reporting radiologists it is clear at a glance what work requires to be done, since all "done" examinations are displayed on his personal RIS-worklist. The radiologist then reports the examination, which status changes after typing and verification to "written" and "verified", respectively. Finally, the signed report and all relevant information is automatically sent back to the HIS via the same interface. The referring physician at the ward can now initiate treatment as he has obtained all relevant information at his HIS terminal and all relevant images at his viewing workstation.

Benefits of digital radiology

Digital radiology allows the functional integration of physically separated systems, centralized archiving and image display, rapid access to images from multiple locations and effective image communication.

Since the beginning of this new digital era in radiology in 1992, some years have passed and it is now possible to show and prove the benefits that evolve from the implementation of these digital technologies. Computerized diagnostic equipment provides new capabilities for radiologists. It provides improvement of the workflow within the department, of the exchange of information between radiologists and referring physicians, and the exchange of information between radiologists specialized in specific diagnostic procedures. This exchange of information is possible locally within the department, between different departments even between widely separated buildings in different hospitals.

Eliminating film as the radiological medium with all its well-known limitations was only possible due to the development of diagnostic monitors with high contrast and brightness and high resolution formats with which the radiological consoles are equipped.

Digital radiography separates the acquisition medium and the viewing medium and permits different image representations by insertion of computerized processes (pre-processing, postprocessing) between the actual radiograph at the acquisition medium and the radiograph represented on a hardcopy or a monitor. It also implies advantages directly related to the generation and production of plain x-rays, using photostimulable phosphorplates, which have a much wider latitude than conventional films and thus allow more tolerance in the exposure parameters, resulting in a more consistent image quality without the need of avoidable re-examinations. Depending on the diagnostic question it is also possible to reduce the exposure dose, in particular if dynamic investigations are performed, where spatial resolution is not that important and some image noise may be tolerated. (For questions where high spatial resolution is necessary, e.g. in searching subtle signs for arthritis, dose reduction in digital radiology is less possible.) Furthermore another great advantage is the possibility to alter window and level of an x-ray, so both soft tissues and bone structures can be assessed at the same image, whereas in a film-based system 2 exposures would be necessary. The same is true for the elimination of re-takes due to lost films.

The faster access to image information and the elimination of the need to search for old films have resulted in increased departmental efficiency. The quality of diagnosis depends not only on its accuracy but also on its time of delivery, to initiate the correct treatment as early as possible. This way, digital radiology contributes to the quality of health care in so far as a faster report cycle time means better treatment (Fig. 10). Although an exact amount is not measurable, digital radiology is certainly an essential part in arriving at the reduction of average length of stay in hospital. In comparison with other Austrian hospitals the Danube Hospital has the lowest hospitalization time of 7.1 days (Table 7). The average cost of radiology services is also remarkably low compared with other Austrian hospitals (Table 8).

Furthermore, the advantages of the digital archive, over a conventional, cause savings in

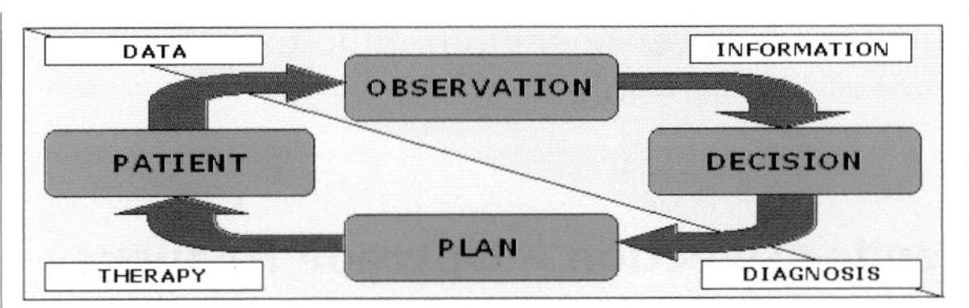

Fig. 10. The diagnostic-therapeutic cycle

Table 7. Average length of stay and average cost per in-patient, comparison of major hospitals in Vienna (source: WrKAV-Leistungsbericht 1998)

Hospital	Systemized beds	Average length of stay	Average cost per in-patient
Danube Hospital	933	7.1 days	52,834 AUT
KFJ Hospital	735	8.5 days	61,311 AUT
Lainz Hospital	1,040	7.6 days	52,610 AUT
Rudolfstiftung Hospital	775	7.6 days	56,329 AUT
Wilhelminen Hospital	1,178	8.3 days	59,082 AUT

Table 8. Average cost of radiology services (excluded: CT, MR), comparison of major hospitals in Vienna (source: Basisdatenauswertungen 1998 des Bundesministeriums für Arbeit, Gesundheit und Soziales)

Hospital	Average cost per service
Danube Hospital	1.411 AUT
KFJ Hospital	1.662 AUT
Lainz Hospital	1.539 AUT
Rudolfstiftung Hospital	1.706 AUT
Wilhelminen Hospital	1.962 AUT

Table 9. Advantages of a digital archive

	Digital archive	Conventional archive
Space	10 m^3	900 m^3
Loss of films	–	5–20%
Image access	fast / easy	↑
Communication	on-line	–
Costs	↓	↑
Staff	↓	↑

material, room and personnel, which are not measurable but obvious.

Finally, the fact that the increase of the number of patients and services in our department, did not result in or require an increase of staff, shows that the stepwise implementation of newer technology resulted in an increase of efficiency.

Integrating the transdanubean healthcare enterprise

The transdanubean healthcare enterprise provides medical and social services assuring a global health

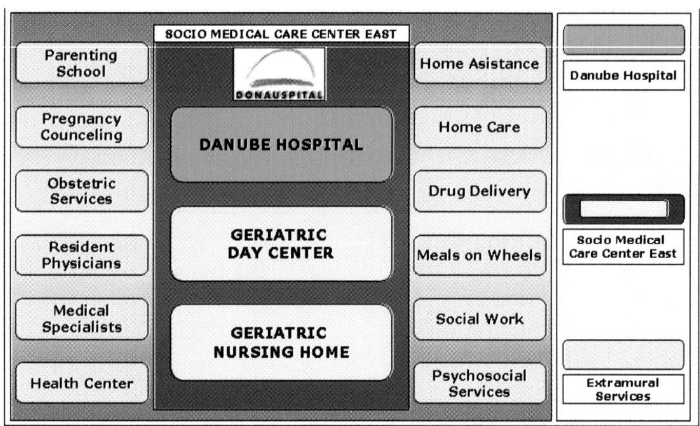

Fig. 11. Integrating the transdanubean healthcare enterprise

care for all patients in eastern Vienna and it forms a supplement or an extension of the cooperation convention of the hospital network (KAV) with the MA 47. The core of this healthcare enterprise also known as the "Regional Alliance/Donaustadt" is the Danube Hospital at the Socio Medical Care Center East of the city of Vienna (SMZO). The project-target of integrating this healthcare enterprise is to provide global healthcare through a close network comprising of the Danube hospital, the health center of the district, the resident physicians and all attached extramural services (see Fig. 11).

The project is divided into four sub-sections. Each of the sub-sections is functionally effective by itself, their synergetic effectiveness however exceeds their singular effectiveness by far:

A. Optimization of the admissions to the hospital
B. Optimization of the dismissals from the hospital.
C. Coordination of the extramural services.
D. Electronic networking of all institutions and services.

The importance of competent support

The technical support of a digital radiology system is divided into two prime areas, namely user support and system support. In our department two designated help-lines (one for PACS and one for RIS) are functional during normal office hours and supply competent solution to whichever user or system problem thinkable. The two system-administrators manning these help-lines are assured in frame of the service contract with the vendor.

Users have to be always trained to compete with the effective operation of every user surface functionality needed. After initial training, which is performed in small groups, further training is provided "on request" to refresh the acquired knowledge and to keep up with meantime effective system modifications.

Routine system support and monitoring is needed to guarantee a frictionless operation. Therefore, the functions of the entire installation are constantly monitored and searched for minor malfunctions. This way, various smaller discrepancies, which are sometimes inevitable, can be detected and recovered to the major part, before they can lead to a workflow impairment. If not so, the system-administrators are immediately informed and depending upon the weight of the disturbance a graded reaction pattern is started. Most system-dependent errors can be recovered within a short time by the administrators. If not so, an expert team is always reachable at the vendor's help-line. The vendor's hotline as well as the hospital EDP hotline are also available outside normal office hours 24 hours a day, 7 days per week.

Due to the high system stability and the competent technical support, workflow impairments of 20 minutes during office hours or 40 minutes during night or weekend are already considered critical. The trauma center's radiology naturally has a higher priority with 15 and 30 minutes, respectively. Finally it is significant to mention that, during 2003 the system-downtime was under 0.1% (75% of which was planned and announced service downtime), during which the clinical operation of the department was never ever impossible.

Vendor selection – Upgrade frequency

Since any digital radiology system is definitely not a "plug and play" system, the selection of the vendor has to be made under consideration of project responsibility, standardization, compatibility, easy upgrading and updating as well as service and maintenance.

Over the last years, rather frequent systems upgrade proved to be not only necessary, but also cost and efficiency effective. The choice of a major vendor was an advantage, both in the development of new technology and in its service and maintenance.

To assure a frictionless clinical operation in the radiology department for the next decade, a competitive bidding is in preparation. The chosen vendor has then to provide software, hardware, modalities and services in an all-inclusive manner for the following ten years.

Conclusion

The main advantage digital radiology offers is reliable and fast access to all relevant medical information. This saves time, speeds up the report turnaround process and results in better diagnosis, considering the timeliness of delivery of the diagnostic outcome being an integral part of its importance, besides its accuracy.

The last decade has proven that digital radiology is an excellent working clinical tool for improving health care. Furthermore, it has now the potential to become successful, since the focus shifts from saving film to increasing productivity and efficiency.

References

[1] Hruby W, Mosser H, Urban M, Rüger W (1992) The Vienna SMZO-PACS project: the totally digital hospital. Eur J Radiol 16: 66

[2] Mosser H, Urban M, Dürr M, Rüger W, Hruby W (1992) Integration of radiology and hospital information systems with PACS: requirements of the radiologist. Euro J Radiol 16: 69

[3] Mosser H, Urban M, Hruby W (1994) Filmless digital radiology – feasibility and 20 month experience in clinical routine. Med Inform 19 (2): 149–159.

[4] Hruby W, Maltsidis A (2000) A view to the past of the future—a decade of digital (r)evolution at the Danube hospital. In: Hruby W (ed) Digital (R)evolution in radiology. Springer, Vienna, pp 81–95

[5] Hruby W (Ed) (2000) Digital (R)evolution in radiology. Springer, Vienna

Digital history of radiology

A. Maltsidis[1] and W. Hruby[2]

[1]Senior Consultant, Siemens AG Austria, MED SYS, Vienna, Austria
[2]Professor and Chairman of the Radiology Department, Danube Hospital, Vienna, Austria

Introduction

The continual evolution and enhancement of digital technology in all realms of industrial development has in recent years become increasingly noticeable in health care. Of particular significance has been the impact of digital technology in radiology.

The history of radiology and thus also the history of digital radiology consists of a continuous series of innovations and starts relatively early with the discovery of X-rays. Since the beginnings of the last century X-rays were used also for diagnosis. A rapid evolution of technology, shortly after the Second World War, led to the development of nuclear medicine and ultrasound. In further consequence and at the same time with the development of the first computers, computed tomography (CT) and magnetic resonance imaging (MRI) became reality. Since these modalities generate digital pictures, the logical consequence was to also handle and store these pictures digitally. The digital handling of images and information in radiology was at the beginning more a vision than reality. Now "digital radiology" is reality and has affected the whole range of diagnostic and therapeutic procedures. The short but eventful past of digital radiology can be declared as history, a history which forces us to learn from the past and allows us to make considerations about the future, briefly it is a view to the past of the future.

From X-rays to digital modalities

According to a famous historian, "the history of the world is but the biography of great man". This statement is especially true for the development of technology in the last centuries and very true for the beginnings of radiology.

X-rays

On Friday, November 8, 1895, **Wilhelm Conrad Roentgen**, a German physicist, made a simple observation that catapulted him to international fame (Fig. 1). While experimenting with an electrical

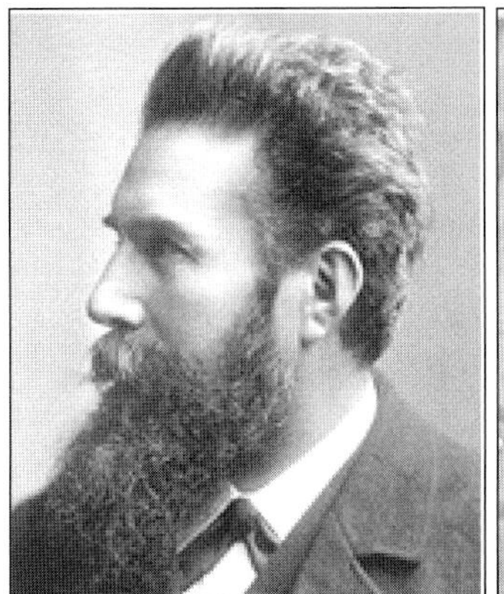

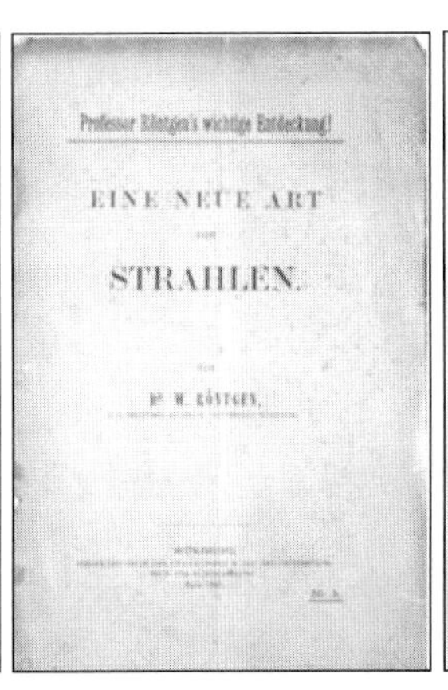

EINE NEUE ART

STRAHLEN.

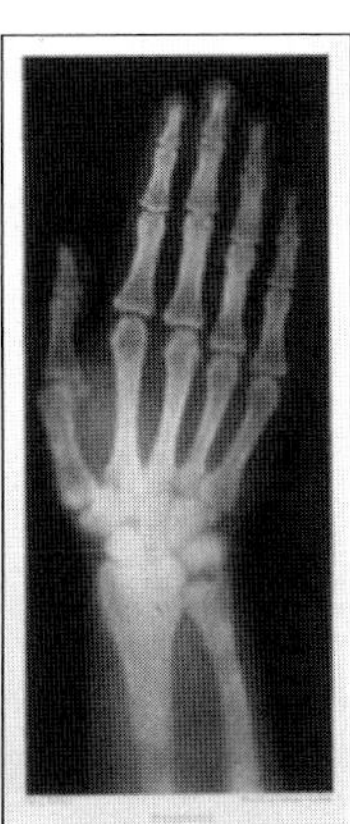

Fig. 1. Wilhelm Conrad Roentgen, publication and early x-ray

discharge tube connected to an induction coil, he noted that a nearby screen coated with barium platinocyanide was caused to fluoresce. He named his new rays with the mathematician's symbol for the unknown: X. On the same day he made the first medical application of his discovery, an X-ray photograph of his wife's hand. Roentgen's observation was remarkable, not only because of its tremendous implications, but because it had been made using simple, standard equipment that was readily available to almost anyone. As a result of this discovery, Roentgen became professor of physics at Hohenheim, Strasbourg, Giessen, Wuerzburg and Munich and was the recipient of the first Nobel Prize for Physics, in 1901.

Ultrasound

The story of the development of ultrasound applications in medicine should probably start with the history of measuring distance under water using sound waves. The underwater SONAR (Sound Navigation and Ranging), the RADAR and the ultrasonic Metal Flaw Detector are all technologies of the Second World War and each, in their unique ways, precursors of medical ultrasonic equipments. The modern ultrasound scanner embraces the concepts and science of all these modalities.

The use of ultrasound in medicine began during and shortly after the Second World War in various centres around the world. The Austrian psychiatrist and neurologist **Karl Theodore Dussik** published in 1942 the first work on the medical use of diagnostic ultrasound (Fig. 2). He was trying to locate brain tumors with a new method consisting of an ultrasound emitter at one end and an ultrasound receiver at the other. The patient stayed between the two devices. He measured the ultrasound beam transmission through the patient's head. The outbound ultrasound beam power was known and he calculated the receiving power, defining ultrasound attenuation and reinforcement. He also tried to visualize the cerebral ventricles by measuring the ultrasound beam modification through the head. Dr. Dussik published his technique in 1942 with the name of "hyperphonography of the brain."

Many workers can be cited as pioneers of medical ultrasound from then on. The work of Professor **Ian Donald** and his colleagues in Glasgow, in the mid 1950s, however, was a major contribution and facilitated the wider use of ultrasound in medical practice in the subsequent decades.

Computed tomography

Johann Radon, an Austrian mathematician, discovered the principle of the C.A.T. scanner in 1917 (Fig. 3). Radon was the first to prove that a two- or three-dimensional image can be reconstructed uniquely from the infinite set of all its projections. Ordinary tomographic images or "slices" through the body have been made since 1922 by using an X-ray source which moves in one direction while a piece of X-ray film moves simultaneously in the other direction. Radon's tomographic method, considerably more complex, could only be applied in practice with the arrival of the modern computer.

Allan M. Cormack, an American physicist developed the theoretical foundations that made computerized axial tomography (CAT) scanning possible using a reconstruction technique called the Radon transform. He published his results in two papers in 1963–64, but these generated little interest until the first C.A.T scanner, built under the leadership of the British engineer **Godfrey N. Hounsfield**, was introduced in 1972 and used in the United States at the Mayo Clinic in 1973. For their independent efforts, Cormack and Hounsfield shared the 1979 Nobel Prize in Physiology or Medicine.

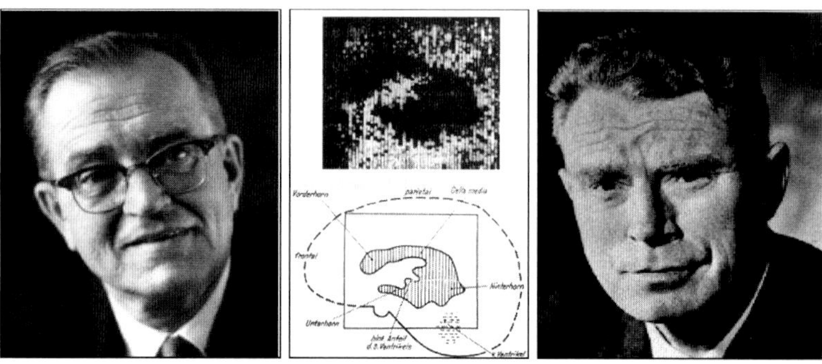

Fig. 2. Karl Dussik, a "hyperphonography of the brain" and Ian Donald

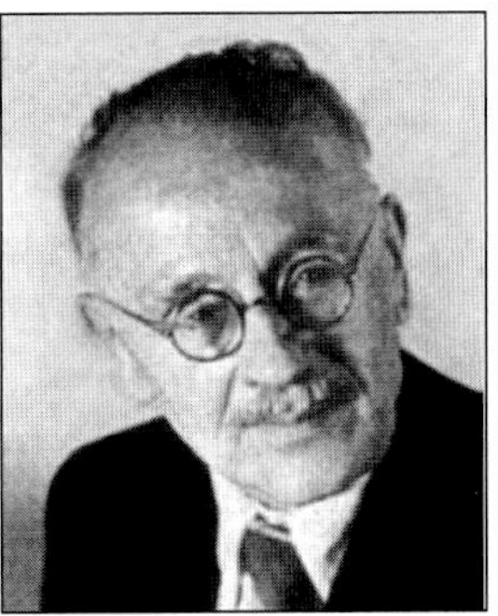
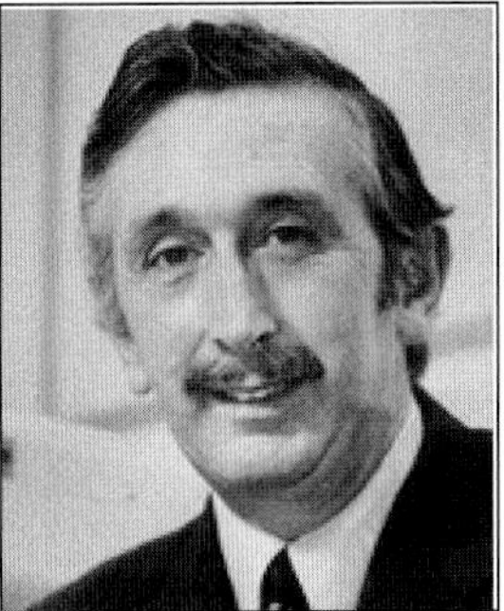
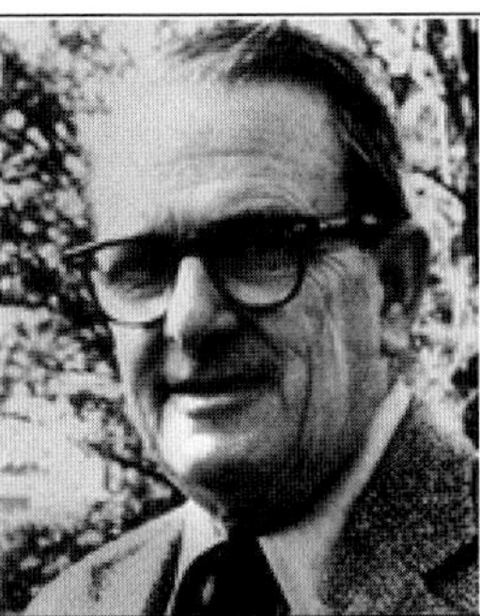

Fig. 3. Johann Radon, Sir Godfrey N. Hounsfield and Allan M. Cormack

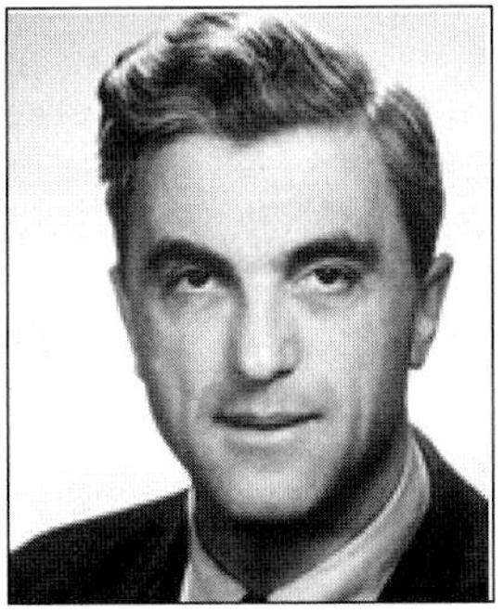
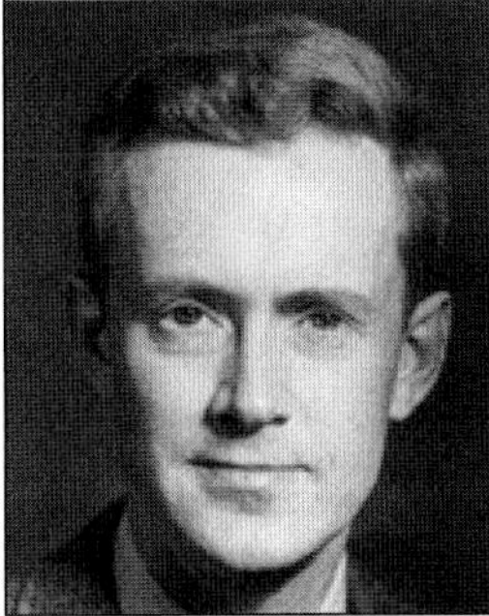
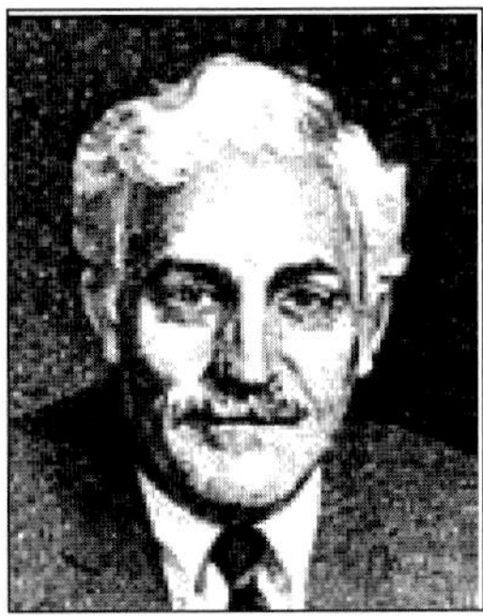

Fig. 4. Felix Bloch, Edward M. Purcell and Raymond Damadian

Magnetic Resonance Imaging

Felix Bloch, a Swiss physicist, found out in 1946 that the nuclei of different atoms absorb radio waves at different frequencies (Fig. 4). In 1952, Bloch and Purcell received the Nobel Prize for their discovery of what was referred to as Nuclear Magnetic Resonance. **Edward M. Purcell**, a American physicist, was also a historic figure in the development of physics in the twentieth century and made independently to Bloch in 1946 the discovery of Nuclear Magnetic Resonance. Raymond Damadian an American medical doctor and research scientist found out in 1970 that the structure and abundance of water in the human body was the key to magnetic resonance imaging. A patent was granted in 1974, it was the world's first patent issued in the field of MRI. By 1977, Dr. Damadian completed construction of the first whole-body MRI scanner, which he dubbed the "Indomitable."

Waiting for better computers

In 1943, the Moore School of Electrical Engineering at the University of Pennsylvania was contracted to construct the Electronic Numerical Integrator and Computer (ENIAC) (Fig. 5), the first electronic computer with design specifications to calculate 5,000 operations per second.

The following citation helps to understand the humble expectations of the time: "Where a calculator on the ENIAC is equipped with 18,000 vacuum tubes and weighs 30 tons, computers in the future may have only 1,000 vacuum tubes and perhaps weigh 1.5 tons." (Unknown, Popular Mechanics, March 1949).

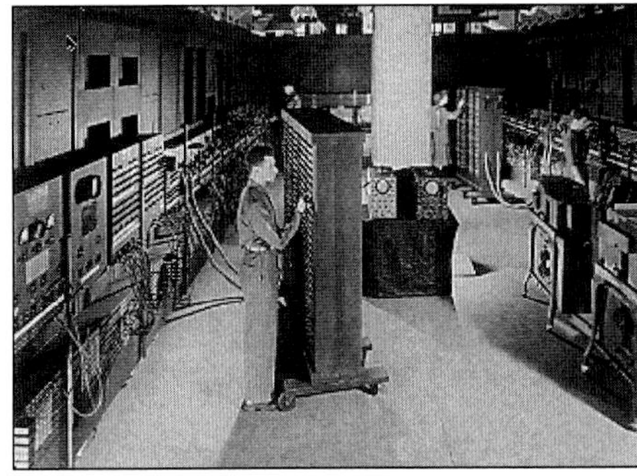

Fig. 5. The Electronic Numerical Integrator and Computer (ENIAC)

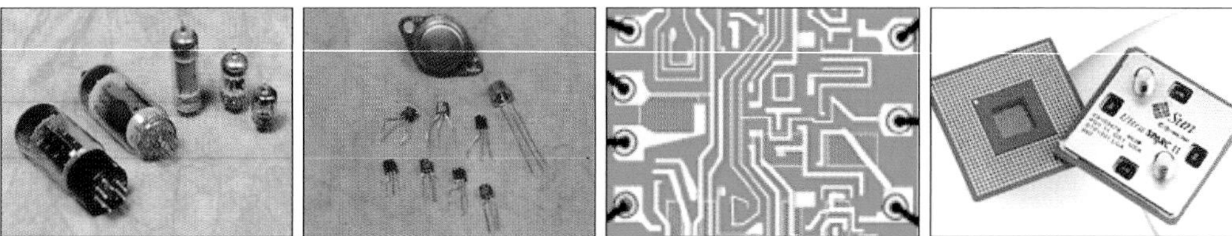

Fig. 6. Four generations of computers: Vacuum tubes, transistors, integrated circuits, microprocessors

The development of computer technology, from after World War II till today, is commonly described in terms of ''generations''. First generation computers (1946–1958) used **vacuum tubes** for circuitry (Fig. 6). They were huge, slow, expensive, and often undependable. In second generation computers (1959–1964), vacuum tubes were replaced by the faster, smaller and more reliable **transistors**. In third generation computers (1965–1970), huge numbers of transistors were packed onto single wafers of silicon, referred to as semiconductor chips or **integrated circuits**. Since the invention of integrated circuits, the number of transistors that can be placed on a single chip has doubled every two years, shrinking both the size and cost of computers even further and further enhancing its power.

What really triggered the tremendous growth of computers and its significant impact on our lives is the invention of **microprocessors** in fourth generation computers (1971–Today), where thousands of integrated circuits were built onto a single silicon chip. Fifth generation computing devices are still in development and will probably use superconductors and/or nanotechnology to make artificial intelligence a reality.

Components of digital radiology

To understand the development of digital radiology during the last three decades, a short description/definition from today's point of view is necessary:

''Digital radiology is a global system comprising and dependant of:

- Hospital Information System (HIS)
- Radiology Information System (RIS)
- Picture Archiving and Communication System (PACS)
- Digital Networking
- Digital Archiving
- Digital Reporting
- Digital Communication & Interfaces
- Digital Modalities

with the physician acting as an interface to the patient.''

Today, ''digital radiology'' is reality and has affected the whole range of diagnostic and therapeutic procedures. The short but eventful past of digital radiology can be declared as history, a history which forces us to learn from the past and allows us to make considerations about the future, briefly it is a view to the past of the future.

First steps of digital radiology

Some of the earliest applications of computers in radiology focused on administrative functions such as patient registration and billing. This focus led to the development of the first Radiology Information Systems (RIS) in various academic centers around the world during the 1970s. In parallel, some hospitals started with the implementation of the first commercial Hospital Information System (HIS).

The first modalities/disciplines, which used computers for imaging and/or generated digital images, were ultrasound, nuclear imaging and digital subtraction angiography (DSA). These were followed by computed tomography (CT) in the 1970s and magnetic resonance imaging (MRI) in the 1980s. At this time, most images in radiology were still analogical and those that were inherently digital – like CT and MRI – were available in analogical versions only, either as printouts or as second-capture images i.e. as frame-grabbed copies taken from the monitor.

The first theoretical concepts of digital radiology were developed and described by various researchers. Dr. T. Iinuma described some first considerations in 1974 in his article ''Image processing in clinical medicine – considerations of a system''. Also in the early 1970s, Dr. P. Capp introduced the term ''digital radiology'' and Professor Heinz U. Lemke, of the Technical University of Berlin, described concepts of digital image communication and display.

The first concepts of digital radiology concentrated on visions of picture archiving and communication systems (PACS). The idea of the PACS was roughly: (i)

Table 1. Overview of the first PACS conferences

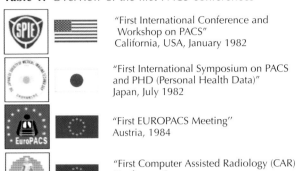

Conference
"First International Conference and Workshop on PACS" California, USA, January 1982
"First International Symposium on PACS and PHD (Personal Health Data)" Japan, July 1982
"First EUROPACS Meeting" Austria, 1984
"First Computer Assisted Radiology (CAR) Conference" Germany, June 1985

to transmit images from modalities to a digital archive and (ii) to allow communication of images from the archive to workstations in the hospital. However, lack of technological development to support the necessities of digital radiology, did not allow the concept to become popular until the 1980s.

First PACS conferences

In 1982, pioneers like Ronald Arenson, A.J. Duerinckx, Samual Dwyer III, H.K. Huang, Gerald Q. Maguire Jr. and M.P. Zeleznik, invited to the first "International Conference and Workshop on Picture Archiving and Communication Systems" in Newport Beach, California (Table 1). This meeting was sponsored by SPIE (the International Society for Optical Engineering), was later combined with the Medical Imaging Conference and became an annual event.

Also in 1982, the "First International Symposium on PACS and PHD (personal Health Data)" was held in Japan. This meeting was sponsored by the Japan Association of Medical Imaging Technology (JAMIT), was later combined with the Medical Imaging Technology meetings and became also an annual event.

In Europe, the EuroPACS society had its first annual meeting in 1984 and the „First Computer Assisted Radiology (CAR) Conference" was held in 1985. These European events later closely coordinated their activities and have since then been a driving force in European PACS development.

Early PACS approaches

Among the earliest research projects related to PACS were approaches in the U.S.A sponsored by the U.S. Army (Table 2). A teleradiology-project was initiated in 1983 and led to the installation of a Digital Imaging Network and Picture Archiving and Communication System (DIN/PCS) at two university sites in 1985, with contribution of Philips Medical Systems and AT&T. These sites were the University of Washington in Seattle, and the Georgetown University/George Washington University Consortium in Washington, D.C. Also in 1985 a project named "Multiple Viewing Stations for Diagnostic Radiology" was initiated at the UCLA.

In Europe, different approaches were initiated more or less independently (Table 3). In **Great Britain**,

Table 2. Overview of early PACS approaches in the United States

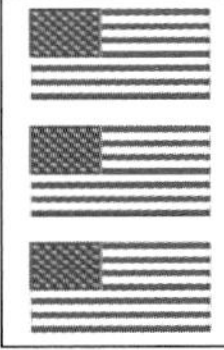

1983 Tele-radiology project sponsored by the U.S. Army
1985 DIN/PCS at the University of Washington in Seattle & Georgetown University in Washington D.C.
1985 PACS-related research project at UCLA, Multiple Viewing Stations for Diagnostic Radiology

Table 3. Overview of early PACS approaches in Europe

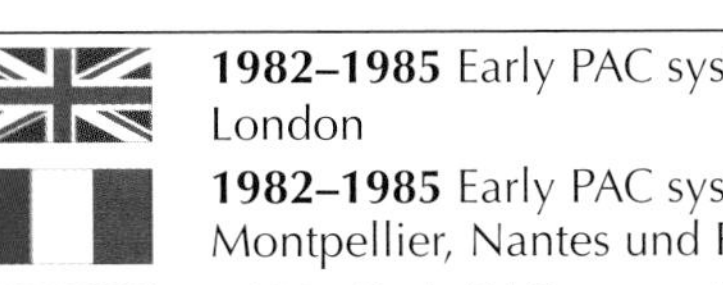

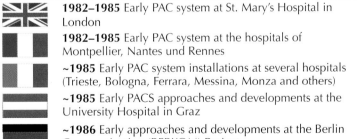

1982–1985 Early PAC system at St. Mary's Hospital in London
1982–1985 Early PAC system at the hospitals of Montpellier, Nantes und Rennes
~1985 Early PAC system installations at several hospitals (Trieste, Bologna, Ferrara, Messina, Monza and others)
~1985 Early PACS approaches and developments at the University Hospital in Graz
~1986 Early approaches and developments at the Berlin Communication (BERKOM) Project
~1986 Start of multivendor PACS approach at University Hospital of Brussels together with PRIMIS

at St. Mary's Hospital in London, plans to implement digital radiology were followed by a request for funding in 1982 and the initiation of a feasibility study in 1983. It became clear throughout 1985 that vendors were unable to supply the required technology and that it was impossible to continue with the project, at this time. All these preparations facilitated the later planning and implementation of digital radiology at Hammersmith Hospital in the mid 1990s.

In **France**, early PACS approaches – also in the early 1980s – were reported from independent sites. The Hôpital Lapeyronie in Montpellier was on of the first PACS sites by Siemens Medical. The Hospital of Nantes and the University Hospital of Rennes also started with small–scale PAC systems. All these attempts did not really achieve their set goals.

In **Italy**, AT&T and Philips installed their CommView PAC system at several hospitals in the mid 1980s. One of the larger of these installations was at the University Hospital of Trieste. Somewhat later, pioneering research activities started at the University of Florence on the use and validation of teleradiology.

In **Austria**, the first PACS project was initiated at 1985 as a cooperation of the Department of Radiology in Graz with Siemens Medical Systems. Many basic concepts of PACS have been developed, implemented and tested in clinical routine at this site. The availability of these concepts prepared the way for the later installation (in 1992) of the first filmless radiology department in the Danube Hospital (also known as SMZO) in Vienna.

In **Germany**, the Berlin Communication Project (BERKOM), initiated in 1986, served as a test bed for future development of broadband networking, radiological workstations and applications. Other early PACS approaches were reported from the University of Hamburg, the University of Berlin, and the Rudolf Virchow University Hospital.

In **Belgium**, the University Hospital of Brussels (ULB) together with the Pluridisciplanary Research Institute for Medical Imaging Science (PRIMIS) at the University of Brussels started a multi-vendor installation PACS project and concentrated very early on workflow and dataflow issues.

First commercial PACS installations

Many of the early PACS approaches started more or less as demonstration projects in academic institutions. Most were initiated in radiology departments in close cooperation with biomedical engineering or informatics laboratories at universities. All early PACS installations began to explore the digital vision of radiology from different points of view and facilitated the development of commercial systems. However, hardware limitations like the speed and capacity of disk drives, standard network protocols, and the limited resolution and contrast of electronic displays were very real barriers to clinical operations at this time. Another long-term barrier of these academic approaches was that they were mostly independent in-house developments and thus one-of-a-kind systems.

The progressive substitution of secondary-capture with first-capture digital images, which could be received directly from digital modalities, increased the clinical and organizational value of PACS installations. The increasing theoretical value for customers and the rather optimistic publications from early PACS installations, forced the industry to develop first commercial solutions. At the beginning of the 1990ies, only Siemens Medical Systems and AT&T/Philips Medical Systems had developed their first commercial PACS-software and shared a great deal of the market. The rest of the PACS approaches had multi-vendor system concepts as a basis or were still home grown.

Bauman, Gell and Dwyer give us the best worldwide overview of the first large PACS installations in the first half of the 1990ies. In a survey (actually it was their second), published in 1996, they identified the 23 first "large" commercial PACS installations (Table 4).

Most of these first large scale installations were initiated earlier and many of them were facilitated by other earlier successful or even unsuccessful approaches. Like with PACS conferences the centers of development were in Western Europe, in North America (mainly U.S.A) and in Eastern Asia (mainly Japan). The probably first PACS with could be given the predicate filmless hospital, was the installation in the 1992 newly built Danube Hospital in Vienna.

Only two years after their second world-wide survey, a third large-scale follow-up survey of Roger Baumann and Gunther Gell shows the speed with which PACS technology spread till 1998 (Fig. 7). The most striking response of this survey was that 97% of the users would at that time recommend PACS to others.

According to the initiative Integrating the Healthcare Enterprise (IHE), by the year 2002 over 50 companies with PACS offerings were active in a fast growing market. It is quite difficult – if not impossible – to say how many PACS installations there exist today. If somebody would start a survey now, the numbers would probably be outdated before it gets published. Apart from that, a survey would only be reasonable today, if global definitions were used to

Table 4. Overview of the first large PACS installations (Source: Bauman, Gell & Dwyer)

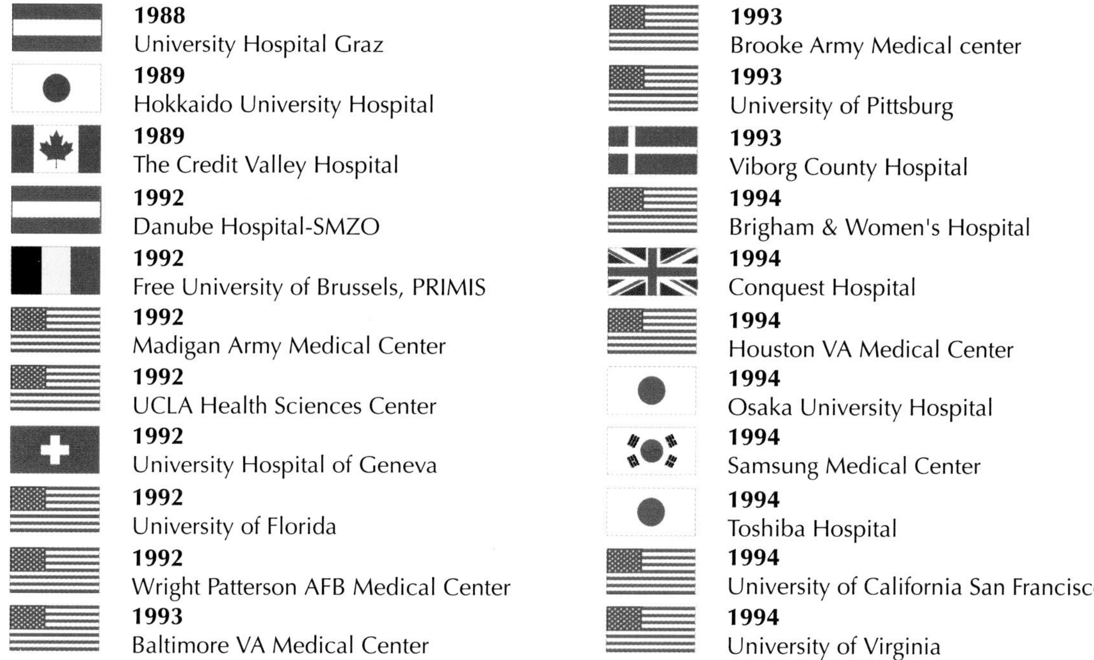

Year	Installation
1988	University Hospital Graz
1989	Hokkaido University Hospital
1989	The Credit Valley Hospital
1992	Danube Hospital-SMZO
1992	Free University of Brussels, PRIMIS
1992	Madigan Army Medical Center
1992	UCLA Health Sciences Center
1992	University Hospital of Geneva
1992	University of Florida
1992	Wright Patterson AFB Medical Center
1993	Baltimore VA Medical Center
1993	Brooke Army Medical center
1993	University of Pittsburg
1993	Viborg County Hospital
1994	Brigham & Women's Hospital
1994	Conquest Hospital
1994	Houston VA Medical Center
1994	Osaka University Hospital
1994	Samsung Medical Center
1994	Toshiba Hospital
1994	University of California San Francisco
1994	University of Virginia

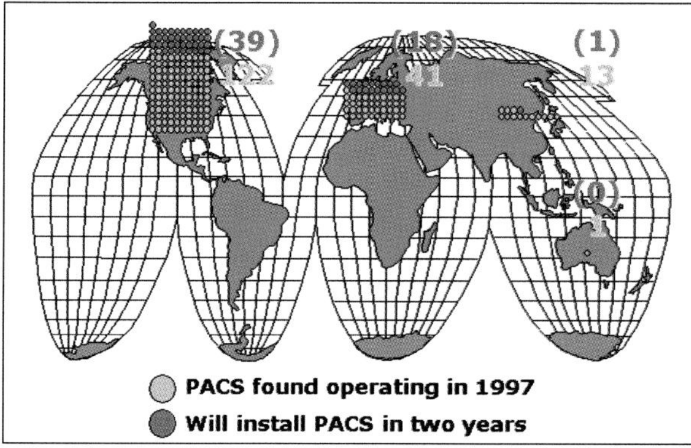

Fig. 7. Overview of PACS installations in 1997 (Source: Bauman & Gell)

answer simple questions like "what counts as a PACS installation".

Milestones that saved digital radiology

Several technological obstacles since the 1980ies had to be overcome in order to make digital radiology practicable, effective and affordable. Development of technology had to catch up with the theoretically existent concepts of digital radiology. The most significant of these milestones can be grouped into three categories: Standards, Technology and Integration.

Standards: The DICOM standard

Leaving out technological factors, the lack of standards was definitely the greatest challenge in early PACS approaches and in many cases also the main reason for failure. Data and image communication between acquisition modalities of different manufacturers was initially almost impossible, because of the heterogeneous image formats and communication standards.

In 1982, the American College of Radiology (ACR) and the National Electrical Manufacturers Association (NEMA) created a committee, which published its first standard in 1985. This standard defined an image file format and a point-to-point communication protocol. A revised version of the standard, known as ACR-NEMA 2.0, was published in 1988. Further changes became necessary, because of the fast developments in network technology and the need to support the respective standards and protocols. The new version of the standard was called the Digital Image Communication in Medicine (DICOM) Standard 3.0. It was presented at the Radiological Society of North America (RSNA) annual meetings in 1992 & 1993 and was voted and passed by members of NEMA in late 1993. The DICOM Standard continues to evolve as new technologies, e.g. imaging modalities, image compression, are being developed.

From today's point of view, it can be said that the DICOM Standard saved digital radiology from a

Babylonian catastrophe. Although many manufacturers still do not maintain strict DICOM representations in their systems internal databases, they all must provide a "conformance statement" that describes how DICOM has been implemented for external communication and what services are supported.

Standards: The HL7 standard

Digital radiology does not only exist and apply in the radiology department but in the whole hospital. Patient demographics, information such as admission, discharge and transfer (ADT) and examination requests are typical examples of inbound communication to a radiology department (and RIS-PACS). Radiological images, reports and billing information are typical examples of outbound communication from radiology (and RIS-PACS).

Founded by healthcare providers, the HL7 Working Group has met approximately every 3–4 months since March 1987 to develop and review the HL7 Interface Standard. The mission of the HL7 Working Group was and is to: "To provide standards for the exchange, management and integration of data that support clinical patient care and the management, delivery and evaluation of healthcare services. Specifically, to create flexible, cost effective approaches, standards, guidelines, methodologies, and related services for interoperability between healthcare information systems." Health Level Seven (HL7) was accredited as a Standards Developing Organization by the American National Standards Institute (ANSI) in 1994, all versions after that were considered international standards.

Similar to DICOM within the radiology department, HL7 was a significant milestone for intra-hospital communication of IT-systems and thus also for digital radiology.

Technology: The imaging plate

Fuji Film made a substantial contribution to progress in digital radiology by introducing its imaging plate, a giant leap in increasing the possibilities for X-ray imaging (Fig. 8).

Announced in 1981, this computerized X-ray system created a medical sensation. The Fuji Computed Radiography (FCR) records the X-ray image on a highly sensitive imaging plate carrying photostimulable phosphor; the image is then read by laser, processed by computer, and reconstructed with enhanced diagnostic information. Using this imaging plate, the radiation dosage for the patient was drastically reduced, while the digitized images were finally available for digital archiving and communication. Digital radiography separates the acquisition medium and the viewing medium and permits different image representations by insertion of computerized processes (pre-processing, post processing) between the actual radiograph at the acquisition medium and the radiograph represented on a hardcopy or a monitor.

Technology: The flat panel detector

About 1990, researchers recognized that the development of a flat panel X-ray detector would be a foremost technological breakthrough in radiological imaging, since it has the potential of direct digital imaging with no need of additional read- out devices (Fig. 9). The development and production of arrays of X-ray detector elements on a two-dimensional surface soon began and was facilitated because of the similarities with the production of arrays of thin film transistors (TFT's) in liquid-crystal display (LCD) screens. A paper presented at the 1995 Radiological Society of North America meeting reported a selenium-based direct-conversion flat panel X-ray detector for static images and attracted

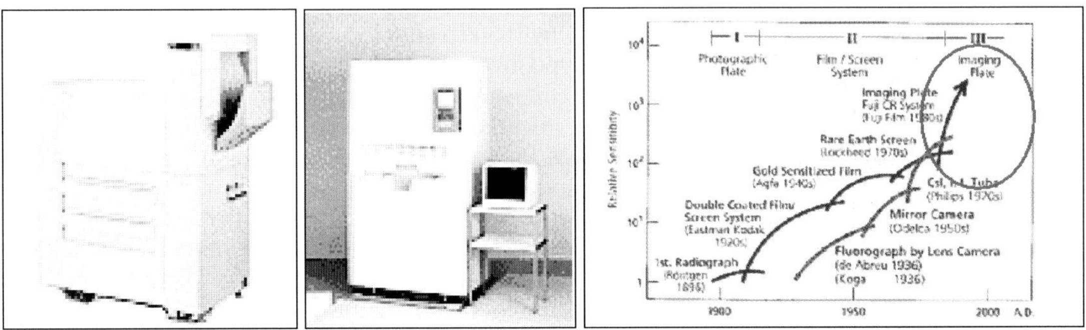

Fig. 8. Fuji Computed Radiography systems; graph of higher relative sensitivity

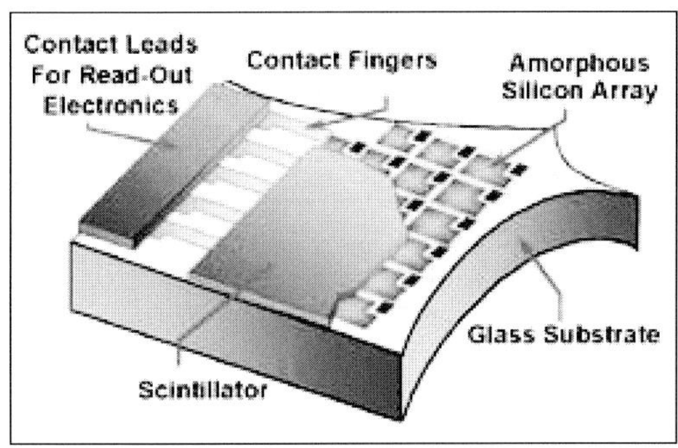

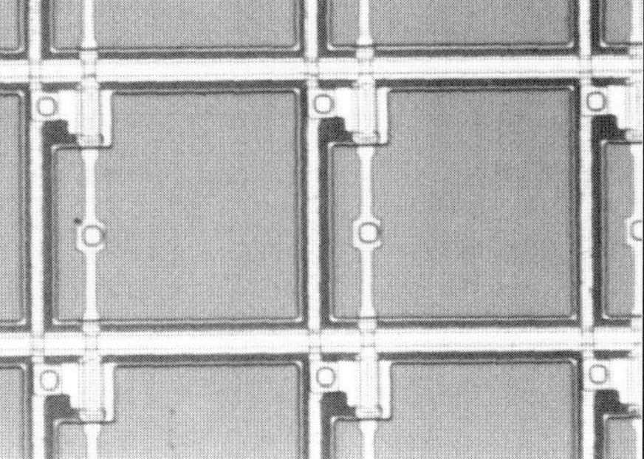

Fig. 9. Structure of a digital flat panel detector and thin film transistors (TFTs)

a great deal of attention. In 1997, the development of an indirect-conversion flat panel X-ray detector for static images was reported.

The development of flat panel detectors closed the digital gap in chest and skeletal radiology. Today, flat panel detectors seem to be a very promising technology for high-quality digital radiography. They offer most advantages of storage phosphor radiography and seem to have advantages in handling and image quality. Since the readout mechanism is integrated in the detector, there is no need for cassette handling and the time to obtain a first readout is much shorter than with storage phosphor radiography, which contributes to reduced examination times and increased productivity.

Technology: The monochrome monitors

The first letter in the acronym PACS stands for "Picture" and the obvious actions someone can perform with pictures is display and viewing. Since pictures in radiology are mostly black and white, special monochrome monitors are needed for display and viewing.

High quality monochrome monitors still contribute only a small segment to the whole computer display market (Fig. 10). If the industry had not developed high quality monochrome CRT monitors (with acceptable luminance range, contrast, contrast sensitivity and spatial resolution), then digital radiology as known today, would not have been possible. Today, high quality flat panel monochrome monitors – with high contrast and brightness and a resolution of up to 5 MegaPixels – allow for significantly reduced space and weight requirements, combined with reduced power consumption and longer display life.

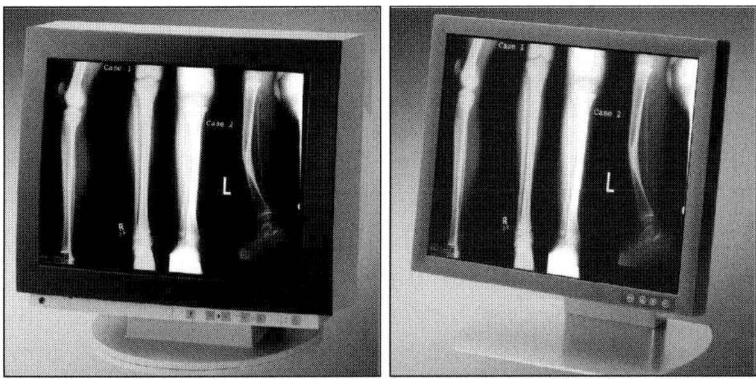

Fig. 10. Modern monochrome CRT and flat panel monitor

Technology: The archive media

The second letter in the acronym PACS stands for "Archiving" and the usual components needed for this task are digital archives and archive media. Archives for digital radiology must be able to handle large amounts of data (Table 5). The amount of data depends roughly of the average number of studies, the average number of images per study and the average size of one image. The size of an image depends further on of the spatial resolution and the pixel depth (i.e. contrast sensitivity and dynamic

Table 5. Capacity of various types of secondary storage

Device	Capacity
CR–RW	640 MB
DVD	15 GB
Magneto-Optical	2.6–5.6 GB
DVD	4.7–17 GB
DLT	35 GB
AIT 1	25 GB
AIT 2	50 GB
AIT 3	100 GB

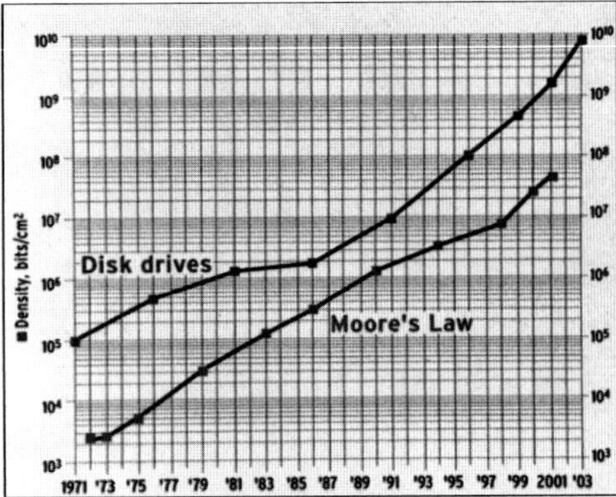

Fig. 11. Moore's Law for bit density on transistors vs. disk drives

range). Since newer imaging modalities produce examinations with both more data per image and/or more images per study, the amount of data for one study often approaches or surpasses 50 megabytes.

A remarkable aspect of computer technology has been the increase in computer speed and the reduction in the cost of memory. According to a widely quoted version of Moore's Law (Gordon Moore, Intel, 1965), "the number of transistors per square inch on integrated circuits doubles every eighteen months" (Fig. 11). Today, the bit density of disk drives is growing even faster than the transistor population of microprocessor chips. A similar growth seems to apply also for other types of secondary storage (CD-R, DVD, Optical Disks, Tape Storage and so on) and also contributed to the success of digital radiology.

Technology: The network

The third letter in the acronym PACS stands for "Communication" and the usual component needed is a digital network. The second most widely acknowledged law in IT is Metcalfe's Law, propounded originally by Robert Metcalfe, the inventor of Ethernet in 1973. Metcalfe's Law states that the usefulness, or utility, of a network equals the square of the number of nodes or users connected to it.

The use of a standardized network technology was a prerequisite for digital image communication (Table 6). The need for high network speed and archive capacity has escorted digital radiology from its beginnings till today. Due to the restrictions of then-existing technologies, proposing attempts were made in the early 1990s to develop specialized network technologies for medical image communication, but the market of medical imaging is too small to set standards in the field of networking.

Table 6. Common communication technology and the need for speed

Communication technology	max. bandwidth	approx. real time to transfer 50 MB
ISDN	128 Kbps	1–2.1 hrs
ADSL (average)	460 Kbps	18–36 min
Ethernet	10 Mbps	50–100 sec
Fast Ethernet	100 Mbps	5–10 sec
ATM	155 Mbps	3–6 sec
Gigabit Ethernet	1 Gbps	0. 5–1 sec

Considering that the amount of data in digital radiology is increasing, limitations in network capacity and archive capacity were always and are still potential bottlenecks. Today, Ethernet is the world's most pervasive networking technology; the remaining network connections are a combination of Token Ring, Fiber Distributed Data Interface (FDDI), Asynchronous Transfer Mode (ATM) and other protocols. Gigabit Ethernet is the latest version of Ethernet and offers 1000 Mbps (1 Gbps) raw bandwidth.

Integration: Integrating the Healthcare Enterprise

In the 1990ies, the lack of consensus by various HIS, RIS, PACS and modality vendors on how to use the existing standards, notably DICOM and HL7, has threatened the integration between these information systems. The integration between these systems was, of course, a prerequisite for the establishment of an efficient routine digital radiology workflow.

Integrating the Healthcare Enterprise (IHE, http://www.vsna.org/IHE) is an initiative undertaken by medical specialists and other care providers, administrators, information technology professionals and industry to improve the way computer systems in healthcare share information. The IHE initiative began in 1998 as a joint effort of the Radiological Society of North America (RSNA) and the Healthcare Information and Management Systems Society (HIMSS), with the goal to promote the coordinated use of established communications standards such as DICOM and HL7 and to address specific clinical needs in support of optimal patient care. The first demonstration was held at the RSNA annual meeting in 1999 and again at the 2000 annual meeting of HIMSS. Since then, system vendors have rapidly become strong supporters of the IHE effort and come together each year to demonstrate the way in which actual products could support this next level of integration. By the year 2002 over 50 companies with PACS offerings relating to the IHE integration profiles were active in a fast growing market.

Today, the focus moves from technological issues to workflow, progress understanding and organizational change. Technology requirements begin to be a non-issue since transmission bandwidth, archive size and processing speed begin to be more than enough for whatever applications are to come. Improving the delivery of healthcare both in a quantitative and qualitative sense will depend on the continuous improvement in the management of digital information not only within but also among healthcare institutions. The evolution of web technology holds great promise for the future of digital radiology, tele-radiology and worldwide knowledge transfer; it will also be a great challenge regarding standardization and integration.

Conclusion

During the last decades, many scientists, physicists, researchers, hardware and software engineers and, last but not least, many radiologists have contributed to the digital (r)evolution in radiology. In that period of time, technical developments related to all components of digital radiology (e.g. Picture Archiving and Communication System, Radiology Information System, Hospital Information System, digital modalities, digital networks) have evolved and matured in different ways and with varying success. As usual for evolution, only the most successful survived and their standardized applications are reflected in many thousands of installations all over the world. Today, it is considered as proven that digital radiology is an excellently functioning clinical tool, which improves radiological services for both the patient and the clinician.

Digital radiology today is the result of the convergence of technologic and financial factors. Furthermore, digital radiology opened Pandora's box in clinical information technology, because the needs of radiology were so enormous and demanding in terms of storage and speed that other applications and information systems were easily accommodated.

References

[1] Andriole KP (1999) Anatomy of picture archiving and communications systems: nuts and bolts – image acquisition: getting digital images from imaging modalities. J Digit Imaging 122: 216–217

[2] Andriole KP (1999) Computed radiography overview. In: Seibert JA, Filipow LJ, Andriole KP (eds) Practical digital imaging and PACS, Vol. 25, Medical Physics Monograph. Medical Physics Publishing, Rohnert Park, CA

[3] Andriole KP (1999) Computer and digital radiography. In: Hangiandreou NJ, Young JWR, Morin RL (eds) Electronic radiology practice – Technical and practical. Oakbrook

[4] Arenson RL, Andriole KP, Avrin DE, Gould RG (2000) Computers in imaging and health care: now and in the future. J Digit Imaging 13: 145–156

[5] Asahina H: Selenium-based flat panel x-ray detector or digital fluoroscopy and radiography, found at http://www.toshiba-europe.com/medical/Materials/Visions/Asahina.pdf

[6] Bauman RA, Taaffe JL (1991) Evolution of picture archiving and communication systems – 1989. J Digit Imaging 4: 37–42

[7] Baumann RA, Gell G, Dwyer SJ III (1996) Large picture archiving and communication systems of the world – Part 1. J Digit Imaging 9: 99–103

[8] Baumann RA, Gell G, Dwyer SJ III (1996) Large picture archiving and communication systems of the world – Part 2. J Digit Imaging 9: 172–177

[9] Bauman RA, Gell G (2000) The reality of picture archiving and communication systems (PACS): A survey. J Digit Imaging 13: 157–169

[10] Boland GWL (1999) Teleradiology: Another revolution in radiology? Clin Radiol 52: 547–553

[11] Bryan S, et al (1999) The benefits of hospital-wide picture archiving and communication systems: a survey of clinical users of radiology services. BMJ 72

[12] Channin DS (2001) Integrating the Healthcare Enterprise: A Primer – Part 2. Seven Brides for Seven Brothers: The IHE Integration Profiles. Radiographics 21: 1343–1350

[13] Channin DS, Parisot C, Wanchoo V, Leontiev A, Siegel EL (2001) Integrating the Healthcare Enterprise: A primer – Part 3. What Does IHE Do for ME? Radiographics 21: 1351–1358

[14] Dreyer KJ, Mehta A, Thrall JH (eds) (2002) PACS: A guide to the digital revolution. Springer, New York

[15] Filipow LJ, Phil D (1999) Picture archiving and communications systems – an overview: In: Seibert JA, Filipow LJ, Andriole KP (eds) Practical digital imaging and PACS, Vol. 25, Medical Physics Monograph. Medical Physics Publishing, Rohnert Park

[16] Foord K (2000) A powerful tool in advancing healthcare – picture archiving and communication system, The World Medical Association, Business Briefing - Global Healthcare 2000: http://www.wma.net/e/publications/pdf/2000/foord.pdf

[17] Health level Seven (2000) Application protocol of electronic data exchange in healthcare environments, Version 2.4, HL7

[18] Health level Seven: HL7 official homepage, found at: http://www.hl7.org

[19] Hruby W, Mosser H, Urban M, Rüger W (1992) The Vienna SMZO-PACS project: the totally digital hospital. Eur J Radiol 16: 66
[20] Hruby W, Maltsidis A (2000) A view to the past of the future – a decade of digital (r)evolution at the Danube hospital. In: Hruby W (ed) Digital (R)evolution in radiology. Springer, Vienna
[21] Hruby W (ed) (2000) Digital (R)evolution in radiology. Springer, Vienna
[22] Huang HK, Andriole K, Bazzill T, Lou SL, Wong AW, Arenson RL (1996) Design and implementation of a picture archiving and communication system: the second time. J Digit Imaging 9: 47–59
[23] Huang HK (1999) PACS – Basic principles and applications. John Wiley & Sons, New York
[24] Huang HK (2002) Medical Image Management in Healthcare Enterprise, The World Medical Association, Business Briefing – Global Healthcare http://www.wma.net/e/publications/pdf/2002/huang.pdf
[25] Inchingolo P (2000) Picture Archiving and Communications Systems in Today's Healthcare, The World Medical Association, Business Briefing – Global Healthcare: http://www.wma.net/e/publications/pdf/2000/inchingolo.pdf
[26] Kotter E, Langer M (1998) Integrating HIS-RIS-PACS: the Freiburg experience. Eur Radiol 8: 1707–1718
[27] Kotter E, Langer M (2002) Digital radiography with large-area flat-panel detectors. Eur Radiol 12: 2562–2570
[28] Lee DL, Cheung LK, Jeromin L (1995) A new digital detector for projection radiography. SPIE 2432: 237
[29] Lehrer S: Explorers of the body, found at http://stevenlehrer.com/explorers/
[30] Lemke HU (1979) A Network of Medical Work Stations for Integrated Word and Picture Communication in Clinical Medicine, Technical Report, Technical University Berlin
[31] Lemke HU (1991) The Berlin Communication System (BERKOM), Picture Archiving and Communication Systems (PACS) in Medicine, H.K. Huang, Series F Computer and Systems Science Vol. 74, Springer, New York
[32] Lemke HU (1992) European picture archiving and communication systems projects, Editorial Review. Curr Opin Radiol 4
[33] Lemke HU, et al (2000) Medical imaging 2000: Early developments of PACS in Europe. Proceedings of SPIE. 2000: 3980
[34] McGehee HA (1976) Adventures in medical research. Johns Hopkins University Press, Baltimore
[35] National Electrical Manufacturers' Association (1996) Digital Imaging and Communication in Medicine (DICOM), NEMA, PS3.1–1996–3.13–1996
[36] O'Brien WD Jr.: Assessing the Risks for Modern Diagnostic Ultrasound Imaging, found at: http://www.brl.uiuc.edu/Projects/Bioeffects/Assessing.php
[37] Radiological Society of North America/Healthcare Information and Management Systems Society: IHE technical framework, year 3, version 4.6, RSNA, 2001
[38] Radiological Society of North America/Healthcare Information and Management Systems Society: IHE official homepage, found at: http://www.rsna.org/IHE
[39] Reiner BI, Siegel EL (2002) Technologists' productivity when using PACS: Comparison of film-based versus filmless radiography. AJR 179: 33–37
[40] Reiner BI, Siegel EL, Sidiqqui K (2003) Evolution of the digital revolution: a radiologist perspective. J Digit Imaging 16: 324–330
[41] Siegel EL, Channin DS (2001) Integrating the healthcare enterprise: A primer – Part 1. Introduction. Radiographics 21: 1339–1341
[42] Siegel EL, Reiner BI, Abiri M, et al (2000) The filmless radiology reading room: A survey of established picture archiving and communication system sites. J Digit Imaging 13: 22–23
[43] Talbott JH (1970) A biographical history of medicine. Grune & Stratton, New York
[44] Webb S (1988) In the beginning. In: Webb (ed) The physics of medical imaging. Adam Hilger, Bristol
[45] Woo J: A short History of the development of Ultrasound in Obstetrics and Gynecology, found at: http://www.ob-ultrasound.net/history.html

Medical image archives

M. W. Vannier[1,3], E. V. Staab[2,3], and L. C. Clarke[3]

[1]University of Chicago, Chicago, IL, USA
[2]Wake Forest University, Winston-Salem, NC, USA
[3]Cancer Imaging Program, National Cancer Institute, National Institutes of Health, Bethesda, MD, USA

Abstract

Most medical images are stored in databases, and creation, expansion, and integration of these archives has become central to advancement in many fields, including radiology, pathology, and dermatology. Image archives are important for clinical practice, education, and research in medicine. Clinical imaging modalities, such as digital radiography, computed tomography, ultrasonography, PET/SPECT, optical and magnetic resonance imaging produce large amounts of data that are managed, archived, and reported using picture archiving and communications systems (PACS) in an integrated healthcare enterprise (IHE) infrastructure.

However, typical PACS and IHE systems are closed to ensure privacy, security and confidentiality. These systems are organized to support image interpretation and viewing transactions, with limited capabilities for population-based research or integration of ancillary data. Sharing of clinical medical image databases is relatively uncommon, despite the widespread prevalence of open public archives for other types of biological data, especially in genomics and proteomics.

Current medical image archives are surveyed, and several applications are identified. The limitations of current systems are discussed, especially metadata creation and integration of heterogeneous data sources. Some of the most important future trends are delineated.

Key words: Archive, image database, repository, metadata.

1. Introduction

Public libraries of printed works have evolved into open access repositories of documents, images, and media, sometimes known as digital libraries [1–3]. New computer technologies for these open archives [4] have been developed, often using very large databases [5]. The basic biological sciences, especially molecular biology, have adopted open standards and data sharing for gene sequences and related data. Major peer-reviewed journals, such as Science [6] and Nature [7], enforce sharing of primary data by requiring authors to deposit their molecular sequence and related supporting data in a publicly accessible database prior to publication. Every January, the prominent peer-reviewed journal Nucleic Acids Research publishes a special issue on databases [8], and beginning in July 2003, this journal will devote a special issue to web-based software tools that use these databases [9].

Harold Varmus, a Nobel Prize winner and former director of the National Institutes of Health who now serves as President of the Memorial Sloan-Kettering Cancer Center in New York, observed that, "all modern biologists using genomic methods have become dependent on computer science to store, organize, search, manipulate and retrieve the new information. Thus biology has been revolutionized by genomic information and by the methods that permit useful access to it." [10]

Biomedical signal databases have been constructed for open access to the academic community [11]. Recently, the concept of shared results from medical research has expanded beyond sequence and signal information to include all forms of data that may be reused by other investigators. In February 2003, the National Institutes of Health announced its data sharing policy [12]. In keeping with these trends, several shared medical image archives are being developed, notably the National Cancer Institute's Lung Image Database Consortium (LIDC) [13], RSNA Medical Imaging Resource Center (MIRC) [14–17] and other image repositories that will be introduced in this paper.

2. Medical image access policy

Access to medical images stored in repositories is essential for investigators who do not possess the resources to collect data of their own, for standardized comparisons of image analysis methods tested with the same input data, for regulatory review of new medical devices, to develop new methods, and potentially for use in clinical decision support. Recently, new data sharing policies have been developed that govern access to medical data, including images. The creation of open archives for imaging research has been encouraged to open the field of imaging science to rapid advancement and reduce duplication of effort [18].

2.1 NIH data sharing policy

Data sharing promotes many goals of the National Institutes of Health's (NIH) research endeavor. It is particularly important for unique data that cannot be readily replicated. Data sharing allows scientists to expedite the translation of research results into knowledge, products, and procedures to improve human health. The NIH issued a statement on data sharing that expects and supports the timely release and sharing of final research data from NIH-supported studies for use by other researchers. Investigators submitting an NIH application are required to include a plan for data sharing or explain why data sharing is not possible. This statement applies to extramural scientists seeking grants, cooperative agreements, and contracts as well as intramural investigators [19]. A draft policy on data sharing has been developed by the U.K. Medical Research Council [12].

2.2 Background

There are many reasons to share data from research studies. Sharing data reinforces open scientific inquiry, encourages diversity of analysis and opinion, promotes new research, makes possible the testing of new or alternative hypotheses and methods of analysis, supports studies on data collection methods and measurement, facilitates the education of new researchers, enables the exploration of topics not envisioned by the initial investigators, and permits creation of new data sets when data from multiple sources are combined. By avoiding the duplication of expensive data collection activities, the NIH is able to support more investigators than it could if similar data had to be collected de novo by each applicant.

NIH-supported basic research, clinical studies, surveys, and other types of research produce data that may be shared. However, NIH recognizes that sharing data about human research subjects presents special challenges. The rights and privacy of people who participate in NIH-sponsored research must be protected at all times. Thus, data intended for broader use should be free of identifiers that would permit linkages to individual research participants and variables that could lead to deductive disclosure of individual subjects. Similarly, NIH recognizes the need to protect patentable and other proprietary data and the restriction on data sharing that may be imposed by agreements with third parties. It is not the intent of this statement to discourage, impede, or prohibit the development of commercial products from federally funded research.

There are many ways to share data. Sometimes data are included in publications. Investigators may distribute data under their own auspices. Some investigators have placed data sets in public archives while others have put data on a web site, building in protections for privacy through the software while allowing analysis of the data. Restricted access data centers or data enclaves facilitate analyses of data too sensitive to share through other means. All of these options achieve the goals of data sharing. A web-based image archive was developed at the NIH Center for Information Technology to support data sharing [20]. However, the NIH also recognizes that in some particular instances sharing data may not be feasible. For example, studies with very small samples or those collecting particularly sensitive data should be shared only if stringent safeguards exist to ensure confidentiality and protect the identity of subjects while recognizing the contribution of the investigators who designed the protocol and collected the data.

2.3 National Cancer Institute – Biomedical Imaging Program (BIP)

The National Cancer Institute (NCI) is the component of the NIH that investigates, develops and applies new methods for patients with cancer. The Biomedical Imaging Program (BIP) in the Division of Cancer Treatment and Diagnosis at NCI is the principal resource for oncologic imaging for the full range of applications from the molecular level to intact patient [21]. The NCI BIP funds the American College of Radiology Imaging Network (ACRIN) to conduct multicenter trials of cancer imaging [22, 23].

2.3.1 ACRIN image access policy

ACRIN archives the images collected in cancer clinical imaging trials under its protocols. For example, the Digital Mammographic Imaging Screening Trial - DMIST [24] will collect digital mammograms from almost 50,000 patients, and the National Lung Screening Trial – NLST performs low dose CT scans on a large population of asymptomatic older adult smokers. Both of these large screening trials place all data (including images) in an electronic archive [25]. ACRIN has developed a policy [26] under NCI guidance for sharing image data after completion of its clinical trials, by allowing access to qualified investigators who were not involved in recruiting subjects or performing examinations [27].

2.3.2 Lung Imaging Database Consortium (LIDC)

Preliminary clinical studies show that spiral CT scanning of the lungs can improve early detection of lung cancer in high-risk individuals. However, more clinical data are needed before public health recommendations can be made for population-based screening. Image processing algorithms have the potential to assist in lesion detection and characterization on spiral CT studies, and to assess the stability or change in lesion size on serial CT studies. The use of such computer-assisted algorithms could significantly enhance the sensitivity and specificity of spiral CT lung screening, as well as lower costs by reducing physician time needed for interpretation. The LIDC initiative [13] receives BIP support for a consortium of five institutions to develop consensus guidelines for a spiral CT lung image resource and to construct a database of spiral CT lung images. The investigators funded under this initiative will create a set of guidelines and metrics for database use and develop a database as a test-bed and showcase for those methods. The database will be available to researchers and users through the Internet and will have wide utility as a research resource [28].

2.3.3 BIP image archive study

The NCI BIP has studied image archives and tracked the technological progress in this field with the assistance of experts in a variety of fields. The results are summarized in reports and on the World Wide Web [29–32]. This work continues with open communications to all interested parties through a public listserver, archive-comm-l, moderated by the authors [33]. Comments on this paper and related matters are encouraged and may be entered in the listserver by sending e-mail to archive-comm-l@list.nih.gov.

3. Medical image archives

Many fields of science have created large databases of images, especially astronomy and geoscience [34] and astronomy [35–37]. These pioneering efforts in organizing and implementing shared database resources have developed technologies that are applicable in other domains, including medical imaging [38–40]. Open medical image archives have been created for teaching biomedical science [41,42], dermatology [43–47], anatomic pathology [48–51], and neuroscience [52–55]. Software has been developed to facilitate shared information resources for researchers, such as Axiope [56].

The applications of publicly available data sets include research, both basic and clinically applied, on the development, testing and standardization of algorithms and heuristics for computer assisted diagnosis, for example [18]. Data mining of clinical databases [57], especially those richly invested with images, may be beneficial in producing quantitative image-based metrics and biomarkers for disease presence, staging, treatment selection and planning, prognosis, and monitoring. The technical requirements for construction of publicly accessible medical image archives that are well suited to exploratory data analysis, synthesis and testing of diagnostic and prognostic quantitative image analysis methods, biomarker and surrogate endpoint testing, and computer aided diagnosis include

Table 1. Medical (and other) Image Databases described in this chapter

Title	Acronym	Reference(s)
Sloan Digital Sky Project	SDSS	[36, 39]
Biomedical Informatics Research Network	BIRN	[72–74]
National Digital Mammography Archive	NDMA	[68–71]
Grid-based standardized mammography database	eDiamond	[71]
Craniofacial image archive		[75]
Digital Mammographic Imaging Screening Trial	DMIST	[24, 76]
National Lung Screening Trial	NLST	[77]
Lung Image Database Consortium	LIDC	[13, 28]
Medical Image Research Center	MIRC	[14–17]
Dartmouth fMRI Data Center	fMRIdc	[78, 79]

access to images and the context in which they were obtained.

DICOM, the Digital Image Communications in Medicine, standards have been developed by the National Electrical Manufacturers Association in conjunction with industry and academia [58–60]. These standards are effective in assuring interoperability of image creation, display and storage systems used in a clinical environment. A further set of standards for the Integrated Healthcare Enterprise (IHE) aids the management of image workflow for entire organizations operating at a single or multiple facilities [61–66].

The organization of clinical image archives as DICOM-based entity-attribute-value repositories is effective for transaction-oriented applications, such as interpretation of radiology examinations. In research applications, however, definition of standardized metadata, use of relational database and data warehouse technology that can accommodate heterogeneous and evolving data while facilitating more general analyses is needed. A brief survey of biomedical image repositories is provided. Important issues in biomedical databases, including sharing, metadata, and future applications are discussed.

Interoperability of heterogeneous databases, including those that contain images, is achieved by one of three approaches: data warehousing, information linkage, and information integration [67]. These technologies are in development, with demonstration projects that involve medical images. For example, digital mammography is the basis of large multi-institutional projects in the USA as the National Digital Mammography Archive [68–70] and in the UK as eDiamond [71].

3.1 BIRN – Biomedical Imaging Research Network

The BIRN is an NIH National Center for Research Resources (NCRR) initiative aimed at creating a testbed to address biomedical researchers' need to access and analyze data at a variety of levels of aggregation located at diverse sites throughout the USA [72–74]. The BIRN testbed brings together hardware and develop software necessary for a scalable network of databases and computational resources. Issues of user authentication, data integrity, security, and data ownership are being addressed.

The testbed is focused on neuroimaging research to take advantage of the relatively advanced level of sophistication of this community in the use of information technology. An essential feature of the testbed is creation of infrastructure that can be deployed rapidly at other research centers throughout the country, including research emphases outside of neuroimaging. This means that in addition to scalability, the software/hardware must be reusable and extensible.

The BIRN testbed is based on the next generation internet, Internet2 [80–84], funded by the National Science Foundation. Many institutions have joined BIRN consortia on functional neuroimaging and neuromorphology, using information infrastructure in the context of ongoing neuroimaging research projects. Support for "system integrators" that coordinate network, grid, and data mining software development as well as hardware configurations has been included.

To contain the scope of the testbed, the BIRN initiative is initially focused on neuroimaging and is supporting several virtual neuroimaging research centers, each of which spans multiple leading academic and clinical institutions.

3.2 Craniofacial image archive

The Craniofacial Imaging Laboratory at the Cleft Palate and Craniofacial Deformities Institute, St. Louis Children's Hospital, Washington University Medical Center, has developed an electronic archive for the storage of computed tomography image digital data that is independent of scanner hardware and independent of units of storage media (i.e. floppy disks and optical disks) [75]. The archive represents one of the largest repositories of high-quality computed tomography data of children with craniofacial deformities in the world. Archiving reconstructed image data is essential for comparative imaging, surgical simulation, quantitative analysis, and use with solid model fabrication (e.g. stereolithography). One tertiary craniofacial center's experience in the establishment and maintenance of such an archive through three generations of storage technology is reported. The current archive is housed on an external 35-GB hard drive attached to a Windows-based desktop server. Data in the archive were categorized by specific demographics into groups of patients, number of scans, and diagnoses. The Craniofacial Imaging Laboratory archive currently contains computed tomography image digital data for 1827 individual scans. Storage of CT image data in a digital archive allows for continuous upgrading of image display and analysis software and facilitates longitudinal and cross-sectional studies. Internet access for clinical and research purposes is feasible, contingent on protection of patient confidentiality and investigator's rights or recognition.

3.3 Radiology teaching files and RSNA's MIRC

The importance of electronic images for teaching medicine and especially radiology has been enhanced by linkage to PACS [17] and the AFIP collection [51]. The Radiological Society of North America (RSNA) is developing a Medical Imaging Resource Center (MIRC). The goal is to develop a central repository for medical images, as well as related text, in support of projects related to research, education, and clinical care. PACS vendors should provide much more sophisticated tools to create and annotate teaching file images in an easy to use but standard format (possibly RSNA's MIRC format) that could be exchanged with other sites and other vendors' PAC systems. The privilege to create teaching or conference files should be given to the individual radiologists, technologists, and other users, and an audit should be kept of who has created these files, as well as keep track of who has accessed the files. Vendors should maintain a local PACS library of image quality phantoms, normal variants, and interesting cases and should have the capability of accessing central image repositories such as the RSNA's MIRC images.

4. Conclusion

Sharing medical image data on public repositories is expected to facilitate the development of image analysis tools and results. Several examples of new policy guidelines for electronic access to images from repositories were given to illustrate how these archives are organized and operated. Many more examples exist, and new medical image archive initiatives are announced each year. In time, we can measure the impact of this fundamental change in the culture of medical imaging research. Importantly, the current format standard for this data is DICOM [59,60] and electronic images may be useful for regulatory purposes in FDA review of new drugs and devices.

Images are ubiquitous in biomedicine, and their importance will continue to grow with better technology – new modalities and combinations of existing ones, advances in displays and computers, faster networks and increased storage capability. Images are readily appreciated by human observers, and they can readily be quantified, reproduced, analysed, validated, and archived. Images are an essential component of biological knowledge, with utility in many aspects of basic sciences, translation projects and clinical medicine.

References

[1] D-Lib Magazine: http://www.dlib.org/. Accessed 21 Apr 03
[2] Prey JC, Zia LL (2002) Progress on educational digital libraries: Current developments in the National Science Foundation's (NSF) national science, technology, engineering, and mathematics education digital library (NSDL) program. Digital Libraries: People, Knowledge, and Technology, Proceedings 2555: 53–66
[3] Hoffman E, Fox EA (2002) Building policy, building community: An example from the US National Science, Technology, Engineering, and Mathematics Education Library (NSDL). Digital Libraries: People, Knowledge, and Technology, Proceedings 2555: 299–300
[4] Open Archives Initiative. http://www.openarchives.org/. Accessed 21 Apr 03
[5] Very Large Data Base Endowment Inc. (VLDB): VLDB Journal. http://vldb.org/. Accessed 21 Apr 03
[6] (AAAS). (2003) Information for contributors. Science 299: 124–125
[7] Nature publication policies: 6. Materials and data availability. http://www.nature.com/nature/submit/policies/index.html#6. Accessed 21 April 2003
[8] (Anon) (2003) Editorial – Special issue on databases. Nucl Acids Res 31: i
[9] Baxevanis AD (2003) The molecular biology database collection: 2003 update. Nucl Acids Res 31: 1–12
[10] Varmus H (2002) Genetic empowerment: The importance of public databases. Nature Genetics 32: 3
[11] Cohen A, Korhonen I (eds) (2001) Biomedical signal databases, special issue. In: IEEE Engineering in Medicine and Biology Magazine 2–85
[12] UK Medical Research Council (MRC): Draft MRC statement on Data Sharing and Preservation policy. http://www.mrc.ac.uk/index/strategy-strategy/strategy-science_strategy/strategy-strategic_implementation/strategy-data_sharing/strategy-data_sharing_policy-link. Accessed 24 April 2003
[13] Clarke LP, Croft BY, Staab E, Baker H, Sullivan DC (2001) National Cancer Institute initiative: Lung image database resource for imaging research. Acad Radiol 8: 447–450
[14] RSNA Medical Imaging Resource Center (MIRC) http://mirc.rsna.org/ and http://rsna.org/mirc/. Accessed 21 Apr 03
[15] Siegel E, Channin D, Perry J, Carr C, Reiner B (2002) Medical Image Resource Center 2002: An update on the RSNA's Medical Image Resource Center. J Digit Imaging 15: 2–4
[16] Siegel E, Reiner B (2001) The Radiological Society of North America's Medical Image Resource Center: An update. J Digit Imaging 14: 77–79
[17] Siegel E, Reiner B (2001) Electronic teaching files: Seven-year experience using a commercial picture archiving and communication system. J Digit Imaging 14: 125–127
[18] Vannier M, Summers R (2003) Sharing images. Radiology (in press)

[19] National Institutes of Health: Final NIH statement on sharing research data. http://grants.nih.gov/grants/guide/notice-files/NOT-OD-03-032.html. Accessed 24 April 2003
[20] Suh EB, Warach S, Cheung H, et al (2002) A Web-based medical image archive system. In: Siegel E, Huang HK (eds) Medical imaging 2002: PACS and integrated medical information systems: design and evaluation. San Diego, CA, pp 31–41
[21] Sullivan DC (2002) The NCI Biomedical Imaging Program: Five-year progress report. Acad Radiol 9: 122–125
[22] Hillman BJ, Gatsonis C, Sullivan DC (1999) American College of Radiology Imaging Network: New national cooperative group for conducting clinical trials of medical imaging technologies. Radiology 213: 641–645
[23] Hillman BJ (2002) The American College of Radiology Imaging Network and the mission of radiologists. Radiology 223: 602
[24] ACRIN: Digital Mammographic Imaging Screening Trial. http://www.dmist.org. Accessed 21 April 2003
[25] Galen B, Staab E, Sullivan DC, Pisano ED (2002) Congressional update: Report from the Biomedical Imaging Program of the National Cancer Institute. American College of Radiology Imaging Network: The digital mammographic imaging screening trial–an update. Acad Radiol 9: 374–375
[26] ACRIN: Policy on requests for access to ACRIN archived images. http://www.acrin.org/archpolicy.html. Accessed 21 April 2003
[27] Hillman BJ (2002) Opportunities for research with the American College of Radiology Imaging Network (ACRIN) image database. Acad Radiol 9: 996–997
[28] Biomedical Imaging Program, National Cancer Institute. Lung Imaging Database Resource for Imaging Research. http://www3.cancer.gov/bip/steercom.htm. Accessed 23 April 2003
[29] Staab E, Clarke LP, Baker H, Sullivan D (2001) NCI image archive management workshop: A preliminary report. Acad Radiol 8: 690–691
[30] Image archive steering committee website: http://www3.cancer.gov/bip/steer_iasc.htm. Accessed 21 Apr 03.
[31] Vannier MW, Staab EV, Clarke LP (2003) Cancer imaging informatics workshop report from the Biomedical Imaging Program of the National Cancer Institute. Acad Radiol 10(7): 798–802
[32] Vannier MW, Staab E, Clarke LP (2002) Medical Image Archives – Present and future. In: Lemke HU, Vannier MW, Inamura K, Farman AG, Doi K, Reiber JHC (eds) CARS 2002 – Computer Assisted Radiology and Surgery. Springer, Paris, pp 565–576
[33] NCI-BIP: archive-comm-l listserver. http://list.nih.gov/archives/archive-comm-l.html. Accessed 21 Apr 03
[34] Staudigel H, Helly J, Koppers AAP, et al (2003) Electronic data publication in geochemistry. Geochemistry Geophysics Geosystems 4: 8004
[35] Szalay A, Gray J (2001) The world-wide telescope. Science 293: 2037–2040
[36] Szalay AS, Gray J, Thakar AR, et al (2002) The SDSS skyserver: Public access to the Sloan digital sky server data. In: Proceedings of the 2002 ACM SIGMOD International Conference on Management of Data. Madison, Wisconsin: ACM Press New York, NY, USA, 570–581
[37] The Digital Sky: http://www.cacr.caltech.edu/SDA/digital_sky.html. Accessed 21 Apr 03.
[38] Microsoft Research: Jim Gray web page. http://research.microsoft.com/~Gray/. Accessed 21 Apr 03
[39] Gray J, Szalay AS, Thakar AR, Stoughton C, vandenBerg J (2002) Online scientific data curation, publication, and archiving. In: Szalay AS (ed) Virtual observatories: Proceedings of the SPIE. pp 103–107
[40] Gray J, Szalay A (2002) The world-wide telescope. Communications of the ACM 45: 50–55
[41] University of Bristol: Bristol Biomedical Image Archive. http://www.brisbio.ac.uk/. Accessed 23 April 2003
[42] Gonzalez-Couto E, Hayes B, Danckaert A (2001) The life sciences Global Image Database (GID). Nucl Acids Res 29: 336–339
[43] Todorovski L, Ribaric S, Dimec J, Hudomalj E, Lunder T (1999) Organization and dissemination of multimedia medical databases on the WWW. Stud Health Technol Inform 68: 557–561
[44] Kaboli F (2003) Dermatology Image Atlas-Johns Hopkins University. http://dermatlas.med.jhmi.edu/derm. Occup Med (Lond) 53: 151–152
[45] Eysenbach G, Bauer J, Sager A, Bittorf A, Simon M, Diepgen T (1998) An international dermatological image atlas on the WWW: Practical use for undergraduate and continuing medical education, patient education and epidemiological research. Medinfo 9 Pt 2: 788–792
[46] Diepgen TL, Eysenbach G (1998) Digital images in dermatology and the Dermatology Online Atlas on the World Wide Web. J Dermatol 25: 782–787
[47] Bittorf A, Krejci-Papa NC, Diepgen TL (1995) Development of a dermatological image atlas with worldwide access for the continuing education of physicians. J Telemed Telecare 1: 45–53
[48] Division of Informatics: Department of Pathology. University of Pittsburgh Medical Center. Anatomic pathology informatics, imaging and the internet. http://apiii.upmc.edu/. Accessed 23 April 2003
[49] Sinard JH, Morrow JS (2001) Informatics and anatomic pathology: Meeting challenges and charting the future. Hum Pathol 32: 143–148
[50] Trelease RB (2002) Anatomical informatics: Millennial perspectives on a newer frontier. Anat Rec 269: 224–235
[51] Williams BH, Mullick FG, Becker RL, Kyte RT, Noe A (1998) A national treasure goes online: The Armed Forces Institute of Pathology. MD Comput 15: 260–265
[52] Shepherd GM (2002) Supporting databases for neuroscience research. J Neurosci 22: 1497
[53] Toga AW (2002) Neuroimage databases: The good, the bad and the ugly. Nat Rev Neurosci 3: 302–309

[54] Toga AW (2002) Imaging databases and neuroscience. Neuroscientist 8: 423–436
[55] Mazziotta J, Toga A, Evans A, et al (2001) A four-dimensional probabilistic atlas of the human brain. J Am Med Inform Assoc 8: 401–430
[56] School of Informatics, University of Edinburgh. AXIOPE. http://www.axiope.org/. Accessed 21 April 2003
[57] Cios KJ (ed) (2001) Medical data mining and knowledge discovery. Physica, New York
[58] Bidgood WD, Jr, Horii SC (1992) Introduction to the ACR-NEMA DICOM standard. Radiographics 12: 345–355
[59] DICOM website: http://medical.nema.org. Accessed 21 April 2003
[60] Mildenberger P, Eichelberg M, Martin E (2002) Introduction to the DICOM standard. Eur Radiol 12: 920–927
[61] Siegel EL, Channin DS (2001) Integrating the Healthcare Enterprise: a primer. Part 1. Introduction. Radiographics 21: 1339–1341
[62] Channin DS (2001) Integrating the Healthcare Enterprise: a primer. Part 2. Seven brides for seven brothers: the IHE integration profiles. Radiographics 21: 1343–1350
[63] Channin DS, Parisot C, Wanchoo V, Leontiev A, Siegel EL (2001) Integrating the Healthcare Enterprise: a primer: Part 3. What does IHE do for ME? Radiographics 21: 1351–1358
[64] Henderson M, Behlen FM, Parisot C, Siegel EL, Channin DS (2001) Integrating the healthcare enterprise: a primer. Part 4. The role of existing standards in IHE. Radiographics 21: 1597–1603
[65] Channin DS, Siegel EL, Carr C, Sensmeier J (2001) Integrating the healthcare enterprise: a primer. Part 5. The future of IHE. Radiographics 21: 1605–1608
[66] Channin DS (2002) Integrating the healthcare enterprise: a primer. Part 6: the fellowship of IHE: year 4 additions and extensions. Radiographics 22: 1555–1560
[67] Ben Miled Z, Li N, Kellett GM, Spies B, Bukhres O (2002) Complex life science multidatabase queries. Proceedings of the IEEE, 90
[68] Beckerman BG, Schnall MD (2002) Digital information management: A progress report on the National Digital Mammography Archive. In: Vo-Dinh T, Benaron DA, Grundfest WS (eds) Biomedical diagnostic, guidance, and surgical-assist systems IV, pp 98–108
[69] University of Pennsylvania: National Digital Mammography Archive. http://nscp01.physics.upenn.edu/ndma/. Accessed 24 April 2003
[70] Wu M, Zheng Y, North M, Pisano E (2002) NLM tele-educational application for radiologists to interpret mammography. Proc AMIA Symp, pp 909–913
[71] e-Diamond: Improving diagnostic confidence with a standardised mammography database. http://www.gridoutreach.org.uk/docs/pilots/ediamond.htm. Accessed 24 April 2003
[72] Biomedical Informatics Research Network (BIRN). http://www.nbirn.net/ and http://birn.ncrr.nih.gov/. Accessed 21 April 03
[73] Martone ME (2001) Biomedical Informatics Research Network to improve understanding of brain disorders. EnVision, pp 1–5
[74] Santini S, Gupta A (2003) Role of internet images in the Biomedical Informatics Research Network. In: Santini S, Schettini R (eds) Internet imaging IV. Proceedings of the SPIE. SPIE, pp 99–110
[75] Perlyn CA, Marsh JL, Vannier MW, et al (2001) The craniofacial anomalies archive at St. Louis Children's Hospital: 20 years of craniofacial imaging experience. Plast Reconstr Surg 108: 1862–1870
[76] Welsh CR, Young B, Gopalakrishnan V, et al (2002) ACRIN digital mammographic imaging screening trial informatics infrastructure. In: Lemke HU, W. VM, Inamura K, Farman AG, Doi K, Reiber JHCe (eds) Computer aided radiology and surgery – CARS 2002. Springer, Paris, pp 503–508
[77] Hillman BJ (2003) Economic, legal, and ethical rationales for the ACRIN national lung screening trial of CT screening for lung cancer. Acad Radiol 10: 349–350
[78] Van Horn JD, Grethe JS, Kostelec P, et al (2001) The Functional Magnetic Resonance Imaging Data Center (fMRIDC): the challenges and rewards of large-scale databasing of neuroimaging studies. Philos Trans R Soc Lond B Biol Sci 356: 1323–1339
[79] Van Horn JD, Gazzaniga MS (2002) Opinion: Databasing fMRI studies towards a 'discovery science' of brain function. Nat Rev Neurosci 3: 314–318
[80] Bunk S (2003) Internet2: The virtual sequel. Scientist 17: 14–14
[81] Internet2: http://www.internet2.edu/. Accessed 24 April 2003
[82] Rabinovitch E (1998) Internet2 [Your Internet Connection]. IEEE Communications Magazine 36: 17–18
[83] Teitelbaum BH, S Dunn L Neilson R Narayan V Reichmeyer F (1999) Internet2 QBone: Building a testbed for differentiated services. IEEE Network 13: 8–16
[84] NLM Home Page for Next Generation Internet (NGI): http://www.nlm.nih.gov/research/ngiinit.html. Accessed 24 April 2003.

Storage and networks

W. Rueger

Siemens Medical Solutions, USA

Abstract

Technologies used for PACS have made tremendous progress within the last decade. The article shows trends and discusses cost, availability and clinical requirements for image storage, primarily based on RAID. Strategies for image data migration are following. In closing, the application of network technologies to image management is explained.

The "A" in PACS

Over the last decade, almost every acronym and the associated storage technology has found it's way into a PACS archive somewhere. The base technologies are magnetic tape, optical disks, and magnetic disks which all come in myriades of derivatives. Differentiators are form factors, capacities, speeds, life cycles and prices.

Prices per data unit stored are highest for magnetic disks, followed by optical and tape media. The same sequence applies to speed performance. Storage systems based on magnetic disks (also hard disks) are the fastest, outperforming the other technologies by 5-10:1. Access is quasi immediate. Capacities for magnetic disks are (2004) up to 300 GigaByte, optical disks up to 30 GigaByte and tapes up to 200 GigaByte. Magnetic disks are grouped in RAID arrays such as SAN (Storage Area Network – disk array is attached via fibre channel, NAS – Network attached storage disk array is attached to the Local Area Network by server).

Tape and optical media are organized in cabinets; data rates are increased by using multiple drives. Price ratios between fast magnetic disks (FibreChannel) sub-systems and tape sub-systems are about 10:1 for the identical storage capacity. On the low end, disk sub-systems based on SATA or equivalent drives (used in desktop PCs) will rival the price of tape subsystems in the near future. Speed performance ratios are more difficult to compare. For tapes and optical disks, there are a "mount" delays by placing the medium into a drive. There is an additional delay for tapes winding it to the position of the desired image file. Once positioned, data can be streamed at speed levels approaching that of low end magnetic disks. Therefore, it makes sense to structure the image archive according to the immediacy of image retrieval. Images needed with immediate access should be stored on magnetic disk, otherwise on tape/optical media.

Legal archiving requirements in most states in the US are to retain images of adults for 7 years and 21 years for adolescents. De-archiving needs: radiologists need immediate access to prior cases when reading the new exam. 90% of the time, they won't need to go back more than 2 years. For oncology, the period is about 3 years.

Thus, Image Archives were designed in 2 storage blocks – A fast short/mid term-storage using magnetic disks and a long-term archive with slower albeit more affordable optical media or tapes. Prior images needed for comparison, so the theory, would then be moved from the slower storage to the fast storage the night before (prefetching). A typical image archive shown in Fig. 1. Archives installed a few years ago have a comparatively small RAID component (down to 2 weeks capacity for active patients) and a large tape/optical disk storage block covering all the images acquired [1].

In contrast, modern archives depend largely on RAID at least for the first 1–3 years and storing older data with tape/optical media. The cost of magnetic disk based storage continues to decline faster than the other technologies. As result, RAID will not only be used for the entire primary archive but will also find it's way into back-up archives as well.

RAID – DAS – SAN – NAS

Grouping drives in a Redundant Array of Inexpensive Disks (RAID), first described in [2], allows for a

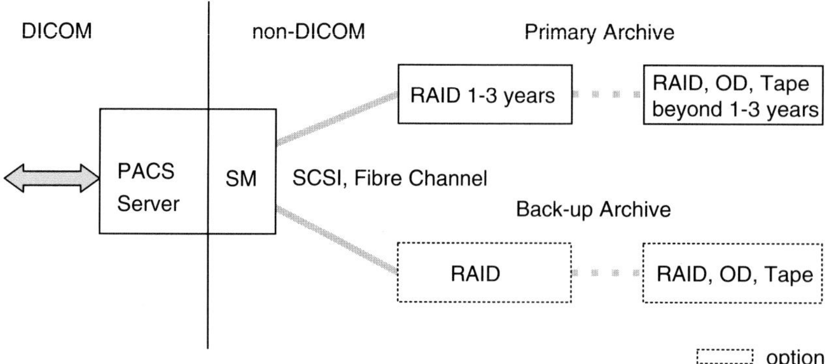

Fig. 1. Image Archive. Images are transferred via PACS server and Storage Management (SM) that coordinates usage of the various storage technologies, usually magnetic disks for fast access for mid-term archiving and either optical disks or tapes for long-term archiving

higher capacity storage sub-system with increased reliability and speed.

Different configurations are known as RAID levels. There are about 10 of them, with only levels 1 and 5 relevant for PACS. Level 1 means duplicating each disk (mirroring), levels 2–5 introduce one additional redundant disk for a group of each eg. 4 disks. The most common level used for PACS is RAID level 5. Data and the error correction code are "striped" in adjustable chuncks across the disks in the group. A faulty drive can be replaced without disrupting operation.

Drives have MTTF (Mean Time To Failure) of 600,000 hours = 70 years or more. Note, that's not the useful life of a single drive. It indicates that a system of 600 drives will run for 1,000 hours before a drive fails (on average). The probability of one drive failing in a group of n drives within the specified time T is P(T) = 1-exp[-n T/MTTF] which is approximately P(T) = n T / MTTF. One drive by itself has the probability T/MTTF of failing which is 5/70 = 7% during its useful life of 5 years. Now that brings a different perspective to 600,000 hours MTTF ! Conversely, the Availability of the drive A = 1 – P = 1 – 7% = 93% during the 5 years.

For a group of 5 drives, the probability of 1 drive and thus the group to fail during the useful life is P_{group} = 57% = 35%. If one of the 5 drives becomes the redundant one to store the error correction code, the probability of 1 drive to fail is still 7%. However, 1 failed drive does not impact system operation at all as long as a 2nd drive doesn't fail during the repair period. That probability is P_{repair} = (n –1) MTTR/MTTF. Assuming 24 hours for MTTR (Mean Time To Repair), P_{repair} = 4 24/600,000 = 1/6,250 = 0.016%. Then the probability for the RAID to fail becomes P_{RAID} = P_{group} P_{repair} = 35% 0.016% = 0.0011%, reduced by a factor of 6,250 compared to the group of drives! The availability A_{RAID} = 1 – P_{RAID} = 99.998% ("four nines") for the 5 years.

In practice, 2nd failures do occur, thus backing up the data (another RAID or tape) is still warranted. For a complete RAID subsystem, probability of failure of the controller(s) and power supplies need to be included in the analysis.

RAIDs can be Direct Attached Storage (DAS) to a server, be linked thru FibreChannel [3] as a Storage Area Network (SAN) to a server, or be linked to a network via a server as Networked Attached Storage (NAS). The term "network" in SAN is misleading. Multiple RAIDs can connect to a server or cluster of servers thru FibreChannel connected to switches but only in the limited area of a data center. NAS connect thru standard Ethernet. For block transfer of data such as database applications (querying for a patient), SAN or DAS are best. For file transfer such

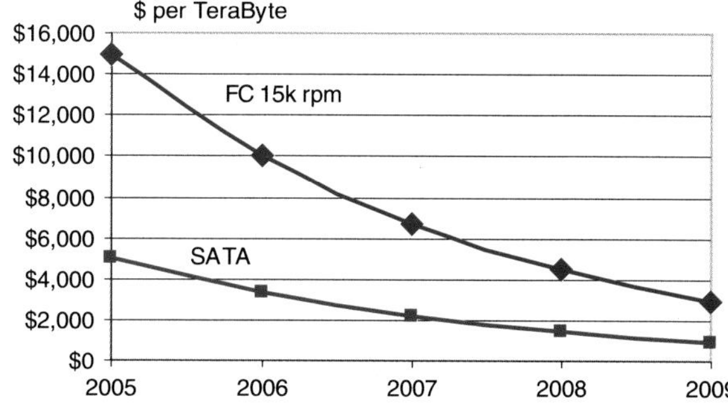

Fig. 2. Projected price per TeraByte for RAIDs with fast 15k rpm FibreChannel (FC) and slower SATA 7.5k rpm disks (used in regular desktop PCs) at 33% annual decline. In comparison, the price per TB for tape archives is $1,000 to $2,000.

as transferring images thru a server to a PACS workstation, SANs or NAS can be used. With SAN, there is typically higher speed peformance associated.

For the PACS buyer, differentiating between SAN and NAS is not all that relevant. It is more about the design of the RAID (redundancy of controllers, power supplies) and the type of drives used which influences price. Figure 3 shows the projected price per TeraByte for systems with fast 15k rpm FC drives and slower but more affordable 7.5k rpm SATA drives [4] (rpm – revolutions per minute the disk is spinning). In the past 5 years, prices declined 50% annually. For a conservative estimate, a 33% decline was projected.

The price differential for both types is 3:1, the speed performance differential for large files (medical images) less than 30%. That clearly favors SATA based RAIDs for image storage. For writing/reading small chuncks of data as needed for databases, high speed FC drive based RAIDs are superior. Both drives can be mixed in one RAID allowing to optimize price, capacity (very small for database, very large for images) and speed.

Prices per TB for optical media are already higher than SATA RAIDs and the trend will continue. Thus, optical media will play much less of a role in PACS in the future. Price per TB for tape archives are still somewhat below RAIDs, so there is a place for tape for long term storage and certainly for backup.

For a projection of drive capacities, see Fig. 3. SATA drives are expected to grow faster in capacity vs high speed FiberChannel drives.

More images per exam

Across imaging in radiology, the average size per exam was 20–25 MB in the early 1990's. It grew to 50MB per exam in 2004 as a result of more x-ray procedures displaced by CT/MR, reduced slice thickness for CT/MR, increased matrix sizes, the proliferation of multi-row CT and the introduction of DR replacing CR (18MB instead of 8MB per image). Increasingly, mammography gets added – no small feat at 200MB per exam. And the exam sizes will still get larger in the future with new storage hungry modalities. Figure 4 shows projections at different growth rates.

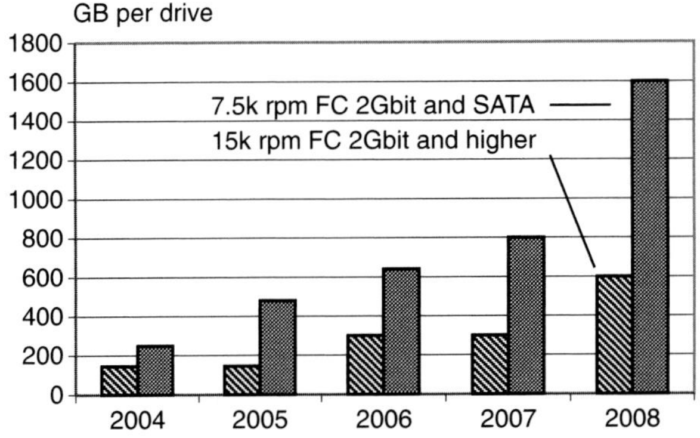

Fig. 3. Projected disk drive capacities for fast and slower FC (FibreChannel) and SATA drives

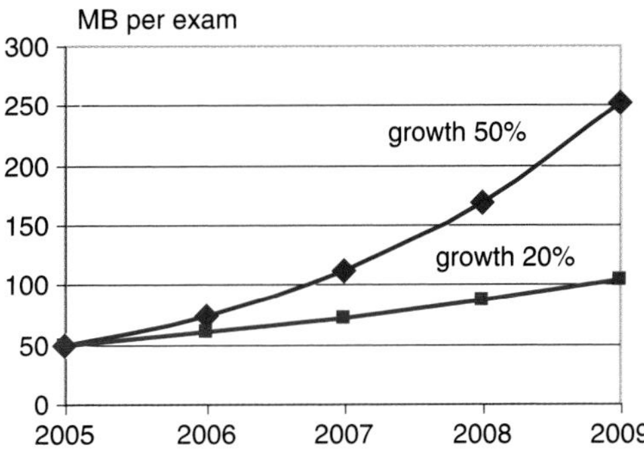

Fig. 4. Expected sizes for the average digital radiology exam for different annually compounded growth

These growth rates will have more impact on required archive capacity than the growth in procedure volume which is currently at around 5% annually in the US.

Planning storage capacity

Considering price erosion, technology obsolescence and budgeting cycles, it makes sense to plan for about a 3 year timeframe. Figure 5 shows pricing trends for a 3 year RAID for a facility with 100,000

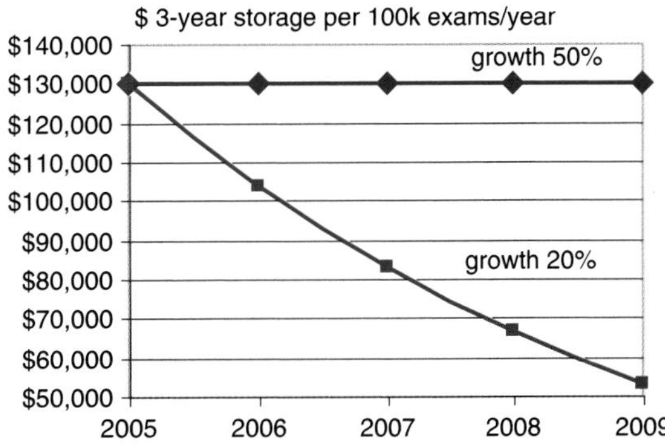

Fig. 5. Price for 3 year storage per 100,000 exams/year considering price erosion of RAID (Fig.2) and growing exam size (Fig. 4). Note, 50% growth is exactly reciprocal to 33% decline in price

exams/year, factoring in pricing declines of Fig. 2 and exam growth of Fig. 4. Note that a growth of 50% is reciprocal to a decline of 33% (1/1.5 = .67). Thus, at a 33% annual reduction in price, the overall price for a 3 year archive remains the same if image data volume (combined between exams size and procedure volume) grows by 50% annually. With growth below the 50% mark, RAID prices will decline.

Compression

For radiology images, an average 2:1 compression ratio, rarely exceeding 3:1 for some images, can be achieved without loss of information. There are "lossy" algorithms (wavelet) that allow much higher compression ratios, eg 10:1 for CT/MR and 20:1 for CR. It is based on the idea is to remove irrelevant information, especially noise. The process is irreversible. While wavelet compressed images with the above ratios can't be discerned from the original by radiologists, also referred to as "visually lossless" compression, there is still reluctance for legal reasons not to be able to reproduce the original when needed. For the foreseeable future, 2:1 compression is expected to be the method of choice for archival, cutting the required storage capacity in half. Lossy compression is frequently employed for transmitting images thru a slow network connections (DSL) to physicians for review, but not for interpretation.

Image data migration

The life cycle of a PACS (or the related contract) is 4–8 years. In the US, many of the early adopters, especially large academic medical centers, are already procuring their 2nd generation PACS. Switching vendors or not, image data migration is always a challenge when moving on to a new technology platform. While database content eg. when migrating RIS can be migrated to a new system comparatively quickly, images can't. The size gets in the way.

DICOM does not specify how to store images on an archive (DICOM Interchange Media applies only to some removable media). See also Fig. 1. Thus, the only way extracting the images is thru the network using DICOM query/retrieve. That puts additional load on an already aged and probably overloaded system. The following elements should be considered in a migration strategy:

a) radiologists should to have access to 2 years of images
b) install the new archive while using the old PACS. Modalities should send to both systems. Some facilities adjust the exams on so called quality check workstations (QCWS). In that case, the adjusted images need to be sent to the new archive.
c1) if the prior images can be prefetched on the old PACS and moved quickly enough to the new PACS (eg pre-fetching initiated by the RIS and automatically forwarding to the new server), the new system can be installed immediately.
c2) Otherwise, the old PACS needs to be utilized until a total of 2 years of images have been collected, both from sending new images (modality, QCWS) and retrieving prior images.
d) retrieving prior images with "foreground load", when the old PACS is still fully utilized, is a tedious process. Experienced speeds are between migrating .5 and 1.5 archived days per day. This applies to archives based on tape/optical media. Thus, factoring in step b), conversion will take a year or more.
e) the old archive needs to be kept until all the images are migrated. Since daily production is now on the new system, migration speeds will increase drastically to 3 or more archived days per day.

What is still left, is cleaning up the records. A good percentage of image headers will be incomplete, incorrect or images will be duplicated. The methodology is explained in [5].

Networks

Ethernet has been, is and continues to be the undefeated champ in the world of networking. It extends to 10Gbit/sec [6] and pretty soon to everyone's doorstep with EFM – Ethernet in the First Mile [6,7].

Common for PACS workstations are currently 100 Mbit/sec (within a building) and 1.5 – 10 Mbit/sec when connected over a Wide Area Network (WAN), such as the internet.

Eventually, 1Gbit/sec will become available on workstations while 10Gbit/sec will only be used for backbone and data center applications.

Transfer rates are shown in Table 1. It is assumed the 70% of the nominal bandwidth can be used for image transfer.

There are two different scenarios for image transfer.

Table 1. Effective transfer rates for uncompressed CT and CR images for different bandwidths

Mbit/sec	0.1	0.5	1.5	3	10	45	100
Example	ISDN	DSL	T1, DSL	DSL	Eth, WiFi	T3, WiFi	Ethernet
CR (8MB) seconds/image	914.3	182.9	61.0	30.5	9.1	2.0	0.9
CR (8MB) images/second	0.00	0.01	0.02	0.03	0.11	0.49	1.09
CT (0.5MB) seconds/image	57.1	11.4	3.8	1.9	0.6	0.1	0.1
CT (0.5MB) images/second	0.02	0.09	0.26	0.53	1.75	7.88	17.50

Table 2. Effective transmission times for uncompressed CT and CR exams

Mbit/sec	0.1	0.5	1.5	3	10	45	100	
CR – 3 images	2743	549	183	91	27	6	3	seconds
CT – 200 images	11429	2286	762	381	114	25	11	seconds

- modality to server; acceptable transfer times for an exam are between 5 min (on campus) and 20 min (from remote location to center).
- physician retrieves images from the server; retrieval times should not exceed 10–20 seconds per exam.

Table 2 shows the minimum acceptable network bandwidth for both cases.

For case a), T1 bandwidth at 1.5 Mbit/sec is the minimum. With compression 2:1, the bandwidth can be cut in half accordingly. For the 5min transfer time, 10Mbit/sec are sufficient. For case b), a 100 Mbit/sec link between client and server are required (with 2:1 compression, 45Mbit/sec).

For viewing purposes (at home) across DSL connections (0.5 –3 Mbit/sec), even 10:1 compression results in 38sec or higher transfer times which is pushing acceptance limits of referring physicians. Thus, the flagging/marking of relevant images by the radiologist becomes important.

Home connections to the internet will improve with the proliferation of Ethernet in the First Mile (EFM), delivering speeds of 5–15Mbit/sec over regular phone wiring.

It is also apparent that there is not much use for bandwidths in the ISDN or (wireless) modem range at around 0.1 Mbit/sec.

Wireless networks (WiFi – wireless fidelity [8]) with bandwidths of 11 and 54 Mbit/sec will find applications within OR/ER/ICUs delivering images to mobile viewing stations.

References

[1] Hruby W, Mosser H, Urban M, Rueger W (1992) The Vienna SMZO project: The totally digital Hospital. Eur J Radiol 16: 66–68

[2] Patterson D, Gibson G, Katz R (1988) A case for redundant arrays of inexpensive disks (RAID). Proceedings of ACM SIGMOD'88, pp 109–116

[3] http://www.fibrechannel.org/

[4] http://serialata.org

[5] Redfern RO, Stremitzer A, Goldszal A, Morton D, Rueger W, Horii SC (2004) PACS data conversion using automatic matching algorithm. Proceedings SCAR, Vancouver

[6] http://www.ieee802.org/3/

[7] http://www.efmalliance.org/

[8] http://www.wi-fi.org

Applications using new digital technologies

Reporting from monitors

R. Mayrhofer and G. Pärtan

Department of Radiology, Danube Hospital Vienna, Austria

During the last two decades medical imaging has moved more and more toward digital technology. At one hand, digital imaging has become a widely used replacement for conventional film in radiography, at the other hand the primarily digital cross sectional modalities contribute an ever increasing part of medical imaging.

Filmless radiology with digital archiving and image communication requires reporting from workstations with high quality electronic display devices, as will be shown below.

Full information content of digitally acquired images can be utilized by interactively working with image data on diagnostic workstations, improving diagnostic quality.

To realize this potential benefits certain technical quality requirements of the display device on the one hand and sophisticated software functionality of the reporting workstation on the other hand have to be fulfilled. Additionally simple ergonomic considerations, for example ambient light are more important for workstations than for film based reading, however are sometimes underestimated.

Digital imaging has comprehensively changed radiologists' workplace compared to working with conventional films viewed on lightboxes and paper printed clinical information. Integration of digital imaging system, radiology information system, and clinical information in digital form by means of information technology enables the radiologist to optimize diagnostic workflow.

Quality of electronic display devices

Principally, quality of single digital images displayed on monitors is currently still typically less compared to printed films, although advantages of using sophisticated software tools of the reporting workstations for interactive viewing and the ability to apply postprocessing algorithms in general compensates this deficit by far.

Nevertheless the combination of printed films and lightbox, which most radiologists are used to deal with, can display higher spatial resolution and more gray scale levels simultaneously than currently available electronic displays. Thus, when planning or evaluating a digital radiology system it is important to give special attention to the core components of the reporting workplace the monitor and software viewing tools of the reporting workstation.

Image perception

The human visual system is part of the imaging chain from image acquisition to perception and contributes to the overall performance of the display system.

Perception of the whole content of a digital image is limited by the confined capabilities of the eye-brain system and the quality of the display. Knowledge about the human visual system from psychovisual experiments can be used to establish criteria for optimized electronic displays that stimulate the visual system of the observer over its full range of response. For an ideal display system technical parameters of the viewing device – which also include the surrounding conditions – should be adjusted to the characteristics of the eye-brain system [1].

Luminance range – Contrast – Contrast sensitivity

Luminance is related to what is perceived as brightness, although correlation is complex and not how might be expected linear. Luminance is a photometric quality reflecting the intensity of a defined small region on a display surface. The SI unit is candela [cd] per square meter or foot-lambert where one cd/m^2 is equal to 0,2919 foot-lambert.

Luminance range is defined as the ratio L_{max}/L_{min} where L_{min} is the minimal and L_{max} the maximal luminance a device is capable to display. In general displaying images by using a wide luminance range results in improved quality due to high physical contrast.

Contrast sensitivity of the human visual system can be determined by carrying out observer experiments. The ratio $\Delta L/L_{mean} = (L - L_{mean})/L_{mean}$ is called the contrast threshold where L is the luminance of an object that is just noticeable in front of a background with an average luminance L_{mean}. In psychophysics contrast sensitivity is a measure of the probability that a standard observer can detect the object and is defined as the reciprocal value of the contrast threshold.

To determine the physical contrast required to detect an object (the contrast sensitivity function) depends on luminance and but is as well influenced by the test pattern, its size, shape and frequency content, the background, the noise and its structure.

With the model developed by Barten [2] contrast sensitivity can be calculated particularly for a sinusoidal variation over a uniform background. At a frequency of 1 cycle (equivalent to 1 line pair) per mm where the human visual system has a good response contrast threshold is nearly constant for medium to high luminance but increases below 10 cd/m^2. In this range the transition from photopic vision to scotopic vision (transition from viewing with the central retinal cones to the peripherally located rods) occurs and contrast sensitivity deteriorates approximately according to $L^{1/2}$.

Display devices with the same luminance range but different maximum luminance will differ in the number of just noticeable differences. For example devices with a maximum luminance of 1,200 cd/m^2 and a minimum luminance of 5 cd/m^2 theoretically are associated with 680 just noticeable differences (JND), display devices with L_{min} of 1 cd/m^2 and L_{max} of 240 cd/m^2 would be capable of displaying only 530 JND, despite having the same luminance range of 240 [3].

These figures are ideal values to illustrate properties of the human visual system. Under realistic viewing conditions the number of perceivable grayscales is less than 250, these mainly due to ambient light and image structure.

When medical images are displayed the image values are modified by display processing e.g. window and level operations to produce presentation values, which are converted into digital driving levels to establish the luminance of each pixel. At high luminance where the contrast threshold is constant a display function where the logarithm of luminance is proportional to the presentation values will produce uniform contrast. However for many display systems the dim regions are in a luminance range where contrast sensitivity of the observer is poor.

This non-linearity in the response of the human visual system requires an also nonlinear mapping of presentation values to digital driving codes. Adapting a specific display function can maximize number of perceivable gray levels for a given luminance range. Based on the Barten model or on other observer experiments a display function can be found that perceptually linearizes the display.

An image presentation device is said to be perceptually linear when equal increments in digital input (presentation values) produce equally perceived differences in luminance throughout the entire range of digital input values.

There are several display functions in the discussion, the one based on the Barten model is proposed by the DICOM working group XI as display function standard. Besides maximization of the dynamic range, perceptual linearization should provide similarity in perceived gray scale of complex images even when absolute luminance and luminance range differ between individual display devices [4].

Spatial resolution

In general, the smaller an object, the less visible it is. Physiology and size of the retinal cone cells limit spatial resolution to about 30/degree. Thus even for a relatively short viewing distance of 40 cm the size of the smallest perceivable object is 120 microns. This corresponds to a maximum of about 2600 TV lines that would make sense for a display height of 30 cm (21 inch landscape monitor) [5] assuming ideal viewing conditions and an optimal adaptation of the observer.

Although printed radiographic film is typically associated with a pixel array of about 4,000 × 5,000 for a 35 × 43 cm size (14 × 17 inch), for electronic display devices with 30 × 36 cm size 2,500 × 3,000 pixels is sufficient and combined with a regional zoom function could be called a high fidelity workstation [2]. However, currently available monitors are limited by a tradeoff between size of the pixel matrix and luminance, i.e. in common monitors with an extremely high resolution are only capable of display with lower luminance unless constancy and longevity of the monitor tube is accepted to be limited.

Spatial resolution should never be discussed without contrast capabilities of a display system. The visual contrast sensitivity is a strong function of spatial frequency. Neither contrast nor size alone determine if an object is visible. To be perceived, an object has to exceed physiological threshold both in size and in contrast.

The relationship between contrast sensitivity and target size is often referred to as Contrast-Detail curves. In general the minimum visible contrast level increases as the object size decreases. An interesting characteristic of the human visual system is the contrast-detail curve for cyclic targets. For typical viewing distances, the response is best at a frequency of about 0.5–1.0 cycles per millimeter (lowest contrast threshold). Sensitivity is reduced for smaller objects and for large objects causing the observer to back away from an image to get a better impression of large features.

However luminance of the display system might remain the key factor for display quality because contrast sensitivity and perceived image quality increase up to approximately 3,500 cd/m^2. At present, luminance levels of computer monitors are in the range of 200 to 800 cd/m^2 and therefore considerably below the optimal values.

For a comprehensive judgement of the overall quality of a display system some other remaining important factors have to be taken into account. Maybe the most important is ambient light reflection.

Ambient light

The luminous intensity of extraneous light in the reading room and its spatial distribution have significant influence on image quality because of back scattering of ambient light in the direction of the viewer. With films these reflections are highly dampened by the coating on the front surface. High quality electronic displays should provide emission of image signals with a broad viewing angle and minimal ambient light reflections. Reflections can be reduced by dark glass of the face plate and a contrast panel. Display reflections can be distinguished in diffuse superposition and structured components (e.g. lamps, windows). The diffuse component is responsible for an additional uniform background luminance which effects contrast sensitivity in the low luminance regions of an image. In general diffuse ambient light reflections should contribute no more than 20% of L_{min}. With low background light levels which can be achieved in diagnostic reading rooms there should be no significant effect on contrast in image regions with a luminance above 5 cd/m^2. This is realistic with a diffuse reflection coefficient of 0.025 cd/m^2 per lux. For higher ambient light levels as typically found in patient care areas (above 100 lx) very low reflection coefficients are required or an adaptation of L_{min} is necessary. Therefore an ambient light sensor which adjusts luminance levels to the extraneous light in the reporting room is of essential value especially if conditions change (e.g. with daylight).

To reduce extraneous light from the digital image itself, also blank areas (collimated areas when viewing in "white bone" mode) should be properly masked, setting them at the lowest luminance level, e.g. with a "shutter" software function. The software controls on the display (toolcards, soft-buttons) also must be of rather low luminance and contrast to avoid a potential source of veiling glare and irritation for the observer.

Structured luminous patterns from light sources which superimpose onto the radiological image can affect the detection of diagnostic features and contribute to visual fatigue. This should be avoided by a proper setup of the reporting room with diffuse lightening and positioning of the monitor in a 90 degree direction to the light source. In addition most medical display devices now have rough surfaces or antireflective coatings, which also reduce static charge of the display surface.

Monitor technology

Cathode ray tubes

Until recently, monitors based on cathode ray tubes (CRT) provide the most advanced available technology for electronic displays. Technical principals have been well known for a long time and components are produced with high quality in great numbers for a relatively moderate price.

Currently only few other applications exist for high quality monochrome monitors as required for reporting medical images from electronic displays. Aviation control is one example, where high luminance is also very important because ambient light levels are high in the control towers.

However, until recently worldwide about 30,000 to 40,000 high quality monochrome monitors are sold, contributing only a small segment to the whole CRT computer display market. Nevertheless basic construction principles and many components for color and monochrome monitors are the same or at least very similar, resulting in synergy effects for development and production.

In a CRT, electrons are accelerated within the vacuum bulb with a high voltage of up to 30 kV and the focused beam which is deflected by magnetic fields excites the luminescent phosphor line by line in a raster fashion. In a monochrome CRT the more or less flat faceplate of the monitor consists mainly of relatively thick glass with the phosphor powder layer and a very thin aluminum coating on the rear side and an antireflective structure or coating on the front side. The aluminum layer conducts the electrons to the phosphor and reflects the light emitted by the phosphor to maximize toward the viewer.

Mainly two different types of cathodoluminescent phosphor are used for monochrome CRTs: P-104 which has a higher luminous efficiency compared to P-45 (approximately 30% less). This means that higher tube currents are needed in P-45 phosphor systems to achieve the same brightness and improved electron beam focusing optics have to be employed to provide sufficient spatial resolution. On the other hand P-104 has a more limited lifetime especially in high luminance systems and a high granularity because it consists of a mixture of phosphors with different colors. In medical CRT systems P-45 is the preferred phosphor because of the naturally emitted broader spectrum of light and the longer lifetime without major decline of brightness.

The pixel size of a CRT is limited by the spot size of the electron beam. The beamspot increases linearly as the square root of the beam current. The minimum diameter to which the spot size can be reduced is given by the beam current required to produce acceptable luminance. Therefore, there is a trade-off between spatial resolution and maximal luminance.

Another intrinsic property of emissive display devices is veiling glare that is caused by multiple scattering processes within the layers emitted light has to pass from the phosphor grain where it originates to the display surface. The effect is a low frequency degradation of image quality perceived as contrast reduction especially in areas around high luminance structures. Light diffusion in the multiple layers of the emissive structure can cause noticeable effects in a distance of up to 20 cm from a point source.

A practically useful definition of veiling glare ratio is the luminance of a full bright field to luminance of a central dark spot of a given diameter.

Active-matrix liquid crystal displays

Recently, active matrix liquid crystal display (LCD) monitors have become the display media of choice for personal and portable computers on a large scale, because of their ergonomic advantages in terms of shorter depth, lower weight, power consumption and heat output. These advantages of LCD monitors have not gone unnoticed by the medical imaging professions and are therefore increasingly used for reviewing imaging studies and also for control panels of imaging devices.

Molecule orientation within a liquid crystal determines its optical characteristics, especially the transmission of polarized light. Application of an electric field changes the molecule orientation. This electro-optical effect is used in liquid crystal displays (LCD) to modulate light transmission.

From a strong source at the back of the device light is directed to the front through polarizer films and the liquid crystal layer. In an active matrix LCD the electric field for each liquid crystal cell is controlled by a thin film transistor deposited onto a glass substrate. Therefore the whole display consists of multiple layers and overall light transmission is rather poor, ranging from about 8% for color LCDs and up to 24% for monochrome designs. High efficiency backlights are necessary to provide acceptable luminance and production of large area (high resolution) design with millions of elements is expensive.

In addition the emission distribution of active matrix LCDs strongly depends on viewing angle due to anisotropy of the liquid crystal cell. Several technical improvements during the last years brought major improvements. Color and monochrome displays with up to $2{,}500 \times 2{,}000$ pixels, a maximal luminance of 250 cd/m^2 and acceptable viewing angles (of about 170 degree) have been developed.

For the future flat panel display technology is likely to replace CRTs for medical imaging applications because of the substantially higher potential for quality improvement. Own experiences and experiments with color and monochrome active matrix LCDs (see below) suggest that diagnostic performance with LCD monitors shows no significant difference compared to monochrome CRTs.

Diagnostic performance of monitor reporting

The most important differences between monitor and hardcopy display are:

- high luminance of conventional viewboxes (2,000 cd/m^2) vs. relatively low luminance of the currently used monitors (about 200–800 cd/m^2);
- fixed grayscale of the hardcopy with relatively limited dynamic range (see beyond) vs. possibility of changing window and level on monitor and thus getting access to the higher contrast resolution of the phosphor storage plate, the dose-brightness response of which is linear over a range of more than 1:10 000.

Luminance seems to be of great importance for high diagnostic performance; a minimum of 170 cd/m^2 is considered as necessary [6]. In the studies addressed below, monitor luminance is given with 200–260 cd/m^2; it would be important to clarify, if this only specifies the highest technically possible luminance of these monitors (the use of which would lead to very fast aging of the display and therefore almost never should be chosen in practice), or if this is the measured luminance used for the image reading in these studies. Many studies investigating diagnostic performance of image evaluation from monitors used digitized film-screen images which are in many ways subject to the same restraints as the film-screen technique itself, especially concerning the limited dynamic range of radiographic film (1:100–500) [7]. Some of these papers reported equivalent performance of monitor compared to digital hardcopy respectively conventional film [8,9,10]. One study [11] reported equivalent performance of monitor compared to hardcopies, but both performed less than the original film-screen images. Some studies found deterioration of diagnostic performance when using monitor compared to film-screen images [12] or to hardcopies [13]. Of studies using primarily digital phosphor storage images, one found approximately comparable performance of monitor and hardcopy [14]. Elam et al. [15] reported a smaller sensitivity for the detection of pneumothoraces on electronic viewing consoles; in an other study [16], Thaete reported significantly poorer diagnostic performance for interstitial disease and pneumothoraces with monitor and hardcopy display of phosphor storage chest radiographs compared to conventional film, although this study was performed with a high resolution (4 K × 5 K × 12 Bit) prototype storage phosphor system. In contrary, in the study of Krupinski et al. [17], reported statistically significantly better performance in detection of pneumothoraces with monitor reading. In an own ROC-study [18], we found a slight, statistically significant advantage when reporting 45 phosphor storage bedside chest images from monitor without edge enhancement compared to large-format contrast harmonized hardcopies concerning pneumonic infiltrates, but no significant differences with pneumothorax, pulmonary nodules, and hilar or mediastinal mass lesions. Most authors comparing conventional film-screen resp. storage phosphor hardcopies with monitor display either used unenhanced images on the monitor [8–12] or compared the same enhancement algorithms on monitor and hardcopy [14,15]. In the study of Krupinski [17] edge enhancement options were available on monitor but only used sporadically. In 1990, Rosenthal et al. [19] reported comparable performance with reporting edge-enhanced and nonenhanced chest images from a workstation, but these images were acquired by digitizing conventional chest radiographs.

Whereas many of the studies mentioned above used high-resolution monitors with an about 2,000 × 2,000 pixel matrix, the monitors used in our study only have a resolution of 1,280 x 1,024 pixel, so that access to the original resolution of the phosphor plate is only possible by using a magnification function, i.e. scrolling through 1/4th of the original matrix. Although some studies lead to the conclusion that for most tasks in chest radiography a 1K matrix is sufficient [20], readers were advised to use this function as often as possible. This is comparable with viewing a film-screen image from different distances, which is recommended for improving diagnostic performance on chest radiology [21].

Otto et al. [22] compared monitors of different quality with hardcopy and found statistically inferior diagnostic performance with subtle pulmonary abnormalities viewed on 1,024 × 1,024 monitors without magnification compared to hardcopies. Once more results for a low luminance (85 cd/m^2) device were below a higher luminance monitor (250 cd/m^2) and high resolution 2,560 × 2,048 monitor (250 cd/m2) without magnification improved performance which was slightly significantly below hardcopy reading. Interestingly, when monitors were used with magnification function only the low luminance 1 K monitor showed minimally statistically significant inferior results whereas the other two monitors and hardcopy performed equal.

Similarly a study of Herron et al. [23], although not performed with electronic displays (no magnification or windowing), suggests that with luminance ranges and spatial resolution as provided by high quality monochrome monitors, diagnostic accuracy is not likely to be affected by the quality of the display. Furthermore it confirms that the effect of image luminance on observer performance is grater than that of spatial resolution.

Considering flat screen LCD displays, it has been proven that reporting of radiographic and CT studies from high-performance LCD monitors is feasible without significant detriment to diagnostic performance [24,25].

Besides diagnostic quality, also time requirements for reporting are an issue when reporting from soft copies is regarded. Whereas in the beginning of digital radiology reporting from monitors has often been considered as cumbersome and time consuming, more recent studies and practical experiences from well set-up PACS systems have shown that report time is not lengthened by the introduction of the PACS, and as an additional benefit more historical images are viewed when a PACS is in use [26]. Moreover, even though also in another study no time differences were found between reading conventional studies on the monitor or as soft-copy, after introduction of PACS, 85.9 % of all cases compared to 41.2 % before could be interpreted on the day of the examination, and 87.2 % of the reports were completed the day after the examination [27].

In conclusion published data from studies, investigating the influence of contrast and resolution on observer performance with digital radiographs, seem to be task specific, and, to a large extent, study design affects the results in a substantial manner. Some studies investigating spatial resolution do not provide clear data about luminance range and gray-scale mapping. Routine use of windowing and magnification functions of the reporting workstation has significant influence on observer performance and can compensate lower spatial and contrast resolution of monitors compared to hardcopies even for subtle findings. Altogether, compared to conventional film-screen systems, complete digitalization of a radiology department including soft copy-reporting is time saving at nearly all steps of the workflow, with expected positive effects on the workflow quality of the entire hospital.

Viewing tools of reporting workstations

One major advantage of digital radiography is the ability to process acquired images with a variety of algorithms. Image processing can roughly be divided in detection (including "preprocessing") and display (including postprocessing). The first step is performed when the detector medium is read out and information transferred into digital form resulting in a basic image compensated for degradation and varying exposure conditions (preprocessing). The information contained in this basic image typically exceeds display capacity of either monitor or film display.

To display the information contained in the read out data and to optimize image presentation for diagnostic reading postprocessing is performed, resulting in an image with modified appearance.

More complex postprocessing algorithms e.g. edge enhancement, unsharp masking, contrast enhancement by specific non linear gradation curves or multiscale contrast amplification are normally applied automatically with predefined parameters for different examinations and are not changed routinely by the reporting radiologist and therefore not considered in detail in this chapter.

Window and level

Selecting grayscales of digital images to be printed on film by defining a "window" is a procedure radiologists are familiar with since the introduction of computed tomography in the 1970's. The information content of a digital image is typically between 8 and 12 bit for each pixel, therefore up to 4096 shades of gray would be necessary to present the whole information simultaneously. But neither the computer screen or film are capable of displaying the full range of gray-scales nor can the human visual system distinguish them. As discussed above even under good viewing conditions we can see only a maximum of about 500 of different gray levels. Under realistic conditions as found in reporting rooms and due to image structure this number falls to approximately 100.

When reporting from workstations the radiologist is no longer limited to one or few fixed window settings but can easily access the whole dynamic range. Because window and level operation is a very basic and essential postprocessing step it can be performed interactively and in real time, preferably with mouse action. The selected grey-level range is distributed over the entire dynamic range of the display monitor. The center of this interval is called the level value, and the range is called the window value or width. Thus, using a smaller window value will increase the contrast in the resulting video image. Gray levels present in the image outside the selected window will be displayed either as black when below or white when above the interval. This function is usually controlled by the radiologist via a mouse or trackball. For example pressing a mouse button and moving the mouse in the vertical direction controls the level value and the horizontal direction controls the window width. Most reporting workstations additionally provide functions to set the window to predefined values with configurable softkeys and to quickly reset the window to a standard value for example by a double click on a mouse button.

Zoom and pan

Because of the limited pixel matrix of computer monitors digital radiographs can not always be displayed with full spatial resolution of about 2 K but have to be fit into a defined segment. Only relatively expensive high end monitors with the maximum currently available pixel matrix of 2,500 × 2,000 are capable of displaying the full size of a CR chest image without reducing spatial resolution. Developments in digital image acquisition especially in the field of flat panel detectors with increased pixel matrix of 3 K and more would not allow to present full size and quality of resulting images simultaneously for softcopy reading using currently available technologies. Therefore it is necessary to find a compromise between overview with reduced matrix and full resolution of an image segment. But even when displaying full resolution of the whole image is possible, it makes sense to use a zoom function to view a region of interest (ROI) without surrounding patterns. As discussed before bright regions can deteriorate image quality in the neighboring regions substantially, mainly due to veiling glare and influence on adaptation of the eye.

For perception of the whole information content the observer has to switch between these two modes routinely. The workstation should be equipped with a spectrum of different software magnification tools to suit individual needs. Examples for functions which according to our experience are most often used in daily routine are:

- Soft buttons for switching between full resolution and full image size with the ability to easily pan the image with the mouse in the magnified mode.
- Drawing a rectangular ROI with the mouse which is magnified to fill the full screen segment with additional automatic masking of the areas outside the chosen ROI.
- Simulation of a magic glass magnifying the region around the mouse pointer without changing the rest of the image.

Soft buttons for fixed zoom factors (e.g. × 2, × 4) or entering a zoom factor via keyboard would be alternatives.

Image arrangement – "hanging protocol"

In conventional radiology departments films are prepared for reading by hanging them on the display in a certain manner and order. For sectional imaging such as CT, MR and ultrasound sorting of images by series, by time of acquisition, by anatomic location or by pulse sequence for MR is of great importance and often done by the technologist as the examination is filmed.

Especially for plain radiograph images there are more or less fixed rules for image arrangement, which have come to be called the "hanging protocol", which the person who is responsible for that task is aware of. For example films of patients with multiple images in one study or multiple studies of different anatomic regions or previous studies for comparison, are arranged in the appropriate manner considering all these factors.

Compared to a conventional lightbox or an alternator panel computer monitors provide a limited area to display images. Nowadays most reporting workstations are equipped with one to four monitors according to the type of examination which is usually reported on the particular workplace. In the early days of PACS when user interfaces were designed mostly by imitating the conventional way of working with films, workstations with six and even more monitors where built trying to maximize display size and display as many images as possible simultaneously. Size and order of images where more or less fixed.

More recent software generations are highly customizable and allow free definition of size and number of screen segments for any display mode. Furthermore rules can be defined for which display mode is automatically used according to number of studies, modality and anatomic region of the examination to be displayed.

With these new features and the development of a specific way to handle images when reporting from monitor, using interactive tools like stack mode and cine mode viewing or magnification functions, much less screen area is required compared to light boxes and no more than four monitors are required. Today for most workplaces two monitors are considered to be enough.

Controls and displays in general could benefit the user if they where customizable. Display modes, the window width and level preset values, and even the location and arrangement of on screen controls and function key definition should all be based on who logs in, so that personalized "user profiles" are automatically set.

Nevertheless standard setups of workstation software should be prepared according to the requirements and the experience of the users before installation of a digital radiology system and support for individually optimizing personal setups should not only be provided in the initial phase.

Cine/stack mode reading

In fluoroscopy and especially in angiography dynamic studies are documented in image series of the same anatomic region. Presenting image of a series sequentially, virtually arranged in a "stack" with the ability to interactively scroll through the images with the mouse [28], producing a cine effect can help to visualize and dynamic processes.

For sectional modalities "stack mode" viewing is not used to give an impression of changes over time, but to support three dimensional (3D) orientation. Interactively navigating through an image stack which represents a scanned volume facilitates perception of structures running perpendicular to the image plane. Tubular structures (e.g. vessels) can be followed and differentiated easier from spheric structures (nodules) than on hardcopies [29].

Multiphasic studies performed on subsecond spiral CT or multi-slice CT scanners and fast MR imaging, often result in a volume of image data, which can hardly be handled by printing on films. Due to the increasing number of images per examination the extended capabilities of softcopy reading like simultaneously scrolling through two image series (stacks) displayed side by side yield more and more benefit. Comparing pre- and post contrast series or different pulse sequences of the same organ in MRI is easier on a reporting workstation providing automatically synchronized and interactive navigation through image series than on hardcopies. Softcopy reading for CT and MRI has replaced conventional reporting from printed films in many otherwise conventionally organized departments and is often the first step when introducing a PACS system.

Interactive real-time multiplanar reformation

Multiplanar reformations of sectional images are available on most CT and MR scanners and have become standard postprocessing for some types of examinations. For example sagittal reformats of spinal CT are considered mandatory for trauma diagnosis. Even experienced radiologists benefit from a second plane perpendicular to the source images for diagnostic reading of complex structures (e.g. temporal bone, cervical spine). Spiral CT and especially multislice technique allow for thin slice collimation over wide ranges and resolution in the z-axis improves considerably. Small reconstruction intervals with overlapping slices further reduce step artifacts of reformatted images and z-axis resolution comes close to acquisition plane resolution resulting in nearly isotropic voxels.

Development of hardware performance and software components for 3D applications during the last years made real time interactive multiplanar reformation available on "standard" reporting workstations. Simultaneously viewing 3 planes (axial, coronal sagittal) and the possibility to interactively navigate through the images help the observer to understand complex structures within the scanned volume easier and faster than with a single plane. For special purposes oblique, double oblique and curved reformats can be obtained with few mouse clicks. Furthermore additional functions like 3D measurement of distances and angles become available.

The advantage of other 3D techniques like maximum intensity projection or shaded surface display is to give an overview of complex structures in a single projection or multiple views from different angles. Main application is visualization e.g. in CT or MR-angiography, further diagnostic information is hardly added to multiplanar sectional images.

For visualization of complex structures prior to surgery and for therapy planning dedicated 3 D workstations providing more advanced 3D reconstruction algorithms like perspective volume rendering or virtual endoscopy have been proved to be useful. Perspectives corresponding to the surgeons' view when operating on the patient can influence surgical planning and are likely to improve quality of therapy. Computer aided surgery, already routinely used in neurosurgery, is an emerging field of application for 3D image data sets beyond diagnostic purposes.

Conclusion

From theoretical considerations based on properties of the human visual system under ideal viewing conditions, together with the limitations of the complex scenario of realistic diagnostic workplaces, it can be concluded that state of the art reporting workstations equipped with high quality electronic displays fulfill the requirements for adequate image presentation in digital radiology.

As discussed above softcopy reading involves interaction with the reporting workstation and thereby differs from reading hardcopy films.

For all imaging modalities but especially for sectional imaging reporting from monitors offers new ways to access information contained in the acquired image data.

The key to optimize electronic image presentation on radiologists' workplace is integration of high quality hard- and software components considering all relevant factors influencing perception of the observer.

References

[1] Wang J, Langer S (1997) A brief review of human perception factors in digital displays for picture archiving and communications systems. J Digit Imaging 10: 158–168

[2] Barten PGJ (1992) Model for the contrast sensitivity of the human eye. Proc SPIE 1666: 57–72

[3] Flynn M, et al (1999) High-fidelity electronic display of digital radiographs. radioGraphics 19:1653–1669

[4] Blume H, Hemminger B (1997) Image presentation in digital radiology: perspectives on the emerging dicom display function standard and its application. RadioGraphics 17: 769–777

[5] Mertelmeier T (1999) Why and how is soft copy reading possible in clinical practice. J Digit Imaging 12: 3–11
[6] Gur D, Fuhrmann CR, Thaete FL (1993) Requirements for PACS: users perspective. RadioGraphics 13: 457–460
[7] Oestmann JW, Greene RE (1992) Components and system layout for digital radiography. In: Greene RE, Oestmann JW (eds) Computed digital radiography in clinical practice. Thieme Medical Publishers, New York
[8] Franken EA Jr, Berbaum KS, Marley SM, Smith WL, Sato Y, Kao SCS, Milam SG (1992) Evaluation of a digital workstation for interpreting neonatal examinations; a ROC study. Invest Radiol 27: 732–737
[9] Razavi M, Sayre JW, Taira RK, Simons M, Huang HK, Chuang KS, Rahbar G, Kangarloo H (1992) Receiver-operating-characteristic study of chest radiographs in children: digital hardcopy film vs. 2K × 2K soft-copy images. AJR 158: 443–448
[10] Hayrapetian A, Aberle DR, Huang HK, Fiske R, Morioka C, Valentino D, Boechat MI (1989) Comparison of 2048-line digital display formats and conventional radiographs: an ROC study. AJR 152: 1113–1118
[11] Slasky BS, Gur D, Good WF, Costa-Greco MA, Harris KM, Cooperstein LA, Rockette HE (1990) Receiver operating characteristic analysis of chest image interpretation with conventional, laser-printed, and high-resolution workstation images. Radiology 174: 775–780
[12] Ackerman SJ, Gitlin JN, Gayler RW, Flagle CD, Bryan RN (1993) Receiver operating characteristic analysis of fracture and pneumonia detection: comparison of laser-digitized workstation images and conventional analog radiographs. Radiology 186: 263–268
[13] Cox GG, Cook LT, McMillan JH, Rosenthal SJ, Dwyer III SJ (1990) Chest radiography: comparison of high-resolution digital displays with conventional and digital film. Radiology 176: 771–776
[14] Frank MS, Jost RG, Molina PL, Anderson DJ, Solomon SL, Whitman RA, Moore SM (1993) High resolution computer display of portable, digital, chest radiographs in adults: suitability for primary interpretation. AJR 160: 473–477
[15] Elam EA, Rehm K, Hillman BJ, Maloney K, Fajardo LL, McNeill K (1992) Efficacy of digital radiography for the detection of pneumothorax: comparison with conventional chest radiography. AJR 158: 509–514
[16] Thaete FL, Fuhrmann CR, Oliver JH, et al (1994) Digital radiography and conventional imaging of the chest: a comparison of observer performance. AJR 162: 575–581
[17] Krupinski EA, Maloney K, Bessen SC, Capp MP, Graham K, Hunt R, Lund P, Ovitt T, Standen JR (1994) Receiver operating characteristic evaluation of computer display of adult portable chest radiographs. Invest Radiol 29:141–146
[18] Pärtan G, Mosser H, Tekusch A, Mathiaschitz U, Augustin I, Hruby W (1994) Reporting digital bedside chest radiographs from monitor vs. hardcopy – a clinical ROC study. RoFo 161(4): 354–360
[19] Rosenthal MS, Good WF, Costa-Greco MA, Miketic LM, Eelkema EA, Gur D, Rockette HE (1990) The effect of image processing on chest radiograph interpretations in a PACS environment. Invest Radiol 25: 897–901
[20] Mosser H, Pärtan G, Urban, Hruby W (1993) Routinely reporting from monitor: is 2K resolution really necessary? (abstract)
8th European Congress of Radiology, Vienna, Austria
[21] Fraser RG, Paré JAP, Paré PD, Fraser RS, Genereux GP (1977–1988) Perception in chest roentgenology. In: Fraser RG, Paré JAP, Paré PD, Fraser RS, Genereux GP (eds) Diagnosis of diseases of the chest 2nd edn. W.B.Saunders, Philadelphia, pp 291–296
[22] Otto D, et al (1998) Subtle pulmonary abnormalities: Detection on monitors with varying spatial resolutions and maximum luminance levels compared with detection on storage phosphor radiographic hard copies. Radiology 207: 237–242
[23] Herron J, et al (2000) Effects of luminance and Resolution on observer performance with Chest Radiographs. Radiology 215: 169–174
[24] Kim AY, Cho KS, Song KS, Kim JH, Kim JG, Ha HK (2001) Urinary calculi on computed radiography: comparison of observer performance with hard-copy versus soft-copy images on different viewer systems. Am J Roentgenol 177: 331–335
[25] Partan G, Mayrhofer R, Urban M, Wassipaul M, Pichler L, Hruby W (2003) Diagnostic performance of liquid crystal and cathode-ray-tube monitors in brain computed tomography. Eur Radiol 13(10): 2397–401
[26] Bryan S, Weatherburn G, Watkins J, Roddie M, Keen J, Muris N, Buxton MJ (1998) Radiology report times: impact of picture archiving and communication systems. AJR Am J Roentgenol 170(5): 1153–9
[27] Langen HL, Bielmeier J, Wittenberg G, Selbach R, Feustel H (2003) Workflow improvement and efficiency gain with near total digitalization of a radiology department. Rofo 175(10): 1309–16
[28] Gur D, et al (1994) Sequential viewing of abdominal ct images at varying rates. Radiology 191: 119–122
[29] Seltzer S, et al (1995) Spiral CT of the chest: Comparison of cine and film-based viewing. Radiology 197: 73–78

Medical reporting using speech recognition – The KFJ solution (Kaiser Franz Josef Hospital, Vienna, Austria)

T. Ybinger, W. Appel, and W. Kumpan

Kaiser Franz Josef Hospital, Vienna, Austria

Introduction

The wish to control machines by means of speech is older than the ancestors of our computers. But only a few years ago computers have gained the power to turn this dream into a useful tool for our daily work. There are different types of speech-controlled systems today: for example, some systems simplify the lives of handicapped people by operating lights or electrical appliances with the human voice. Other systems enable text to be entered into word processors; these speech recognition systems may be combined with speech-control functions, e.g. to enable the computer to recognize commands such as "Print" or "Save" during dictation.

Speech recognition systems (SRS) have been spreading rapidly ever since some fundamental problems were solved. Among the first professions to recognize the advantages of this revolutionary technology were lawyers and medical doctors. In the beginning there were also different software packages for surgical reports, general medical reports, neurologists, cardiologists, internists, orthopedists, and other medical areas [2, 3, 4, 6]. The latest software releases can be used not only for radiology but for all medical reporting and dictation purposes in multi-workstation networks and 23 different languages.

The underlying technology

Speech recognition poses a great challenge for computers, since there are many and various problems to be solved. First, the relationship between written letters and spoken words is only a very indirect one. Every language has its own set of sound units, the so-called phonemes. This means that the computer must analyze the sound vibrations recorded by a microphone according to an "acoustic model" and convert these into individual phonemes; these phonemes are then combined into sets and assigned to suitable words taken from a large database. However, recognizing phonemes is not as easy as it may look. On the one hand, unwanted background noise such as ringing telephones or banging doors must be recognized and suppressed. On the other hand, people have different voices, accents and, above all, speaking styles. For every spoken word, the software chooses the most likely entry from several entries stored in the electronic dictionary, and then compares the word combinations found in the text with a "language model". This model reflects the fact that certain words frequently appear together in medical reports while other word combinations are extremely unlikely. Only after this analysis the final transcription can be performed by the speech recognition software [7, 8].

Finally, varying speaking speeds must also be taken into consideration. The first systems required the speaker to pause between one word and the next [5], which made speech quite unnatural. Advanced software programs allow natural dictation without artificial pauses, and even strongly varying speaking speeds are no problem. Alternating speaking volumes, however, may still cause difficulties, and the distance between microphone and mouth as well as the volume should be kept constant during dictation. The system in use at the Department of Radiology/Kaiser-Franz-Josef Hospital allows us to choose between several adapted environment settings during dictation, e.g. a setting for (loud, busy) day-time and another for (quiet) night-time conditions. If the job permits, wearing a headset with a microphone holder in front of the speaker's mouth could help to keep the microphone at the same distance, but for practical reasons this tool is not in use in our department.

Most systems use individual speech reference files (acoustic models) for every user. This requires an initial training of only a few minutes during which every user must read a standard text. Although the newest software release used in our department requires principally no training, it is recommended. The advantage is that the individual pronunciation is analyzed. The resulting individual analysis has a decisive influence on recognition (as anyone knows who has accidentally used somebody else's user login to dictate a report).

There are single-user systems but also complete network solutions where dictation, recognition, editing, electronic validation and automatic transmission of the reports may be performed on any computer in the network. Our software also offers a choice between online recognition, where the recognized text is displayed in real time on the screen, and background batch recognition, which takes place at a central speech recognition server. There are different approaches to the integration of speech recognition software into a computer system: implementing it into a word processing program via an API or ActiveX control, using DLL technology interfaces or an HL/7 interface to a HIS (Hospital Information System).

Aims and requirements of the speech recognition system at the KFJ Hospital

The Kaiser Franz Josef Hospital (KFJ), operated by the City of Vienna, is an 800-bed tertiary care clinic. The totally digitized Department of Radiology offers examinations with direct digital technology (FD), digital fluoroscopy and angiography, ultrasound, CT, MRI, FFD-Mammography and Interventional Radiology. More than 145.000 services are performed every year.

One of the most important motives for installing a speech recognition system at our department was to accelerate the turnaround time of x-ray reports in order to shorten the therapeutic reaction time [2, 6, 8]; this was achieved by integrating a HIS/RIS (Hospital Information System / Radiology Information System) and a PACS system (Picture Archiving and Communicating System). The main goal was to realize a faster and more effective therapy which would in turn shorten the hospital stay of patients. We also wanted to reduce the workload of our secretaries (transcriptionists). On Monday mornings they were usually faced with piles of dictated tapes collected over the weekend which often took one or two days to transcribe. This delay was hard to catch up during the week. Although reports on acute cases were of course produced immediately (as short reports), we aimed at shortening the turn-around time of reports – for medical and economical reasons, but also as a service to our patients and the referring physicians – thus contributing to shorter hospital stays.

We wanted to replace preliminary or hand-written reports, and so far as possible any diagnostic information provided via the telephone, which is a potential legal risk. Our goal was to issue final, validated and legible clear report documents immediately, with constant accuracy around the clock [4, 5].

The correction of speech recognition errors and the formatting and layout of documents should still be done by the secretaries (transcriptionists) during their office hours (on weekdays, from 7.30 a.m. to 6.00 p.m.); the doctors themselves were to do it only during night shifts, on weekends, public holidays and in cases of emergency.

Another important aim was a high recognition rate of dictations as well as quick and user-friendly text editing. The working habits were to change as little as possible. The system should be easy to use for everyone and require only little additional administration effort.

To make the speech recognition software well accepted and usable as a matter of routine, it has to be completely integrated into the RIS and support all required procedures within this environment [4, 7].

The speech recognition system also needs to be easy to administrate, stable and tolerant of user errors, thus allowing the creation of report documents with a clear identification of the patient at any time.

Table 1. Goals

Goals for the SRS at the KFJ
• Faster creation of reports • Shorter therapeutic reaction time • No preliminary reports • Productivity increase • Legible reports around the clock (independently of a secretary's time schedule)

Table 2. Requirements

Requirements
• High recognition rate • Easy to use • Stable system with low maintenance effort • Minimal change of working habits • "Dual principle" – networking capability

Aspects of product selection

When the invitation to tender for our project was made (1996), the market offered only a few speech recognition systems for radiological reporting which were functional and could be completely integrated into a HIS/RIS/PACS. One of our essential requirements was the support of a "dual working principle". This concept requires that the secretaries edit and format the recognized texts during routine office hours, while the reporting radiologists take over these tasks during the nights or on weekends. This implies that the working procedures of doctors do not change essentially during regular office hours; even the handling of tapes is no longer required. We think that this workflow has contributed significantly to the good acceptance of our system because, in the long run, a system will only succeed if it makes the doctors' work easier instead of harder. This fact and other aspects, such as the extent of the radiological vocabulary and the ease of integration, finally led to the selection of a speech recognition software solution which did not require additional special hardware components.

Another crucial aspect is the complete networking capability of the system. Dictation, correction and electronic validation should be possible independently on every PC in the speech recognition network. The vocabulary, including newly learned words, and the "list of ConTexts" are up-to-date available for all workstations in a central database.

Software solution, integration, working method

The speech recognition system (SpeechMagic™ from Philips) was installed at the KFJ as a completely integrated component of a new installation of a HIS/RIS/PACS system (Radiology Information System MagicSAS® and Picture Archiving and Communicating System Sienet®, both from Siemens) in the spring of 1998, the first installation of its kind worldwide. The hospital's HIS/RIS interface makes it possible for referring departments to retrieve and print radiology reports directly on their HIS terminals, and to check on the current status of the examination and the report. Since the introduction of the speech recognition system more than 500.000 reports of one or more examinations were produced and transferred in this way. The integration of speech recognition into the newly installed RIS/PACS system was characterized by efficiency and high synergy. The speech recognition software is now used by all 15 radiologists and 7 residents routinely. In the meantime 35 staff and guest doctors have worked with the system.

Although not absolutely necessary, every new user should perform an initial training of only a few minutes by reading a short given text. The phonetic material collected during this training is then automatically processed by the system, resulting in an acoustic reference file adapted to the speech characteristics of the individual user.

Users dictate with their normal, individual speech rhythm and natural pronunciation. Thanks to the individual reference files, different accents or dialects are no problem. There is no need to speak more slowly or with exaggerated pronunciation; on the contrary, this has a negative impact on speech recognition.

Factors of influence for a high recognition rate are a constant volume during dictation and the same distance to the microphone (about 3 to 10 inches). This takes a little while to get used to, but with some discipline in microphone handling, the recognition rate can be quickly optimized.

The system can also be adapted individually to background noise. A special software tool can be used to determine optimal values for the recording and playback volumes, the microphone input level and the recording threshold level. With help of this tool three profiles for different background noise levels can be stored in the RIS for every user and workstation (e.g. low, normal and high background noise). The tool has the distinctive advantage that it eliminates the sometimes very sensitive disruptive influence of different sound card properties. This is automatically compensated by varying the amplification of input signals.

Hardware requirements and operating system

In the beginning we used only Pentium® 166 MMX™ PCs for our reporting workstations and Pentium® II PCs for our three speech recognition servers. This configuration was sufficient. However, since it was not possible to use sound file compression algorithms which require higher computing power, the transfer time between speech recognition server and correction PC was prolonged, and the network was heavily loaded. These PCs also became quite slow when handling large sound files for multiple reports. After upgrading our hardware to Pentium® III, and a few months ago to Pentium®IV systems, performance increased significantly, thus making the workflow much faster. Now there are no considerable delays when proofreading reports while listening to the sound files, which in turn "boosted" the motivation of users because the "hourglass" would be especially nerve-wrecking in stress situations. These computers are also well suited for online recognition where the dictation can (optionally) be recognized locally on the reporting PC, without transfer of sound files to the central speech recognition server. The operating system for our speech recognition and RIS network is Windows 2000®.

We use a special, commercially available microphone, which has buttons like a dictation device as well as a small, built-in loudspeaker, trackball and mouse buttons (SpeechMike™ from Philips). A headset may be used as an alternative. Theoretically we could also use small mobile dictation devices, which would not bind us to a PC while making a report. However, this would complicate the RIS workflow in our institute, because during dictation we emphasize a strong link between a sound file, the corresponding examination and patient identification (as guaranteed by the complete integration of speech recognition into HIS/RIS/PACS). In a pure speech recognition and text processing system, however, mobile dictation may be quite useful.

During editing, listening to the dictation is possible by means of earphones or the built-in PC loudspeakers. Secretaries may also use the traditional foot pedals or just the PC mouse for synchronizing speech and text.

Handling and workflow

In the case of an existing HIS/RIS system with several reporting workplaces, the speech recognition system should be completely integrated rather than planned as a stand-alone solution. In our hospital, the request for an x-ray examination is entered via HIS by the referring clinical department and automatically transferred to RIS. This induces a set of consecutive actions based on individual worklists, starting with the request for the patient's transport, afterwards the examination, and finally the patient's return transport. After a quality check by the doctor, the radiographer receipts the examination or individual services performed. In this way, the patient appears in the room or organ worklist for reporting; these lists are user-specific and can be retrieved and edited on every RIS PC [4].

After the examination requested for the patient has been selected – simply by clicking an entry in the worklist – dictation/reporting with the speech recognition system can be activated. The radiologist starts the dictation using the special microphone as described above. As with all types of dictation devices, the doctor can stop the dictation during reporting, listen to the recording, and correct it by re-recording. As with digital dictation devices, sentences or text passages may be inserted or deleted at any position of the dictation (Fig. 1). Punctuation and formatting commands may also be dictated; these are processed by the system. Standard report text components or autotext entries can be integrated in addition to speech recognition, depending on the range of diagnoses.

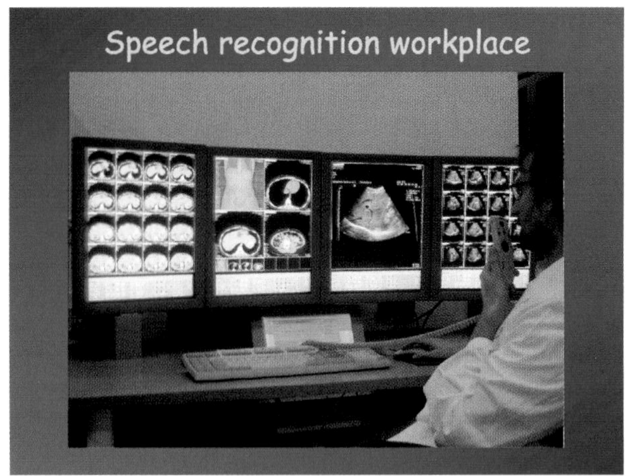

Fig. 1. Reporting and speech recognition workplace

As soon as the dictation is finished, the recorded sound file is automatically transferred to the recognition process at one of our three central speech recognition servers. The time needed for batch recognition depends on the length of the dictation, but also on the current load on the speech recognition server by simultaneously dictating colleagues; usually we dictate several reports one after the other, and it takes less than 60 seconds for the first to complete the recognition process. During editing of the first the following will also have passed the recognition process and are therefore available without delay.

The text document can then be retrieved at any speech recognition workstation and corrected with or without simultaneously listening to the sound file. It is essential to correct the document carefully because the speech recognition system is able to learn and expand its vocabulary. In contrast to some other systems, the changes are analyzed automatically, and incorrectly recognized words do not have to be dictated again. During correction, only recognition errors of the system may be corrected; sentences or words which were not dictated may not be inserted during this correction process. This would lead to an incorrect matching with phonetic sequences, and thus decrease the recognition rate of the respective user.

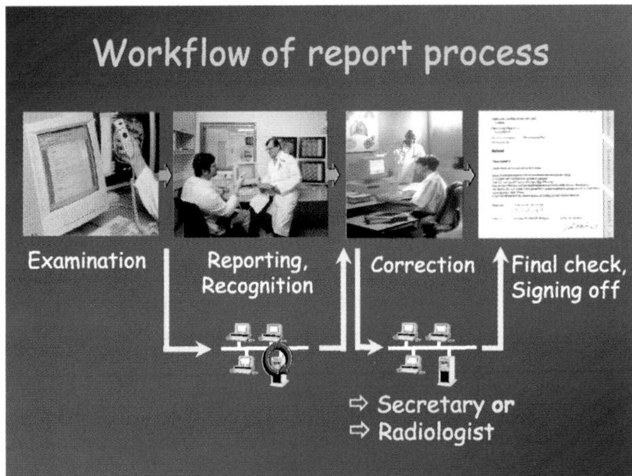

Fig. 2. Workflow of report process

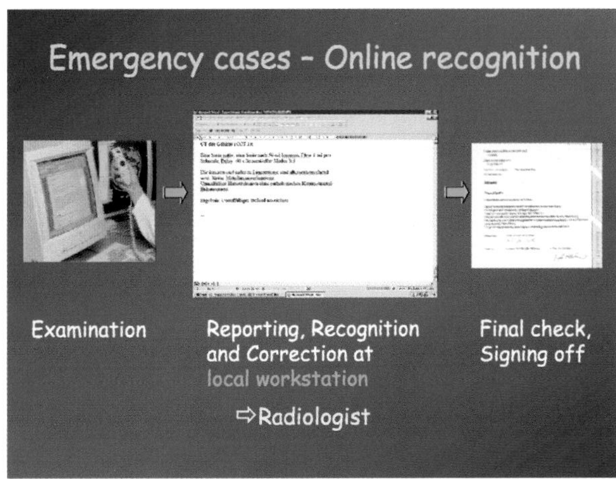

Fig. 3. Workflow with online speech recognition

After correction is completed, the text document is copied automatically into a new Microsoft® Word document based on the appropriate report template into which the patient's data and referral information are automatically inserted. Now is the time, if required, for adapting the lay-out, adding text, changing word order or replacing words. If the radiologist has corrected the recognized dictation himself, he now can validate the report by automatically adding his scanned signature, provided that he is authorized by the system to sign this type of examination. The reporting and validation rights are updated every month and assigned to individual persons. After the report has been validated, it is automatically transferred via the HIS/RIS network to the referring clinical department where every authorized doctor can display and if necessary print it on a HIS PC. At the same time, the validated report is stored in the common RIS/PACS database. If a secretary has made the correction and finalized the layout, the patient's report appears in the worklist of the doctor who has made the report. He can then update it, if required, and perform validation as described above (Fig. 2).

A validated report cannot be changed; if an addendum is needed, an additional, clearly marked corrected report must be made and validated in the usual way.

Newer software releases of this professional system also include the possibility of online recognition, where the recognized text is displayed in real time on the screen (Fig. 3); this feature is very useful in emergency cases by improving workflow. However it should only be an option, because for routine patients, we do not think that doctors should take over the secretaries' work. Neither we want the speech recognition process to distract us from our real work (i.e. reading images and making diagnosis). Furthermore, space on the RIS monitors, which are set up besides the PACS terminals, should continue to be reserved for previous reports and other medical data.

Continuous maintenance tasks

During correction of the recognized reports the individual acoustic reference files are continuously adapted by comparing the saved sound files with the corrected texts. The new acoustic reference files are better than the initial acoustic reference files which were created after initial training, this improves the recognition rate considerably [1, 2].

Our system administrator has the small task (altogether 30 minutes) of training new users, which includes initial training and the creation of an individual acoustic reference file, entering the individual user rights into the RIS system, and applying software updates. The system administrator is also responsible for supporting the entire RIS/PACS, speech recognition and the HIS interface.

The speech recognition system has an active vocabulary of up to 128,000 words, and about 500,000 words in a background dictionary. Depending on the amount of dictations, the active vocabulary is adapted approximately once every week. During this process, the system automatically adds words to the vocabulary which have been entered by secretaries or doctors during correction and which are unknown to the system. After control-reading by our secretaries to sort out spelling mistakes, they are available for all users. During ConText Adaptation the user-specific language model is also updated. In this way, the vocabulary is constantly enlarged.

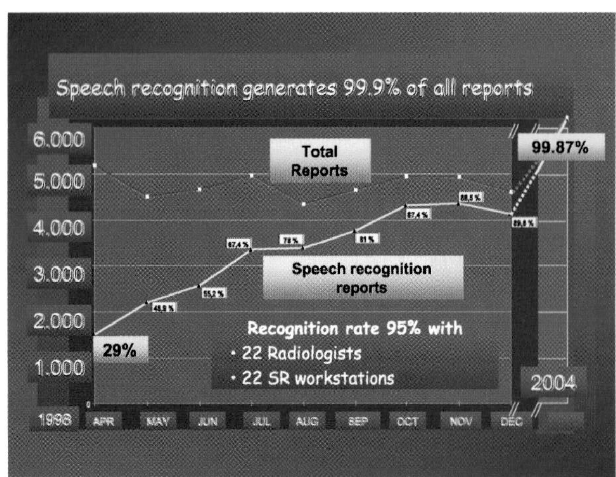

Fig. 4. Reports made with speech recognition

Results

The speech recognition system was installed in March 1998. During the first few weeks about one third of reports were generated using speech recognition. From the beginning the system was used on a voluntary basis, which means that every doctor was free to work with either the speech recognition software or traditional tapes. Originally the aim was to use the technology for about two thirds of all reports. During the first few months the system became more and more popular, so that the target was already exceeded in July 1998. 99.9% of all reports are now generated by means of speech recognition (Fig. 4). Currently the average recognition rate of all 22 dictating doctors is 95%!

To test the efficiency and productivity increase due to the software, we performed numerous measurements of the time required to generate the reports. These measurements proved that in our department speech recognition helped to shorten the average time between end of dictation and electronic validation of the signed report with automated electronic distribution from 10.5 to 6.5 hours, which means that 95% of reports are completed within one day. Our colleagues in the clinical departments appreciate this time gain very much, because in many cases it reduces the therapeutic reaction time and thereby often shortens the average hospital stay of patients.

The productivity increase of secretaries was also investigated. We tested secretaries who had more than 20 years of transcription experience at our institute. Even so, they were 40% faster using this technology compared to typing reports from dictations recorded on tape. As a result, at least one of the five persons, who had worked in the typing pool, is now available for other important administrative tasks in our department.

Table 3. Results

Results
• Used for 99.9% of all reports • Average recognition rate 95% (22 doctors) • Average time from dictation until validation shortened from 10.5 to 6.5 hours • 95% of reports sent out within one day • Transcription/correction time decreased by 40%

Acceptance

After the speech recognition software had been implemented and thoroughly tested, all users of the system were questioned anonymously by independent interviewers. 18 out of 20 radiologists said that they preferred speech recognition to traditional dictation. They especially appreciated that there was no need to handle tapes, referrals and paper-reports any more as well as to be able to produce final reports instantly and independently from secretaries, especially during nights and weekends. The users however also mentioned a small additional effort for radiologists because the introduction of the RIS system required them to carry out administrative tasks on the PC, such as selecting an examination for reporting or marking a report after dictation. On the other hand RIS also makes work much easier by providing legible referrals, clearly arranged worklists, and instant access to additional patient data and previous reports.

All five secretaries also preferred editing after speech recognition to traditional typing! Although they voiced vague fears that this technology might lead to loss of jobs, they were not afraid of losing their own job. They appreciated their new job profile and considered their work to be more interesting. Physical complaints such as back pains and tense shoulder muscles due to hours of typing have improved dramatically due to the new method in which reports were mainly proofread with the help of the recorded dictations and corrected if required. Not least, the secretaries appreciate the reduced stress level because they do not find hundreds of dictations to be typed out urgently after weekends or busy night shifts.

Conclusion

The production of reports by means of speech recognition has become daily routine at our department.

It works flawlessly and stable, and has so far proved itself with more than 500.000 reports of one or multiple examinations. The system is easy to operate and does not force users to change their dictation styles significantly. Above all, doctors can dictate reports as quickly as before, and if necessary produce final reports independently of a secretary's or transcriptionist's time schedule. The productivity of our secretaries has increased while working conditions have improved significantly. This technology has drastically shortened the time until completion of our reports, which means better service for our customers (patients and referring physicians) and raised the quality of our department's work. Acceptance is excellent, both by radiologists and secretaries. We are convinced that speech recognition is state-of-the-art technology right now.

References

[1] Arndt H, Petersein J, Stockheim D, Gregor P, Hamm B, Mutze S (1999) Anwendung der digitalen Spracherkennung in der radiologischen Routine. Fortschr Röntgenstr (Stuttgart New York) 171: 400–404

[2] Hundt W, Stark O, Scharnberg B, Hold M, Kohz P, Lienemann A, Bonel H, Reiser M (1999) Speech processing in radiology. Eur Radiol (Berlin Heidelberg) 9: 1451–1456

[3] Kumpan W, Karnel F, Brüll T, Nics G, Rödler H, Wolffhardt R, Zolles C (1999) Handling a growing workload with natural speech recognition. In: ECR'99 Scientific Programme and Abstracts Supplement 1 to Vol. 9 European Radiology. Springer, Berlin Heidelberg, pp 335–336

[4] Kumpan W, Karnel F, Nics G (1999) 18 months experience with an integrated radiology system: HIS-RIS-SPEECH-PACS. In: Lemke HU, Vannier MW, Inamura K, Farman AG (eds) CARS'99 Computer Assisted Radiology and Surgery Proceedings of the 13th International Congress and Exhibition, Elsevier Science B.V., Amsterdam Lausanne New York Oxford Shannon Singapore Tokyo, pp 524–528

[5] Mrosek B, Grünupp A, Keppel E, Kunzmann S, Moese G, Mohr K, Stargardt A, Günther RW (1993) Computergestützte Spracherkennung und Ausdruck von Röntgenbefunden. Fortschr Röntgenstr (Stuttgart New York) 159 (5): 481–483

[6] Rosenthal DI, Chew FS, Dupuy DE, Kattapuram SV, Palmer WE, Yap RM, Levine LA (1998) Computer-Based Speech Recognition as a Replacement for Medical Transcription. AJR 170: 23–25

[7] Schwartz LH, Kijewski P, Hertogen H, Roossin PS, Castellino RA (1997) Voice recognition in radiology reporting. AJR 169: 27–29

[8] Teichgräber UKM, Ehrenstein T, Lemke M, Liebig T, Stobbe H, Hosten N, Keske U, Felix R (1999) Digitale Spracherkennung bei der Erfassung computertomographischer Befundtexte. Fortschr Röntgenstr (Stuttgart New York) 171: 396–399

[9] Ybinger T, Kumpan W, Karnel F, Bruell T (2002) Long-term experience with speech recognition of more than 300,000 dictations. Radiology [Suppl] 225: 504

Physiological tests and functional diagnosis with digital methods

R. Rienmüller and U. Reiter

Department of Radiology, Graz University Hospital, Austria

Introduction

The introduction and the continuous improvement of digital imaging techniques as digital radiography, computed tomography, magnetic resonance and ultrasound with permanent shortening of the image exposure time enable not only qualitative morphological statements but also functional analysis as quantification of function, bloodflow and perfusion basically of all organs. It may be expected that the simultaneous evaluation of morphological structures and their function may improve not only our understanding of organ function and disease mechanism but may also contribute to the earlier recognition and better staging of various organ disorders as it was already mentioned by Sir Arthur Keath in 1918: "Structure is a sure guide to function. There is no understanding of the function as long we don't understand all parts of the structures" (and vice versa) [8].

As the above named imaging methods are based on different physical processes, they may differ in the quality of morphological statements but they are, however, similar in their potential of functional information. Therefore, in the following we will concentrate on the evaluation of functional statements available by the application of just one imaging method as electron beam tomography and here again on the functional status of the lung and the heart where the authors do have most practical experience.

Principle of electron beam tomography

In contrast to conventional, spiral, multi-volume and multi-detector CT systems, the Electron Beam Tomography does have 4 stationary X-ray tubes and 2 detectors and therefore it is possible to achieve single images by 50 and/or 100 ms exposure time with a frequency up to 34 images per second (real time imaging) [4,17].

Pulmonary function

The introduction of High Resolution CT-studies (HRCT) of the lungs in the daily clinical work-up dramatically improved the sensitivity and specificity for early detection and identification especially of diffuse pulmonary disease.

However the qualitative detection and identification of the diseased lungs and the reproducibility of the assessment of pulmonary CT-values may be hampered by inconstancy of lung inflation because of varying inspiration levels of the patients [3,13]. This problem may be overcome by applying a spirometrically defined and controlled constant level of inspiration during HRCT-scanning of awake patients.

Because of the short exposure time using EBT it is additionally possible to scan patients lung during breathing activities and at exercise (stress) tests.

Theoretical remarks

As most CT-voxels consist of various amounts of air, lung parenchyma, blood, lung fluid, interstitial tissue and sediments (Fig. 1) the measured CT-values represent "effective" CT-values, implying the need for histogram CT-value analysis. Comparative evaluation of the histograms of CT-values distribution versus pulmonary functional data reveal that it is possible to identify four CT-value intervals [14,15] (Table 1).

Interval A showed the best positive correlation with pulmonary Total Gas Volume, Interval B the best positive correlation with pulmonary O_2-Diffusion Capacity, Interval C showed no correlation with any of the pulmonary functional tests and Interval D showed negative correlation with pulmonary O_2-Diffusion Capacity (opposite to interval B). Thereby Interval A is reflecting the percentage of free air as an "Index of Emphysema", Interval B the percentage of "normal" lung parenchyma, Interval C the percentage of lung fluid and Interval D the percentage of interstitial tissue, described as "Pulmonary, Fluid and Interstitial Index".

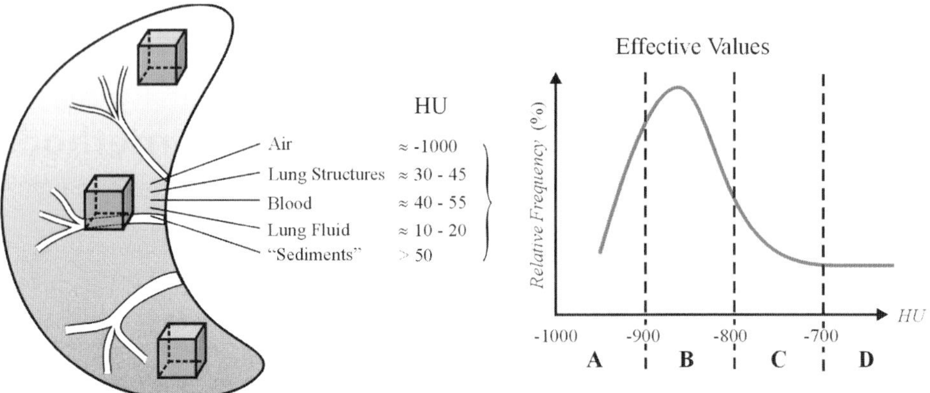

Fig. 1. Relationship between CT values and CT histogram of the lung [14]

Table 1. Significant correlation of lung function data with mean CT-density value and frequencies of CT-density values at defined intervals A, B, C and D

		Vital capacity (% pred.)	Diffusing capacity (% pred.)	Exercise PaO_2 (mmHg)	Intrathoric gas volume (% pred.)	Specific resistance (kPa s)
Mean CT-density Value (HU)		r = −0.57	r = −0.34	r = −0.44	r = −0.54	r = n.s.
Frequency (%) of CT-density value at intervals						
A	<900 (HU)	r = n.s.	r = n.s.	r = n.s.	r = −0.73	r = −0.48
B	−899 ⋯ −800 (HU)	r = 0.69	r = 0.63	r = 0.68	r = n.s.	r = n.s.
C	−799 ⋯ −700 (HU)	r = −0.26	r = n.s.	r = −0.34	r = −0.39	r = n.s.
D	>−699 (HU)	r = −0.56	r = −0.4	r = −0.47	r = −0.43	r = n.s.

Obstructive pulmonary function is characterized by a histogram curve showing increase of CT value frequencies in interval A and a reduced CT value frequencies in interval B. Restrictive pulmonary function is characterized by a histogram curve showing increase of CT value frequencies in interval D and a reduced CT value frequencies in interval B. A combination of obstructive and restrictive pulmonary function is characterized by a histogram curve showing increase of CT value frequencies in interval A and D and a reduced CT value frequencies in interval B. CT value frequencies in interval C is increased by pulmonary fluid overload causing a shifting of the histogram curve from left to right and vice versa depending on the amount of pulmonary fluid.

Method

For HRCT studies of the lungs with histogram analysis the following protocol [3,7,15] is used in our department:

1. HRCT of the lungs.
2. Spirometrically controlled scans of the upper lungs (5 cm above the carina, at 50% of the actually measured vital capacity) the middle lungs (at the level of carina, at 20, 50 and 80% of the actually measured vital capacity) and the lower lungs (5 cm below the carina, at 50% of the actually measured vital capacity) and additionally at any level of interest.
3. Spirometrically controlled breathing cycle from maximal expiration to maximal inspiration to maximal expiration with time defined scanning.
4. Spirometrically controlled scans of the middle lungs at 50% of the actually measured vital capacity at rest, after putting legs up, at treadmill-test at 0, 50 and 100 W.

Clinical examples of functional impairment

The following three examples should demonstrate that by using digital imaging technologies and applying the method of CT value measurements and histogram analysis it is possible to identify fluid overload at rest and stress test to distinguish between dyspnoe caused by emphysema or left heart failure and to identify those parts of lungs which participate on breathing and that way on gas exchange from

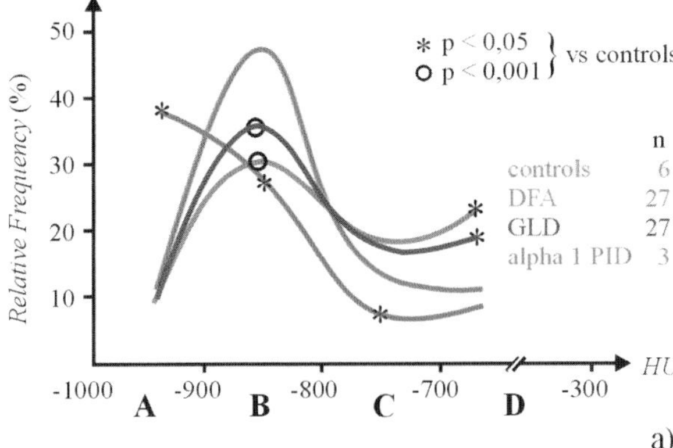

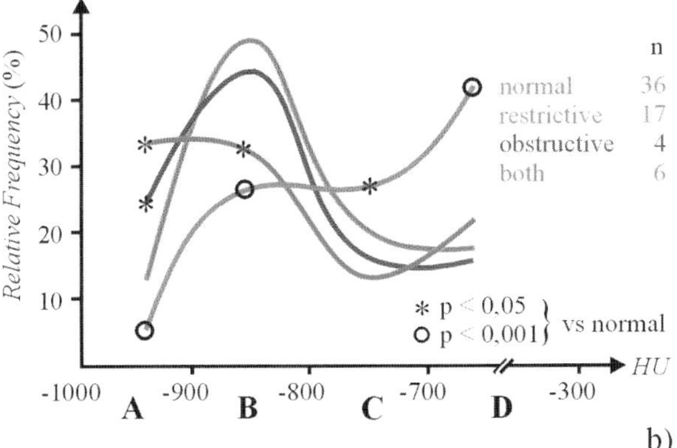

Fig. 2. Distribution of CT-values (HU) in inspiration at 50% of vital capacity [15]; **a** in man with different, however morphologically well defined pulmonary disease; **b** at various pulmonary functional status in man

those which don't and to contribute to the differential diagnosis of the various causes of the reduced diffusing capacity.

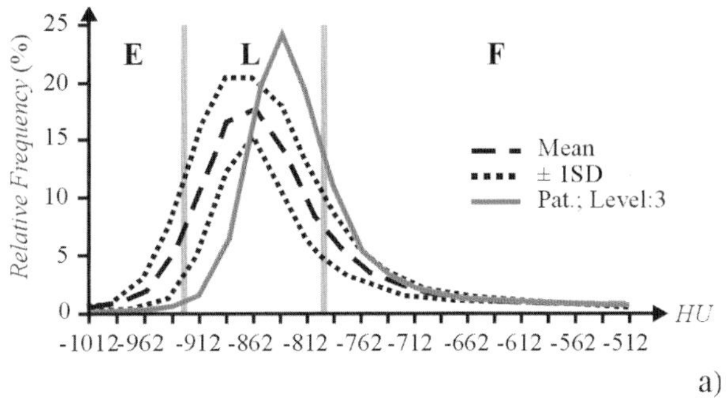

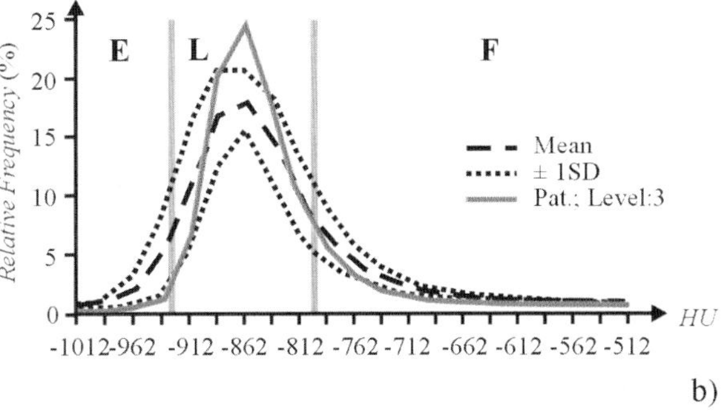

Fig. 3. CT-histogram of the lung [13] (healthy normals: VC ≥ 80% predicted, SR ≤ 1 kPa s); **a** patient before hemodialysis and **b** after hemodialysis with a lost of 2.5 l of fluid

The first female patient after left sided lung transplantation because of bilateral severe bullouse emphysema was studied by CT in high resolution mode at 50% inspiration of the actually measured vital capacity. The HRCT image 5 cm above the diaphragm is morphologically showing diffuse bullouse emphysema at the right side without any interstitial changes. At the left side there is

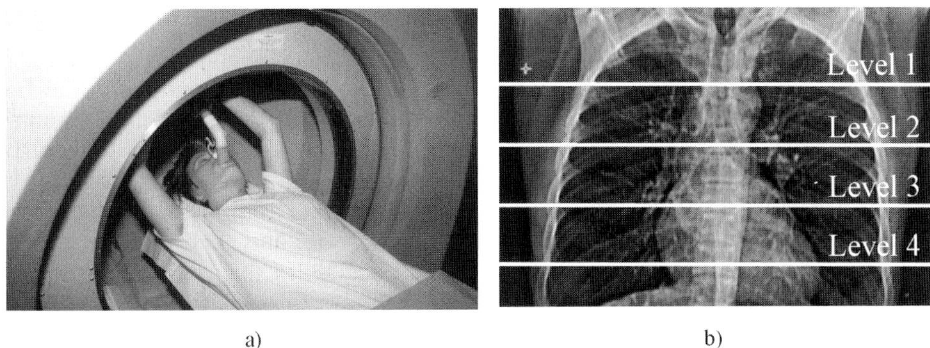

Fig. 4. **a** CT study with spirometrically controlled inspiration level; **b** scan levels at the carina, 5 cm above and below and an additional 4th level because of thorax oversize [7]

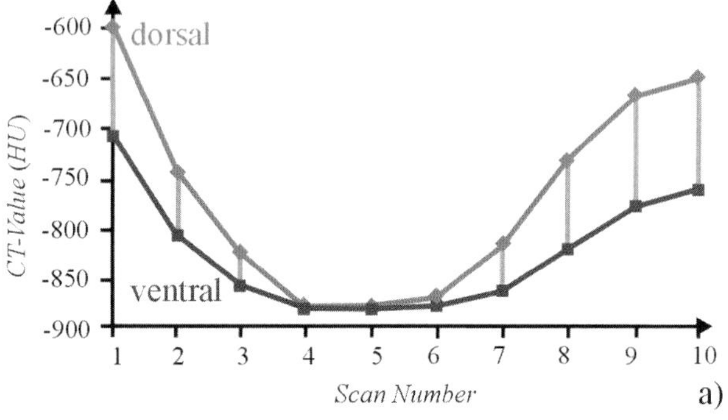

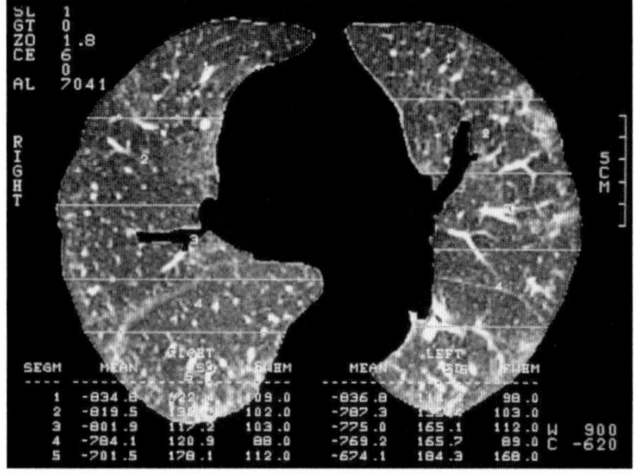

Fig. 5. CT-values during spirometrically controlled breathing cycle in the anterior and posterior segments of the lungs; **a** CT scan of the lungs at the level of carina after segmentation of non pulmonary structures with defined anterior and posterior segments of the lungs; **b** from maximal expiration to maximal inspiration to maximal expiration

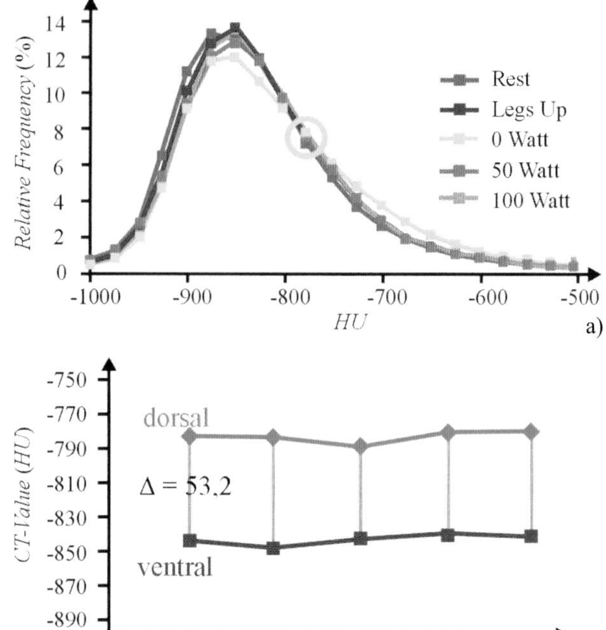

Fig. 6. a CT-histograms of the lung in healthy adults in inspiration at 50% of the actual measured and controlled vital capacity at rest and after stress tests. **b** Dorso ventral difference of CT values of the lung at rest with legs up, 0, 50 and 100 W stress test

an increase of the number and diameter of the pulmonary vessels and of the amount of pulmonary fluid increasing from the ventral to the posterior (dependent) part of the lungs. Also the interlobulary septum is thickened because of fluid overload. 60.9% of the right sided lung are emphysematically changed. The amount of normal lung parenchyma is reduced to 30.3% and there is no evidence of volume overload or interstitial disease as the index is reduced to 9.1% (Fig. 7b). After transplantation the left sided lung is showing normal index of emphysema (3%). The index of normal lung parenchyma increased from previous 30% to 43.5%. This just slight increase of the normal parenchyma increase is compromised by blood volume overload of approximately 40% (see Fig. 7b and 7c: 53.5–9.1%). There is no increase of interstitial indices or tissue.

As a second example a 65 years old male with known severe emphysema and dyspnoe at rest, who started to complain about increasing dyspnoe and discomfort at usual physical activities is demonstrated. The three HRCT images of the lungs, shown in Fig. 8a, performed 5 cm below the carina at 20%, 50% and 80% inspiration level of the actually measured vital capacity don't show any morphological changes of the pulmonary structures and also nearly no changes of pulmonary CT values because of severe emphysema. With putting legs up and with physical stress tests with 0, 50 and 100 W the ECG did not show any ST-segment changes as could be expected in coronary heart disease. In the simultaneous performed CT study of the chest the dorso ventral CT gradient was found to be enlarged at rest because of the known severe emphysema. However, already by putting legs up, and even more by treadmill-stress test, CT values of the ventral part of the lungs were found to decrease. As the volume of the lungs did not change, the decrease of the CT values is suggesting an increase of the pulmonary blood volume. This increase of blood volume may be explained by looking at the CT image at the same level

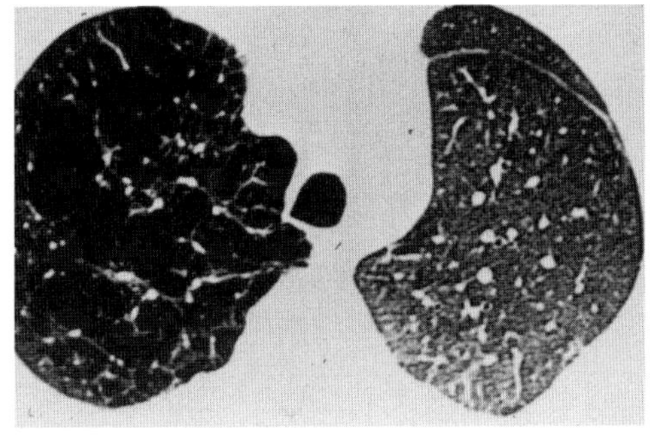

a)

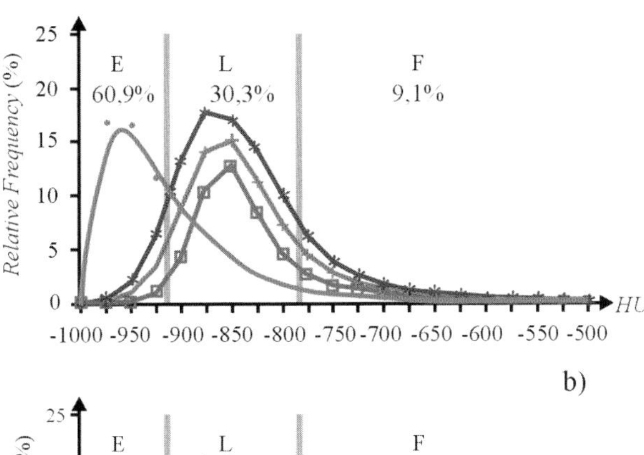

b)

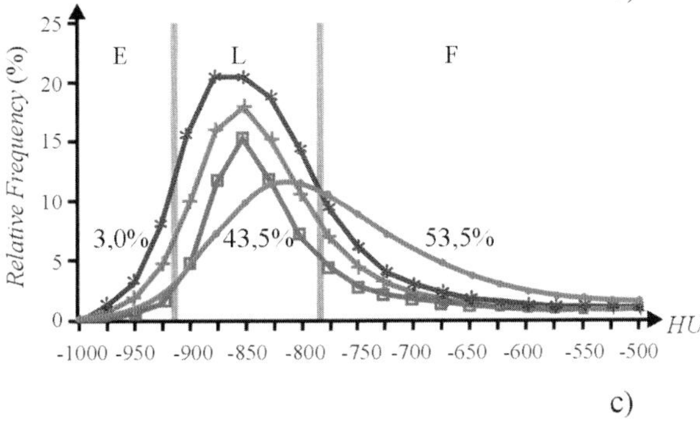

c)

Fig. 7. Patient after left sided lung tansplantation because of severe bilateral pulmonary emphysema. **a** CT 5 cm above carina at 50% inspiration level of the actual VC. **b** Histogram analysis of CT value distribution of the right lungs with severe emphysema. The blue curve represents the histogram of the patient, the three other curves are the reference curve of healthy volunteers (red curve) and the area of a single standard deviation (green/dark blue curve). **c** Histogram analysis of CT value distribution of the left lungs after lung transplantation

in mediastinal window showing calcified LAD as a symptom of coronary heart disease (Fig. 6b).

The last example shows a 68 years old patient with left heart failure, bilateral pleural effusion, emphysema and progredient reduction of diffusing capacity. The CT scans 5 cm below carina at 50% inspiration level of actual measured VC in pulmonary

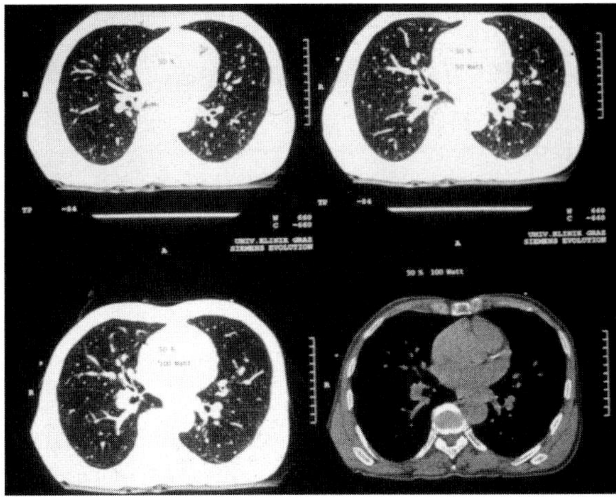

a)

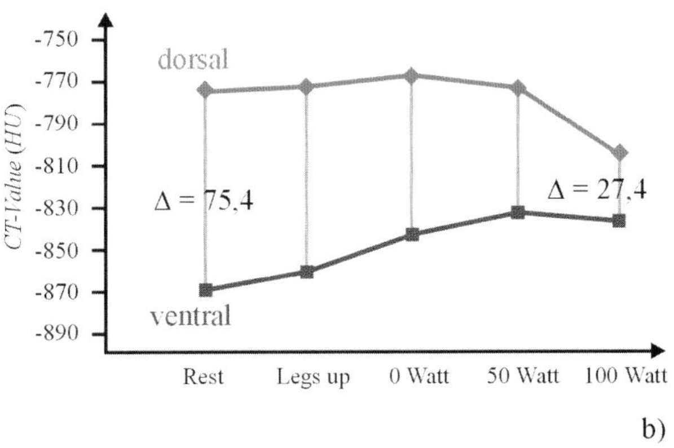

b)

Fig. 8. 65 years old male with dyspnoe and chest pain at stress **a** CT scans 5 cm below carina at 20, 50 and 80% inspiration level actual measured VC in pulmonary window and in mediastinal window showing calcified LAD. **b** Dorso ventral difference of CT values of the lung at rest with legs up, 0, 50 and 100 W stress test showing pulmonary emphysema and increasing fluid overload at stress (see for comparison Fig. 6b)

window is showing inhomogeneous distribution of mainly bullouse emphysema and pulmonary venous congestion with calcified LAD and circumflex and bilateral pleural effusion.

The dorso ventral CT value difference is diminished at maximal expiration from 200 HU (see Fig. 5a) to 100 HU and does not reach zero CT value difference at maximal inspiration (see Fig. 9b). This is caused in part by pulmonary volume overload and in part by emphysema (see Fig. 9b).

Three days later (see Fig. 9c), with increasing volume overload due to progredient left heart failure, the CT value in the dorsal parts of the lungs don't change over the respiratory cycle. This means that the dorsal part of the lungs do not participate in

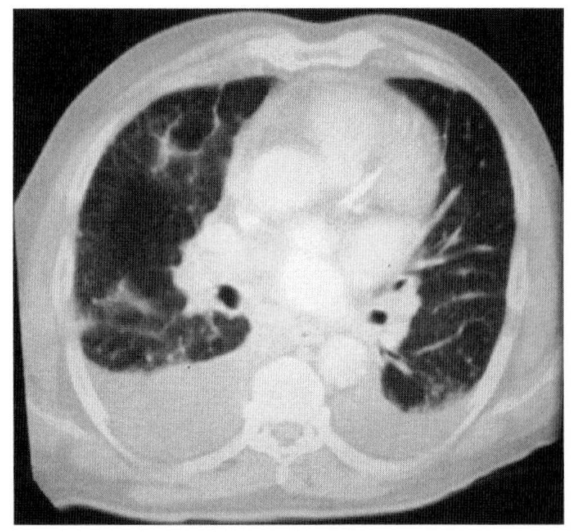

a)

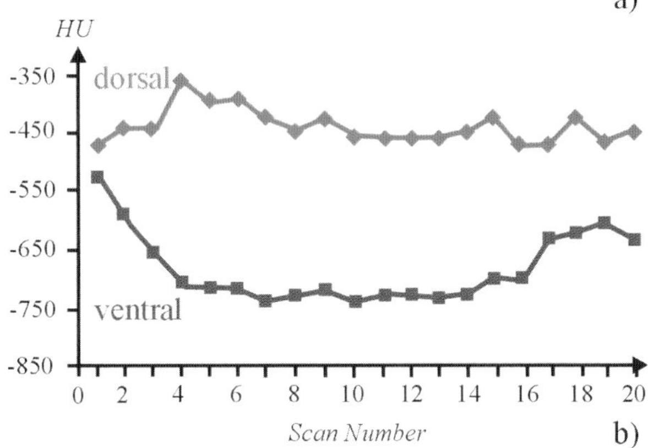

b)

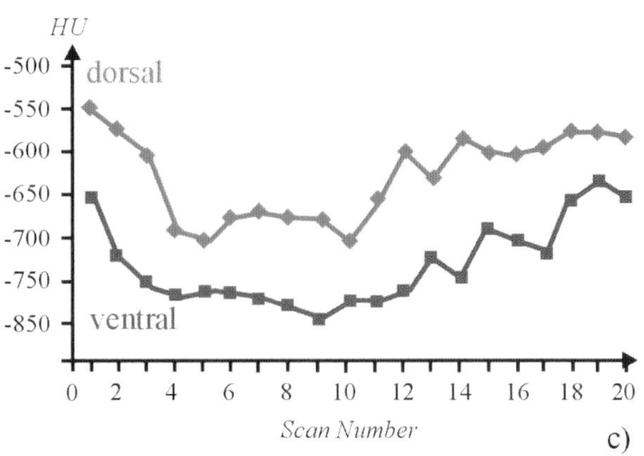

c)

Fig. 9. 68 years old patient with severe left heart failure and bilateral pleural effusion. **a** CT scans 5 cm below carina at 50% inspiration level of actual measured VC in pulmonary window. **b** Dorso ventral difference of CT values from maximal expiration to maximal inspiration to maximal expiration. **c** Dorso ventral difference of CT values from maximal expiration to maximal inspiration to maximal expiration 5 days later showing no CT value changes in the dorsal part of the lungs because of increasing left heart failure with pulmonary volume overload in the dependent part of the lungs (see for comparison Fig. 5c)

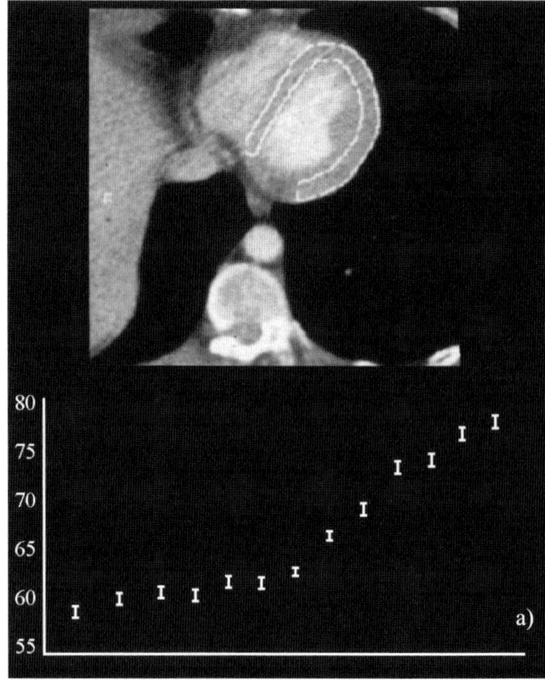

$$\text{Perfusion (ml/min/cm}^3\text{)} = \frac{\text{Max. Slope Myocardium Enhancement (dHU/dt)}}{\text{Max. ventricular Enhancement (dHU)}}$$

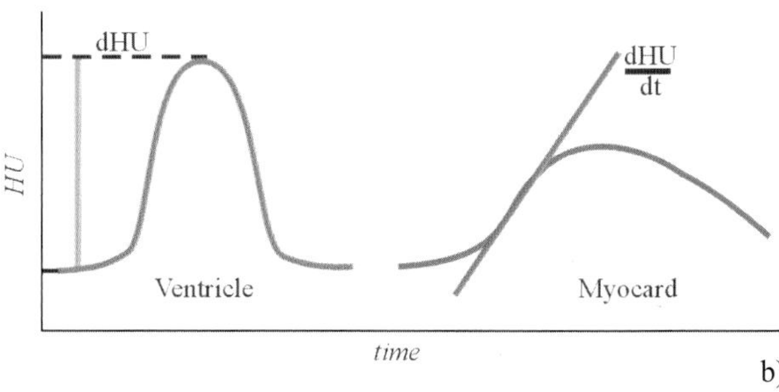

b)

Fig. 10. Myocardial blood flow measurement by EBT. **a** 50 ms EBT image at the left midventricular portion after i.v. contrast agent application. The region of interest drawn in the myocardial wall and the graph below shows the increase of CT values in the myocardial wall over time. **b** Principle of measuring and calculation of myocardial blood flow in ml/min/cm^3. The applied formula is based on a relationship given by Miles [10]

breathing, and therefore there is nearly no gas exchange explaining the reduction of the diffusing capacity, which is caused by volume overload as seen by the very high CT values of approximately −400 HU. Only the ventral part of the lungs show CT value changes over the respiratory cycle. That means only this part of the lungs participate in breathing activities. However, also here the gas exchange is reduced as this ventral CT value curve now is similar

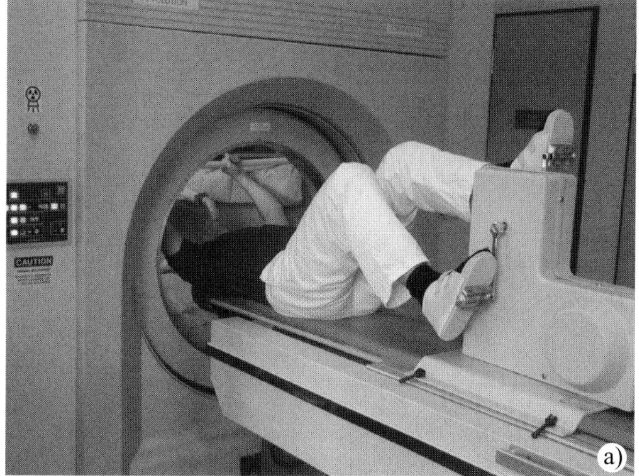

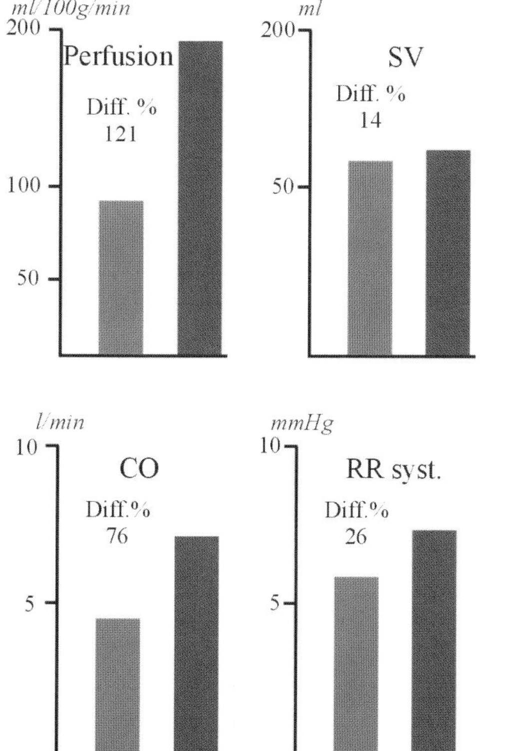

Fig. 11. Change of cardiac parameters in healthy volunteer before and after treadmill-stress test by doubling the heart rate. **a** EBT machine with patient at treadmill-stress test. **b** Cardiac parameters at rest and after stress test

to the one of the dorsal part of the lungs three days before (Fig. 9b).

Conclusion

Spirometrically standardized and controlled HRCT-studies of the lungs enable to quantify the amount of emphysema, of normal lung parenchyma, of pulmonary fluid and of interstitial tissue. The quantitative histogram analysis of these pulmonary CT-values provide objective quantitative data in the early diagnosis and staging of patients with diffuse pulmonary disease reflecting not only changes of pulmonary structures but also of pulmonary function impairments as obstruction, restriction and combination of obstruction and restriction. The analysis of CT values changes over the respiratory cycle enables to distinguish between various causes of reduced diffusing capacity of the lungs. As in patients with left heart failure the percentage of CT values for interstitial index and fluid index increases and the dorso ventral CT value difference decreases, this phenomenon may be used as a sensitive test for early, non invasive detection of left heart failure.

Cardiac function

Cardiac function is a complex process depending on nonlinear relationship of functional and morphological parameters. The functional parameters consist of preload, afterload contractility and heart rate which further depend on coronary blood flow, myocardial perfusion, myocardial metabolism and on morphological parameters as the state of peri-, myo- and endocardium, cardiac valves and coronary arteries as well as on form and content of cardiac cavities. A variety of systemic diseases, and/or thoracic processes may also influence cardiac function. Additionally extra- and intracardiac endocrine and neurohumoral mechanisms play also an important role [12].

The essential task of the heart is to maintain the pulmonary, the systemic and the cardiac circulation. As an organ the heart is able to compensate acute and chronic events or processes by using a variety of individually different adaptive, morphological and functional mechanisms. For this reason it is not surprising, that generally it is not sufficient to evaluate just one or only a few of the functional and morphological parameters [11].

Method

A four steps diagnostic approach was developed at the University of Graz, to study patients with suspected or known coronary heart disease. This protocol consists of:

1. Native single slice scan, 100 ms exposure time to identify and to measure the extent of coronary calcification.

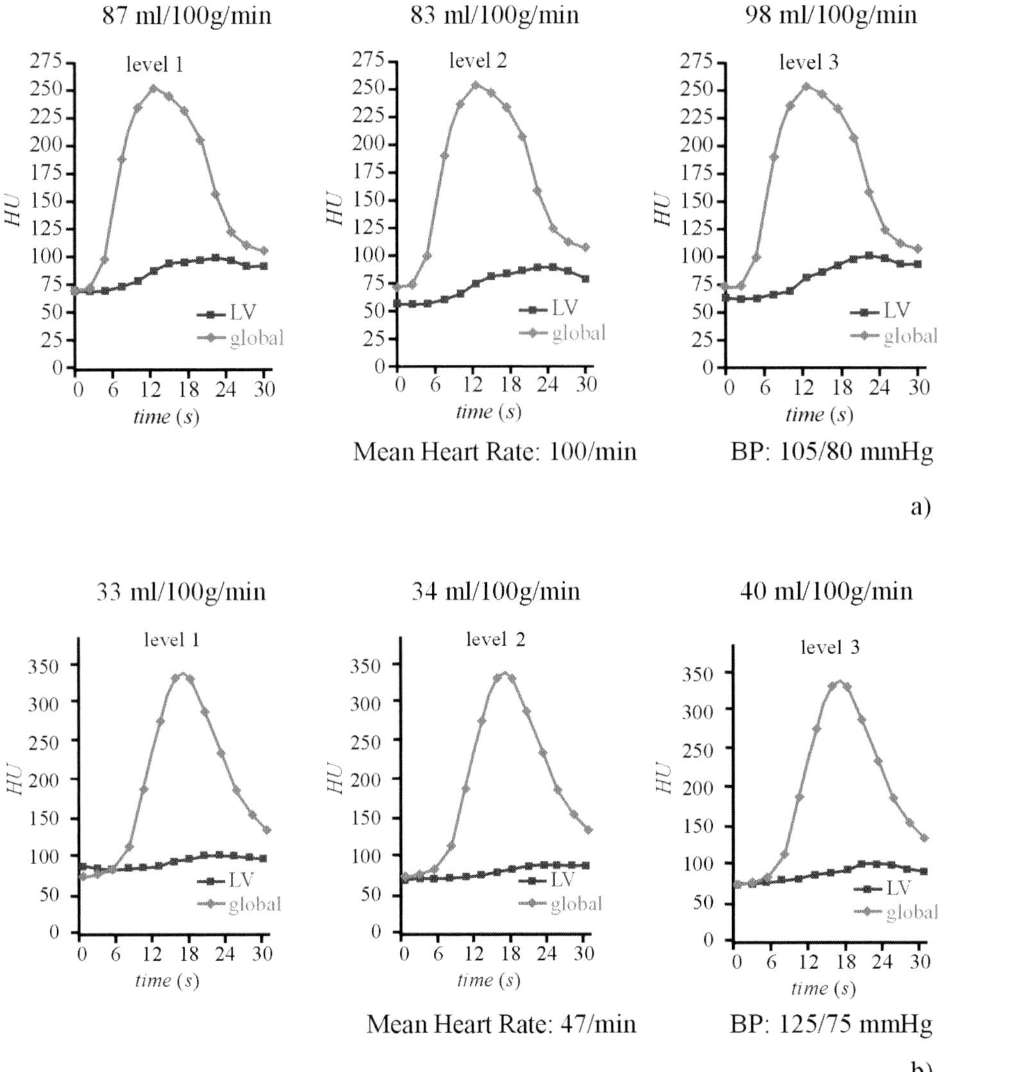

Fig. 12. Global myocardial blood flow at 3 different levels; **a** in a patient with diffuse coronary arterie disease and tachycardia; **b** in a patient without coronary heart disease and bradycardia

2. Multi slice scan, 50 ms exposure time and intravenous contrast agent application to measure myocardial blood flow.
3. Multi slice scan, 50 ms exposure time and intravenous contrast agent application to measure functional determinants as enddiastolic and endsystolic volumes, ejection fraction, left ventricular muscle mass and global and regional wall thickness changes over the cardiac cycles.
4. Single slice scan, 100 ms exposure time and intravenous contrast agent application to evaluate the morphological state of the proximal 4–6 cm of the subepicardial coronary arteries.

The EBT study of the individual patient to measure coronary calcification lasts approximately 5 min. The complete protocol of the EBT study lasts up to 30 min with an effective radiation dose of approximately 9 mSV and a need for up to 200 ml of intravenously applied contrast agent.

General statements about functional and morphological parameters of the heart as determined by EBT

Coronary atherosclerosis: In various studies it was shown that coronary artery calcification as seen by

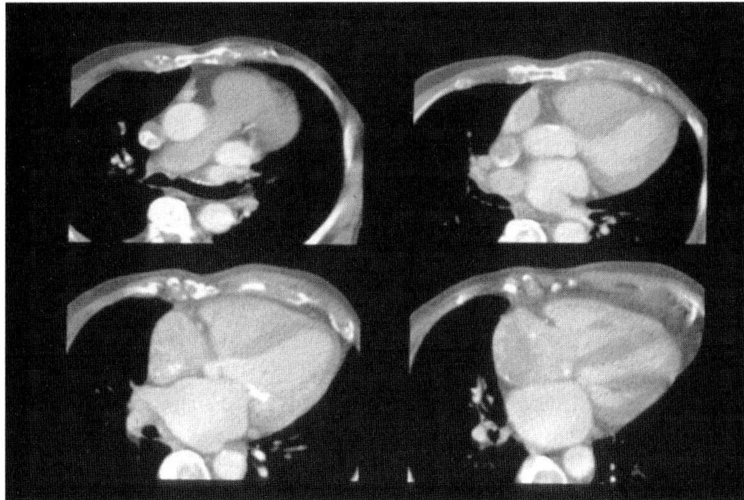

Fig. 13. 50 ms EBT images at 4 different cardiac levels for calculation of left ventricular volumes

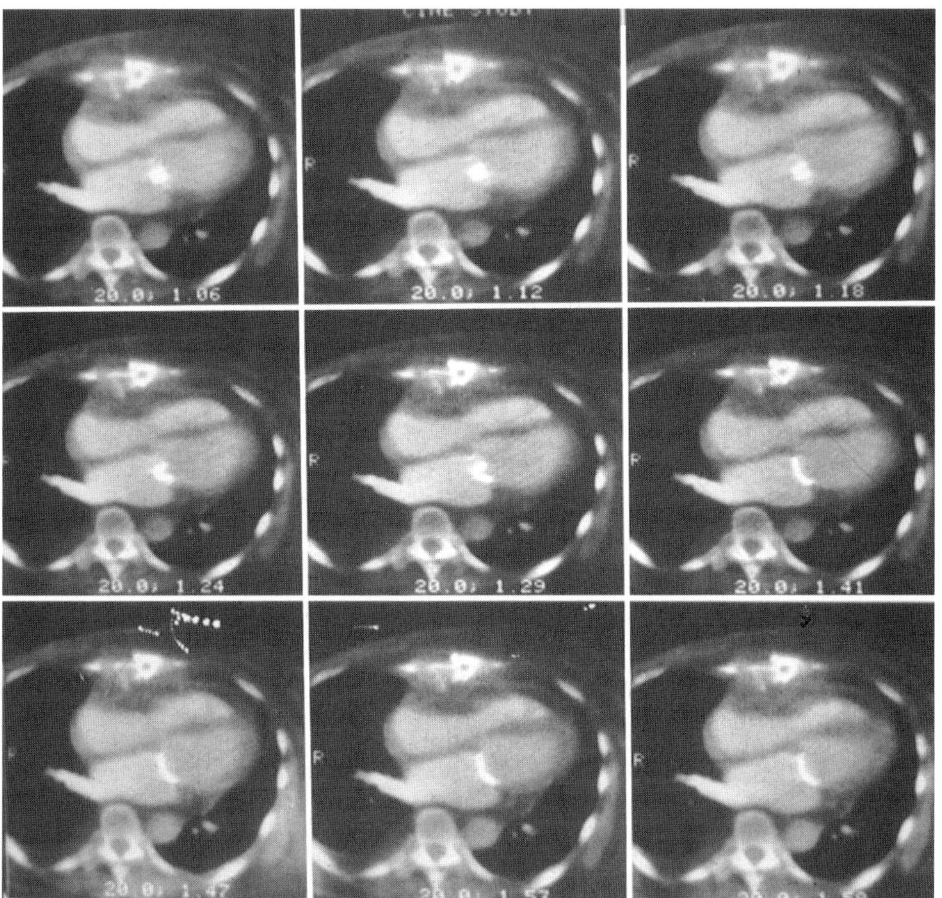

Fig. 14. Patient after mitral valve replacement imaged in multislice mode with 50 ms exposure time showing opening and closing of the mitral valve

EBT is always associated with coronary wall atheroma. Several studies demonstrated that the increasing amount of coronary calcification (Coronary Calcium Score) is accompanied by a parallel increase of the amount of "soft" atherosclerotic plaques. In our and in other studies was shown that independently of patient's age, with increasing coronary calcification score the probability having coronary artery stenotic lesions above 50% is continuously increasing. In patients after dilatation of coronary stenotic lesions the coronary calcium score predisposes to higher restenosis rate [18].

Myocardial blood flow: In experimental studies it was shown that there is a linear relationship between the myocardial blood flow measured with the bubble method versus EBT after intravenous contrast agent application [2,16].

In clinical studies (n > 1600) we could show:

- that it is possible to measure myocardial blood flow in a daily routine work
- the mean value of the "normal" myocardial blood flow at rest is 75 ± 10 ml/100 g/min
- by doubling the heart rate using treadmill test in "healthy" patients there is an increase of myocardial blood flow of about 100%
- in presence of just one coronary stenotic lesion above 50% (i.e. LAD) regional reduction of myocardial blood flow is frequently seen
- in patient with several diffuse stenotic lesions above 50% the myocardial blood flow may be in normal range if there is tachycardia and/or increase of cardiac output and/or increase of blood pressure
- in patients with bradycardia and/or low cardiac output and/or low blood pressure, reduced myocardial blood flow at rest may be found even with normal coronary arteries
- in patients after successful dilatation of significant LAD stenosis there may be an increase or decrease or no change of myocardial blood flow.

Left ventricular functional determinants: In experimental and in clinical studies it was shown that it is possible to measure enddiastolic volume, ejection fraction and left ventricular muscle mass in comparable quality as by cardiac ventriculography. Selecting the one level on the left ventricle showing the largest enddiastolic circumflex we can calculate the volumes using the formula of a rotating ellipsoid (2-Axis-Method).

$$\mathrm{EDV}\ [\mathrm{ml}] = \frac{\pi}{6}\mathrm{LM}^2 \qquad (1)$$

$$\mathrm{EF}\ [\%] = \frac{\mathrm{EDV} - \mathrm{ESV}}{\mathrm{EDV}} 100 \qquad (2)$$

$$\mathrm{LVMM}\ [\mathrm{g}] = (\mathrm{Total\ LV} - \mathrm{EDV})1.05 \qquad (3)$$

Coronary arteries: In our institution as well as in others it was demonstrated that after intravenous contrast agent application it is possible to evaluate the proximal 5–6 cm of the subepicardial coronary arteries (with regard to minimal changes, stenotic lesions above or below 50% and occlusion) with a quality comparable to coronary angiography. The negative predictive value for coronary stenotic lesions above 50% revealed to be 91–100% for EBT [1].

Clinical examples of functional impairment

The following two examples should demonstrate some of the real routine possibilities of fast digital technologies in studying two different "cardiac patients":

First one, after mitral valve replacement because of severe mitral stenosis. The images performed at the midventricular level (four chamber view) are showing not only the opening and closing of the artificial mitral valve but also the changes of the volume of both ventricles and of both atria as well as the changes of myocardial wall thickness over the cardiac cycle.

The second patient is a 73 years old man after myocardial infarction. The native scan showed coronary calcification at the LAD with a coronary calcification score of 142. After intravenous contrast agent application the complete heart was imaged again ECG gated with 100 ms exposure time at the 80% R–R-interval. A stenotic lesion above 50% at the proximal part of the LAD close to the above mentioned coronary calcification is visualised at Fig. 15a. In the "four chamber view" both ventricles and both atrias are of normal size and the left myocardial wall is showing normal wall thickness of the septum as well as of the anterior and posterior wall (Fig. 15b). At the cardiac level close to diaphragm there is still normal wall thickness of the septum and of the postero lateral wall of the left ventricle. However, at the apex there is no myocardium visible because of a small transmural myocardial infarction. The hemodynamic parameters received using the multi slice mode with 50 ms exposure time revealed normal endiastolic and stroke volume, normal ejection fraction and normal cardiac output. Left ventricular muscle mass was at upper limit and mass volume relationship increased. The global myocardial blood flow was in normal range regionally however reduced at the anterior wall to 60 cm^3/100 g/min (it is normal to have highest blood flow at the postero lateral wall and somehow lower at the septal wall

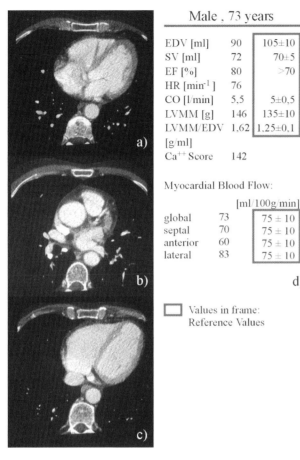

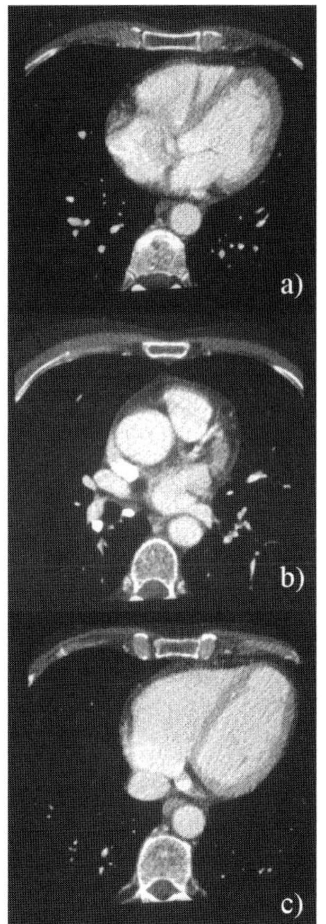

Male , 73 years

EDV [ml]	90	105±10
SV [ml]	72	70±5
EF [%]	80	>70
HR [min^{-1}]	76	
CO [l/min]	5,5	5±0,5
LVMM [g]	146	135±10
LVMM/EDV [g/ml]	1,62	1,25±0,1
Ca^{++} Score	142	

Myocardial Blood Flow:

		[ml/100g/min]
global	73	75 ± 10
septal	70	75 ± 10
anterior	60	75 ± 10
lateral	83	75 ± 10

d)

☐ Values in frame: Reference Values

Fig. 15. Patient with solitary stenotic lesion above 50% at the proximal LAD after transmural apical infarction. **a** Coronary calcification and stenotic lesion above 50% at the LAD. **b** Transmural apical infarction of left ventricular myocardium. **c** Normal wall thickness of interventricular septum anterior and posterior myocardial wall. **d** Functional parameters showing regional decrease of myocardial blood flow in the anterior myocardial wall

which is parallel to the different extent of wall thickness changes). This example demonstrates that by using digital technology with short exposure times it is possible to study the morphological and functional determinants of the heart under clinical conditions routinely as a "One-Stop-Shop".

Conclusion

Based on more than 1600 cardiac EBT studies using the above mentioned protocol it is possible like in an *"One-Stop-Shop"* to assess the extent of coronary atherosclerosis as Coronary Calcium Score (first part of the definition of coronary heart disease) to evaluate the degree, location and number of stenotic lesions in the proximal 5–6 cm of the coronary arteries, to determine the severity of coronary heart disease by measuring the global and regional myocardial blood flow (second part of the definition of coronary heart disease) and to measure the functional left ventricular parameters giving the information if they are still in normal range or changed either as a sequel of the coronary heart disease or as a compensatory mechanism to keep myocardial blood flow as adequate as possible with respect to the balance of oxygen supply and demand [5,6,9].

Conclusion

The demonstration of the functional results obtained by EBT with respect to pulmonary and cardiac function clearly demonstrate the progress which was achieved by shortening of the exposure time and by increasing the number of images per second. The simultaneous visualization of pulmonary and cardiac structures without overlapping reveals especially to be advantageous in comparison to projection radiography, giving the possibility to evaluate simultaneously the morphological determinants of pulmonary and cardiac function. These widely unexpected extremely positive EBT results till the year of 1998 in the early recognition of functional organ disorders encouraged and forced the manufacturers to look for further improvement of conventional CT and MRI technologies.

The present progress and developments in the area of EBT, of fast multi-volume multi-slice CT technology and in fast MR imaging techniques (diffusion, perfusion) are so dramatic that in the very near future these methods will completely revolutionize and change the approach of disclosing, proving and staging of functional and morphological changes in most of the human organs.

This will cause a complete change of the understanding of present radiology and present radiologists and will require profound knowledge of physiology and pathophysiology with direct access to treatment and to modeling of organ diseases combined with new forms of interdisciplinary collaborations.

Acknowledgements

The authors would like to thank Prof. Harnoncout for plenty of very helpful discussions in pneumological questions, Prof. Klein and Prof. Rigler for excellent collaboration in cardiac and cardio-surgical topics and Prof. H. Hutten and his coworkers for continuous technical advice and input. Further we would like to emphasize the important role of our "radiological team", especially Prof. Gröll, Dr. Schröttner, and Dr. Kern in daily clinical and scientific work.

References

[1] Aschauer M, Groell R, Schafhalter I, Rienmueller R, Graif E, Simbrunner J, Ebner B (1995) Coronary arteries: contrast enhanced elektron beam computed tomography (EBCT) versus conventional coronary angiography in the evaluation of stenosis. Card Interv Radiol 18 [Suppl 1]: 56

[2] Baumgartner C, Rienmüller R, Bongaerts A, Kern R, Harb S, Weihs W (1996) Measurements of myocardial perfusion using elektron beam computed tomography. Am J Card Imaging 10 [Suppl 1]: 8

[3] Beinert Th, Behr J, Mehnert F, Kohz P, Seemann M, Rienmüller R, Reiser M (1995) Spirometrically controlled quantitative CT for assessing diffuse parenchymal lung disease. Diseas J Comput Assist Tomogr 19 (6): 924–931

[4] Boyd DR, Lipton MJ (1982) Cardiac computed tomography. Proceedings of the IEEE 71: 298–307

[5] Canty JM (1993) Measurement of myocardial perfusion by fast computed tomography. Am J Card Imaging 7: 309–316

[6] Georgiou D, Wolfkiel CJ, Brundage BH (1994) Ultrafast computed tomography for physiological evaluation of myocardial perfusion. Am J Card Imaging 18: 151–158

[7] Kalender W, Rienmüller R, Behr J, Seissler W, Fichte H, Welke M (1992) Quantitative CT of the lung with spirometrically controlled respiratory status and automated evaluation procedures. In: Fuchs WF (ed) Advances in CT. Springer, Berlin Heidelberg New York London Paris Tokyo Hong Kong, pp 85–93

[8] Keath Sir A (1918) Br Med J 1: 361

[9] Ludman PF, Coats AJS, Burger P, Yang GZ, Poole-Wilson PA, Underwood SR, Rees RS (1993) Validation of measurement of regional myocardial perfusion in humans by ultrafast X-ray computed tomography. Am J Card Imaging 7267–7279

[10] Miles KA (1991) Measurement of tissue perfusion by dynamic computed tomography. Br J Radiol 64: 409–412

[11] Rienmueller R, Kern R, Baumgartner C, Hackel B (1997) Electron-Beam Computertomographie (EBCT) des Herzens. Radiologe 37: 410–416

[12] Rienmüller R (1990) Computertomographie versus Kernspintomographie in der klinischen Diagnostik kardialer Erkrankungen. Internist 31: 321–332

[13] Rienmüller R, Schulz H, Mehnert F, Heilmann P, Hillebrecht A, Behr J, Brand P (1992a) Quantitative analysis of CT value changes of the lung with different respiratory volumes. In: Fuchs WF, Langer M (eds) Advances in CT II. Springer, Berlin Heidelberg New York London Paris Tokyo Hong Kong Barcelona Budapest, pp 13–16

[14] Rienmüller R, Schulz H, Mehnert F, Heilmann P, Hillebrecht A, Behr J, Brand P (1992b) Evaluation of CT histograms determined by spirometrically standardize high resolution CT studies of the lung in man. In: Fuchs WF, Langer M (eds) Advances in CT II. Springer, Berlin Heidelberg New York London Paris Tokyo Hong Kong Barcelona Budapest, pp 17–24

[15] Rienmüller R (1991) Standardized quantitative high resolution CT in lung diseases. J Comput Assist Tomogr 15 (5): 742–749

[16] Rumberger JA, Bell MR, Feirung AJ, Behrenbeck T, Marcus ML, Ritman EL (1995) Measurement of myocardial perfusion using electron beam (ultrafast) computed tomography. In: Marcus ML, Schelbert HR, Skorton DJ (eds) Cardiac imaging, 2nd edn. Saunders, Philadelphia

[17] Stanford W, Rumberger J (eds) (1992) Ultrafast computed tomography in cardiac imaging: principles and practice. Futura Publishing Company, New York

[18] Weixler L, Brundage B, Crouse J, Detrano R, Fuster V, Madedeahi R, Rumberger J, Stanford W, White R, Taubert K (1996) Coronary artery calcification, pathophysiology, epidemiology, imaging methods and clinical implications. A scientific statement for health professionals from the American Heart Association. Circulation 94: 1175–1192

eHealth: The economic perspective[1]

E. R. Reinhardt

Member of the Board Siemens AG and CEO, Siemens Medical Solutions, Erlangen, Germany

Abstract

People's desire is quite simple: They want to stay as healthy as possible. The aim of healthcare is to help make this desire a reality. Innovations have substantially supported healthcare providers' in their efforts to increase the quality of care. To continue to make significant improvements – even under difficult socio-economic circumstances – healthcare must now become more process-oriented throughout the complete care process, i.e. from early detection to cure. Modern information and communication technology, i.e. eHealth, is the key to optimize processes within the entire healthcare system and to provide higher quality care at less cost. Quantifiable proven outcomes that clearly demonstrate the efficiency of eHealth are being realized. Action and co-operation between all healthcare players is necessary to structure and enable healthcare in a way that allows all people to benefit from the tremendous potential for progress that information technology offers to healthcare.

Continuous improvement of care through innovation

During the last decades, innovative technologies have made significant contributions to the quality of healthcare. With the discovery of x-rays 100 years ago it became possible to take images from inside of the body without the need for invasive procedures. Since then, there have been continual and significant improvements in radiology. Today, it is not only possible to receive an x-ray image, but a digital 3-D movie with high spatial resolution revealing anatomic structures up to a resolution of 0.5 millimetres. Very innovative techniques allow incredible details to be displayed. At the same time, acquisition times have become significantly shorter and x-ray exposure has been greatly reduced.

This example is meant to illustrate how innovative technologies contribute to improvements in the quality of diagnosis. However, innovative technologies also often bring new challenges, e.g. in this case how to effectively and efficiently interpret the tremendous amount of data that is now being generated. Computer aided diagnosis will likely prove to be an effective tool to do this, e.g. when it comes to diagnose state of the art computed tomography examinations with a volume of 2,000 images per 20 seconds. In much the same way, eHealth has the same potential to improve the quality of care in the entire healthcare system.

Focus on quality

General healthcare discussions, unfortunately, are not focused on the quality improvements that can be achieved with innovative technologies. They are typically focused on cost reduction. Indeed, healthcare expenditures have greatly increased, as shown below [1].

What is driving this increase? Are expenditures being driven by so-called high-tech systems? The answer is very clearly, no. If one considers investments in high-tech equipment, e.g. Computed Tomography, Magnetic Resonance, or Angiography, it accounts for only 0.2% of total annual healthcare expenditures. Even taking all electro-medical equipment into account, just 1% is being invested. And including all reimbursement fees, running costs only account for an additional 4%.

We should not only focus on the cost aspect, but also on the quality aspect. If the quality of diagnosis improves, if treatments are more specific and more comfortable for the patient, these are aspects that need to be considered. Innovative technologies are able to provide tremendous improvements in the quality of care.

[1]Adapted from a contribution originally published in "E-Health: Current situation and Examples of Implemented and Beneficial E-Health Applications", IOS Press (2004)

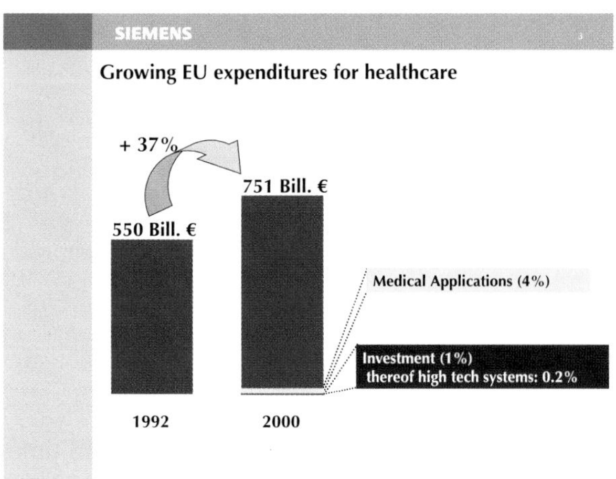

Fig. 1. The increase of healthcare expenditures from 1992–2000 in European countries was 37%. However, the share of investment in medical equipment is just 1%

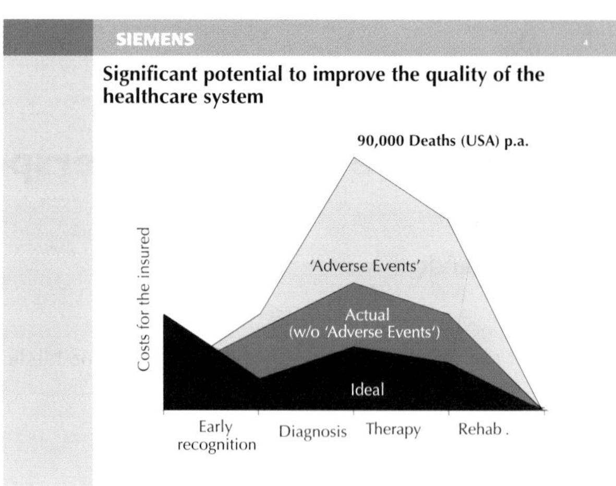

Fig. 2. The costs for the different steps in the healthcare process depend on quality assurance and early recognition. The current healthcare process differs from the ideal course. In the case of "adverse events", costs explode

Quality assurance and early recognition safes cost

From a quality perspective, we have to understand the complete healthcare process from early detection to diagnosis, therapy, care, rehabilitation, and home care. In the ideal case, where diseases are detected at an early stage, the burden for patients is lower and the chances for a complete recovery are much greater. Costs for treatment and rehabilitation are also minimized. This can be seen in Fig. 2:

Today, however, diseases are most often detected at a rather advanced or acute stage, with negative effects on cure and costs. Furthermore, if unintended "adverse events" occur, the situation is even worse. Besides the highly negative effects on costs, "adverse events" are a very serious quality issue. The Institute of Medicine (IOM) published a report in 1999 [2] that stated medical errors cause about 90,000 deaths in the United States every year. Sceptical people may say that this number is exaggerated, but even assuming that it is half, it is still a very significant number. It is in our interest to develop products and solutions that enable us to move from the light blue curve in Fig. 2, "adverse events", to the dark blue curve, the ideal scenario. This is how industry can contribute to improving the quality of healthcare while at the same time reducing cost.

Levers for improving healthcare

If we agree that there is a need to increase efficiency in healthcare, how do we do this? The main objective must be to increase the quality of healthcare while reducing costs. At the same time, this must be accomplished in a patient-centred healthcare system, i.e. one in which the patient is in focus and patients' values guide all decisions. In compliance with the position of the IOM [3], Fig. 3 gives an overview:

First, it is important to understand what industry calls "process-driven concepts". What does "process" mean? In healthcare, process is clinical workflow, which involves three categories: prevent, cure, and care. Let's take the case of cure: workflow starts when a person gets injured and finishes when a person is well again. Each and every step in between has to be optimized in a way that healthcare services become qualitatively better, less expensive, and

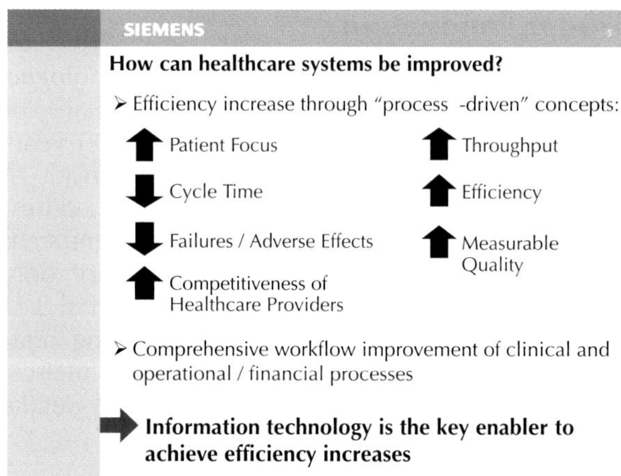

Fig. 3. Healthcare delivery involves complex processes and different aspects have to be considered simultaneously

more comfortable for the patient. This is what we mean by process optimization. Therefore, with the patient always in focus, we have to reduce cycle time, failures, and adverse events. We also have to increase throughput and efficiency, and it is essential to establish more competition between healthcare providers. Finally, we have to define parameters that allow us to measure the quality of the care being delivered. In summary, we have to comprehensively improve the workflow, the clinical and operational / financial processes, in the healthcare system. Information technology is the key enabler to do this.

Time is brain for stroke patients

Let's look at an example of how eHealth can make a significant improvement in a highly time-sensitive workflow, stroke management in an emergency room.

About 600,000 US citizens suffer a stroke each year. A study from 1995 [4] concluded that thrombolysis, if administered within the first three hours after the symptoms occurred, would have a significant impact on the patient's quality of life. 45% of all patients arrive in the emergency room within three hours, one would say "in time", and frequently have a therapeutic window less than one hour. Nonetheless, only 2% currently receive the thrombolysis they need in time. In this case, "time is brain".

However, ensuring treatment is a complex process. Different departments must work closely and flawlessly together. This is a perfect situation for an intelligent eHealth solution, a so-called "workflow engine". It can actively support the management of stroke patients (Fig. 4).

When the patient arrives at the hospital, the tasks that must be performed are immediately defined and the time remaining for treatment is assessed. All necessary steps are then aligned to the goal of delivering the patient the appropriate infusion on time. However, the "workflow engine" does more than define the various rules, it actively pushes tasks and monitors their status. At the beginning of the process, all of the departments receive a task list. If a task is not completed on time, there is an alarm. If the alarm does not help, a back-up solution is immediately initiated. The impact is significant, making sure that all participants know what they have to do and by when.

Proven outcomes: measurable, tangible results through eHealth

Optimizing processes, i.e. clinical workflow and operational/financial workflow, with the support of eHealth is key. The effectiveness and efficiency of eHealth solutions is relatively easy to describe, but only real results can convince. Quantifiable proven outcomes validate our message and motivate us to achieve more. "Proven outcomes" means having tangible and measurable efficiency improvements. In the following pages, seven eHealth proven outcomes are described and demonstrate that eHealth is already making a contribution to high quality, patient-focused care with optimized processes.

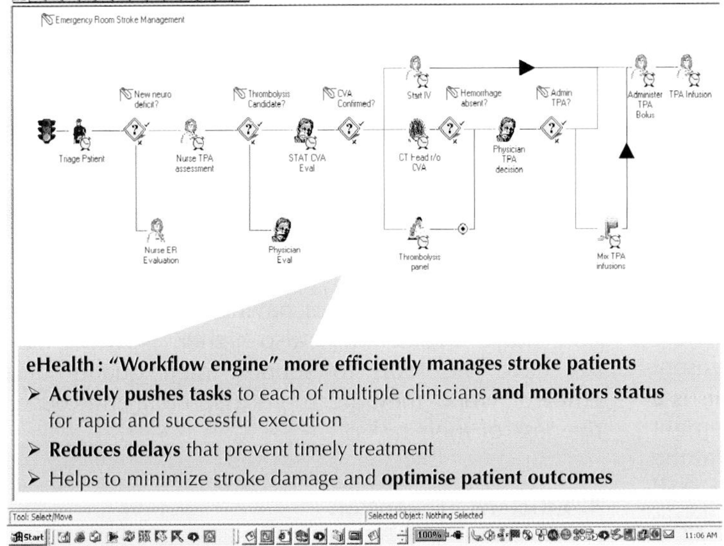

Fig. 4. Screen shot of an eHealth-managed stroke patient

1. Optimised data management

At Bethesda Healthcare System, USA, report turnaround time was significantly reduced, from 16.5 to 4 hours, through electronic archiving and distribution (Fig. 5). As a consequence, information is available quicker and decisions makers are more informed, thus allowing therapy to start earlier and hospital stays to be reduced. This has significant impact on the total clinical process [5].

Another case can be found at the Deaconry Hospital in Germany, where a restructuring and optimization of both clinical and operational workflows using eHealth improved resource utilization in the radiology department (Fig. 5). With nearly the same number of people and the same equipment, 80% more examinations could be done.

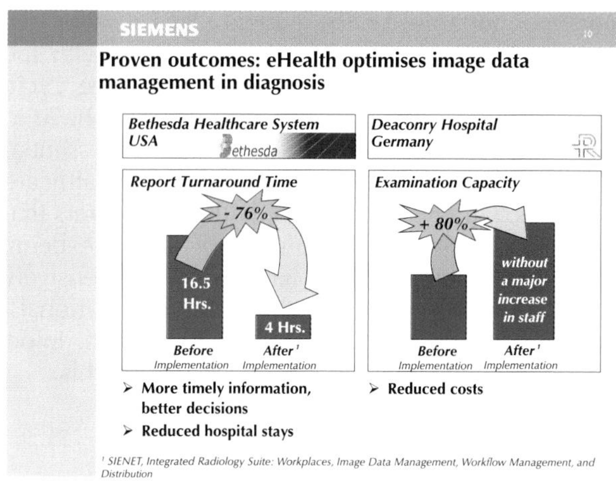

Fig. 5. eHealth supports timely and cost efficient information exchange and workflow

2. Faster processes

eHealth is not only able to synchronize processes in one department, but also among referring physicians in the healthcare enterprise. For example, at the South Carolina Heart Center, post-procedural report turnaround time was greatly reduced (Fig. 6). Reports that previously took up to 2 days to turnaround, are now available in a matter of minutes. And through the additional procedures allowed by the this time savings, the return on investment on the system was less than one year.

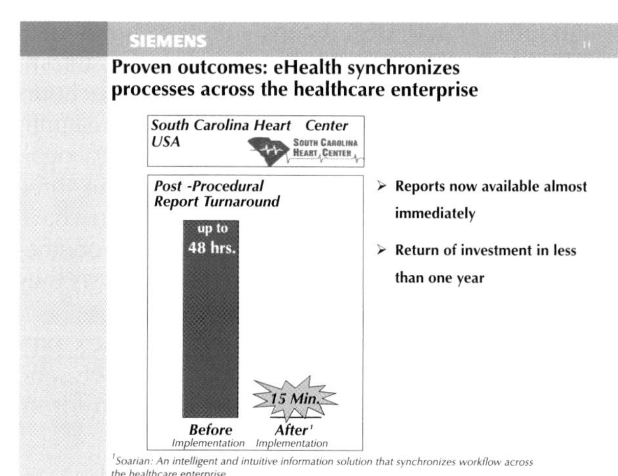

Fig. 6. eHealth accelerates processes across the healthcare enterprise

3. Faster administration of medication and reduction of medication errors

The aforementioned Institute of Medicine report also concluded that about 7,000 patients die in US hospitals annually due to medication errors. This has resulted in enormous efforts to optimize the medication process and reduce failure rates. The application of an automated Physician Order Entry (POE) system has led to significant efficiency improvements at the Ohio State University Health System (OSUHS), USA [6] and Soedersjukhuset, Sweden [6] (Fig. 7).

In the first case, the medication turnaround time (from physician order entry to medication administration) was reduced by 64% at OSUHS, where the system has been running for more than one year. Medication now arrives significantly earlier at the point of care and, often, the nurse who was present when the drug was prescribed, is still there. This is a significant advantage in order to ensure that the right medication is administered to the right patient at the right time in the right dose. In terms of the overall medication process, it is now easy to verify, to obtain and/or provide additional information, and to document the different steps.

The second case, in Sweden, shows that the medication error rate was greatly reduced. And not only are erroneous or incomplete prescriptions the source of medication errors, but they often also cause time consuming investigations. Besides the obvious patient benefit of having the right medication, nurse satisfaction is also higher. Now, as nurses have the tools to support high quality and efficient work, they are more assured in the effectiveness of their tasks.

4. Efficient prevention

When considering clinical processes, we cannot forget prevention. eHealth also supports this growing

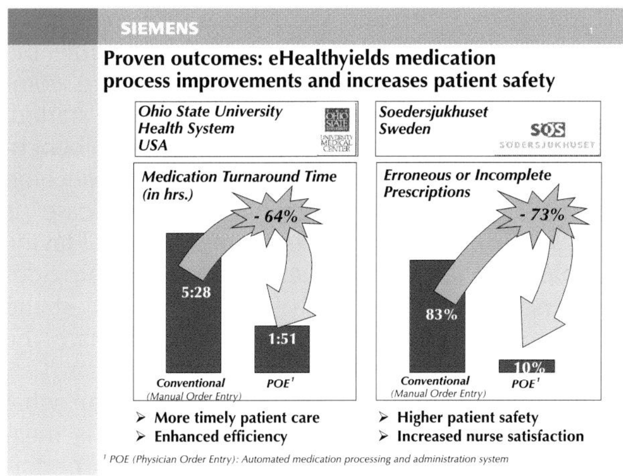

Fig. 7. eHealth reduced the medication process cycle time and medication errors

area of healthcare. An example for efficient prevention with eHealth is the project "t@lking eyes", shown in Fig. 8. The aim of the project is to identify individuals to be at a higher risk for stroke or heart attack. Images of blood vessels in the back of the eye, which are considered to mirror blood vessels in the brain [7], are easily produced using a laser-camera that can be located anywhere, for instance at an employer. Images are taken and transmitted via internet to a specialized center. There, experts evaluate the images and then place a report on a secure server accessible to the participant.

7,000 individuals participated in the first phase of this project. Therefrom, 20% were identified to be at a higher risk for stroke. These people are offered a disease management program that investigates the cause of their vascular abnormalities and educates them on measures to minimize the risk of a stroke or heart attack.

5. Reduced investments

Through the use Application Service Providers (ASP), healthcare providers no longer have to invest in their own hardware, no longer have to maintain their own IT department, and no longer have to operate their own data center. All of this can be effectively outsourced and centrally hosted. The healthcare provider pays per use and receives all the applications via the net. This results in significant economies of scale (Fig. 9):

ASP is real business today. In our data center in the United States [8], we already serve more than 1,200 customers with 200,000 physicians conducting 137 million transactions every day. If each of these 1,200 customers would maintain their own IT department, each of them would need at least two people during three shifts for seven days a week. In total, they would have at least 7,200 people. Our data center does the same work for them with 75 people. This should only illustrate how eHealth can be harnessed to improve the efficiency and to significantly reduce investment in healthcare.

Political requirements to provide the basis for ehealth

The eHealth concept is already being successfully realized and delivering proven outcomes. The question now is: What can we do on a political level, what do we have to do, in order to utilize all of the potential of eHealth for the benefit of people? This is

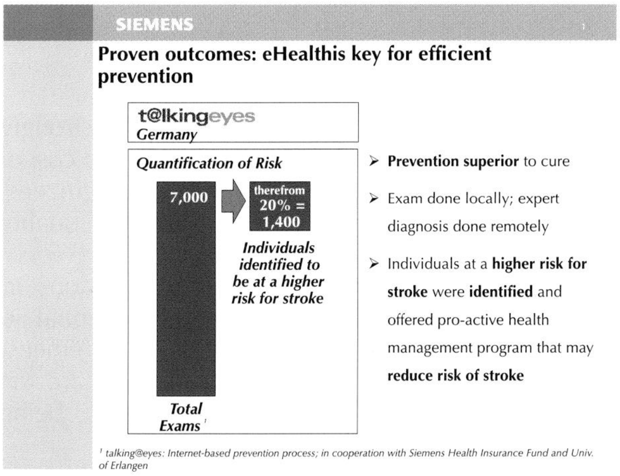

Fig. 8. eHealth can efficiently identify individuals at a higher risk for stroke

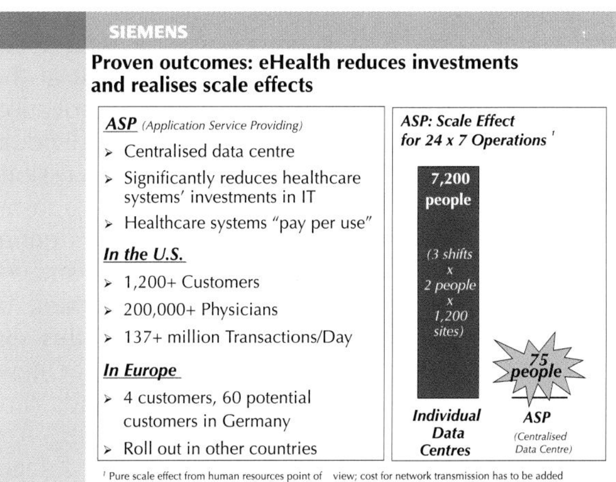

Fig. 9. eHealth can centralise and scale healthcare transactions

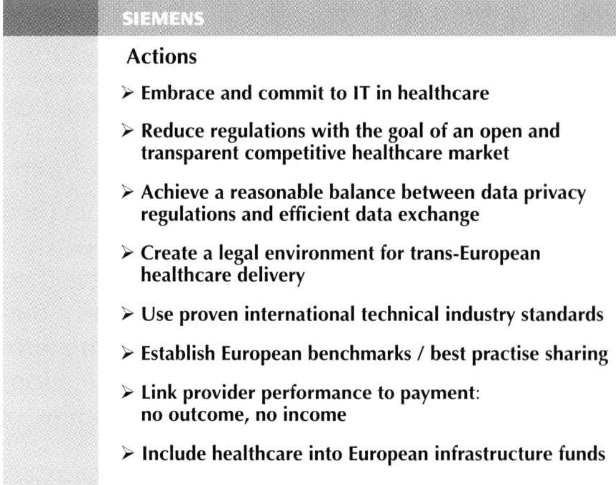

Fig. 10. Eight actions to build an integrated, transparent and efficient healthcare system for the benefit of citizens

summarized in the following eight action points (Fig. 10):

First: Fully embrace and commit to IT in healthcare. It is fundamentally necessary to have the key participants understand the tremendous benefits that information and communication technology has for healthcare.

Secondly, it is essential to reduce regulations and create a more open and transparent competitive healthcare market. It needs to be determined what should be regulated and what should be open to competition, as well as what should be publicly financed and what should be the financial responsibility of the individual. One thing is for certain, a market open to competition will be marked by quality, innovation, and cost improvements.

Thirdly, a reasonable balance between data privacy and efficient data exchange has to be implemented. Specifically defined rights for data access and sophisticated procedures for data security can ensure that data is kept private, but at the same time that it be harnessed to drive innovation and improve the quality of care. For the individual there are significant advantages to data accessibility, e.g. avoidance of redundant exams and a faster and more accurate diagnosis. For the entire healthcare system there are also major advantages of data accessibility, such as the development of proven of evidence-based care paths. On this extremely important topic, we should strive to achieve international and European agreements and standards.

The fourth action is also in this context: a legal environment for trans-European healthcare delivery should be created. This is, incidentally, a good opportunity for integrating the EU countries.

Action five: eHealth should use proven international technical industry standards and utilize the information in existing systems to minimize complexity. Here, a lot of work has already been started.

Next action point: establish European benchmarks and share best practices. We need to develop a common understanding of what "quality of care" is and define clear parameters to measure it. Having databases to exchange such information provides answers to questions such as "Who is doing best and why?". Let's learn from each other and share the different competencies.

Now the seventh step: once it is clear what "quality of care" means and performance is measured, we have the basis to link provider performance to payment. "No outcome, No income" is natural and successful in other industries, so let's introduce this self-regulating instrument in healthcare, too.

Finally, acceding countries have a lot to accomplish in order to reach the standards of the associated countries of the EU. Therefore, a large budget has been provided to further develop their respective infrastructures. However, healthcare has not been included in these development funds. As is investment in transportation, energy, and telecommunication infrastructure, investment in and the continual development of an effective and efficient healthcare system is important. It is important for a country's economy and is a pre-requisite for the fast harmonization of healthcare standards that will be required through accession. Accession countries have a unique opportunity to set up a modern healthcare system right from the start. However, the success of their accession and integration will be greatly affected by the level of investment that is made in IT infrastructure and medical technology.

A promising future with eHealth

Without a doubt, eHealth will continue to strongly contribute to improvements in the quality and cost of healthcare. This is absolutely in line with the citizens' desire to stay healthy and to receive high quality care.

Industry can make significant contributions to help develop eHealth and realize the potential in healthcare systems. And industry is not only Siemens. Our competitors are also investing here, as are the large IT companies. Proven outcomes are being achieved.

Healthcare delivery is a common task in Europe, so it should be accomplished together. Now, a European Institute of Medicine has been established.

In close cooperation with the European Parliament, all the different players have been brought together to synchronize the efforts to provide high quality care in Europe.

If there is a real commitment of all of these players, Europe has the opportunity to become an eHealth trendsetter. The technology is available, as are very talented and committed people. We have everything we need. Now, it's just up to us!

References

[1] OECD Health Care Data 2002

[2] To Err Is Human: Building a Safer Health System, Institute of Medicine (IOM), 2000

[3] Crossing The Quality Chasm: A new Health System For The 21st Century, Institute of Medicine (IOM) 2001

[4] NEJM The National Institute of Neurological Disorders and Stroke rt-PA Study Group (1995) Tissue plasminogen activator for acute ischemic stroke. 333:1581–1587

[5] Proven Outcomes Case Studies 1, p.8; Siemens Medical Solutions, Order no. A91100-M-B135-10-7600

[6] Baldauf-Sobez W, et al (2003) How Siemens Computerized physician order entry helps prevent the human error. electromedica 71(1): 2–10

[7] Wong T Y, et al (2001) Retinal microvascular abnormalities and incident stroke: the Atherosclerosis Risk in Communities Study. Lancet 358: 1134–40

[8] Emig D, Kijewski J (2001) The application service providers in healthcare. electromedica 69 (1): 2–4

Image fusion

W. Backfrieder[1], R. Hanel[2], M. Diemling[1,3], T. Lorang[4], J. Kettenbach[2], and H. Imhof[2]

[1]Department of Biomedical Engineering and Physics, University of Vienna, Austria
[2]Department of Radiology, Vienna University Hospital, Austria
[3]Department of Nuclear Medicine, PET Centre, Vienna University Hospital, Austria
[4]Department of Medical Computer Science, University of Vienna, Austria

Introduction

In modern radiology imaging modalities for three-dimensional medical visualisation of anatomy and function are in clinical use. Various physical quantities measured by the interaction of e.g. X-rays, magnetic fields or ultra sound with the human body provide modality inherent information about the human body, in general information is complimentary.

For instance, a 3D map of physiological processes is reconstructed in positron emission tomography (PET). Specific radio-chemicals label metabolic processes by the emission of positrons (β^+-particles). The positrons are localised by the detection of the coincident photons emitted in opposite directions after electron–positron annihilation.

Magnetic resonance imaging (MRI) uses nuclear spin interaction with the magnetic field and resonance phenomena to generate an image of the tissue of the human body.

Computed tomography (CT) uses the absorption of X-rays on its way through the body to reconstruct a 2D image of the absorption coefficients within an axial slice. Stacks of slices are used to get a fully 3D image of the body.

PET however shows physiological processes but little anatomical information, MRI in general proton densities of the human body and CT highly detailed anatomical information on the distribution of absorption coefficient, with high contrast in bone but little in soft tissue.

Image fusion is applied for local integration of complimentary information in multi modality images for use in diagnostics and therapy planning. For example, to add anatomical information from MR to the physiological information of PET, or to add information on the soft tissues from MRI to the information on bony structures from CT.

Possible applications are comparing pre- and post-therapeutic images in order to evaluate treatment or image fusion in image-guided surgery, where the surgeon's view is overlaid by a preoperatively prepared feature model. This allows the surgeon to look beyond the skin, or to control immediately the performance with respect to the preoperatively planned surgery.

The problem which image fusion faces, assuming consistent reconstruction, disregarding problems coming from distortions in medical imaging, is how to align the 3D data sets accurately. Depending on the modalities and the anatomy in the region of interest, alignment is obtained manually or automatically. Both means to compare the grey values of volume elements (voxels) in each modality, which allow the computation of the appropriate matching transform. The simplest case to consider is rigid misalignment, which can be compensated by translation and rotation of the rigid volume. Most likely the situation is more sophisticated, as for instance the physical volumes that are mapped in diverse modalities cannot necessarily be aligned by rigid transforms, since the patient most likely is not in the same position during both acquisitions or the post operative anatomy has changed. This may lead to deformations of tissue, which have to be considered in the image matching algorithm, either as a linear or non-linear model.

Principles of image fusion

The representation of complimentary information in multi-modality imaging, is achieved by fusion (registration). Respective anatomical structures are matched against each other to visualise for example functional information from PET together with anatomical structures from MRI. Generally image volumes acquired in different modalities have different slice positions and orientation, furthermore corresponding tissue types in general differ in grey values or are not visible at all. Thus simple comparison of plain image slices is not possible. Complex mathematical algorithms are used for image fusion under user control or fully automated applications were developed for special anatomical sites and modalities.

A registration procedure is considered as a four steps procedure.

- Identification of relevant features in both volumes to be matched (segmentation, classification)
- Minimisation/maximisation of a cost function indicating the degree of alignment between the images. The cost function is defined using the identified features.
- Transformation (reformatting) of the data sets to match each other in scale and position.
- Representation of data.

The human interpreter needs a presentation of registered images in an intuitive way. There exist various display methods optimised for diagnosis, biomedical image evaluation, surgical planing and navigation. Application dependent relevant features are emphasised or both image data are shown in full detail without any abstraction.

As an example for the above registration scheme the matching of two rectangles, as shown in Fig. 1, is discussed. A simple matching method, point-to-point matching, is used. Three corresponding points at the corners of each rectangles are defined as features and

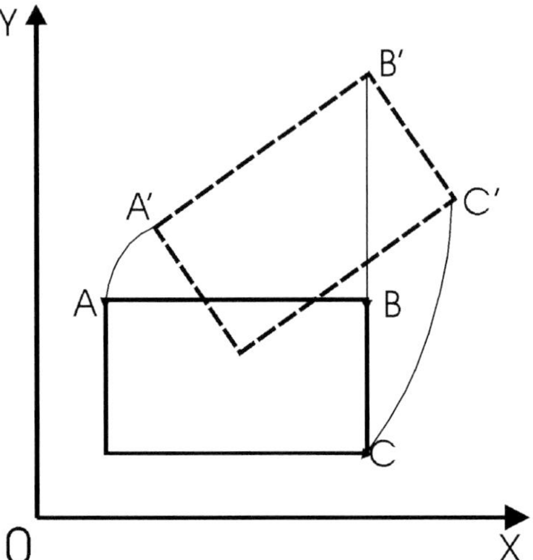

Fig. 1. Registration of two rectangles. Point pairs at the corners of the rectangles are matched by a point-to-point matching algorithm using a rigid body transform

ordered into pairs (A,A′), (B,B′) and (C,C′). Each of the pairs contains one point on both rectangles. In this case the cost function is the sum of the distances of the point-pairs. There exist various methods to solve the problem. In this simple case the parameters for rotation and translation are estimated in one step, solving a system of mathematical equations. The iterative estimation of the matching parameters provides an alternative solution to the problem. Alternating incremental translations and rotations are performed before the evaluation of the cost function. Optimal registration is given when an extreme value of the cost function is found. A multi-scale approach could speed up the procedure. There a coarse parameter estimate is refined in every iteration step. Iteration is terminated when a tolerance limit is reached.

With the matching parameters a transform matrix is computed, reflecting the mathematical relation between the base and matching image. The matching image is transformed to the grid of the base image using this matrix. Since reformatted pixels of the matching image generally lie between the grid points of the base image interpolation is necessary. Linear interpolation is fast and mostly provides sufficient accuracy. For high image quality spline or windowed sinc interpolation is used at the cost of higher computational efforts and interpolation artefacts, e.g. distortion of sharp edges due to over oscillation.

In this simple case it is sufficient to show the base and reformatted matching image side by side on the screen or together with a transparent overlay of both. For more complex anatomical sites or in surgical planing and navigation an abstract three dimensional (3D) display is generated. Organs (objects) from both image volumes are merged and the image volume is rendered in transparent 3D mode.

Segmentation

In a way the concepts of image fusion or registration need reliable definition of image inherent features. These features are prepared by segmentation or classification. In the simplest case features are landmarks, where at least three distinct landmarks are needed to register two image volumes in 3D. These are minimum requirements, since inaccurate definition of even one landmark inevitably leads to registration errors. To achieve redundancy more than three landmarks are chosen, what is done in simple manual registration procedures.

There is no general solution for segmentation of medical images. It is reported, that manual segmentation has large variability [11,26]. Warfield and Kikinis report 15% variability in the segmentation of cortical grey matter of the brain doing segmentations by five different experts. Kaus reports 15–20% variability in segmentation of brain tumours by multiple experts. Automated segmentation techniques, designed for special problems, would decrease operators bias in segmentation results, as for instance in applications developed for neuro radiology [15].

There is a great variety of segmentation algorithms [16], incorporation different levels of automation: manual thresholding, semiautomatic region growing, morphological operations and multi-spectral methods like clustering methods or neural networks [20]. Since multi spectral methods require registration of spectral images, these algorithms are implemented using an iterative procedure. In each iteration images are classified and registered until sufficient overlay is achieved [2]. Classification algorithms need prior information from training sets of each tissue type. These training sets are defined either manually or by a rough preclassification, e.g. a geometrical model.

After segmentation features are extracted for input into the registration algorithm. In general results of automated segmentation are reproducible, since most algorithms are deterministic. From grey level images anatomical structure have to be extracted like a human expert would do. Due to restrictions inherent to the imaging modality, e.g. resolution, imaging artefacts, partial volume effect, image inhomogeneities, external information has to be implemented [4]. This external or a priori information is either structural or functional and is called domain information. With segmentation techniques under operator control decisions employing domain information on complex anatomical features are implicitly drawn by the human expert. But in an automated procedure this domain knowledge needs to be formulated by a mathematical rule set.

Knowledge based algorithms incorporate domain information to achieve further automation. Questions are answered checking some model in the knowledge domain [28]. Questions on the grey-level distribution of some structure within the image are checked using intensity models [22]. Questions on the characteristics of the imaging modality, that was used to acquire the image, are checked by imaging models [28]. Shape models, dealing with questions of shape, like the average curvatures of anatomic features in the healthy adults, are used for biasing predictors [21]. Finally there are geometric models for the description of spatial relationship in structures, like "where feature **A** branches feature **B** is expected to be in near vicinity" [7].

A simple intensity model is the Gaussian classifier. The likely-hood of a voxel being a member of a specific tissue class is estimated by evaluating Gaussian probability distributions derived from representative grey values for each tissue type from predefined training sets. More sophisticated models will include higher orders of stochastic relations between not only voxels but contiguous regions [29].

The imaging models have to contain information on geometrical distortions of the image intrinsic to the acquisition device as well as reconstruction artefacts and the grey value bias that may systematically be superimposed on images. Commonly the procedures needed for dealing with these kind of phenomena are not included in the segmentation task, but are performed in an preprocessing step [28].

Although recognition of shape cannot be formulated with exact mathematical rules, a class of shape models proofed to be useful during last years: combinations of deformable models and principal component analysis [11,21]. The models are used in general to uniquely segment structures, which were left unclassified by the intensity models.

To achieve "objective" and reproducible segmentation, reducing operator interaction the combination of grey level based classifiers together with sophisticated geometrical models is a prospering field of research.

Registration in clinical applications

In [13] a general framework of medical image registration is given. We want to focus on intra-subject, inter-modality matching, i.e. image data from the same subject acquired in several modalities. There rigid and elastic transforms are of clinical relevance [8,9]. Assuming no deformation of the object the image volumes are related using a model for motion of rigid bodies. A global transform matrix with 9 parameters (respectively 3 for translation, rotation and scaling) is used for matching in 3D space. These methods are computationally fast and show sufficient accuracy, especially in the head region. Machine inherent distortions in MR images are compensated using complex hydro-mechanical models for intermodality matching. There are several application for matching functional EPI images to anatomical T1 weighted images in MR or the fusion of emission CT images with MR [12].

In the following the concepts of two method using rigid transforms are discussed in detail.

Chamfer matching

In the group of rigid transform methods chamfer matching is a surface-to-points matching algorithm. The matching features are the surfaces of the same object in both image volumes. By segmentation these features are identified. The accuracy of the final matching is strongly dependent on careful feature segmentation. There exists no general automated segmentation procedure applicable to all anatomical sites of the human body. Semi-automated, grey level based methods as region growing are commonly used. Under operator control regions of interest (ROIs) are defined around manually selected seed points by adjusting upper and lower thresholds of grey values of pixels contained in the region. Region growing can be controlled by manually drawing limits to separate neighbouring structures with similar grey values. A higher degree of automation can be achieved with morphological operations prior to region growing [10]. By erosion small connections between neighbouring organs with a similar range of grey values are removed. The focused organ is selected by region growing and a final dilation step is applied to compensate for the erosion. This procedure was used for the segmentation of the brain in MR images [17,18].

Defining the cost function, the surface of the segmented organ in the base volume is extracted and a set of random points on the respective surface in the matching volume is selected. The cost function gives the summed distance of the point set from the base surface. Computational efficacy is increased by using a surface to distance map. To every voxel position in the base volume the distance to the closest surface point is assigned. Distances are calculated using the efficient chamfer algorithm [1]. In an iterative algorithm the point set is moved over all possible locations in the distance map. The global minimum of the cost function marks the position of best matching. A multi scale approach further speeds up the matching procedure [14,19].

Mutual information matching

Given the problem of registering two different MR image volumes of the same individual. When perfectly aligned the grey values of corresponding voxels are nearly the same. Differences are due to noise. With multi modality images different tissue types show characteristic ranges of grey values, inherent to the modality. Simple similarity measures as squared difference of voxel values or correlation are not sufficient in that case for use in a cost function. A more general measure, mutual information, reflecting the statistical properties of data, shows the correlation of tissue types in different modalities.

The cost function used for registration of the reference and matching volume maximises the mutual information of all voxels in an image volume. This is a statistical measure, defined in terms of entropy. Entropy can be interpreted as the degree of uncertainty, variability, or complexity in a random variable. If images are in perfect registration every voxel in both images should belong to the same specific tissue type. The co-occurrence matrix (two dimensional histogram) shows distinct clusters for each tissue type. If images are not registered clusters are blurred, since voxels at corresponding locations in both volumes belong to different tissue classes. The degree of blurring is estimated by mutual information. A statistical standard method, Parzen windowing, is used to estimate the entropy density function from the discrete samples in the co-occurrence matrix. Accounting for noisy data in finding the global maximum, noisy derivative estimates are used in the gradient ascension procedure to exclude local maxima [3,5,26]. Accelerating the search for the maximum a multi scale approach is implemented, where the search is done with a coarse to fine method. Maxima found on the coarse grid are used as initial guesses on the finer grid in the next step.

The method works automatically and direct on medical images, in contrast to other methods that require the setting of fiducial markers or some other types of manual interaction for registration. Thus, the algorithm is suitable for intra operative registration, where stability and simplicity are desirable.

Furthermore this type of cost function is flexible to be used with a deformable registration method. Several groups of investigators [6] reported the cost function can be formulated as the sum of a voxel similarity and an elastic regularisation energy term, so that the general problem of registration is to minimise the matching energy function. For elastic deformations the potential energy of the object deformed by an external force is measured.

Clinical applications

Interactive registration of MR and CT volumes

Interactive methods allow physicians to gain complete control over the registration process. Matching volumes may be translated, rotated and scaled with respect to a phase volume. Rotations, translations and scalings of the base volume are mapped to the matching volume. A framework for fast reformatting of oblique slices gives immediate feedback of rigid body transformations to the physician by overlaying transparent images of the matching volume onto images of the base volume in multiplanar reconstructions. This allows for easy correction of patient-related mis-alignment, provided both volumes have the same slice orientation.

Different slice orientations require physicians also to handle image inherent mis-alignments. However, most modern imaging modalities supply header information containing the orientation for each slice; this information is standardised in DICOM 3.0. Further information like pixel dimensions and slice distance, location and thickness allow for an automated registration of equipment related – or series related – geometrical parameters. In this way, axial slices are automatically reconstructed out of volumes composed of sagittal slices, and this reconstructed volume may be registered to a base volume composed of axial slices again. Especially the scaling between both volumes is completely determined by the pixel dimensions in the header information fields.

Interactive registration methods commonly suffer from a subjective validation of registration processes. Their main advantages are intuitive handling, immediate display of results and the fact that they do not need any time consuming pre-processing. Figure 2 shows the user interface of the software developed at the Vienna University Hospital. The result achieved by a registration of an axial MR (256 × 256 × 21, 0.976 mm voxel dimensions) and an axial CT (512 × 512 × 46, 0.625 mm pixel dimensions) are displayed. To visualise the degree of alignment the contour of bones from the CT is overlaid in the MR image.

CT-SPECT registration

Diagnosis and therapy of malignant carcinomas in the oral cavity, e.g. squamous cell carcinoma, is based on accurate information about tumour extension, infiltration of adjacent tissue and metastasises in lymph nodes. Since CT provides detailed anatomical information but no functional information, accurate differentiation of infiltrated cancerous tissue is difficult. In SPECT accumulation of a tumour-specific radioactive marker is imaged. Glands are shown together with pathological changes in tissue. Spatial fusion of CT and SPECT images enables accurate tumour diagnosis.

The example shows a patient with a squamous cell carcinoma of the oral cavity in the head and neck region. 3D-CT image data were obtained on a Philips Tomoscan SR7000 (120 kV, 400 mA), 512 × 512 pixel/slice, 3 mm slice thickness, FOV = 185 mm, using an iodic contrast medium. ^{99m}Tc Sestamibi szintigrams were acquired on a Picker Prism3000, 128 × 128 pixel/slice, 3.6 mm slice thickness, FOV = 46 cm. For spatial registration of the images chamfer matching was used. Semiautomatic segmentation (region growing, manual tracing) was used to define the surface of the glandula parotis and the opposite glandula submandibularis in respective volumes of both imaging modalities. Figure 3 shows the segmented glands in both modalities, red in CT and green in SPECT. Figure 4 shows a semitransparent overlay of the registered CT and SPECT image. Activity is shown in the glands and in the tongue where the tumour is located.

Sufficient registration of anatomical structures and functional information was achieved. The mean distance between corresponding surfaces was about

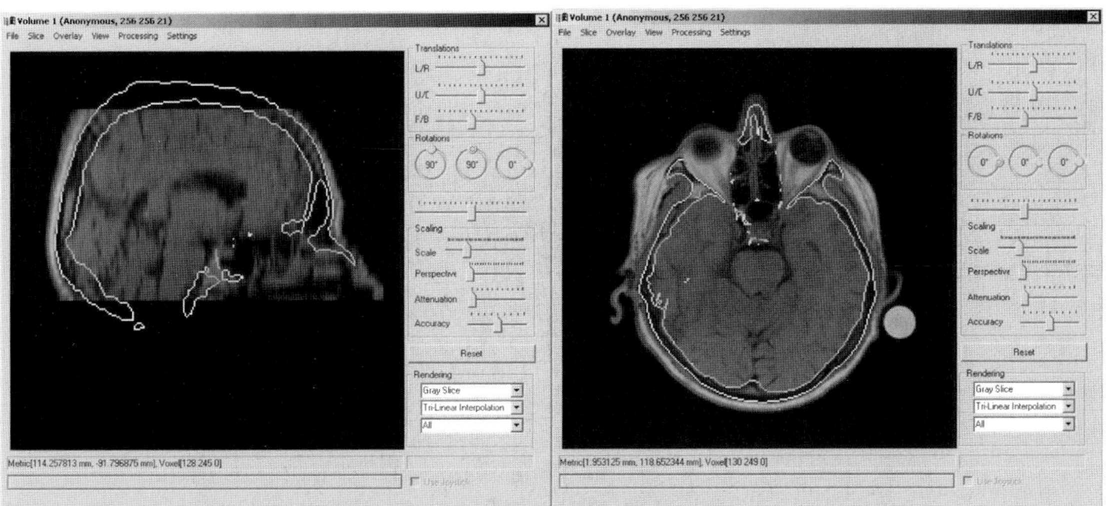

Fig. 2. User interface for manual image registration. A transaxial and sagittal view of the data volume in MR is shown. The overlay shows the contour of the skull bone in the corresponding CT volume. By manual adjustment of rotation and translation images are put to optimal alignment

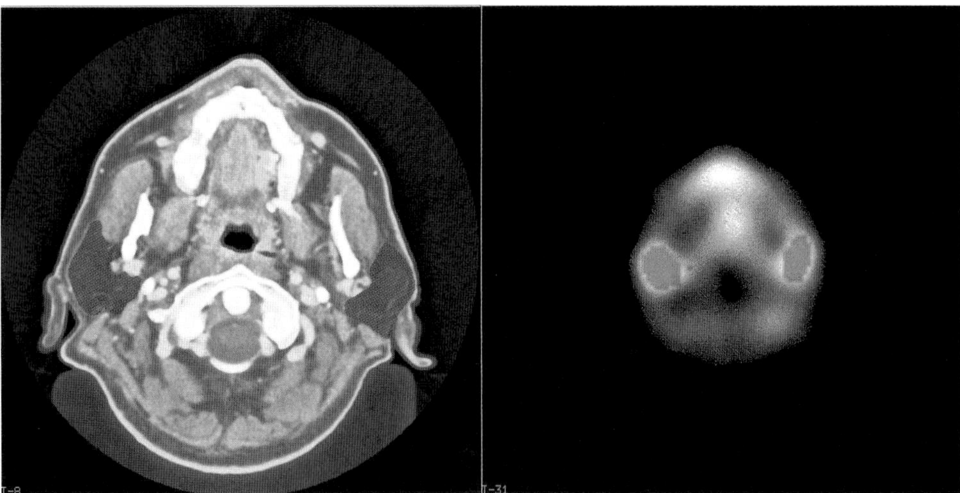

Fig. 3. Semi-automatic segmentation of the parotic glands in CT and SPECT images. The surfaces of the glands are used to register image volumes by chamfer matching

4 pixel, i.e. 2.8 mm. This calculated value is worse than observed spatial overlap, since glands are overemphasised in SPECT, because of imaging artefacts and rigid filtering of reconstructed scintigraphic images.

Semiautomatic registration provides a tool for simultaneous representation of anatomic and functional information and thus improves accuracy in tumour staging in the complex anatomical site of the oral cavity and the neck.

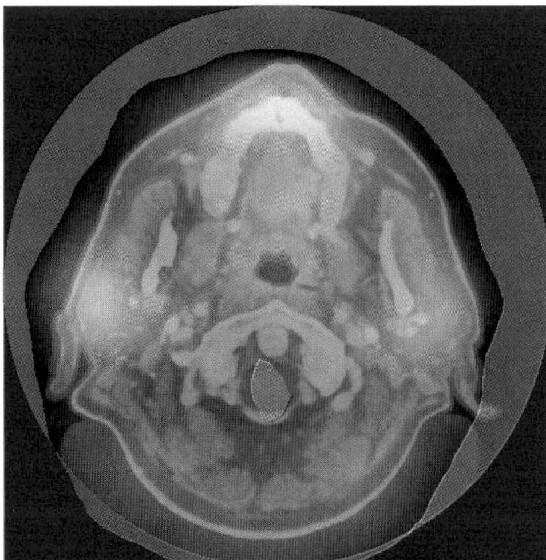

Fig. 4. Semi-transparent overlay of CT and SPECT images for staging of a squamous cell tumour. The CT image shows anatomical details completed by information of the accumulation of radio pharmaceuticals in glands and tumour tissue

MRI–CT registration in ENT surgery

In ear-nose-throat (ENT) surgery minimally invasive methods have been established during the last decade. Since the area of surgery is not open, the surgeon cannot look directly on the surgical target. Optical devices are used to control surgical instruments in small body cavities. Experienced surgeons have to interpret distorted images provided by the fish eye optics of the endoscope. Besides image distortions navigation in the surgical field is complicated by humidity of the patients breath and blood covering the lens. Under these facts sensitive structures like nerves and blood vessels must not be injured to prevent the patient from severe harm.

Modern radiology with high resolution 3D imaging from MR and CT together with medical computer science is the basis for surgical planing and intra surgical navigation. Images from both CT and MR are fused to show both soft tissue, nerves, blood vessels and bone in high detail. Figure 5 shows the fusion of a MR and CT data set. Data are reformatted to the grid of the CT images. A transaxial slice through the head is shown. Bone, invisible in MR, is coloured yellow. Since surgical planing and navigation needs more than in-plane information a 3D display mode was developed. Critical structures were segmented from MR images and imported to the CT volume. Colours were assigned to the anatomical object and the whole scenery was visualised using transparent 3D rendering. Figure 6 shows a transparent gradient shading from a skull. The optical nerve is yellow, the arteria carotis is red and the tumour green. With

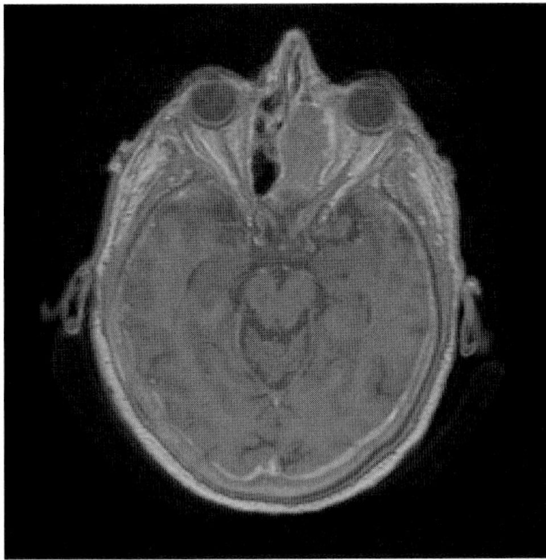

Fig. 5. Fusion of MR and CT images for ENT surgery. The MR image shows high contrast in soft tissue. The matched CT image provides detailed information about bony structures (yellow), which is completely missing in the MR data

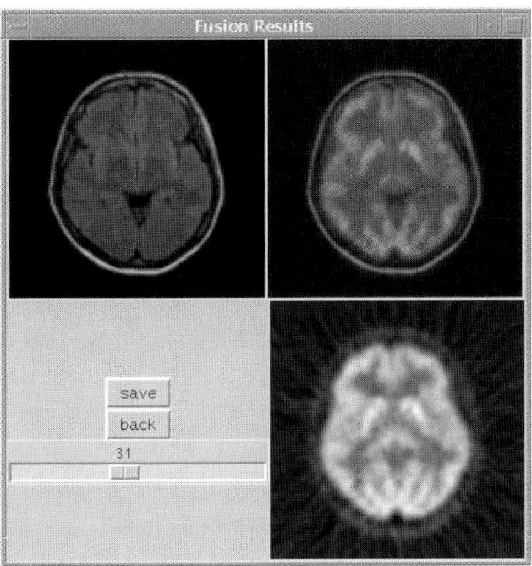

Fig. 7. Three panel display of the results of MR-PET matching. The transaxial MR slice is shown in the upper left position. The reformatted PET slice is shown as a grey level image at the lower right position. An overlay of MR and PET images is shown at the upper right position. To emphasise functional information from PET a colour representation is used

transparent rendering the surgeon can see behind surfaces and gets an impression about the relative distances between objects. With special hardware, like 3D goggles, a real 3D view by stereoscopic rendering can be generated.

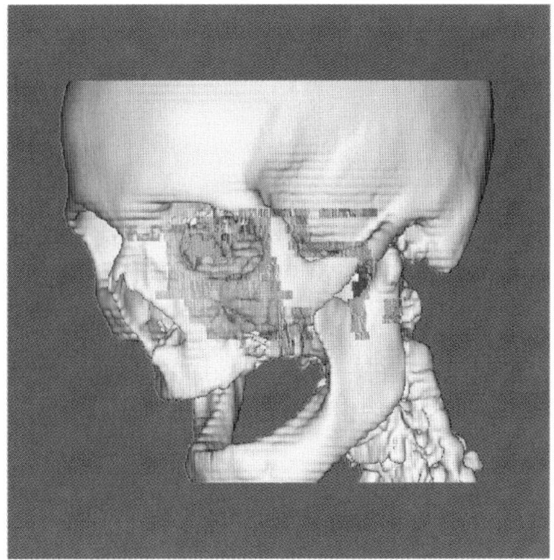

Fig. 6. Three dimensional representation of a registered CT and MR data set for use in surgical planing and navigation. Structures of interest were segmented and rendered in transparent mode. The optical nerve (yellow), the carotid artery (red) and the tumour (green) are shown together with the skull

MRI–PET registration

For the clinical application of multi modal image fusion it is desirable to have tools available that require minimum operator interaction. An application performing multi modal image registration of brain scans without user interaction was developed. It has the advantages of full 3D support and short processing time. The tool is clinically used for the coregistration of PET–MR and SPECT–MR images.

The software presented performs image registration using the normalised mutual information algorithm from the 'AnalyzeAVW' library (Biomedical Imaging Resource, Mayo Foundation, Rochester, MN). This algorithm maximises the degree of dependence of two variables by means of the Kullback-Leibler measure [23,24]. No prior manual segmentation of the volumes is necessary.

Figure 7 shows the input and the output windows of the fusion tool. A MRI scan from a patient suffering from temporal lobe epilepsy was fused to the corresponding PET scan for the anatomical identification of pathological PET foci.

The MR scan was acquired on a Philips Gyroscan at 1.5 T using a FLAIR sequence with a slice thickness of 4 mm, image matrix of 256×256 and a FOV of 23 cm.

The PET FDG image was acquired on a GE Advance, attenuation corrected and reconstructed with a slice thickness of 4.25 mm, image matrix of 128×128 and a FOV of 40 cm. For display, all images are interpolated to $200 \times 200 \times 70$ voxel grid.

As a result of fusion, the two volumes are presented after registration as well as a colour coded overlay of both.

Acknowledgements

Authors would like to thank the Clinic of Nuclear Medicine, the PET Centre, the Department of Neuroradiology and the Clinic of ENT diseases of the Vienna University Hospital for providing image data. This work was partially supported by the grant P12463-MED of the Austrian Science Fund.

References

[1] Borgefors G (1988) Hierarchical chamfer matching: A parametric edge matching algorithm. IEEE Trans Pattern Anal Machine Intell 10: 849–865

[2] Collins DL, Peters TM, Dai W, Evans AC (1992) Model based segmentation of individual brain structures from MRI data. SPIE Proceedings of 1st International Conference on visualisation in Biomedical Computing 1808: 10–23

[3] Collins DL (1994) 3D Model-based segmentation of individual brain structures from magnetic resonance imaging data. PhD thesis, McGill University

[4] Dellepiane S, Fontana F (1995) Extraction of intensity connectedness for image processing. Pattern Recognition Letters 16: 313–324

[5] Gangolli AR, Tanimoto SL (1983) Two pyramid machine algorithms for edge detection in noisy binary images. Information Processing Letters 17: 197–202

[6] Gee JC, Reivich M, Bajcsy R (1993) Elastically deforming 3D atlas to match anatomical brain images. J Comput Assist Tomogr 17: 225–236

[7] Gibbs P, Buckley DL, Blackband SJ, Horsman A (1996) Tumour volume determination from MR images by morphological segmentation. Physics in Medicine and Biology 41: 2437–2446

[8] Hata N (1998) Rigid and deformable medical image registration for image-guided surgery. PhD thesis, University of Tokyo

[9] Hata N, Dohi T, Warfield S, Wells W, Kikinis R, Jolesz FA (1998) Multimodality deformable registration of pre- and intraoperative images for MRI guided brain surgery; http://splweb.bwh.harvard.edu:8000/pages/papers/noby/miccai98/hata192.htm

[10] Höhne KH, Hanson WA (1990) Interactive 3D-segmentation of MRI and CT volumes using morphological operators. J Comput Assist Tomogr 10: 41–53

[11] Kaus M, Warfield S, Jolesz F, Kikinis R (1998) Adaptive template moderated brain tumor segmentation in MRI. Bildverarbeitung für die Medizin. Springer, pp 102–106

[12] Levin D, Hu X, Tan KK, Galhotra S, Pelizzari CA et al (1989) The brain: Integrated three-dimensional display of MR and PET images. Radiology 172: 783–789

[13] Maintz A, Viergever M (1998) A survey of medical image registration. Medical Image Analysis 2 (1):1–36

[14] Mokhtarian, F Suomela R (1999) Curvature scale space for image point feature detection. Proceedings of the International Conference on Image Processing and its Applications, Manchester, UK 206–210

[15] Nakajima S, Atsumi H, Kikinis R, Moriarty TM, Metcalf DC, Jolesz FA, Black P (1997) Use of cortical surface vessel registration for image-guided neurosurgery. Neurosurgery 40 (6): 1201–1210

[16] Pal N, Pal S (1993) A review on image segmentation techniques. Pattern Recognition 26: 1277–1294

[17] Robb RA (1995) Three-dimensional biomedical imaging: Principles and practice, VCH, pp 183–188

[18] Serra J (1982) Image analysis and mathematical morphology. Academic Press

[19] Soltanian-Zadeh H, Windham JP, Chen F (1994) Automated contour extraction using a multi-scale approach, Proceedings IEEE Medical Imaging Conference, Norfolk, VA

[20] Specht DF (1990) Probabilistic neural networks. Neural Networks 3: 109–118

[21] Szekely G, Kelemen A, Brechbuhler C, Gerig G, (1996) Segmentation of 2d and 3d objects from MRI volume data using constrained elastic deformations of flexible Fourier contour and surface models. Medical Image Analysis 1 (1): 19–34

[22] Vannier M, Butterfield R, Jordan D, Murphy W, et al (1985) Multi-spectral analysis of magnetic resonance images. Radiology 154: 221–224

[23] Viola PA (1995) Alignment by maximization of mutual information. Artificial Intelligence Laboratory. Massachusetts Institute of Technology, PhD thesis, Cambridge, MA pp 155

[24] Viola PA, Wells III WM (1995) Alignment by maximization of mutual information. Fifth International Conference on Computer Vision, IEEE, Cambridge, MA 16–23

[25] Warfield SK (1998) Real-time image segmentation for image-guided surgery, http://splweb.bwh.harvard.edu:8000/pages/papers/warfield/sc98/index.html

[26] Warfield S, Jolesz F, Kikinis R (1998) A high performance computing approach to the registration of medical imaging data. Parallel Computing 24: 11345–11368

[27] Wells WM, Viola P, Atsumi H, Nakajima S, Kikinis R (1996) Multi-modal volume registration by maximization of mutual information. Medical Image Analysis 1: 35–51

[28] Wells III W, Kikinis R, Grimson W, Jolesz F (1996) Adaptive segmentation of MRI data. IEEE Transactions on Medical Imaging 15 (4): 429–442

[29] Westin C, Kikinis R (1998) Tensor controlled local structure enhancement of CT images for bone segmentation. Medical Image Computing and Computer Assisted Intervention (MICCAI) 1205–1212

Expanding the digital revolution to physical anthropology

W. Recheis[a,*], G. W. Weber[b], K. Schäfer[b], H. Prossinger[b], R. Eder[a], H. Seidler[b] and D. zur Nedden[a]

[a]Department of Radiology II, Medical University Innsbruck, Austria
[b]Institute for Anthropology, University Vienna, Austria

1. Introduction

Ötzi, the world-famous Iceman from Hauslabjoch was discovered in 1991 by a German couple. Results of anthropological analysis and carbon dating have confirmed that the man lived approximately 5300 years ago during the late Neolithic Age. The body is in an excellent state of preservation and many personal artifacts were found on or near the corpse [1]. This remarkable finding lead various international research groups to work on the Iceman. The radiological examinations were performed at the Department of Radiology II, University Hospital Innsbruck (DRII) and more recently at the Hospital of Bolzano, Italy [2]. These covered digital radiography and computed tomography.

It has to be mentioned that the introduction of new technologies like 3-dimensional reconstructions and stereolithography and their successful application in examining this astonishing corpse acted as a starting point of introducing highly sophisticated approaches into anthropology. However, earlier studies were performed using CT techniques and image postprocessing to investigate anthropological objects [3, 4].

In the case of the Iceman, advanced and novel technology like computer-aided design and rapid prototyping techniques was applied. By these means, a 3D hardcopy of the skull of the precious mummy (Fig. 1) could be produced from CT scans to examine its anatomy. This was the first time that a stereolithographic model was used for anthropological investigations [5]. The model was solely based on the CT data of the frozen mummy. The noninvasive approach allowed subsequent morphologic investigations.

These circumstances spurred various projects that allowed testing some of the new diagnostic and visualization methods within the Iceman research project, including: image processing and analysis, three-dimensional reconstructions, real-time volume rendering, virtual endoscopy, stereoscopic viewing stations and autostereoscopic display, modeling through stereolithography and fused deposition modeling. To get an impression of the impact of these technologies and methods in anthropology, some will be described in the subsequent chapters.

The related research activities promoted new techniques and an intensive collaboration between radiologists and anthropologists that was later successfully transferred to evolutionary studies.

2. Imaging techniques

2.1 Computed tomography in anthropology

Our computed tomography investigations of Ötzi and several fossils (see below) used commercially available scanners situated closely to the respective museums. Siemens Somatom Plus scanners were used in most cases. All scans performed in Innsbruck used a Siemens Somatom Plus S 40 and a Siemens Somatom Plus S 4 scanner. More recent examinations were performed with Multidetector CT, like Siemens Volume Zoom and Siemens Sensation 16. Other scanners included the GE Advantage (Broken Hill), GE PACE (Monte Circeo), and GE 9800 (Atapuerca) and a Siemens ART (Petralona). Contiguous 1mm – and <1mm when available – slices were obtained from each skull to achieve the best spatial resolution.

The matrix size of all scans was 512 × 512 pixels with a pixel size ranging typically from 0.4mm to 0.6mm depending certainly on the field of view. Most fossils were scanned in conventional mode, contrary to the spiral mode which is used normally in

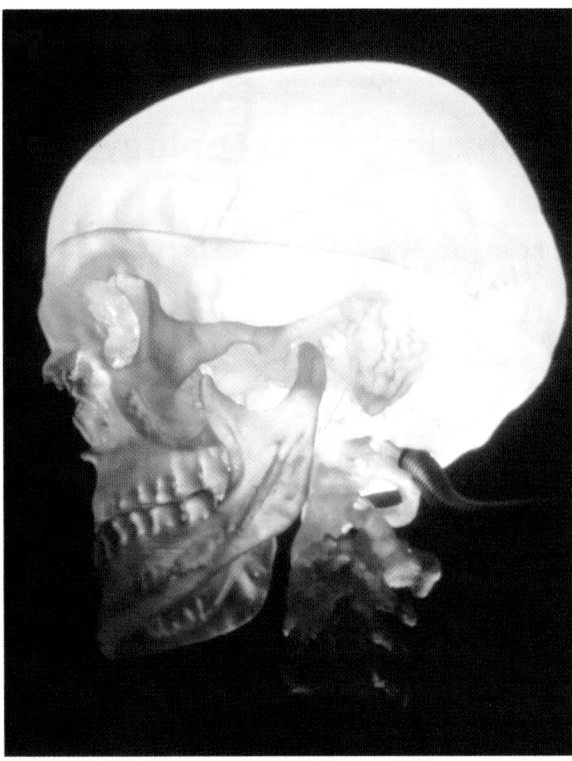

Fig. 1. Stereolithographic model of the cranium of the Tyrolean Iceman, reconstructed in two parts (calotte removable). All structural details are manufactured from the polymer with a resolution of 0.15 mm

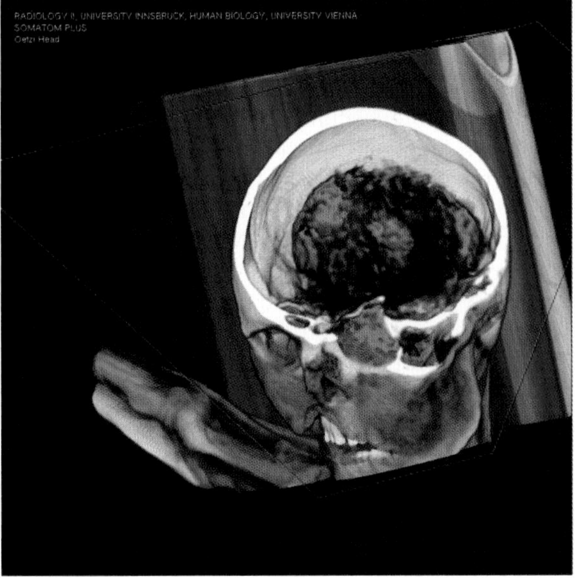

Fig. 2. 3D rendering of the Iceman's skull that demonstrates clearly the shrunken brain

medical examinations. The reason for the conventional protocol lies in the better spatial and contrast resolution. Different filters were used when calculating the image data: depending on the region of interest or the desired outcome soft algorithms were used in order to get an optimal dataset for visualization purposes or modeling. On the other hand, kernels applying more edge enhancement (high resolution kernels and filters) were used to augment small structures like the inner ear. A dental CT protocol was applied to study teeth and teeth structures. The spatial resolution of medical CT scanners clearly is soon at its limits when it comes to study small details – like trabecular structures – in sufficient accuracy. Recent examinations on teeth were performed with a so-called micro-CT allowing for a resolution in the μm scale.

2.2 Micro-CT

With the advent of cone-beam CT scanners or micro-CT another dimension in terms of spatial resolution has been opened. Micro-CT scanners allow a pixel resolution down to 5μm and it is expected that sub-micrometer scanners will be available on market the next few years (however, very rarely there are nano-meter scanners available: in combination with a synchrotron x-ray source in nuclear physics labs). These scanners – originally developed for material sciences and quality control – become more and more interesting in medical research and also in anthropology. The image matrix size goes up to 8000 × 8000 pixels or more. This high resolution allows the investigation of small structure e.g. on human or prehuman teeth [6]. The computational costs are, however, enormous. A 9μm full resolution scan of a 17mm scan length and a 35mm field of view needs up to 60 GB hard drive storage. Performing reasonable 3-dimensional structure analysis requires high end workstations or PC clusters. The constraints of commercially available micro-CT lie in the limited size of the object that can be scanned (typically 70mm – 100 mm field of view as a maximum). Some research facilities have own-built scanners with bigger field of views. Currently, micro-CT is also the tool for medical applications in osteoporosis research, it allows one to look beyond bone density measurements getting access to bone structures [7, 8]. The data allow researchers to predict mechanical properties. The suggested method for studying trabecular structures in patients is also a very promising one for the study of the direction of principal strains in fossilized bones to investigate behavioral patterns of hominids [9].

2.3 Image processing and analysis

Commercially available and free software packages such as 3dViewnix, Analyze (various versions) or ImageJ and others were used for segmenting the CT data and for generating and visualizing the 3-dimensional reconstructions. These software packages allow various kinds of image processing, analysis and visualization. During the segmentation process the interesting parts of the object are identified and defined. This procedure is sometimes difficult to perform because of the limited resolution (gray value dynamics and spatial resolution) of the CT scans, e.g. in the Iceman bony structures are sometimes demineralized or show different densities usually found in CT scans.

In contrast, most of the fossils showed some incrustation caused by stone matrix, having nearly the same Hounsfield Units as parts of interest lying beneath. The skulls of Steinheim, Bodo and OH 9 are prominent examples. There are no easy methods for removing these disturbing incrustations. Sophisticated filters are being designed to gain access to the underlying interesting parts and newly designed algorithms were used to remove the incrustations e.g. of the frontal sinuses of Steinheim. The electronic preparation of CT data is in fact a highly complex but helpful and, in contrast to physical methods, a reversible process that can be also applied to internal structures. These methods led, for example, to a representation of the anterior cranial fossa and paranasal sinuses of the mid-Pleistocene specimen of Steinheim [10]. This approach also offers a second benefit: Preparators sometimes use artificial material to complete a partly fragmented skull. Occasionally, it is difficult for investigators to distinguish (painted) plaster from fossilized bone, primarily because one fears scratching the specimen surface.

The previous examples point out the potential of virtual anthropology for meaningful morphologic analysis by using procedures that are similar to those applied in traditional anthropology. But virtual anthropology also allows for study approaches that are completely novel.

2.4 Geometric morphometrics

Digital 3D data per se are a source of information for morphometric analysis, no matter if they were acquired with CT scans, MRI scans, mechanical surface measuring devices, or by laser scanning. Landmark coordinates, linear and angle measurements, surface areas, and volumes represent quantitative data that validate and document the evolutionary changes of species with hard numbers and permit statistical analysis of form and shape by methods of usual biometry or the methods of geometric morphometrics [11, 12]. The possibility of probing every hidden structure rapidly increases the amount of data generated. For example, a very interesting result only became evident by the recent morphometric analysis of mid-Pleistocene and modern hominids: The forms of the inner and outer aspects of the human frontal bone are determined by completely independent factors [13]. The morphometric analysis also indicated that an unexpected stability in anterior brain morphology was evident during the time when modern human cognitive capacities emerged [13].

3. Rapid prototyping techniques in anthropology

3.1 Stereolithography

During the stereolithographic process a computer-guided laser beam hits the surface of a liquid photo monomer that covers a metal grid by about 0.1 mm. At the incident of the laser beam the monomer hardens by polymerization. After creating the first layer the metal grid is lowered, another layer of liquid photo monomer covers the hardened parts, and the exposure repeats. In this way the laser beam "writes" the contours of the loaded object layer by layer into the liquid surface and thus often very complex 3-dimensional objects are accomplished. Although the principle seems to be simple, some difficult steps have to be performed by a specifically trained engineer. Support structures have to be calculated and set up correctly to prevent distortions of the parts as they harden. After creating a model, post processing is necessary: the so-called finishing of the model. Our models are produced by Zumtobel Staff GmbH (Dept. of Rapid Prototyping / Rapid Tooling). The translucent stereolithographic models also turned out to be helpful for studies concerning endocranial morphology in evolutionary studies. Internal structures like sinusses are visible inside the translucent material and are even accessible if the specimen is replicated in several disassembleable parts. There is a good reason for this expensive procedure: because a rendering on a computer screen is still a two-dimensional projection of a virtual 3D object it is sometimes necessary to have a tangible model to understand the spatial relationships of structures. This is valid for both areas of our application: Clinical and anthropological. Of course, conventional casts of fossil specimens can also be used for morphologic comparison and do contain some information about texture, but they do not provide information about internal features.

3.2 Fused deposition modeling (FDM)

Like stereolithography, the FDM process forms three-dimensional objects from CAD-generated solid or surface models. In this procedure, a temperature-controlled head extrudes thermoplastic material layer by layer. The object emerges as a solid three-dimensional part.

The process begins with the design of a conceptual geometric model on a CAD workstation. The "design" is imported from the segmented CT data into the software, "Insight", which mathematically slices the conceptual model into horizontal layers. Support structures are automatically generated if needed. The generated path-data, which guide the building process, are then downloaded to the FDM system. In effect, it draws the model one layer at a time.

Thermoplastic modeling material feeds into the temperature-controlled FDM extrusion head, where it is heated to a semi-liquid state. The head extrudes and deposits the material in thin layers (0.18 mm) upon a base, directing the material into place with precision; as the material solidifies, each layer is laminated to the one preceding. The support material is water soluble thus making the necessary cleaning process easy by simply dropping a model into a water container.

The University Hospital Innsbruck, DRII was part of an international test program to evaluate the usefulness of this model-making device in clinical environment. The provider – as well as developer – of these systems is Stratasys, Inc. So far, the DRII is the only clinical department in Europe that facilitates a rapid prototyping system as a service for preoperative planning on site.

4. Examined fossils

The finding of the Iceman together with the invention of new technologies opened a new era in physical anthropology. The use of stereolithographic models and 3-dimensional analysis on computer screens has led to totally new perspectives. Extensive research on ancient skulls, with emphasis on endocranial morphology, has offered fascinating insights into the evolution of the human brain. Precious hominid fossils from the middle Pleistocene age (from

Name	Age	Specimen	Locality	Curator
Petralona	250–400 ky	*Homo heidelbergensis*	Petralona, Greece	G. Koufos
Kabwe I (or: Broken Hill)	300 ky	*Homo heidelbergensis*	Kabwe, Zambia	Ch. Stringer
Steinheim	250 ky	*Homo heidelbergensis*	Steinheim, Germany	M. Ziegler
Atapuerca V	300 ky	*Homo heidelbergensis*	Sierra de Atapuerca, Spain	J. L. Arsuaga
Monte Circeo	45 ky	*Homo neanderthalensis*	Rome, Italy	R. Machiarelli
Krapina (more specimens)	130 ky	*Homo neanderthalensis*	Krapina, Croatia	J. Radovcic
Bodo	600 ky	*Homo heidelbergensis*	Bodo, Ethiopia	A. J. H. Mariam
"Mrs. Ples" (STS 5)	2.5 My	*Australopithecus africanus*	Sterkfontein, South Africa	F. Thackaray
STW 505	2.5 My	*Australopithecus africanus*	Sterkfontein, South Africa	F. Thackaray
STS 71	2.5 My	*Australopithecus africanus*	Sterkfontein, South Africa	P. V. Tobias
OH 5 "Nutcracker Man"	1.8 My	*Australopithecus (Paranthropus) boisei*	Olduvai Gorge, Tanzania	C. Magori
OH 9	1 My	*Homo ergaster, erectus*	Olduvai Gorge, Tanzania	C. Magori
AL 129 – 1a + 1b	3.4 My	*Australopithecus afarensis*	Hadar, Ethiopia	Ato Muluneh A. J. H. Mariam
AL 333	3,4 My	*Australopithecus afarensis*	Hadar, Ethiopia	Ato Muluneh A. J. H. Mariam
OMO 1 and 2	130 ky	*Homo sapiens*	Kibish, Omo Basin, Ethiopia	Ato Muluneh A. J. H. Mariam
Mladec 1 and 2	35 ky	*Homo sapiens*	Mladec, Czech Republic	Maria Teschler Nicola

The fossil record examined by our team.

600.000 to 200.000 years old) like the skulls of Petralona (Greece), Kabwe I or - more popular - Broken Hill (Zambia), Steinheim (Germany), Bodo (Ethiopia), Atapuerca (Spain) were examined by the means of computed tomography [3, 4, 14, 15]. Neanderthal specimens such as the skull of Monte Circeo (Italy), [16] and some findings from Krapina (Croatia) were also examined.

5. Some results

5.1 Some findings in the Iceman

Three-dimensional reconstructions of the Icemans skull offered completely new insights regarding the Iceman's body. The skin was intact all over the skull and face, but certain surface abnormalities were apparent. This included the collapsed globes of the eyes, a flattened left malar eminence, a wide space between the maxillary central incisors, and pressure-induced deformities of the lips, nose, and ears. 3-dimensional images clearly show a shrunken brain with separated meninges (Fig. 2).

On the other hand the stereolithographic model (Fig. 1) showed several features like the erosion of teeth and a tripod fracture [17]. The model showed flat surfaces on all the teeth, most likely caused by abrasives in the diet, such as mineral particles that might be added to flour as grain is ground. Furthermore, the stereolithographic model faithfully rendered a tripod fracture of the left maxilla and replicated the amount of fracture fragment displacement and the relationships of the fracture fragments. The model also showed a kind of flattening of the entire left maxillofacial region that could not be visualized on individual CT slices. The asymmetry as well as the fractures are thought to be caused by the pressure due to the weight of the glacial ice. A recent research project has described mathematically the deformations of the Icemańs skull [18]. In 2001 additional CT scans and digital radiographs were obtained in Bolzano. These scans revealed a structure situated between the left scapula and rib cage that is now verified as an arrow head [2], (Fig. 3).

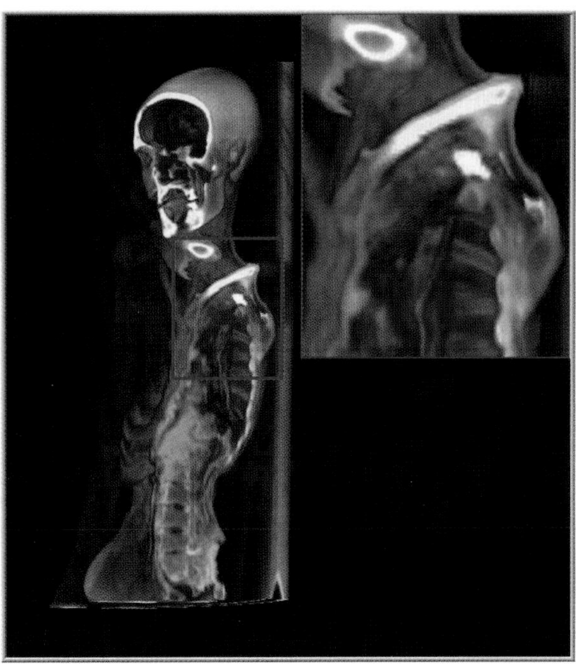

Fig. 3. Visualization made from CT scans of the arrowhead that probably killed the Iceman: The arrowhead is ledged between the ribs and the left scapula

5.2 The skull of Monte Circeo – an example for "virtual anthropology"

A Neandertal specimen called "Monte Circeo" was found in 1939 at Monte Circeo (Latina, Italy). Using various anatomical markers, the endocranial capacity was estimated to be 1550 cm^3. In 1997 a high resolution computer tomography scan was performed. As the original skull has several incrustations, which also can be seen on the CT scans, the data were electronically "cleaned". On the other hand the Monte Circeo finding has major defects on the right temporo-orbital region and at the cranial base. Using medical image processing tools like those described above, the missing part of the temporo-orbital region was modeled as a reversed replica of the intact side. The missing parts of the cranial base were reconstructed using various anatomical landmarks. The software packages allowed the enclosed endocranial cavity to be rendered as a separate 3D object (virtual endocast) and its volume to be calculated directly. The accuracy of this 3D computer modeled endocast has been checked by making the cranial bones transparent in order to visualize the virtual endocast. No obvious incongruity between the original endocast and the volume-rendered endocranial cavity has been recognized. The thus calculated endocranial capacity is about 1350 cm3 [16], (Fig. 4).

5.3 Findings in middle-Pleistocene fossils

Until recently, anthropological examinations were restricted by limited access to these fossils. The validity in digital data processing is going to change this [19]. Although visualization of the internal morphology of the supraorbital torus appears similar

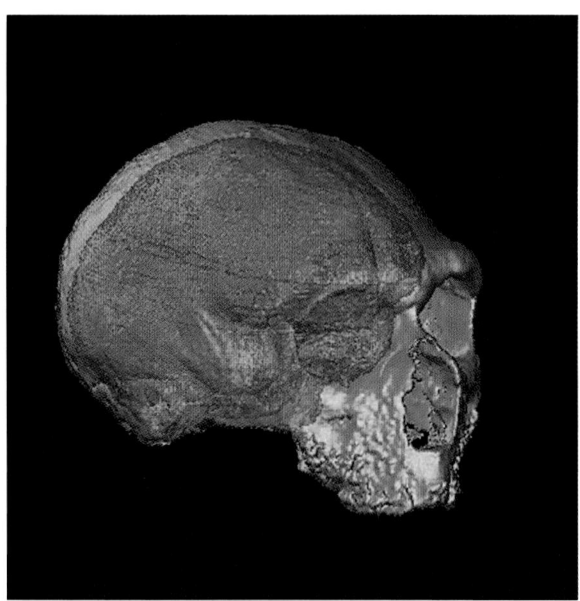

Fig. 4. Semitransparent reconstructions of the skull of Monte Circeo are used to prove the anatomy and morphology of the virtual endocast as well as to perform various measurements

in some ancient fossils, reconstructions performed at the University Clinic of Innsbruck showed differences. 3-dimensional reconstructions and stereolithographic modeling revealed extremely strong pneumatization in Petralona and Broken Hill, whereas Arago 21 shows only minor pneumatizations of the paranasal sinuses. The model of Broken Hill for example reveals corresponding crests that appear less massive than in those in Petralona. It has been shown that the frontal lobes of Petralona and Broken Hill are not only positioned behind the orbits, but are also inclined more steeply in a rostrocaudal direction than in modern humans. The forehead in these two specimens (*Homo heidelbergensis*) is built mainly by the extent of the frontal sinus, while the forehead of modern humans is built by the anteriorly positioned frontal lobes. Impressions and ridges (impressiones digitale) that correspond to *gyri* and *sulci*, respectively, on the orbital surfaces of the frontal lobes are difficult to assess due to destruction in Petralona and are reproduced only faintly in Broken Hill. These features are pronounced in the anterior cranial fossa in Arago 21, as it is also the usual case in modern humans [20]. Astonishingly, these impressions are well developed in Bodo, the oldest representative of *Homo heidelbergensis* (600.000 years). Such impressions have been interpreted as indicating progressive evolution of the basal neocortex. At a first glance, the orbital sulcus patterns, as well as frontal lobe shape, would be needed before one can assess their significance of their fossil shape in middle-Pleistocene hominids.

5.4 Findings in Australopithecines

The cranial capacities for the australopithecines STS 5 ("Mrs. Ples") and STW 505 ("Mr. Ples") were determined to 485 cm^3 and 515 cm^3 respectively. Earlier estimation of the endocranial volume of STW 505 went up to 600 cm^3 [21].

These differences in endocranial morphology and volume between the examined specimens may allow new interpretations in human evolution. The recent measurements on australopithecines, especially STW 505, suggest that current views on the tempo and mode of hominid brain evolution may need to be reevaluated.

Another brain-related research question is that of cranial capacity, which in addition to the structural characteristics of the brain can be an important item of taxonomic classification. Estimating this volume is relatively easy if a skull is almost intact, but the task is more susceptible to observer errors in the case of fragmented skulls. Virtual endocasts of the braincase have been produced electronically in a highly reproducible way and helped to visualize and measure the cranial capacity of Australopithecus africanus specimens or archaic Homo with a minimal error [22, 23], (Fig 5).

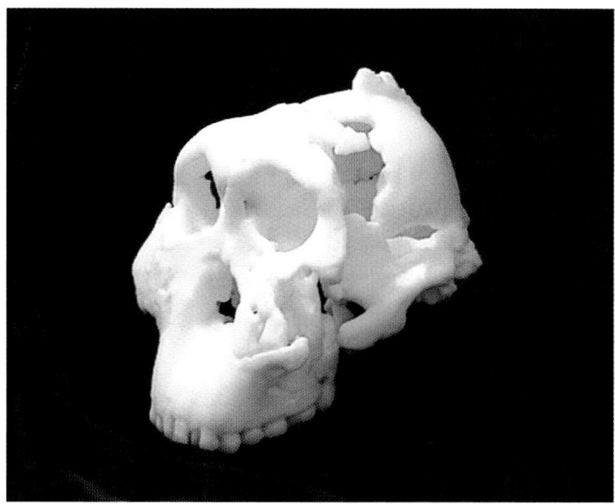

Fig. 5. Model made with "fused deposition modeling" of OH 5 ("Nutcracker Man", Australopithecus boisei, 1.8 million years old)

6. Successful medical applications of rapid prototyping techniques

Plastic surgery and maxillofacial surgery are the most prominent disciplines that took advantage of the results of Iceman research. The first stereolithographic model to be used in preoperative planning was made in 1992 [24]. In the meantime an average of about 40 models per year have been successfully built, since 1999 with our own FDM equipment on site. Normally stereolithography is used to produce a model of a skull or a part of a skull. The models are used in several ways:

- Operation planning: The surgeons can identify osteotomy lines, which have to be cut in the bony skull. Thus the surgeon is able to plan the operation steps days in advance.
- Training: the surgeon is able to practice the operation on the model.
- Surgeons can evaluate new operation techniques on the model at hand before operating on the patient.

The stereolithography model allows better visualization of the skeletal systems thus reducing the surgical risk. The object can be measured and touched thus deepening the feeling for the operation. Healing and growth can be documented optimally. The preoperative skull and the postoperative skull can both be used for teaching purposes.

Operation time can be reduced up to 40 %. This results in an increased wellbeing of the patient. In some cases, the number of follow-up operations could be decreased and as a consequence the overall costs could be reduced, even though the costs of such a model are still relatively high (600–4000 Euro) [25], (Fig 6).

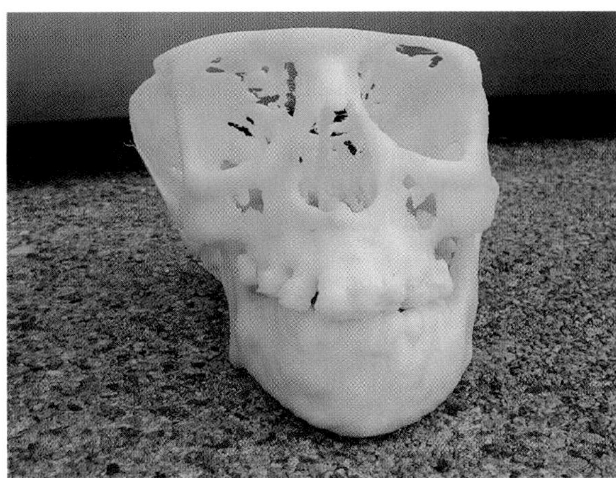

Fig. 6. Model of a patients skull as it is used for preoperative planning in maxillo-facial surgery

A more recent approach to models for medical purposes is the fused deposition modeling (FDM) process. This technique allows the construction of real-sized models on site. The Department of Maxillo-Facial Surgery, Medical University Innsbruck is using this method for preoperative planning routinely. Meanwhile this technology is going to be introduced into neurosurgery. Exact models of intracranial vessels and aneurysms allow to fit coils and clips preoperatively (Fig. 7), and luminal models can be used in basic research of the fluid dynamics in aneurysms and vessels.

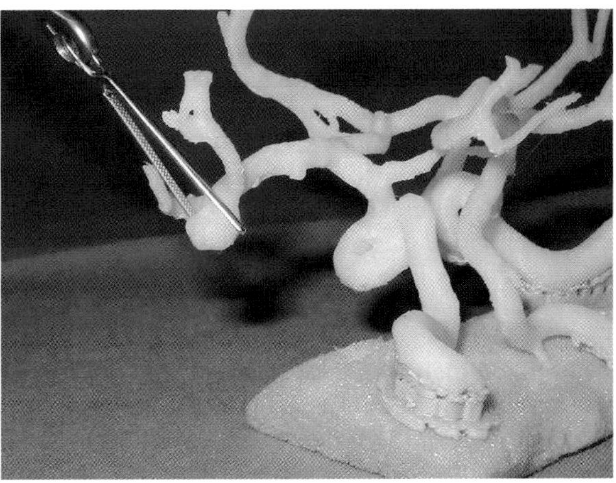

Fig. 7. Fused Deposition Modeling (FDM) of an intracranial aneurysm. This method of preoperative planning is now introduced into neurosurgery

7. Discussion

Ötzi's mummy was examined radiographically. Multiplanar and three-dimensional reconstruction of the available CT scans preserved the head while extracting the necessary anthropological data from the skull. The invention of stereolithography, a very accurate rapid prototyping technique, allowed exact "hardcopies" of the Iceman's skull, copying not only the outer surface but also the cavities and the inner surface. This semitransparent material enables intuitive and direct understanding of anatomical features.

The outer measurements taken from this model proved identical to those obtained directly from the mummy's head. The accuracy (as measured experimentally on either specimen) is + −0.5 mm in derived linear measurements.

The development of new rendering algorithms in combination with fast graphics workstation offers new ways to visualize complex structures like the

Iceman's anatomy and allowing real-time access to large data sets such as "virtual fly-throughs".

These impressive results in the Iceman research have opened a new era in anthropology: The so-called "virtual anthropology" [26]. Precious anthropological objects are examined by the means of computed tomography at the highest resolution. Many measurements of anthropological interest can be performed on computer workstations. Consequently, computer-aided anthropology represents a new and accurate instrument in describing and visualizing precious objects of anthropological interest.

If a model is needed for clearer interpretation of morphological structures, stereolithography seems to be an ideal tool – the "gold standard". But new techniques like Fused Deposition Modeling offer a different quality in making models. The easy handling of the modeling process and the ability to produce models on site seem to be great advantages.

At about the time the Iceman was found, modern imaging and post processing techniques began to be introduced into medicine. Various national and international collaborations were spurred allowing the testing of some of the new diagnostic methods within the Iceman research project. As shown above, anthropological research may profit enormously from virtual anthropology: It enables views into the interior of structures as well as ensures highly reproducible quantitative measurements and easily controllable manipulations. The published data suggest that if skulls resemble each other externally, this does not necessarily mean that they resemble each other internally. In studying this morphology by using virtual fossils and stereolithographic models, some insights were provided that contributed to the interpretation of the origins of modern humans. No doubt, an essential part of studies will have to be carried out not on the real object, but in a computer lab by using various kinds of digital data.

The success of virtual anthropology triggered the clinical applications of techniques presented here – and certainly vice versa. Thus various fields in research as well as clinical routine were opened that gain more and more importance.

References

[1] Seidler H, Bernhard W, Teschler-Nicola M, et al (1992) Some anthropological aspects of the prehistoric Tyrolean ice man. Science 258: 455–457

[2] Murphy WA, Jr, Nedden Dz D, Gostner P, Knapp R, Recheis W, Seidler H (2003) The iceman: discovery and imaging. Radiology 226: 614–629

[3] Vannier MW, Marsh JL, Warren JO (1984) Three dimensional CT reconstruction images for craniofacial surgical planning and evaluation. Radiology 150: 179–184

[4] Conroy GC, Vannier MW (1987) Dental development of the Taung skull from computerized tomography. Nature 329: 625–627

[5] zur Nedden D, Knapp R, Wicke K, et al (1994) Skull of a 5,300-year-old mummy: reproduction and investigation with CT-guided stereolithography. Radiology 193: 269–272

[6] Weber GW (2004) GLL 33. In: Seidler H, Woldeagaray K, Macciarelli R, Bondoli L, Illerhaus B, Kullmer O (eds) Vienna: Institute of Anthropology University of Vienna, DVD Edition

[7] Durand, Ruegsegger P (1992) High contrast resolution of computed tomography images for bone structure analysis. Medical Physics 19: 569–573

[8] Ruegsegger P (2001) Imaging of bone structure, 2nd edn. CRC Press, Boca Raton, pp 1–24

[9] Macchiarelli R, Bondioli L, Galichon V, Tobias PV (1999) Hip bone trabecular architecture shows uniquely distinctive locomotor behaviour in South African australopithecines. J Hum Evol 36: 211–232

[10] Prossinger HGW, Seidler H, Recheis W, Ziegler R, Zur Nedden D (1998) Electronically aided preparation of fossilized skulls: Medical imaging techniques and algorithms as an innovative tool in paleoanthropological research. Am J Phys Anthropol 181

[11] Bookstein FL, Grayson B, Cutting CB, Kim HC, McCarthy JG (1991) Landmarks in three dimensions: reconstruction from cephalograms versus direct observation. Am J Orthod Dentofacial Orthop 100: 133–140

[12] O'Higgins P, Jones N (1998) Facial growth in Cercocebus torquatus: an application of three-dimensional geometric morphometric techniques to the study of morphological variation. J Anat 193: 251–272

[13] Bookstein F, Schafer K, Prossinger H, et al (1999) Comparing frontal cranial profiles in archaic and modern homo by morphometric analysis. Anat Rec 257: 217–224

[14] Zonneveld F, Spoor F, Wind J (1989) The use of CT in the study of internal morphology of hominid fossils. Medicamundi 34: 117–128

[15] Conroy GC, Vannier MW, Tobias PV (1990) Endocranial features of Australopithecus africanus revealed by 2- and 3-D computed tomography. Science 247: 838–841

[16] Recheis W, Macchiarelli R, Seidler H, et al (1999) Re-evaluation of the endocranial volume of the Guattari 1 Neandertal specimen (Monte Circeo). Coll Antropol 23: 397–405

[17] Wilfing H, Seidler H, zur Nedden D, et al (1994) Cranial deformation of the Neolithic Man from the Hauslabjoch. Coll. Antropol 8: 269–282

[18] Prossinger H, Seidler H, Weaver DS, Schafer K, Fieder M, Weber GW (1999) The iceman under pressure (Part I): A description of skull deformations due to

5100 years of glacial action. Coll Antropol 23: 345–367

[19] Weber GW (2001) Virtual anthropology (VA): a call for glasnost in paleoanthropology. Anat Rec 265: 193–201

[20] Seidler H, Falk D, Stringer C, et al (1997) A comparative study of stereolithographically modelled skulls of Petralona and Broken Hill: implications for future studies of middle Pleistocene hominid evolution. J Hum Evol 33: 691–703

[21] Conroy GC, Weber GW, Seidler H, Tobias PV, Kane A, Brunsden B (1998) Endocranial capacity in an early hominid cranium from Sterkfontein, South Africa. Science 280: 1730–1731

[22] Falk D, Redmond JC, Jr, Guyer J, et al (2000) Early hominid brain evolution: a new look at old endocasts. J Hum Evol 38: 695–717

[23] Conroy GC, Falk D, Guyer J, Weber GW, Seidler H, Recheis W (2000) Endocranial capacity in Sts 71 (Australopithecus africanus) by three-dimensional computed tomography. Anat Rec 258: 391–396

[24] Anderl H, Zur Nedden D, Muhlbauer W, et al (1994) CT-guided stereolithography as a new tool in craniofacial surgery. Br J Plast Surg 47: 60–64

[25] Recheis W, Rapid ES (1996) Prototyping and its importance for the successful optimization of production processes. Managing intergrated manufacturing, 105–113

[26] Weber GW, Recheis W, Scholze T, Seidler H (1998) Virtual anthropology (VA): methodological aspects of linear and volume measurements–first results. Coll Antropol 22: 575–584

Metropolitan healthcare networking

H. Grosinger and A. Plihal

Vienna Hospital Association (VHA), EDP-Management and Organisation, Vienna, Austria

Introduction

In Austria as much as elsewhere, the healthcare system, with its multitude of service providers and its many access opportunities and responsibilities, is an essential element in a society that is evolving into an information society. Measures taken by the European Union – for example, the initiatives eEurope, eGovernment and eHealth – show how far society as a whole has changed already. The health system uses modern information and telecommunication technologies and is therefore very much part of this development. In future, all healthcare providers within a fragmented health system are expected to start cooperating more closely by using modern technologies. Hospitals as centres of medical competence and doctors who have set up their own practices are leading this trend. Issues related to medical informatics, health telematics, and standardisation in the context of health communications have therefore become subject to technological development. These developments raise people's expectations – for example, in terms of higher-quality treatment, rationalization, and cost savings – as well as fears – for example, the loss of confidentiality in the use of patient-related information.

For health politics in Austria, these developments have created new responsibilities in terms of coordination and regulation. The first step that the Ministry of Health took was to establish the so-called "STRING Commission" (German acronym for standards and guidelines for the use of informatics in Austria's health service), which worked out the framework conditions for a logical Austrian health data network. The results were communicated as the "MAGDA-LENA-guideline" (German acronym for medical-administrative data exchange – logical electronic network Austria).

In view of the changed conditions, the existing Data Protection Act was expanded and a new health telematics law initiated, which is currently a draft bill.

The initial spark

Health network Donaustadt – a pilot

Still a few years ago, patients who were discharged from hospital often had to wait for weeks for their patient's letters or discharge letter. As a result, domestic care was based on rudimentary information, so that the medical knowledge and information accumulated at that moment could not be used fully. So that hospitals' medical competencies could be used effectively in an extramural setting, the project "Health Network Donaustadt" was initiated in 1998, under the medical director Professor Dr. Karl-Heinz Tragl. The aim of the project was to provide doctors with their own practices, speedily with patient information and thereby improve medical care. In realising this objective, electronic forms of communication – such as the internet and secure emails – played a central part.

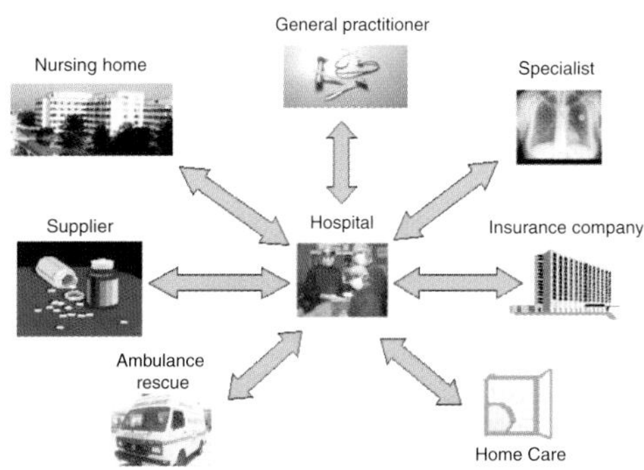

Fig. 1. Transmural electronic communication in the healthcare system

This was the first step towards bridging the gap between hospitals as centres of competence and the extramural sector.

From its very beginning, the new pilot project met with great interest from many social services organisations. In 1999, the municipal authorities department 47 – "Home Care" approached the Danube Hospital to gather information on its own clients. The department selected as its pilot base the health centre of Vienna's 21st and 22nd municipal district. Close collaboration between the pilot base and Danube Hospital subsequently resulted in a Thera Care Report. This report is compiled by the care staff and the physiotherapist and nursing of the hospital to which the patient was admitted, and its purpose is to support home care after discharge (discharge management). The Thera Care Report includes all necessary information that is required for the further care of the patient. In addition, it contains information on ergotherapy, physiotherapy, speech therapy, and dietary and nutritional advice. Shortly before a patient is discharged, the report is transmitted electronically to the Home Care, which then provides services to the patient – ranging from mobile care delivered in the patient's home, household help, and meals on wheels. This collaboration was made official in May 2001.

Since 2003, all Thera Care Report from the Donauspital were delivered to "Home Care".

Reflexion on the Health Network Donaustadt

The work associated with the Donaustadt Health Network's development necessitated a multitude of nationwide adjustments. This close cooperation mainly between the Austrian Medical Chamber, the Vienna Hospital Association, the Federation of the Austrian Social Security Institutions, and many more.

The Health Network Donaustadt parallel to the "MAGDA-LENA guidelines" of the "STRING Commission" and the new health telematics law, three milestones in the enhancement of communication achieved:

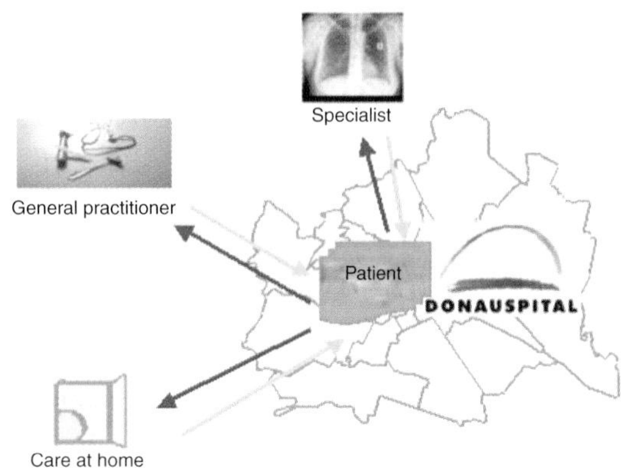

Fig. 2. Health Network Donaustadt

Register of communication partners

During the course of the project, the need for a secure register of partners became obvious. This central electronic register needed to include all potential participants of a "health alliance". Under the aegis of the Austrian Medical Chamber, an "electronic register of healthcare providers" was created.

This register provides the data that are necessary for the electronic exchange of diagnoses in response to automated and individual queries, and it includes only those who are entitled to participate in the communication. In this way, large amounts of health data can be handled in an efficient and economic manner. The entries are maintained by the organisation from which the data originated, with the help of a web-based application. For example: data on doctors are provided by the Austrian Medical Chamber, and the cost centres of Vienna's hospitals by the Vienna Hospital Association etc.

This service is being made available to Austria's health service by the Austrian Medical Chamber and the medical chambers for Lower Austria and Vienna.

Technically, this takes the shape of an LDAP-Server (LDAP = lightweight directory access protocol).

The electronic register is still under construction, and additional health service providers are continually being added.

Standardisation

Electronic communications so far had been shaped by a multitude of different file formats and forms that are used by the information technologic-applications of the communication partners. This made data exchange difficult.

In collaboration with Austria's Standards Institute, the standardisation of medical forms was advanced. Thus far, Austrian norms, which are based on international standards, have become available for three electronic reports.

- Exchange of administrative patient information between hospitals and private insurance companies (K2201)

- Referral/admission (K2202)
- Patient discharge letter, patient's letter, and medical report (K2203)
- Reports for electronic data transfer of cost data between hospitals and private insurance companies (K2201-1/2)

Suppliers can provide the data in a structured format, and recipients (communication partners) can integrate these into their information technologic environment.

Empowerment of the communication partners

A particular challenge lay in providing the technical capability to communication partners to use the established communications channels. This should be achieved by expanding the information technologic infrastructures in the practices of established doctors.

To facilitate this, the initiative "Networking Viennese Doctors" was founded, on the background of the Health Network Vienna, by the Viennese Social-Health Insurance Company, Vienna's Medical Chamber, and the City of Vienna, represented by the Vienna Hospital Association. The project is hoping to entice software manufacturers to integrate a secure, standard-based procedure for the electronic transfer diagnoses and the account with Health Insurance Companies into their medical software packages.

Existing communications channels

With the electronic register, standardising forms, and technical empowerment of the communication partners, several electronic communications of the Vienna Hospital Association were initiated.

Pharmacy

In 2000 the ordering process for pharmaceuticals in the Vienna Hospital Association was modernised. Seven pharmacies located in the main hospitals now register their orders in with software "SAP". About 47,000 orders annually are now handled in this way – which is equivalent to about 250 million euros. Previously, orders had been printed out and faxed to the suppliers. Now they are being sent directly from the SAP-system as faxes and simultanously transmitted electronically to the suppliers.

Radiology

In the last years, individual radiologists whose institutes are in close proximity to the Danube Hospital have been linked up with a secure tunnel link via the internet to the Institute for Radiology at the Donauspital. Exclusively radiological images are transmitted via these tunnel links. These are therefore available to the Danube Hospital's picture archiving communication system.

Neurosurgery

Although the county hospital Klosterneuburg in Lower Austria has modern imaging technologies at its disposal, no neurosurgical procedures or treatment can currently be made at this hospital. For patients who require neurosurgical treatment, however, the images obtained in Klosterneuburg can be transmitted electronically to the neurosurgery department at "Rudolfstiftung" and Danube Hospital. Thus a clarification for the patient can be requested and if necessary transferred to the other hospital.

Collaboration with Vienna Social Fund

On 1 July 2004, Vienna Social Fund was founded, which since then has acted as the successor organisation to Home Care. To support the fund's organisational tasks in caring for its clients, the exchange of administrative patient information data with the Vienna Hospital Association was seen as desirable. The fund wants to receive information on patient admission and discharge from the hospitals as rapidly as possible. The aim is for the fund to control the agreed services more effectively, or to initiate services that will be needed in the future. The information channel is used all across the Vienna Hospital Association.

Cooperation with private health insurance providers – a pilot

In order to facilitate the Danube Hospital's cost accounts for patients receiving additional services, an electronic communication channel with private insurers was established. When a patient with private health insurance is admitted to hospital, an admission note is simultaneously sent to the insurer. The insurance company then returns its declaration to cover the costs for a fixed period. If the patient needs to remain in hospital for a longer period than the insurer has agreed to cover, an extension note is sent to the insurer to extend the period covered. This two-way cooperation is being tested in Danube Hospital in the context of a pilot project; it is planned to become fully operational in late 2004.

Cooperation with mandatory health insurance

In breaking down hospitals' inpatient and outpatient costs, the Federation of the Austrian Social Security Institutions has a pivotal position. If no social insurance body can allocate the administrative data for a particular cost item, these are returned to the hospital for further investigation and clarification. To facilitate this query, the federation has made available a tool to all Austrian hospitals that can be used to run online queries into a patient's insurance status. The queries are run via a secure tunnel link via the internet.

Perspective

The steps taken so far in extending communication channels between individual health service providers in Austria's health system have laid the foundation for efficient cooperation between all partners. The consistently positive response to the services provided has prompted increased efforts: existing communication channels are expanded and new ones added; the many one-way electronic collaborations are transformed into two-way ones; and successful pilot projects are rolled out. All this has resulted in a deeper understanding and increased awareness of problems among the participants.

In addition to the existing communication channels, the following are planned:

Dispatching discharge letters – rollout

Dispatching discharge letters to the extramural sector was limited to the Danube Hospital for the duration of the initial project "Health Network Donaustadt". After a technological adaptation of the word processing used for discharge letters, a rollout to additional hospitals in the Vienna Hospital Association has become possible hospitals "Lainz" and "Rudolfstiftung" as new communication partners can now use the improved communication process for themselves and have initiated the planned expansion process in 2004.

Thera Care Report – rollout

The Thera Care Report that was also developed in the context of "Health Network Donaustadt" has now been updated to state-of-the-art technology. This facilitates its rollout across the entire Vienna Hospital Association. The start of this rollout is planned for early 2005.

Pharmacy

By establishing automated pharmacy ordering for the Vienna Hospital Association, it has now become possible to include hospitals from the private sector into this non-medical ordering process. The following project plan is under discussion at the moment: two privately managed hospitals in Vienna are intending to handle their pharmacy ordering via the Danube Hospital pharmacy. The orders would go to the Danube Hospital pharmacy first and then be faxed by automated fax to the suppliers. The Danube Hospital pharmacy will then deliver the goods to the private hospital.

Radiology

To make individual communications between Danube Hospital and individual radiology institutes in its environs, a new IT project has been started in collaboration with an external radiology institute to place a general usable bases. The aim is to import digital images and the accompanying reports into Vienna Hospital Association. Both, images and reports, will then be made available to the diagnosing physician in the context of the electronic patient history.

Cooperation with Vienna Social Fund

Since the transmission of a patient's admission note to the Vienna Social Fund has become established successfully, it has now become possible to receive, in return, data about that particular patient from the fund. This information is received by the carers in the domestic area and helps the nursing in the hospital to continue patient care more rapidly and targeted. These data are transmitted on the basis of the standardised referral form of the Austrian Standards Institute. The Danube Hospital has volunteered to pilot this communication channel. If the pilot is found to be successful, the project will be rolled out across the entire Vienna Hospital Association.

Experiences with the referral form are also collected, to be used for referrals from doctors with their own practices.

Cooperation with private insurance companies – add on

To complete the existing cooperation with the private insurers (query and declaration that costs will be covered), a further step is required. In individual cases, private insurers may request diagnoses from the Vienna Hospital Association. Currently these have to be sent in the post. As soon as the electronic patient history has been enhanced by a function to send reports, these can be transferred electronically to the respective insurers.

After a positive conclusion to the pilot, rollout across the hospitals in the Vienna Hospital Association is planned.

Austria-wide linking of patient indices

For historical reasons, Austria's health services are very fragmented, and the electronic patient administrations in the public and private organisations use many different patient indices. To enable an efficient exchange of data, relating to a particular patient, a unified communication structure is required. For this reason, the working group "patient index" has been set up in the "IT-Forum of the funding bodies of Austria's hospitals". This group is specifically concerned with this topic and aims at linking existing patient indices.

The first use of such a linkage is to find out about a specific patient whether data about him or her have been captured in a medical care unit, and if so, in which one.

Making these data accessible is planned only as a second step. This will require a general and complete clarification of data protection matters. In this context, the introduction of the so-called "e-card" is of importance. Using this card as an essential access criterion for patient data may be an option, similar to a cash card.

Birth and death certificates

These currently have to be completed by hand. To save parents or relatives unnecessary visits to official bodies and to reduce the administrative effort for the City of Vienna, this procedure will be changed. In future, communications of municipal authorities of City of Vienna, "Citizenship and personal status matters," about births and deaths will be handled electronically. This means that birth and death certificates may be issued with greater speed.

Patient oriented, integrated care management

In July 2002, the sickness fund for the Vienna region and the municipal authorities of City of Vienna have started the model project "patient oriented, integrated care management" in the west of Vienna. The problems relating to the interface between internal and external partners are central themes.

As a result the model project in an initiative was started, to find out whether the transmitted admission and discharge notes of inpatients can contribute meaningfully to optimising the work of doctors in their own practices. Within the project, 10 doctors' practices are provided with the required IT environment and the doctors receive the admission and discharge notes for those patients of the Vienna Social Fund of whom they are the treating physician.

Summary

The fragmentation of Austria's healthcare system makes networking healthcare providers an essential task in future healthcare provision. Under this central challenge, a multitude of initiatives have been started. In the areas of pharmacy, neurosurgery, radiology, administration, care, and patient documentation, essential progress has been made. Further steps initiatives are already in the project stages.

By systematically applying modern project management methods in the IT area, new foundations were created for Austria's healthcare sector, which enable a successful expansion of communications. Essential for success have been standardisation of several working tools, linkage of dispersed identification registers, and the creation of a central register of partners.

References

DSG (2000)
Health telematics law
Ö-Normen K2201 bis K2203

Links

Federal Ministry of Health and Social Security:
http://www.bmgf.gv.at/
CEN – European Committee for Standardization:
http://www.cenorm.be/cenorm/index.htm
DSG – Data Protection Act:
http://www.ad.or.at/office/recht/dsg2000.htm
Health Network Vienna:
http://www.gesundheitsnetzwien.at
Health telematics law:
http://www.marc.co.at/Gesundheitstelematikgesetz.pdf
Vienna Hospital Association:
http://www.wienkav.at/kav/
MAGDA-LENA-guideline:
http://www.bmgf.gv.at/cms/site/detail.htm?thema=CH0015&doc=CMS1038912712944
ON – Austrian Standards Institute:
http://www.on-norm.at/
ÖAK – Austrian Medical Chamber:
http://www.aek.or.at/
Patient oriented, integrated care management:
http://www.univie.ac.at/pik/
WGKK – Wiener Gebietskrankenkasse:
http://www.wgkk.at/
DSG 2000
Health telematics law
Ö-Normen K2201 bis K2203

Teleconsultation in medicine and radiology – theory and legal aspects

W. Hruby

Chairman of the Radiology Department, Danube Hospital, Vienna, Austria

Introduction

Medicine in a network only expresses the use of a network for the purpose of medicine, whereas networked medicine is the optimized application of medical examinations and therapeutic methods with the physician as an interface for the diseased person. Provided it fulfils certain requirements – networked medicine is a valuable enrichment in medical diagnosis and therapy.

In essence, teleconsultation consists of obtaining expert advice from colleagues when the physician is confronted with especially difficult or rare cases. Teleconsultation also denotes the transfer of information concerning a specific patient for the purpose of comparison and for establishing the diagnosis or making decisions in regard of therapy. The transfer of medical data and images to elucidate written medical reports also belongs to the spectrum of teleconsultation.

The major application of telemedicine is the situation in which the treating physician seeks another physician's opinion or advice, at the request or with the permission of the patient. However, in some cases, the patient's only contact with the physician is via telemedicine. The aim of these services is normally to provide guidance to patients as to whether they should seed a face-to-face consultation with a physician, and if so, where and how urgently.

The World Medical Association recognizes that, in addition to the positive consequences of telemedicine, there are many ethical and legal issues arising from these new practices. Notably, by eliminating a common site and face-to-face consultation, telemedicine disrupts some of the traditional principles which govern the physician-patient relationship. Therefore, there are certain ethical guidelines and principles that must be followed by physicians involved in telemedicine.

Teleconsultation in radiology in Austria

As the technical requirements for teleconsultation are particularly advanced, especially in the field of radiology, the Austrian Radiological Society established a work group for current requirements and legal and structural preconditions for teleconsultation. Based on the results of this investigation and a legal expert report, five guiding principles were formulated. A statement of the Ministry of Health underscored and confirmed the opinion of this work group. The purpose of this group was to work on the following subjects:

- List the existing facilities and the experience gained thus far;
- define the legal prerequisites;
- establish professional and minimal technical requirements;
- data protection, data safety, documentation;
- promote communication between in-patient and extramural areas with the help of teleconsultation as a service for patients, and
- goals to be realised, in consideration of the fact that medicine is an immediate service and that investigation and initial reporting constitute a single unit.

Evaluation of significant basic data

In a questionnaire addressed to all members of the Austrian Radiological Society basic data for further actions of the work group were collected. The institution-based percentage of returned questionnaires was more than 20 per cent. The questionnaires showed that the technical requirements for teleradiology are already established to a large extent. The implementation of systems for digital administration of radiographic images and text data is making good progress. Several institutes already use digital radiography, partly with and partly without electronic

Table 1. Application bandwidth of networked medicine

University hospitals, key hospitals
Hospitals for basic care
Practicing physicians
General health services, e.g. mobile nurses
Social services

Table 2. Application bandwidth of teleconsultation in medicine

Lack of qualified personnel on site
Hospitals for basic care without a specialist on duty
Developing countries
Thinly populated areas
Deep-sea vessels
Military missions

networks (PACS). A yet larger number of institutes use systems for digital text data administration (so-called radiology and hospital information systems, abbreviated to RIS and KIS). Regarding connections for external communication, radiological institutes are fully equipped with fax connections and a relatively large number of ISDN, modem and internet connections, which are reflected by the large number of institutes with telemaintenance.

The presence of such a large number of connections is also a critical facet of the safety of patient data. The fact that a large number of respondents mentioned that medical reports are frequently communicated by fax or via internet contradicts the still unresolved legal and data protection aspects of such data transfer.

At the time of the survey 16 institutes (radiology departments) in Austria were already working with teleradiology. In 8 institutes, projects concerning teleradiology were shortly before completion. It may be assumed that, in the meantime, the circle of users has further increased in number. Teleradiology in Austria has grown out of the pioneering stage and is emerging as an aspect of routine radiology. Less than one half of the respondent institutes reported that they intended to introduce teleradiology much later or had no plans in this regard. The pioneer of teleradiology is pursuing this project since 1991 and there has been a consistent increase in the number of users since 1994/95. The majority of institutes transfer sectional images; only a small percentage of the transferred images are plain radiographs (conventional radiographs). Teleradiology is most commonly used to transfer images between radiology departments of various hospitals or between such radiology departments and private practices. Only three users reported exclusive or, to a large extent, image transfer between private practices.

Responses to the question "For what purpose do you use the system?" revealed a percentage of 18.8% and 7.5% for problematic applications such as "replacing the radiologist on call" or "extending the catchment area into those of private practices". In principle, the departments that already use teleradiology believed that this technical option had not reduced the personal contact between radiologists and referring physicians.

Comparing the main areas of work, private practice, hospital/private practice and hospital with the current level of implementation of teleradiology, it becomes evident that radiologists who exclusively work in practices intend not to use teleradiology at all or not to use it in the near future, whereas a large number of physicians who work in practices as well as in hospitals already use teleradiology or plan to use it within the next two to three years. The majority of radiology departments within hospitals also mentioned that they already use teleradiology or intend to use it in the near future.

Obviously, teleradiology has already made its entry into medical practice and appears to be advancing as dynamically as it is in the USA. There seems to be a connection between the extent of radiological activity and the implementation of teleradiology. Our data indicate that the departments which are networked and already active in this field are a step ahead of private practices.

While the majority of responding departments use or intend to use teleradiology for purposes that may be regarded as in improvement of medical services for patients and for the treating physicians, a fairly large number of such installations are being used or planned for more controversial purposes such as replacing the radiologist on call or extending the catchment area of some institutions. Thus, the work group for teleconsultation investigated a subject that not only concerns a hypothetical future but is related to specific, currently existing questions concerning practical imaging diagnostics and therapy.

Considering the widespread and advanced establishment of teleradiology facilities (which was documented by the survey) it seems quite important to procure legal expert reports in this regard, especially concerning:

- professional–legal aspects
- aspects of liability
- legal aspects concerning patients
- legal aspects of data protection and
- cooperation contracts.

The legal viewpoint of the Austrian Medical Society

The Austrian Medical Society entrusted an expert from the legal section (Dr. Th. Holzgruber) with the task of formulating such an expert report. His conclusions are summarised as follows:

Section 22, sub-section 2 of the Medical Law states that a physician may only practice his profession personally and unmediated, if necessary in cooperation with other physicians. The option and permissibility of consulting colleagues is confirmed by the latter part of the sentence. *"However, even in the event of cooperation between physicians it should be remembered that the treatment must be carried out personally and unmediated. Thus, the physician being consulted via teleconsultation is personally, but not unmediated active on the patient. The law of immediacy in treatment may also be interpreted as prohibition of long-distance treatment"*.

Long-distance treatment denotes treatment exclusively based on letters or via telephone. According to the legal expert, however, teleconsultation is not long-distance treatment. The inadmissible form of long-distance treatment signifies that a physician establishes the diagnosis for a patient without an intervening physician being involved in the process.

"In actual teleconsultation a specialist 'only' obtains the advice of a further specialist; the physician responsible for the diagnosis and for any therapy is still the physician asking for advice". Holzgruber raises doubts concerning the concept of trying to compensate the shortage of trained physicians in a hospital by consulting specialists from other hospitals via teleconsultation.

However, Holzgruber concedes that one has to adopt a more generous approach in radiological diagnosis, since images are often interpreted by physicians who have not personally seen the patient. Therefore, it should be of no significance whether the reporting physician is in the same hospital or in a hospital farther away. In order to draw a line of demarcation between "immediacy" and "long-distance treatment" Holzgruber cites a further regulation of the Medical Law.

"According to the Medical Law (also Section 22), treatment may only be carried out in accordance with the standards of medical science and experience. This is a general reference to the rules of medical practice. If the rules of practice are such that a comprehensive diagnosis may be formulated on the basis of an image alone, then the earlier mentioned concept may be regarded as permissible. (Of course, in every case it will be necessary to have trained personnel who are able to take standard images). (....) If the rules of medical practice are otherwise, then this concept must be discarded. In that case, radiological diagnosis would not be carried out in accordance with accepted principles of medical science and practice which, according to the applicable Federal Hospital Law (Section 8, sub-section 2, B-KAG), would be inadmissible".

Finally, Holzgruber also mentions that, according to the Federal Hospital Law, standard hospitals as well as key and central hospitals must have facilities for X-ray diagnosis which also includes the prerequisite of having a sufficient number of specialists. Thus, Holzgruber concludes that a hospital with teleradiology alone would be a violation of Austrian law.

Who is liable in the event of incorrect advice?

As stated in an analogous expert report on teleoperation, those physicians or institutions who (which) implement (or have implemented) the conclusions derived from teleconsultation on the patient are liable. In the event of incorrect or wrong advice, however, the physician consulted via teleconsultation and/or his hospital are liable. *"In accordance with the contract between patient and hospital or practicing physician and patient, in every case the hospital or private physician whom the patient has consulted is liable. This means that they must be billed the charges of the physician being consulted via teleconsultation"*. Of course, the teleconsulted physician is also liable for incorrect advice.

Legal aspects concerning the patient when information is passed on

This primarily concerns informing the patient about teleconsultation. It should be remembered that, in the professional–legal sense, teleconsultation is also subject to the law of professional discretion. When a patient agrees to undergo treatment in hospital he does consent to information about his state of health being passed on to other professionals within the hospital. However, Holzgruber states that this consent of the patient does not include teleconsultation.

Therefore, an explicit declaration of consent from the patient is required. *"Teleconsultation in Austria is still not so common that a patient must reckon with it when he enters into hospital care"*. Since the patient cannot assess the benefits and consequences of teleconsultation, he must be carefully informed about the subject. If he consents to teleconsultation, then the physician's professional discretion towards the physician being consulted is no longer a problem, says Holzgruber. Furthermore, Holzgruber states the following about documentation: "*For reasons of liability alone it should be ensured that every teleconsultation is documented either via image transfer lines or via e-mail*".

If the patient's consent has been obtained and the data are protected such that no unauthorized person can gain access to them, then the data protection aspect should be no problem, says the legal expert.

To provide legal protection for the involved parties, Holzgruber recommends a contractual agreement in case teleconsultation is frequently used. The financial remuneration could also be agreed upon in this contract. However, according to the current remuneration system for hospitals, the legal and insurance aspects of teleconsultation have not been regulated. Accordingly, teleconsultation is not prohibited but is also not included in the scheme of remuneration.

From the insurance point of view, passing on services between private practices is still treated in a restrictive fashion. Indeed, teleconsultation is not regulated at all. In other words, it is not prohibited, but is also not separately remunerated.

Holzgruber concludes as follows: Teleconsultation may well be integrated into the Austrian legal system in accordance with currently applicable laws and in consideration of specific principles, and may therefore be regarded as an admissible institution.

Legal conception of the Ministry of Health

A query addressed to the Federal Ministry of Employment, Health and Welfare about the viewpoint of the Ministry regarding this subject, in August last year, evoked the following statement which conforms with that of the work group of the Austrian Radiological Society and with Holzgruber's expert report:

According to the Federal Ministry of Employment, Health and Welfare, teleconsultation which, in essence, consists of procuring expert advice to clarify a specific case with colleagues via telecommunication, conforms with the currently applicable law, Section 22, sub-section 2 of the Medical law of 1984, according to which a physician has to, if necessary, practice his profession in cooperation with other physicians.

Additional legislative measures are therefore not required. Like Holzgruber, the Health Ministry refers to the immediacy of medical action in the course of treatment and to the subject of responsibility which also applies to telemedicine.

"*The advantage of teleradiology is that, by means of a conference circuit, several expert reports can be procured and discussed fast in case the radiologist is uncertain about the information provided by X-ray images. The advantage of teleradiology is the possibility to monitor and consult/advise colleagues. Teleradiology could well become a fixed aspect of specialized medical training and advanced education.*

One may also consider quality assurance programs which could function in a similar fashion as the ring experiments used for quality assurance within laboratories.

From the legal point of view for hospitals it should be remembered that, according to Section 2, subsection 1, lit. A of the Basic Federal Hospital Law, standard hospitals must have facilities for radiological diagnosis which should be staffed by specialists of the respective specialty. Key hospitals must have facilities for X-ray diagnosis and therapy which should also be staffed by specialists in the respective field of specialization.

As central hospitals must also, in principle, be equipped with the specialized facilities conforming with the respective level of medical science, facilities for medical radiological diagnosis must also be available in such hospitals and must be operated by specialists trained in the respective field".

Thus, for the Ministry of Health it is clear that, in the legal sense, all general hospitals must have facilities for radiological diagnosis which should be operated and manned by suitably qualified specialists. Depending on the purpose of the respective institution and the range of services offered by it, the institution must have facilities for radiological diagnosis.

If such facilities are offered it should be ensured that suitably qualified medical specialists are available, "*since Section 7, sub-section 3 of the Basic Federal Hospital Law refers to the regulations of the Medical Law of 1984 for practicing the medical profession and therefore also include the limitation concerning special disciplines*".

Five guiding principles for an efficient approach

Based on the earlier mentioned conclusions, the work group for teleconsultation formulated five guiding principles in the beginning of 1998:

- telecommunication and teleconsultation improve the quality of medical services;
- teleconsultation is an additional service;

- teleconsultation is no substitute for specialized medical care;
- the immediacy of medical action must be ensured;
- all hospitals must have a specialist (radiologist) on call.

Conclusion

Therapeutic action itself, must always be directly carried out by a physician who must be responsible for it; this also applies to therapeutic telemedicine. The consultant physician gives advice (as a consultant) to the acting physician who is and remains responsible for his actions as the executor of the measure. The former physician gives his advice through the media of telecommunication. Ideally, all patients seeking medical advice should have a face-to-face consultation with a physician, and telemedicine should be restricted to situations in which a physician cannot be physically present within a safe and acceptable time period.

Teleconsultation is only meaningful if it provides more service for the patient. For this purpose it is important to create the basic preconditions for this technology so that it does not deprive its users of the law (freedom) of action.

Socially as well as legally, a physician's action is characterized by immediacy, which should not be jeopardized by this technology. Only if this requirement is fulfilled can "networked medicine" develop to optimize medical diagnosis and therapy for the benefit of the diseased individual.

If telemedicine becomes an end in itself, then the medical profession will have failed.

Application service providing (ASP) – a challenge for the future of medicine. An example: marc – major centre for digital image exchange

W.I. Wieser

Siemens Austria, MED HS, Vienna, Austria

Introduction

Radiology is one of the biggest service providers among the medical specialties. As such, modern radiology is expected to deliver and committed to providing its services to the highest professional and quality standards.

Today, modern radiology is not only equipped with the best modalities – such as computed tomography (CT), magnetic resonance (MR), ultrasonography (US), or digital luminescence radiography (DLR) – to generate medical images, but beyond this function, specialists use picture archiving and communication systems (PACS) in connection with a departmental management system (RIS) for reporting.

This service is now available to users in digital form and at a high professional standard.

All radiology institutes in Europe are legally obliged to archive all radiological images for 10 years. The necessary infrastructure for digital archives is complex, requires high implementation effort, and incurs a high capital expenditure.

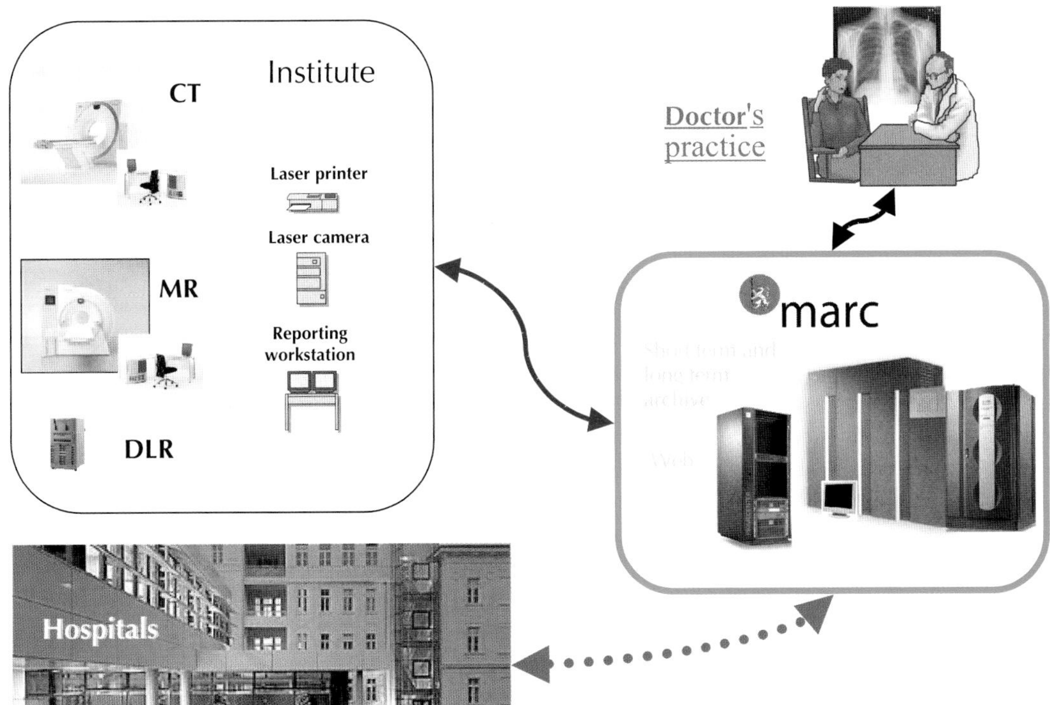

Fig. 1. Graphic representation of the system

The Steiermärkische Medizin Archiv GesmbH (marc) a joint venture of Steiermärkischen Krankenanstaltenges.m.b.H. (KAGes) and Siemens AG Austria, runs archives for radiological images that meet high standards of reliability.

Marc, as an application service provider (ASP), offers central storage facilities for images and management, and includes the connection to the worldwide web for doctors who require this. Images are available at any time and anywhere, to anyone who is authorized to use them. The storage system optimizes the workflow between external institutes, specialists, and hospitals. The rules for storage and communication as regulated by the law and the requirements concerning data protection are guaranteed to be met.

Material and methods

The technical prerequisites for intramural and extramural communication are widely available and accessible today. Up to now now, this was the case only within the context of a hospital or clinical network.

Results

Marc users can devote themselves to their main activity, diagnostic radiology. They have the opportunity to see prior reports and earlier images of the patient, independent of whether these were produced in their own institute or by another marc user.

Discussion

Various activities shape tele-medicine today; these have varying objectives and need varying degrees of input.

Tele-consultations in their simplest form can be carried out worldwide, wherever a telephone is available. The technical requirements of tele-medicine today are rather modest, whereas the cooperative relations network (allocation of responsibilities, remuneration) has to meet more stringent standards.

Radiology enables technology users to see that the way in which the information community processes information is feasible. marc's performance has shown that this is possible.

All countries that want to integrate tele-medical solutions have to have a system for identifying patients that is reversible and unambiguous as well as unique. One possible solution is an identification card for patients, provided that politicians, medical professionals, and the health industry agree on this.

Information Technology (IT) in radiology tele-consultation

W. I. Wieser

Siemens Austria, MED HS, Vienna, Austria

IT systems are increasingly used in radiology to improve and intensify medical communication. The principal areas of application are central diagnosis, expert consultation, and tele-conferencing.

⊕ What does each of these concepts mean:

Central diagnosis (Fig. 1)

The term "central diagnosis," describes the temporary or permanent creation of a central radiological service that assumes the task of evaluating image material acquired at another location without the presence of a radiologist. This is increasingly important, especially for clinics without a radiology service at night or at weekends.

The term "expert consultation," describes a consultation with an expert for the purpose of acquiring a second opinion in the event of an unclear diagnosis. In this way, the judgment of a specialist can be obtained about specific issues.

Expert consultation (Fig. 2)

Tele-conferencing (Fig. 3)

The term "tele-conferencing," describes the cooperative discussion of a case with simultaneous access to the patient's image data. Interactive, simultaneous display of the images is one of the fundamental prerequisites for this.

⊕ New legal regulations in Austria:

The 2000 Data Privacy Law (DSG2000) BGBl. I Nr. 165/1999

1. What is a file (DSG2000 §4 Z6) ?
   A file is a "structured collection of data that are accessible by using at least one search criterion."
2. Basis for the legally correct use of data (DSG2000 §7ff)
   - There must be a legal basis for the use of data (§7 Par. 1)
   - There must a legal basis for the use of the concrete data (§7ff)

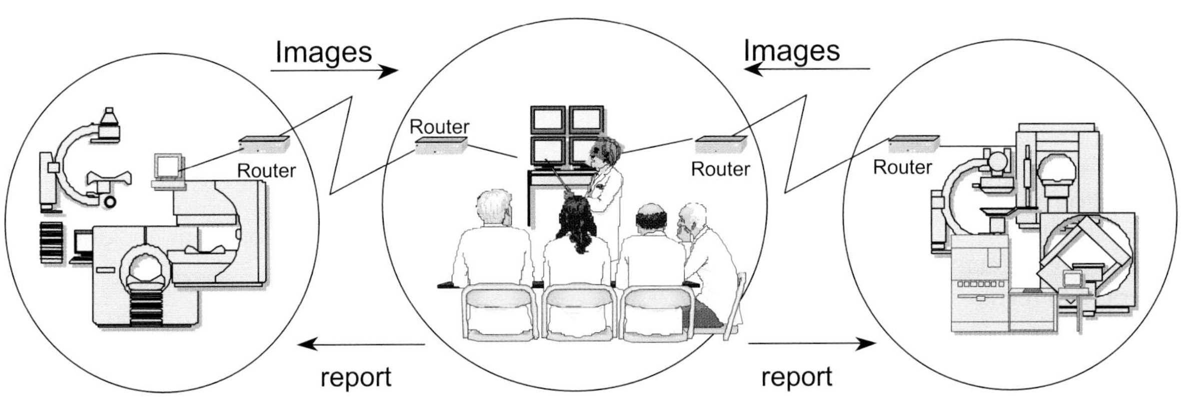

Fig. 1. Scenario: central diagnosis

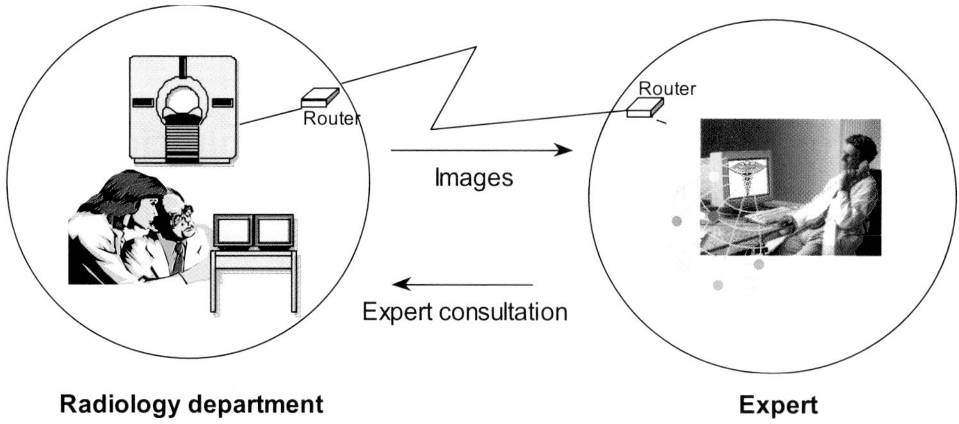

Fig. 2. Scenario: expert consultation

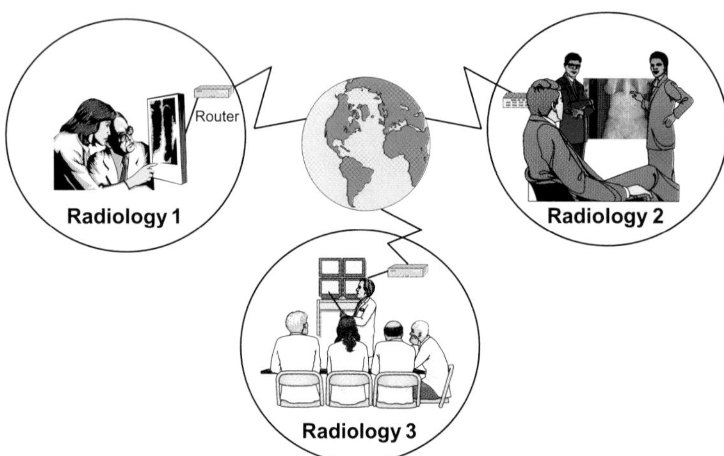

Fig. 3. Scenario: tele-conferencing

The consent of the owner of the data is not a substitute for the legal basis for the use of data.

3. When may data be used (DSG2000 §8, §9)
   - There is an express legal authorization or obligation (§8 Par. 1 Z1)
   - There is an express legal authorization or obligation to safeguard an important public interest (§9 Z3)
   - The person affected has consented and has the right to revoke that consent (§8 Par. 1 Z2; §9 Z6)
   - Vital interests of the person affected are concerned (§8 Par. 1 Z3; §9 Z7)
   - The data have been published in a legally approved way (§8 Par. 2; §9 Z1)
   - The data are only indirectly relevant to persons (§8 Par. 2; §9 Z2)
4. Requirements for security provisions (DSG2000 §14)
   - Corresponding to the state of technology
   - They are financially acceptable
   - An appropriate level of security must be achieved
   - There must be protection from accidental or illegal destruction

There are no specific regulations governing provisions for encryption.

5. Requirements for record keeping (DSG2000 §14)
   - The use of data is subject to mandatory protocol requirements (Par. 2 Z7)

- Unregistered transmissions are subject to mandatory protocol requirements (Par. 3)
- There are restrictions on the use of the data in the protocols (Par. 4, 5)
- The security provisions must be available for staff members to consult at all times (Par. 6)

6. Right to information (DSG2000 §26)
   - Information is to be provided on request (Par. 1)
   - With the customer's consent, the request for information can be submitted verbally (Par. 1)
   - With the consent of the person affected, the information can be provided verbally (Par. 1)
   - The information is to be provided within 8 weeks (Par. 4)
   - To a reasonable extent, the person affected must participate in the information process by means of consultation (Par. 3)
     – Unjustifiable effort is to be avoided
   - Where justified, information can be withheld
   - There is no charge for information about current data
   - Deletion is prohibited

7. Content of information
   The customer must provide information about:
   - The data used
   - Information available concerning their origin
   - Any recipients or groups of recipients of transmissions
   - Name and address of the service provider (on separate request)

8. Deletion / Correction (DSG2000 §27)
   - The customer is obligated to perform corrections
   - The time limit is 8 weeks
   - This also applies to incomplete data
   - Data that were not needed and data that were processed improperly are to be deleted
   - The burden of proof is (with exceptions) on the customer
   - There are alternatives because of financial reasons
     – Temporarily blocking access
     – Furnishing the data with a comment
   - Recipients must be informed of this

⊕ The role of the digital signature when transmitting patient related medical data

1. Cryptograph (encryption)
   - Symmetrical encryption

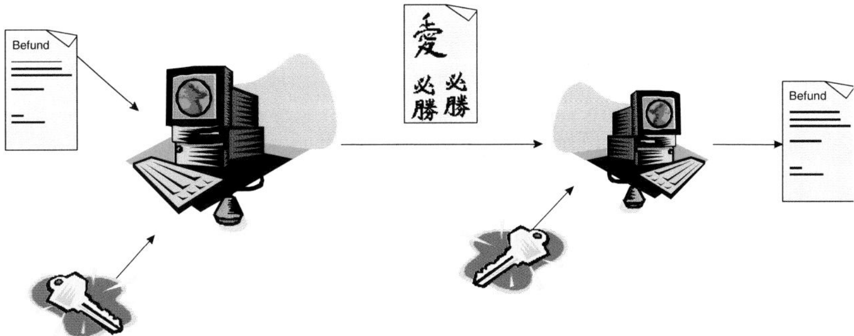

One and the same key for both encryption and decryption short keys (≥128 bits); fast procedure for example, Triple DES, IDEA, AES

   - Asymmetrical encryption

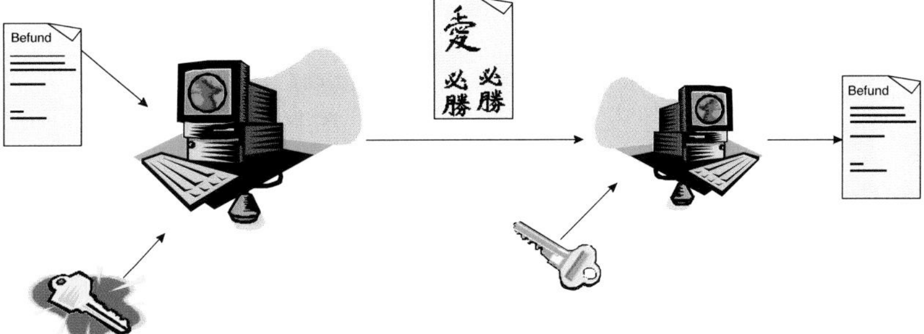

Two different keys for encryption and decryption long keys (≥1024 bits); slow procedure for example, RSA, DAS, DH

- Hash algorithm (fingerprint)

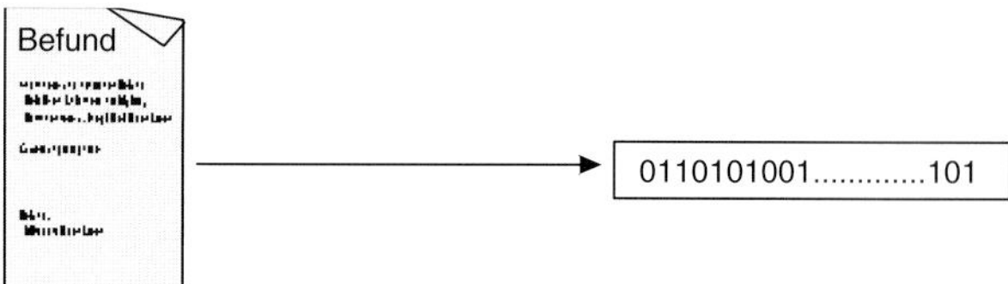

Generates a Hash code out of random data for example, MD-5, SHA-1, RIPE-MD

- Digital signature

- Signature function of the signature generation unit can be released only with an authorization code
- Maximum validity of a certificate: 3 years
- Prescribed minimum lengths for keys:
  - RSA, DAS 1023 bits
  - DAS varieties based on elliptical curves, 160 bits

⊕ Sending diagnoses by email

General

The technical foundation here is traditional email as the most widely used service on the internet. Email is a technically mature service, simple to operate, and relatively cost effective.

At the same time, email solves the problems of

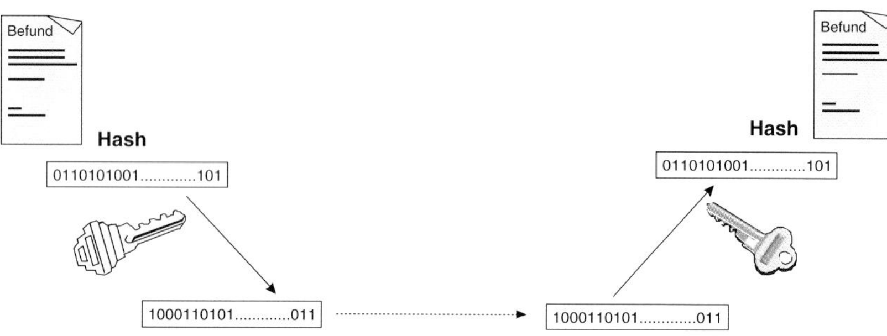

- Certificate

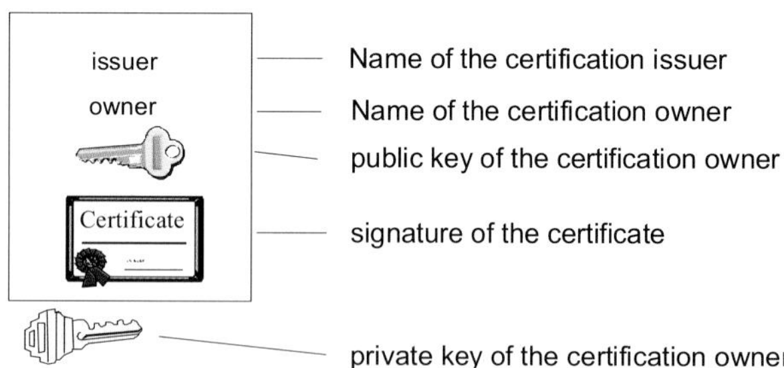

Safeguarding authenticity
Austrian Signature Law (of August 19, 1999)

- Providers of certification service must reliably establish the identity of persons by means of an official picture ID
- The Telekom-Control-Kommission (TKG; telecommunications control commission) is in charge of overseeing this

Austrian Signature Regulation (of February 2, 2000)

Prerequisites for a secure electronic signature

- Completion display of the data to be signed

simultaneous data transmission. In other words, sender and receiver are independent of switch-on times.

The actual information is sent in attachments.

Communication Partners

In the healthcare area, one is usually faced with more than two communication partners: for example, the patient (as the person affected), the sender (= physician, lab, hospital, insurance company...), and the recipient (= physician, hospital, lab, insurance company...), each of them with very different fundamental legal prerequisites.

Communication partners in healthcare are different people and/or organizations. They include physicians in private practice, hospitals, various treatment facilities, public institutions, nursing homes, etc.

One basic prerequisite is that all these persons and/or institutions be uniquely identified and that there be appropriate procedures to ensure their authenticity and authorization.

All the necessary legal requirements—introduced above—must be applied to this communication model.

I would like to point out a few problematic areas:

- The patient and recipient are known, as is in all likelihood the sender. Take as an example

a patient who comes into the hospital and says that he had visited a certain physician, but doesn't know exactly which one.
- The sender can no longer be identified, but information about previous diagnoses or previous treatments is needed.

Prerequisites

Please refer to the documents of the STRING Commission "MAGDA-LENA" (www.akh-wien.ac.at/STRING/MAGDA-LENA.html) for Austria and to the CEN/TC251 procedural model. 25 European Pre-Standards (ENV's) or technical CEN Reports (CR's) have been issued so far. At the national level in Austria, conversion is being advanced in the framework of (among others) the Austrian Institute for standardization (in the "Medical Computing" technical standards committee) and the Austrian Chamber of Commerce (in the "Healthcare" working group at AUSTRIAPRO). Currently, there are Ö-NORMEN (Austrian national standards) that are based on international standards and correspond to three electronic message types: the exchange of administrative patient information between healthcare facilities and private insurance companies (K2201); transfer/admission (K2202); and patients' letters, physicians' letters, and diagnosis reports (K2203).

In Germany (Bavaria), for example, the Health Care Professionals' Protocol (HCP Protocol) is being defined.

The English term "Health Care Professionals' Protocol" was intentionally selected for its similarity to the internet's "hypertext transport protocol" (HTTP), since this proposed standardization too involves decentralized online transmission. Its similarity to the project name "HPC" (health professional card) is also intentional, since those "electronic ID cards" in healthcare will serve as the basis for mutual recognition within the scope of the HCP Protocol. Taking into account current and foreseeable legal circumstances, the goal of this pilot project—a joint project of the Bavarian Association of Panel Physicians (Kassenärztliche Vereinigung Bayerns) and the Bavarian State Physicians' Board (Bayerische Landesärztekammer)—is to take established individual projects and approved skeleton concepts as the starting point for an effort to provide, for the first time in Germany, an evaluation of the practical aspects of a safe, secure, provable, and open comprehensive system for the online transmission of (in the first instance) medical data for decentralized, variously equipped participants.

Avoiding proprietary single-facility solutions, a provable security structure will be developed by using available components and modules, tested, and published. An important element in the project, after validation within the scope of Bayern Online II, is the creation of a new, open standard that creates opportunities for free market development, while at the same time ensuring the interoperability of the individual components used.

Moved as quickly as possible into the public domain, the standards and provisions created should give all manufacturers a chance for their own implementation; the result should be a "ripple effect" whose influence goes beyond the pilot nature of the project and Bayern Online to affect healthcare in its entirety. Critical scientific confrontation with the structure models developed and their effective public presentation, along with an intensive discussion of data privacy, should ensure and strengthen confidence in the new multimedia technology. The protocol that has been developed should then be proposed for standardization at the federal level.

EWOS/EG MED – European Workshop for Open Systems – Expert Group Healthcare EWOS is the European Workshop for Open Systems. It is responsible for defining and drafting profiles for OSI (open systems interconnection) and OSE (open systems environment). Profiles in this context show how sets of related base standards may be brought together for use in real implementation.

EWOS works closely with CEN and CENELEC. On a worldwide level, it liaises with:

- OIW (OSE Implementers' Workshop) in North America
- AOW (Asia-Oceania Workshop for Open Systems) in the Far East

Current EWOS members include a wide range of manufacturers, suppliers, software developers, users, PTTs, network providers, testing houses, consultants, research centers, and academia. Membership is open to all individuals or companies with an interest in open systems.

EWOS/EG MED – Expert Group on Medical Informatics

A major aspect of medical informatics is the transfer of healthcare information between different computer systems. In order for the transfer of information to be meaningful, it is necessary for the disparate computer systems to have agreed means of transfer.

Although several ad hoc (often proprietary) standards are available, it is much easier to achieve full interworking across national boundaries by using internationally agreed standards or "publicly available specifications" (PASs).

For various reasons, standards often have a wide range of options. To make sure that two implementations interwork, it is necessary to select a set of standards and options within those standards to fulfil a particular business requirement. Such a set is known as a "profile". Profiles themselves can be international standards -International Standardized Profiles (ISPs).

The European Workshop for Open Systems (EWOS) is concerned with the development of profiles. The role of its expert group on healthcare (EG MED) is to develop appropriate profiles for the healthcare domain and identify requirements for base standards where appropriate standards do not exist. The user requirements are usually provided by TC 251 working groups.

In many cases, it is expected that these profiles will not differ from those applicable in other contexts. In other cases, specific profiles will be required.

Furthermore, there will be international standards that are of particular relevance to healthcare and for which profiles do not exist. Again, EG MED will undertake such profiles.

The EWOS Workshop meets four times a year, for a week each time, in Brussels. During this week most of the expert groups, including EG MED, meet. EG MED meetings are normally held for three days (Tuesday to Thursday).

The chairman of EG MED attends CEN/TC 251 (medical informatics) meetings as an observer. Similarly, the chairman of CEN/TC 251 attends EG MED meetings. In this way there is very close liaison between the two organizations (especially as EG MED members also attend various CEN/TC 251 working groups as individual experts).

The following standards are taken into account in this protocol:

- European Committee for Standardization CEN/TC251 (Working Group 7, Interoperability), Healthtrust 1 (TTP Functional Specifications).
- International Organization for Standardization (ISO), Authentication: DIS ISO 9798, and Secure Messaging: DIS ISO 7816
- Article 3 (Signature Law, SigG) of the new "Information and Communication Service Law" (IuKdG). The emphasis here is on the effort to harmonize the structure of the "contents of signature-key certificates" (§ 7, SigG) to ensure interoperability across the entire healthcare system.

Conclusion

At present, because of the lack of an EU-wide standard, every computerized solution based on email is an isolated, individual solution, and will have to be adjusted to any new standards that are enacted. The MAGDA-LENA guidelines, products, and use concepts of the service providers involved require that the above prerequisites be met and that additional quality criteria, particularly in the field of data security, be satisfied. Rules and responsibilities for such 'Certification' are currently in preparation.

Multimodality registration in daily clinical practice

R. Bale

Interdisciplinary Stereotactic Intervention- and Planning Laboratory Innsbruck (SIP-Labor), Department of Radiology (Chairman: Professor Werner Jaschke, MD), Medical University Innsbruck, Austria

Introduction

The discovery of x-rays by Wilhelm Conrad Röntgen in 1895 revolutionized medicine. The novel technology permitted to investigate internal structures of the body without surgery in a non-invasive manner. In the meantime many different imaging modalities have been developed allowing for non-invasive and painless examination of the patient. In contrast to plain x-ray images modern tomographic imaging technologies allow to reconstruct cross-sectional images providing superposition-free images. Digital images are generated which can be transferred via internal for external networks and processed and modified by various computer algorithms. Digital images allow for the direct measurement of biological structures and their functions. Accurate quantitative and qualitative information can be extracted.

Two global categories of imaging modalities can be defined: Anatomical modalities depicting primarily information on morphology and functional modalities depicting primarily information on metabolism. The relationship of anatomical and functional information is of major interest for biological science and in particular for medical practice.

Various imaging modalities, including x-ray, CT, MR, PET, SPECT, ultrasound etc. are based on different physical principles thereby often containing complementary information. Each imaging modality possesses special attributes which may contribute to a better understanding of the physiology, abnormality or the disease.

Many patients with signs and symptoms possibly related to a brain tumour undergo different imaging procedures including MRI, CT, SPECT and PET, each of them contributing specific information. CT and MRI provide complementary morphological information. For example MR optimally depicts brain tissue, but bony structures and calcifications are visualized better by CT. In addition many patients with brain tumours undergo radiation therapy necessitating a CT study for calculation of the dose distribution. Nuclear imaging modalities as SPECT and PET provide information about function (e.g. proliferation state with 201Tl or receptor status with somatostatin analogs) and metabolism (e.g. glucose uptake in 18FDG PET). Functional imaging has the capability to differentiate between metabolically active and inactive tissue corresponding to tumour or necrotic tissue.

Multiple 3D – image datasets are usually displayed with a light box side by side. For the clinician it is difficult to mentally integrate information from multiple diagnostic sources and construct a 3D – geometric relationship. Usually the radiologist extracts the useful data from the images and interprets it according to his knowledge. Whenever correlating information from multimodality studies from one patient is considered, the images should represent the same anatomy. However, since the same or different image sets acquired in the same subject may differ in scale, orientation (angle) and position, an integration process is necessary in order to achieve a correct spatial alignment of all study modalities. This procedure is called registration. Recent advances in computer and software technology provide comprehensive capabilities for multimodal image fusion, which is useful in many medical applications in the whole body. Especially for applications in the brain for radiotherapy planning, anatomic mapping of cerebral function and tumour volume response to treatment image fusion was used successfully. After registration, a fusion step is required for the integrated display of the data involved [1]. Multimodality imaging is a synthesis of these different imaging datasets into a single composite image.

Besides multimodality registration monomodality registration is very important for verifying changes over time in order to monitor treatment and to get an idea about the biological features of various structures and pathologies. In addition, differences between individuals and populations are investigated.

In schizophrenia, for instance, subtle changes of certain structures of the brain in comparison to the normal population have been found using registration and quantitative volumetric measurements.

Methods of medical image registration

Excellent survey of publications concerning medical imaging registration techniques were published by van der Elsen [2], Maintz and Viergever [1], and by Hanjal JH et al. [3].

Two different steps of integrating two or more images were defined: First, registration, bringing the modalities into spatial alignment and second, fusion for integrated display of the data. For medical applications usually 3D data is registered to 3D data, however it is also possible to register 2D to 3D data or coregister planar images. Applications of 2D-2D registration include comparison of different portal images at different times in order to evaluate and verify patient positioning during radiotherapy. An example of 2D – 3D registration is the matching of preoperative 3D – CT data with intraoperative fluoroscopy [4].

According to Maintz and Viergever the nature of registration basis can be classified extrinsic and intrinsic image-based registration and non-image-based registration. Extrinsic registration relies on external reference points that have to be introduced into the imaged space reliably in identical relationship to patient anatomy. These reference structures are either invasively of non-invasively attached to the patient. In contrast to extrinsic methods intrinsic methods rely on the patient image data only, thus allowing retrospective co-registration. A set of anatomical landmarks, segmented structures or the voxels itself are used for the registration process.

Extrinsic methods

Invasive extrinsic methods

The gold standard for registration accuracy are invasive stereotactic frames rigidly mounted on the patients skull under local or general anaesthesia by means of pins or screws. These frames are usually applied for stereotactic neurosurgery, neurosurgical biopsies and radiosurgery. Conventional frames have to remain on the patient's skull in the time between the different image acquisitions and surgery, the patient often being anesthetized for a long time. According to this, invasive frames are limited by their short-term only application and not suitable for the purpose of (follow-up) multimodal image fusion.

Table 1

Primarily morphological modalities
x-ray
Portal images
DSA (digital subtraction angiography)
CT (computed tomography)
CTA (computed tomography angiography)
MRI (magnetic resonance imaging)
MRA (magnetic resonance angiography)
US (ultrasound)

Primarily functional modalities
Scintigraphy
SPECT (single photon emission computed tomography)
e.g. intra- and interictal SPECT
PET (positron emission tomography)
fMRI (functional MRI)
Doppler US
EEG (electro-encephalography)

Alternatively, invasive screws can be used as markers or as marker carriers [5,6]. They provide an accuracy comparable to stereotactic frames. However, they may cause patient discomfort and should not be left in place over an extended period of time, thus application of invasive markers is not justified for diagnostic purposes solely.

Non-invasive extrinsic methods

In order to overcome the drawbacks of invasive markers, adhesive, low cost skin markers may be applied [7,8]. However, skin markers have several drawbacks including inaccuracies due to skin shift. If there are no clearly defined points on the skin (naevi, scars, etc.) for precise marker repositioning for the different scans, the markers have to remain on the patient's skin during the time between different scans. This problem may be solved by applying artificial ink landmarks to the skin.

The Laitinen stereoadapter [9] is mounted on the patient's head by means of two ear plugs, a nasion support and a connector plate over the vertex. The repositioning accuracy of this stereoadapter depends upon how tightly the support arms are braced between nasion, external auditory meati and vertex. Unfortunately, such rigid fixation-devices exert pressure on the external auditory canals and can cause patient discomfort and pain.

Attaching markers to mask-based fixation systems [10–12] is an interesting and viable method if one assumes high repositioning accuracy of the underlying anatomy. The accuracy of all mask based systems is however limited by movement of the underlying skin. The patient would also need to be fixated for each imaging procedure.

The systems of Hauser [13], the GTC localizer [14] the Banana Bar system [15] and the VBH mouthpiece [16] are devices based on a dental impression for repositioning a registration device on the patient: Hauser et al. fixate their referencing system on the patient by an upper dental cast, nasion and the external auditory meati. An attached N-box creates external points of reference. It is used for image-guided surgery in the ENT region. The GTC localizer [14] (Radionics Inc., Burlington, Mass., USA) is connected to the patient via an upper dental impression and a head support. Registration rods comparable to other commercially available invasive Stereotactic frames connected to the base ring of the frame provide precisely defined correlation points. The non-invasive relocatable Banana Bar (BB) fiducial marker system consists of a symmetrical U-shaped aluminum bar, sweeping backwards bilaterally along the head. It is held in place by actively biting on a dental impression of both maxillary and mandibular teeth.

The above mentioned devices that are based on dental impressions have two important drawbacks: First, they contain metallic components and therefore they are not suitable for MR exams, second the repositioning accuracy depends on the cooperation of the patient.

In 1994 our group has developed and patented the Vogele-Bale-Hohner (VBH) vacuum mouthpiece (Medical Intelligence Inc., Schwabmünchen, Germany) for computer-assisted ENT surgery and neurosurgery [17,18]. The VBH mouthpiece (Fig. 1) is a simple, non-invasive and rigid device which does not contain any metallic components. Fabrication of the VBH mouthpiece takes 10–15 minutes and is fabricated prior to the initial scan. The form-stable impression material allows for repositioning accuracy of less than 1 mm [16]. In contrast to other systems a vacuum system fixates the VBH mouthpiece on the upper dentition of the patient and in addition, the vacuum pump (Fig. 2) guarantees continuous monitoring of the positioning accuracy. Recently we have developed a universal reference frame, the so-called SIP-Lab Innsbruck frame (Medical Intelligence Inc., Schwabmünchen, Germany) (Fig. 3), to be reproducibly mounted to the VBH mouthpiece. The SIP-Lab frame with its 12 markers is always and objectively in identical relationship to the cranium due to the negative pressure of the MP, irrespective of patient compliance.

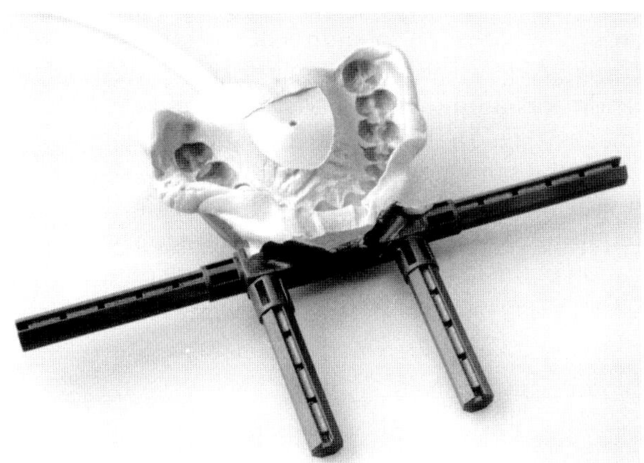

Fig. 1. The Vogele-Bale-Hohner mouthpiece with the vacuum area in the centre. The anterior and lateral rods may be used for the attachment of the reference frame and fixating arms

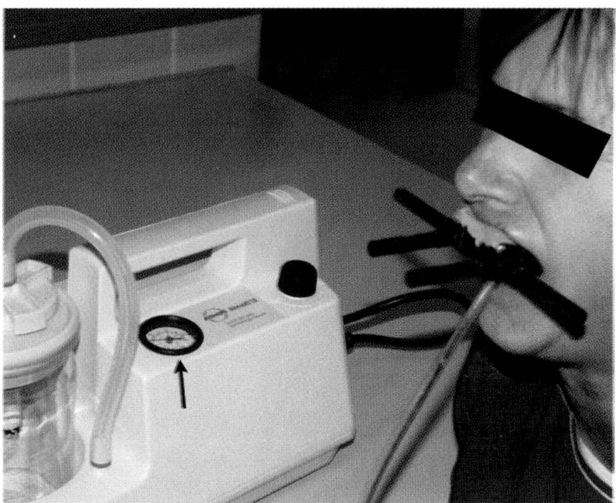

Fig. 2. Patient wearing the VBH mouthpiece: A tube connects the VBH mouthpiece with the vacuum pump. It fixates the mouthpiece on the upper dentition and allows for continuous monitoring of the positioning accuracy. The manometer is indicated by the arrowhead

Our phantom and patient study [19] showed that a high level of registration accuracy can be achieved despite the poor resolution of the scintigraphic images. In contrast to segmentation and voxel based registration methods the actual level of accuracy can be quantified by means of the RMSE value (root mean square error) as calculated by the software. The RMSE represents the mean distance between the matched paired-points after registration. Introduction of the mouthpiece with the frame takes additional 1 minute per CT/MR/SPECT/PET scan.

The localization error increases not only as a function of marker/ fiducial localization error (RSME) but also as the distance from the marker centroid to the point of interest increases [8]. Therefore the SIP-frame curves around the head with the most posterior

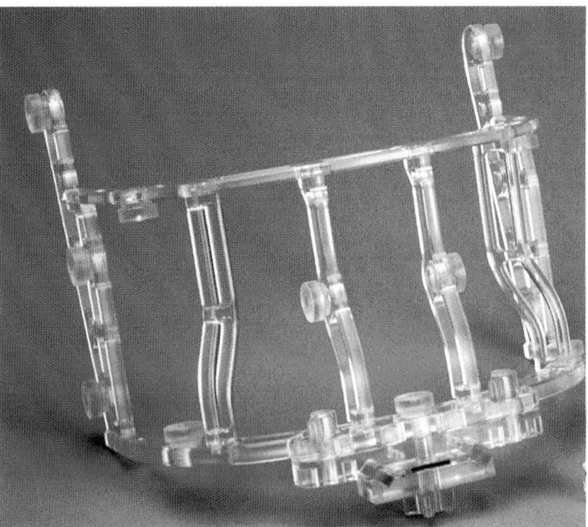

Fig. 3. The SIP-Lab Innsbruck frame contains 12 exchangeable spherical shaped markers. Depending on the imaging modality the respective markers are applied (glass beads for CT, nitrolingual capsules for MRI, ^{241}Am for SPECT, ^{18}F-FDG solution for PET)

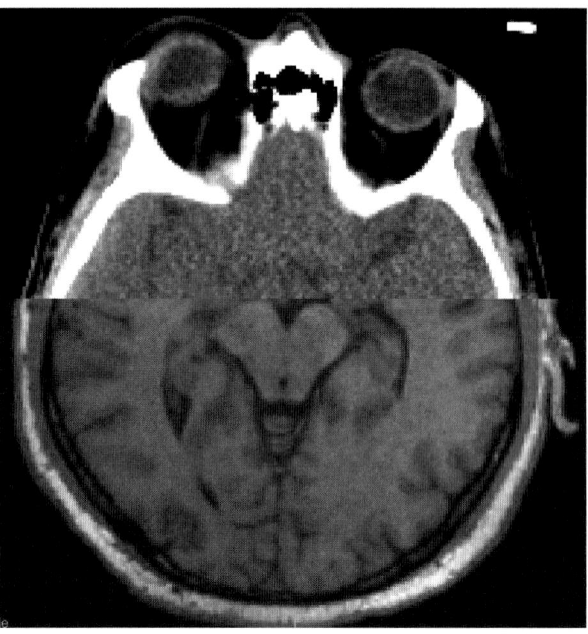

Fig. 4. Visual inspection of CT-MRI registration of the brain based on mutual information algorithm shows a satisfactory result

markers located behind the ear. Since the markers are larger than the dimensions of a single voxel, defining their centre of mass in large magnification allows subvoxel registration accuracy [5]. It has to be noticed that the RMSE error is an indicator of the registration accuracy of the extrinsic reference points (frame), not the intrinsic anatomical structures. Our experiences however confirmed the results of a phantom study conducted at this institution, whereby fiducial (frame) and actual target registration error between CT/MR and CT/SPECT datasets correlated to under 1.5 mm.

We see the usefulness of this method mainly for registration of low resolution images such as SPECT and PET. The reference points on this frame grant completely objective registration using relatively simple and ubiquitous software, independent of a user's capability of defining anatomic landmarks or the varying limitations of more elaborate and costly algorithms. In addition we have developed an algorithm for automatic detection of the spherical markers of the reference frame on CT/MR/SPECT and PET, allowing a fully automatic extrinsic registration [20].

The limitations of the dental based reference systems are that accuracy of registration and repositioning is not reliable in edentulous patients. One important drawback of all extrinsic methods is the prospective character. This requires additional intrinsic methods that allow to performing the registration from the image content itself.

Intrinsic methods

Anatomical landmark-based methods

The simplest method is the use of anatomical landmarks. In the landmark-based registration method three or more appropriate, precisely definable landmarks or features are identified by the user or in an automatic fashion in the different image data sets and correlated to each other. Due to the good anatomical resolution, intrinsic registration methods work well for CT-CT, MR-MR and CT-MR fusion (Fig. 4). Our own experience is in accordance with that of other groups[3] that such anatomical landmarks can be co-registered to about 2–5 mm for CT and MRI. Such landmarks are however hard to define in SPECT/PET images (Fig. 5). It is often difficult to identify precisely the same anatomic features on two studies that reveal the anatomy in complementary fashion [21] requiring skill and practice of the user. The identification of the landmarks should be done or supervised by an experienced radiologist.

Surface-based methods

The "head-hat" method by Pelizzari et al. [22] relies on the segmentation of the skin surface from the different modalities. This method may yield gross misregistrations although the contours align perfectly due to identical axes of symmetry. Different imaging modalities can also provide substantially different

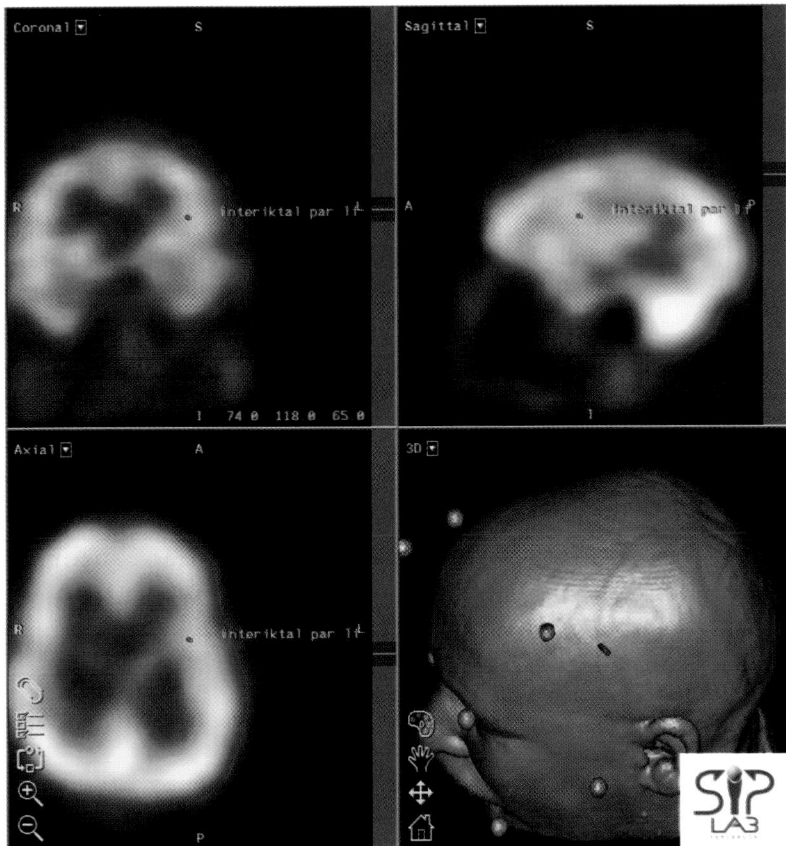

Fig. 5. Due to the low resolution SPECT images appear very blurry and it is very difficult to define (precise) anatomical landmarks as demonstrated in these axial, sagittal and coronal reformatted interictal SPECT data of the brain

image contrast between corresponding surfaces. The registration accuracy is limited to the accuracy of the segmentation step which is especially problematic in SPECT/PET images.

Voxel-property based methods

Voxel property-based registration methods [23,24] rely on the image grey values without prior segmentation, using the full image content for the registration process. In most approaches the registration is performed automatically. The voxel property-based or mutual-information based registration methods are not influenced by segmentation errors or subjective determination of anatomical landmarks. Comparisons of mutual information based registration with external marker based registration of the brain as part of the retrospective evaluation project performed at the Vanderbilt University, TN, USA showed subvoxel accuracy of CT to MR and PET to MR. It is highly robust and does not require segmentation or definition of landmarks. Therefore it is very user-friendly and useful for daily clinical routine.

However, especially in extra-cranial regions problems related to the intrinsic based registration method may occur. In addition, the quality of registration is also influenced by the resolution of the images, modality specific image degradations and artefacts. Due to the intrinsic selective uptake of tracers only in areas with altered metabolism, SPECT images do not sufficiently depict the anatomy. For this reason precise, internal anatomical markers, precise surfaces and comparable voxels are lacking so that image fusion based on intrinsic information may fail.

The result of CT-MR registration can be visually checked by the naked eye. Registration results seem somewhat more satisfying in methods involving SPECT and PET images because the blurry nature of the images seems to allow a larger displacement. The image resolution should not be used to formulate a clinically relevant level of accuracy: SPECT-to-MR or PET-to-MR registration may even require higher accuracy than some instances of CT-to-MR registration, even though the smaller error is more easily assessed by the naked eye in the latter case. The actual level of accuracy is still unknown in many applications, and cannot be quantified accurately, even by the clinicians involved.

Especially in cases where scintigraphic images are implemented in neurosurgery, radiotherapy or other therapeutic interventions high precision of co-registration is paramount.

All the above mentioned algorithms assume the image datasets as rigid bodies.

Non-image based registration

Combined PET-CT or SPECT-CT scanners

Non-image based registration is possible if the coordinate systems of different scanners are calibrated to each other. Combined PET/CT or SPECT-CT scanners provide spatially registered images from the two modalities acquired in a single imaging session.

CT-US Fusion

Another example is a navigated ultrasound system where the ultrasound probe is tracked by a 3D – localization system, the patient being immobilized in the CT-or MR-scanner. Due to a calibration of the ultrasound system with the coordinates of the scanner a real-time registration and fusion of ultrasound images with reconstructed CT/MR images can be performed [25].

In the SIP-Lab Innsbruck a different approach is performed: The patient is scanned in the CT/MR/SPECT/PET with artifical markers attached to the patient, the BodyFix or the SIP-Lab frame. The dataset is sent to the navigation system. The patient is registered in the laboratory or in the OR using the navigation system. A video signal of the tracked ultrasound probe (SONONav, Medtronic, USA) (Fig. 6) is sent to the navigation system and the navigation system reconstructs the respective planes of the CT/MR/SPECT/PET in real time, thus the actual ultrasound image can be superimposed to the pre-operative scan datasets (Fig. 7). The weighting of the ultrasound image over the other modalities can be adjusted via mouse-controlled sliders. This technology has originally been developed for the compensation of brain shift during neurosurgical interventions. However it can be used in the whole body using various immobilization and registration devices.

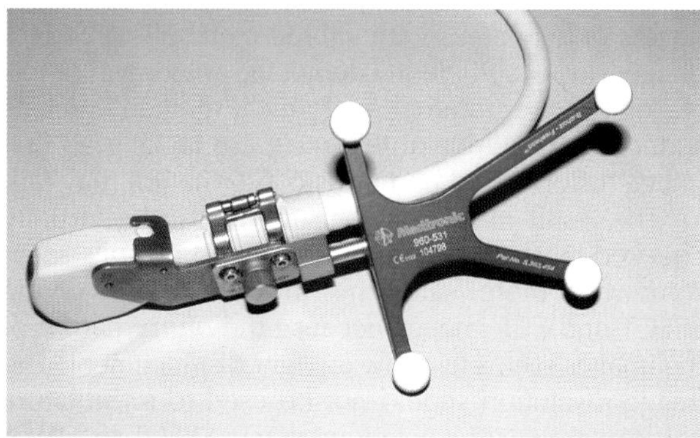

Fig. 6. A dynamic reference frame with 4 reflective markers is mounted to the SonoNav ultrasound probe. The reflective markers are detected by the cameras of the navigation system, which calculated the actual position of the ultrasound probe in 3D space with respect to the patient

Routine application of Image Fusion for diagnosis and interventions at the interdisciplinary Stereotactic Intervention- and Planning Laboratory (SIP-Lab) in Collaboration with the Department of Nuclear Medicine Innsbruck

A few years ago the optical based Treon navigation system (Medtronic Inc., Louisville, U.S.A.) was installed at our interdisciplinary laboratory for image-guided neuro-, ENT- and orthopaedic- surgery. The software module "Cranial 4" is part of the Treon navigation system. It allows for synergistic simultaneous fusion of any combination of CT/MR/SPECT/PET data based on paired-point matching of extrinsic markers or intrinsic (anatomical) markers. In addition, a mutual based fully automatic algorithm for fusion of CT/MR/SPECT/PET data is available.

The "Cranial 4" multimodality software

The CT/MR/SPECT/PET studies respective of each patient are transferred to the Treon via hospital own intranet. The Cranial 4 multimodality software allows the user to correlate more than 10 different image sets of one patient and to display and review the correlated images.

The registration procedure is a one-to-one mapping between the reference and the working image set ensuring that the same anatomical point in both images corresponds to each other. Image fusion software process starts with loading of the reference CT scan, which remains the base standard for fusion with MR/SPECT/PET since it is free of distortion artefacts. After preview and verification of the images the CT dataset is set as a reference, the following CT/MR/SPECT datasets as working image sets. The Cranial 4 software is capable of two different image registration methods; both are rigid-model based:

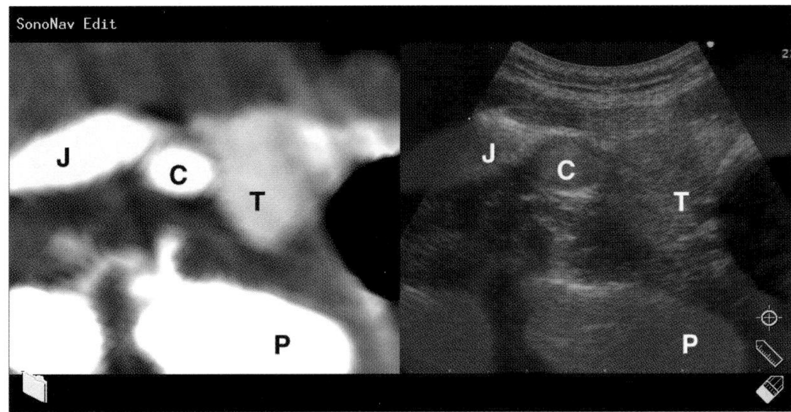

Fig. 7. Sononavigation in the neck area: Left image: reformatted CT according to the realtime-ultrasound image. Right image: 50% superposition of the real-time ultrasound with the real-time reformatted CT. (J jugular vein, C carotid artery, T thyroid, P parathyroid adenoma)

I. Paired-point matching

The registration is performed manually by selecting a minimum of 4 clearly defined corresponding fiducials or anatomical landmarks on both, the reference and the working dataset. The landmarks are selected by pointing-and-clicking the mouse cursor within the image in the highest possible magnification (Fig. 8). Using the SIP Lab Innsbruck frame 4–11 spherical fiducials (external markers) are selected for each registration process (Fig. 9).

When manually registering two data sets, registration accuracy is calculated by the software as the root square mean error (RSME) which is the mean distance of the respective frame-reference points in the two data sets.

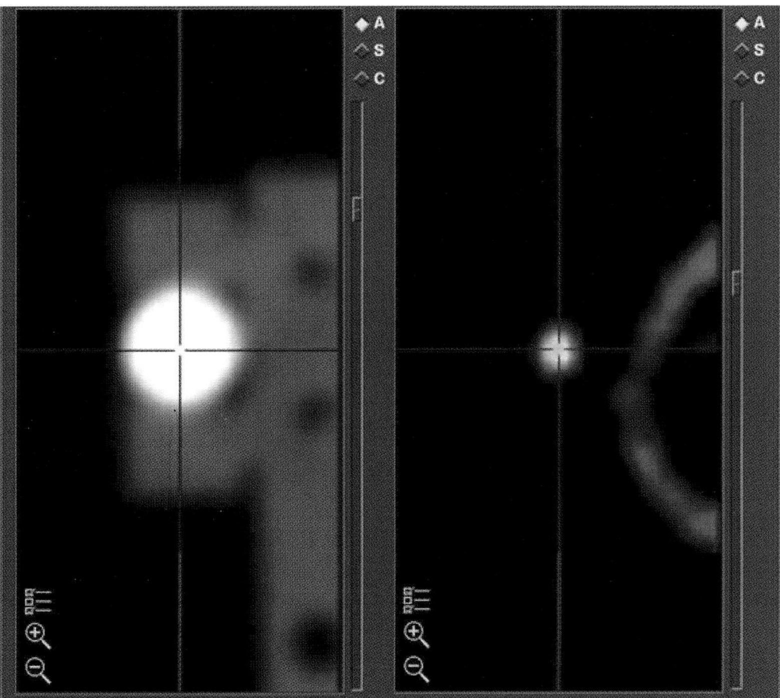

Fig. 8. The centres of the external landmarks in the CT data (left) and SPECT data (right) are selected in the highest possible magnification

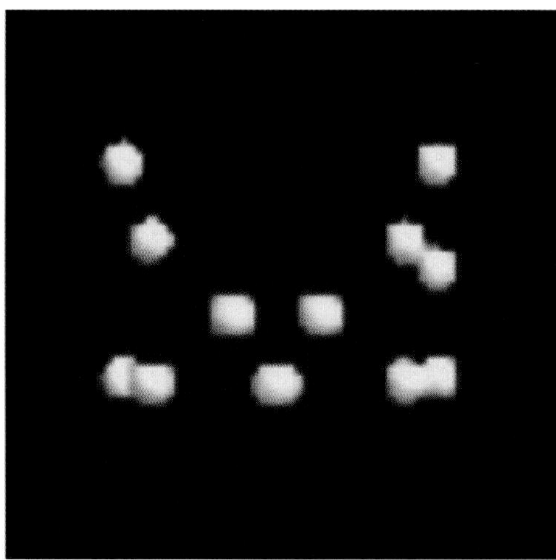

Fig. 9a. Shows a 3D reconstruction of the ^{241}Am markers on the SIP Lab Innsbruck frame based on SPECT data

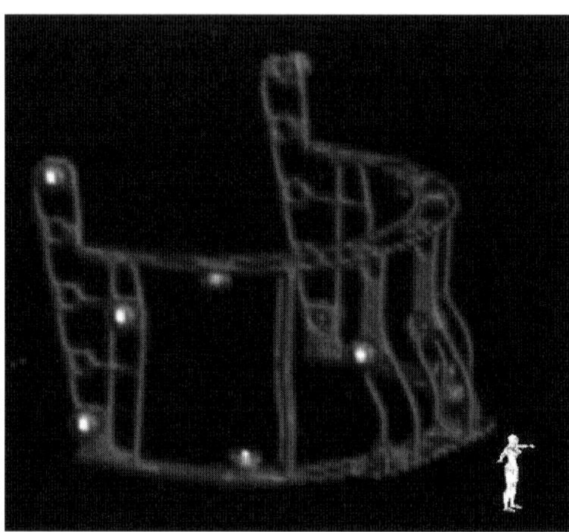

Fig. 9b. Shows a 3D reconstruction of the reference frame with the glass bead markers based on helical CT data

2. Voxel-intensity based algorithm

The fully automatic voxel-intensity algorithm implemented in the Cranial 4 workstation is based on the use of the general notion of mutual information. It allows us to import and co-register the previous CT/MR images, which were obtained without the frame, with the actual multimodal datasets, which are obtained with the frame.

Fusion / display

Once the image set has been registered the Cranial 4 software provides a variety of tools which enable the user to quantitatively and qualitatively compare the registered image sets. The software enables the user

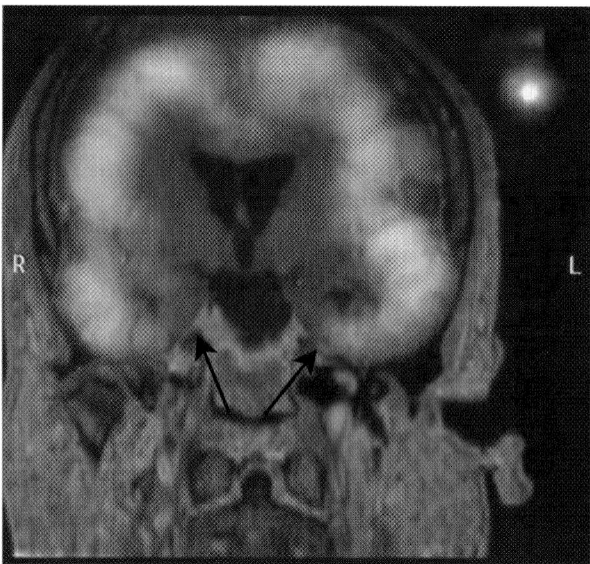

Fig. 10. Figure depicts coronal reconstruction of a fusion (blend mode 50%) of MRI and ^{123}I-Iomazenil - SPECT in a patient with left temporal lobe epilepsy. Note the discrepancy of activation between left and right hippocampus (arrowheads)

to combine the registered image sets by using the blend mode for visual comparison of results (Fig. 10). In this manner, each image modality can be displayed with the others as a combined level of reference and working pixel intensities in three planes (axial, coronal, sagittal). The threshold levels of all image sets as well as the weighting of one modality over the other can be adjusted via mouse-controlled sliders allowing quick visualization of any region in any magnification in three planes (axial, coronal, sagittal). Using interactive linked cursors a pixel to pixel correspondence can be evaluated. More than ten further previously registered studies, be it CT, MRI or functional imaging studies (SPECT/PET), can then be uploaded and compared to each other individually.

Implementation of multimodal image data into image-guided ENT and neurosurgery

Image-guided surgery may be performed on the basis of the multimodal datasets. The tip of the pointer is displayed in real-time on re-sliced 2D and 3D images. A transformation of the coordinate system associated with the pre-operative datasets and the coordinate system of the 3D – localizer is achieved. For such a link structures that are visible on the imaged data and that can be detected by the 3D – localizer must exist. For many neurosurgical procedures high registration accuracies are required which – according to our own experiences in more than hundred ENT cases – cannot be achieved with simple anatomical paired-point matching. Mutual information based registration algorithms can – as a matter of course – not used for registration of imaged space to physical space. Some groups use surface based algorithms by rendering the skin surface of the 3D object and touching at least 30 points on the patient or, alternatively, using a laser to render a 3D – surface of the real patient. As discussed above the accuracy of these methods are sensitive to tissue shift and depend on correct rendering of the skin surface. In addition, an irregular shape of the surface is paramount for an accurate registration. In order to achieve higher degrees of accuracy reliable extrinsic reference points are necessary.

Invasive markers are accurate, but they are cumbersome for the patient and the surgeon. For most image-guided neurosurgical procedures a prospective registration based on skin fiducials is performed, even though this method is sensitive to soft tissue shift which may result in deviations. An additional preoperative MRI has to be acquired, with the skin markers attached to the patient. We routinely use the reference points on the SIP-Lab Innsbruck frame for image-guided neurosurgery (Fig. 11).

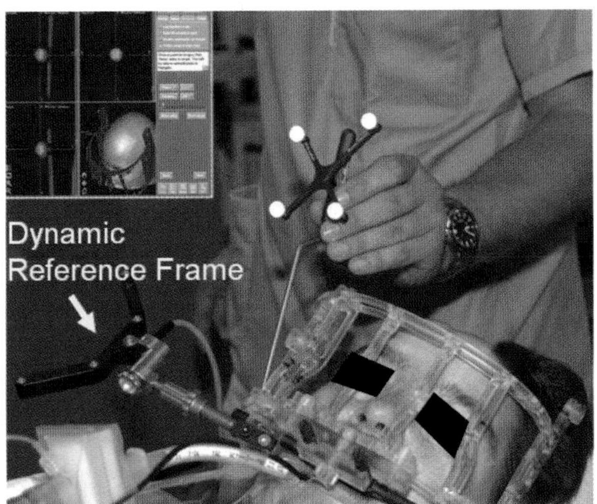

Fig. 11a. Image-guided neurosurgery using the VBH mouthpiece: Fig 11a shows the registration procedure in the OR. The dynamic reference frame and the SIP-Lab frame are attached to the mouthpiece. The markers on the frame are indicated by the probe of the navigation system and the corresponding fiducials are selected on the 3D-image dataset

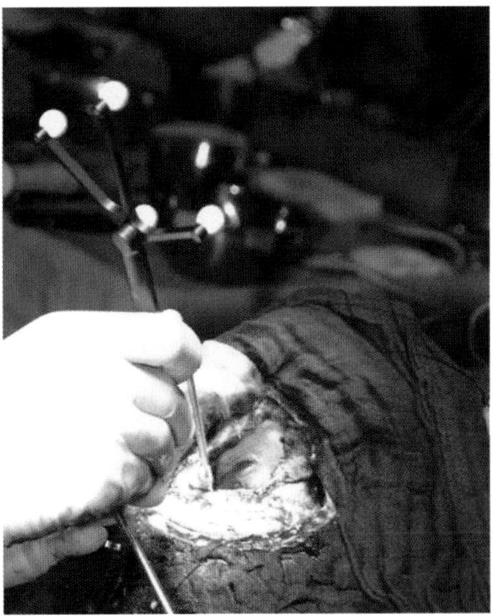

Fig. 11b. After registration the reference frame is removed and the surgeon can use the pointer to navigate during neurosurgery

1. Image Fusion and image-guided surgery in the cranial area

In patients with intact dentition of the upper jaw a VBH mouthpiece is made at initial presentation of a patient presenting with symptoms suspicious of a cranial tumor [26]. The initial 3D CT/ MRI /SPECT / PET data sets can then be registered and used for frameless stereotactic neurosurgery and/or radiation –planning and -treatment [27,28] as well as brachytherapy applications [29], reducing the need for additional scans as the patient proceeds from department to department. Previous anatomical and functional datasets are registered to the current data by voxel-based algorithms or, in selected cases, by choosing intrinsic landmarks.

In edentulous patients the different CT- and MR- and PET- datasets are registered to each other by mutual information or, in some cases, by selecting clearly defined anatomical landmarks. For image-guided surgery in these patients an additional MRI scan of the patient with skin fiducials is performed.

2. Extra-cranial Image-fusion

All the above mentioned algorithms assume the image datasets as rigid bodies. The result of extra-cranial image fusion highly depends on the positioning of the patient in the various scanners. In addition, different filling of the bladder and the gut as well as differences in breathing may cause big deviations. The most

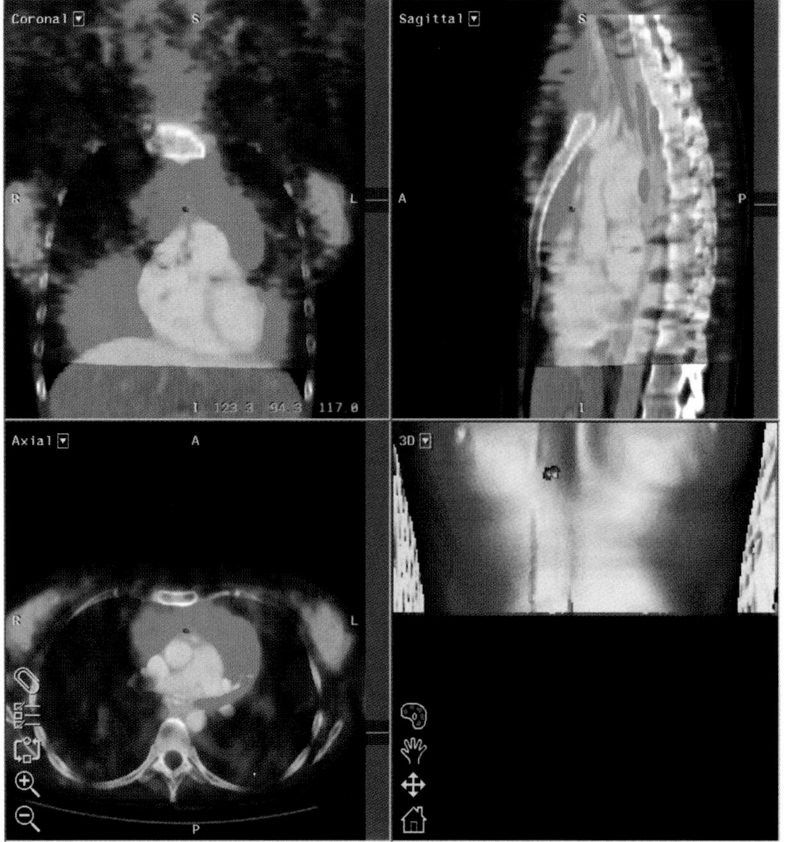

Fig. 12. Visual inspection shows a disastrous result after retrospective CT-PET fusion of the thorax using mutual information algorithm requiring additional registration based on anatomical landmarks

important reason is the different respiration patterns during the different scan acquisitions (up to 5 cm, experience by the author). Frequently we are asked to fuse image datasets in a retrospective manner. Retrospective image fusion of CT/MR/SPECT/PET datasets using mutual information based algorithms provides sometimes disastrous results (Fig. 12) which cannot be applied for diagnostic purposes. In these cases we try to use anatomical landmarks. Every organ near the diaphragm has to be matched separately.

For precise fusion identical positioning and fixation is required. This can be performed by immobilizing the patient in the scanners with an individually formed vacuum mattress. Depending on the type of imaging the respective external markers are attached to the fixation system.

Procedure

An individual mattress from the patient is formed by the radiation technician prior to the image acquisition (Fig. 13). This takes about 5–10 minutes. The vacuum

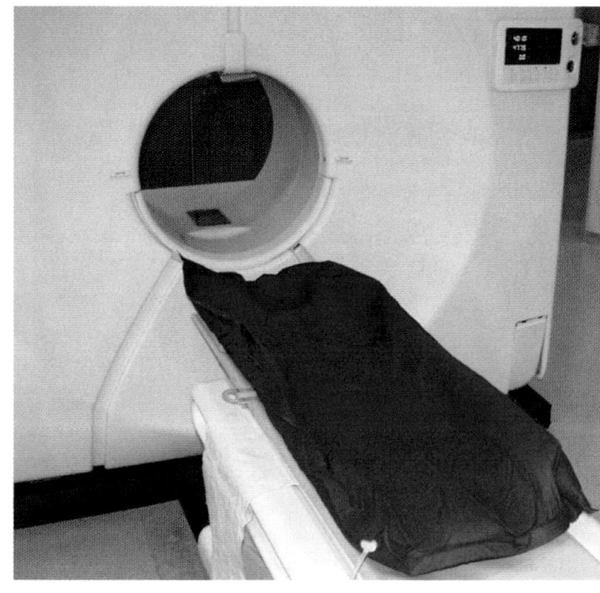

Fig. 13. Individual mattress for CT-PET fusion of the body

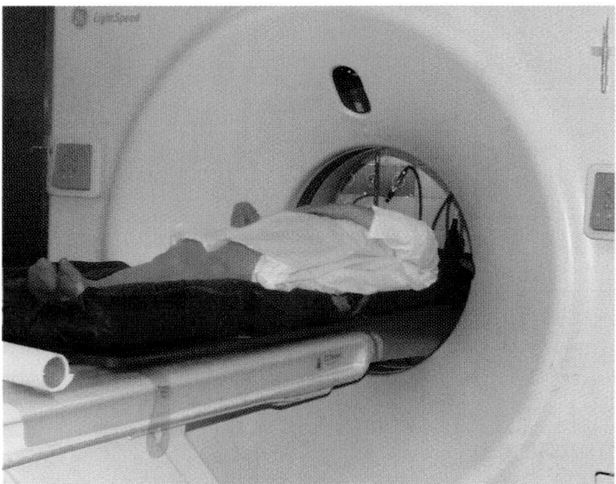

Fig. 14. For imaging acquisition the patient is repositioned into the vacuum mattress and the respective markers are attached to the mattress at identical positions

mattress is stored in the SIP-Lab. For every imaging acquisition (CT/PET/SPECT) the patient is repositioned into the vacuum mattress and the respective markers are attached to the mattress at identical positions (Fig. 14). We use 5 markers per region (thorax, head/neck or abdomen). During the PET and SPECT acquisition the patients breathe normally. For the CT scan the patient has to expire slightly and keep his breath during the scan. In most scanners respiratory triggering for PET and SPECT is not available. Thus the resulting information is a sum of the information provided by different respiratory positions. By our breathing protocol an optimal correlation between the functional data and the anatomical data can be achieved. Using this respiratory triggering the lung and the organs in the upper abdomen are in a similar position according to the "mean position" during the PET/SPECT acquisition. The same breathing protocol should also be used in combined PET/SPECT – CT scanners. The different datasets are sent to the Treon navigation system and registered to each other by means of paired-point matching based on the external markers.

Examples of clinical applications of image fusion that are routinely performed by the SIP-Lab Innsbruck

1. Diagnostic work-up

In most cases image fusion is used in the diagnostic investigation of a variety of pathologic conditions including tumors, inflammations etc. Fusion of SPECT and CT is routinely used in the investigation of hyperparathyroidism (Fig. 15) and neuro-endocrine neoplasm. Fusion of PET with MR/CT is routinely performed in patients with malignant disease (Fig. 16).

2. Epilepsy – Detection of the anatomic origin of the seizure activity

2.1 Fusion of MR – PET – ictal and interictal SPECT

For localization of the origin of the seizure different imaging data are available, all providing different information. For epilepsy patients it is important to have conclusive diagnostic information concerning the origin of the seizure. In patients with a conclusive localization the respective brain area is resected. In a high percentage of epilepsy cases the origin of the seizure is located in the hippocampus. The so-called hippocampal sclerosis can be visualized by MRI and must be confirmed by image fusion with functional imaging (PET/SPECT) prior to surgery (Fig. 17). In addition data from the EEG and videomonitoring are important for the therapeutic decision. In some cases structural abnormalities in other brain areas are responsible for the disease. These lesions may also be detected by MRI and must be confirmed by functional imaging.

2.2 Detection of the focus of seizure activity based on the EEG

In the remaining cases the MRI does not reveal any pathology or anatomical abnormality and the decision for surgery is very difficult. EEG electrodes can be replaced by markers visible in MRI. A 3D – reconstruction of the brain and the skin marker are performed visualizing the region of the brain being responsible for the seizure activity.

2.3 Fusion of two different 3D – objects from different image acquisitions

If the fusion of anatomical data and functional data and the other neurological examinations do not provide enough information about localization of the seizure origin invasive electrodes are implanted on the brain surface or via the foramen ovale inside the basal cisterns. For precise lesion localization it is important to know the actual location of the different electrodes with respect to the brain surface. Therefore two 3D – models have to be reconstructed, one 3D reconstruction of the brain surface and one of the electrodes. After implantation of the electrodes it is not possible to perform an MRI scan due to the

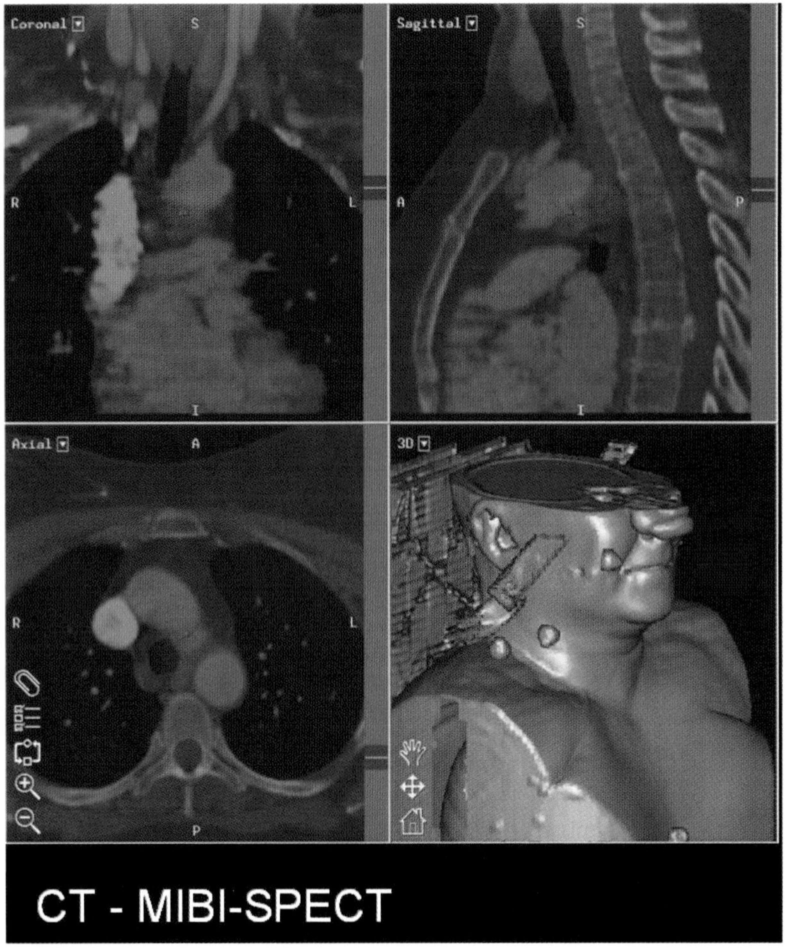

Fig. 15. Fusion of ^{99m}Tc-SPECT and CT in a patient with primary hyperparathyroidism showing an activation in the mediastinum which corresponds to a soft tissue mass visible in the CT scan. Surgery confirmed an atypically located parathyroid adenoma

metallic components. A post-operative CT scan is obtained to reconstruct the electrodes. However due to the artefacts of the electrodes it is not possible to reconstruct the brain surface with sufficient quality. Thus the post-operative 3D – CT dataset is matched with the pre-operative 3D MR dataset. A 3D reconstruction of the brain surface of the MR is then superimposed to the 3D – reconstruction of the electrodes of the postoperative CT. By this means 3D – volume images indicate the positions of subdural and trigeminal electrodes with respect to the brain surface (Fig. 18).

2.4 Subtraction of inter-ictal from ictal SPECT data (between and during seizures)

In some patients the acquisition of a SPECT between and during the seizures is required. By using a subtraction algorithm the active focus remains. By fusing this active focus with an MR scan the anatomical localization of this focus can be visualized.

3. Radiotherapy planning

CT is needed for calculation of the dose distribution, MR is required for precise definition of the treatment volume due to better outlining of the tumour tissue. Accurate CT-MR-SPECT-PET image registration allows for precise definition of active tumour tissue to be irradiated.

4. Follow-up: verification of treatment

Monomodality registration by comparison of pre-and post-intervention images (after radiation therapy,

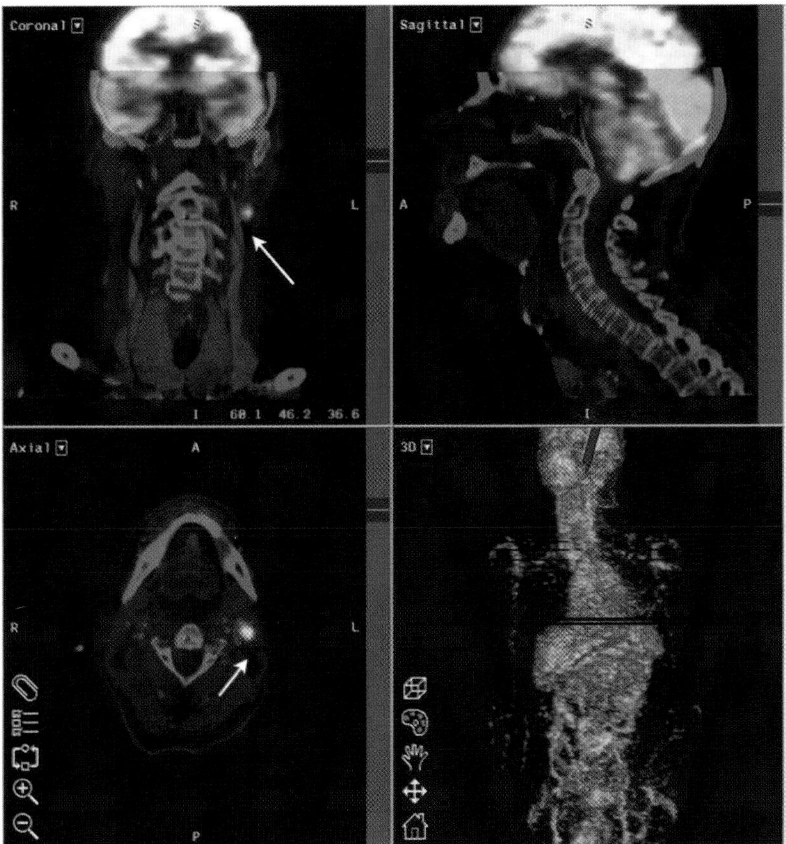

Fig. 16. Follow-up CT-PET image fusion in a patient with Hodgkin lymphoma of the stomach reveals an additional pathological lymphnode in the neck, which was initially not detected in the CT scan

chemotherapy, surgery etc.) is an interesting tool for growth monitoring and treatment verification (Fig. 19).

5. Evaluation of accuracy of image guided punctures

During an image guided puncture an intraoperative CT or MR can be obtained. This dataset can be fused with the pre-operative planning dataset and the actual position of the biopsy needle, the driller or the drill-hole can be superimposed to the planned path (Fig. 20).

6. Sono-navigation

The Sono-navigation tool can be used for diagnostic purposes. We currently use it for the comparison of CT, MIBI-SPECT and ultrasound in the diagnosis of parathyroid adenoma (Fig. 7). Ultrasound can also be used as an intraoperative real-time imaging tool to compensate brain shift.

Conclusion

The most important prerequisite for the application of image fusion is an excellent cooperation between radiologists and nuclear medicine specialists. In our setting the radiation technician from the SIP-Lab fabricates the reference/fixation device, the PET/SPECT data are obtained at the Department of Nuclear Medicine and the anatomical data are acquired at the Department of Radiology. The datasets are fused in the SIP-Lab and all the fused images are discussed in interdisciplinary conferences between radiologists from the SIP-Lab and nuclear medicine specialists.

This article focuses on the methods used in daily clinical practice by the authors. Currently we use only rigid or affine transformations. Elastic deformation algorithms are currently developed and are very interesting for inter-subject and atlas registration. For further information on other registration algorithms in other medical fields see the paper by Lavallee [25] and the review paper by Maintz and Viergever [1].

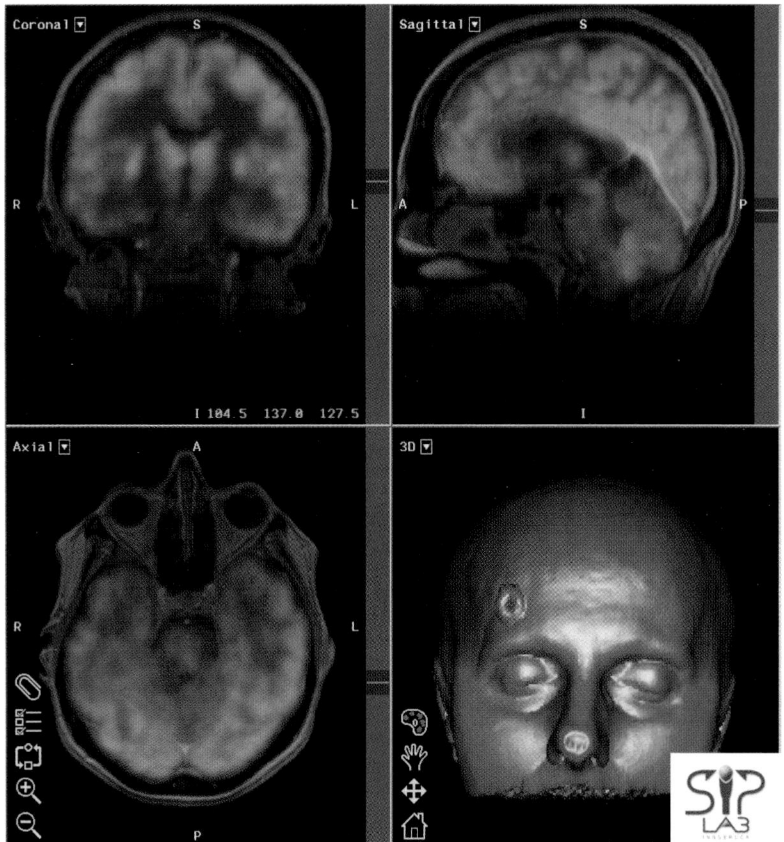

Fig. 17. Patient with right sided hippocampal sclerosis in the anatomical MRI and decrease of activation in the functional PET (blend mode 50%)

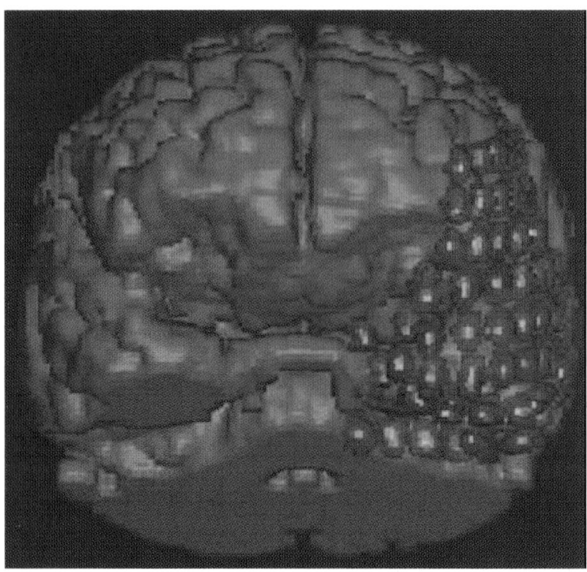

Fig. 18. Fusion of the 3D-surface of the brain from the pre-operative MRI and the 3D-reconstruction of the electrodes from the post-operative CT

Advances in imaging and computer technology should increase and optimize the extraction and quantification of useful inherent information and the application of this information for patient treatment. Effective visualization, synthesis, extraction and analysis of fused 3D biomedical images will be enhanced by continuing improvement of current methods. Multimodality image fusion provides synergistic information about the different imaging data, which might result in a better interpretation of the total imaging data. Hopefully this may result in a more effective diagnosis and treatment of disease.

Acknowledgments

I would like to thank the SIP-Lab team from the Department of Radiology (Prof. Dr. Werner Jaschke): Peter Kovacs, Thomas Bob Lang, Martin Knoflach and Christoph Hinterleithner for their invaluable support in the whole process including fabrication of

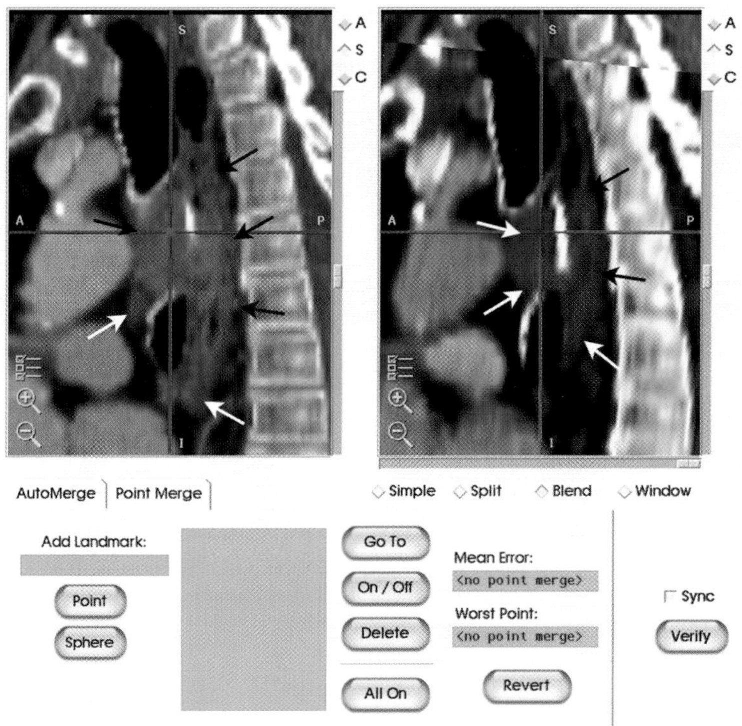

Fig. 19. Sagittal views after fusion of a CT of a patient with oesophageal carcinoma before (left) and after (right) chemotherapy. Monomodality registration allows for precise monitoring (arrowheads) of the growth/treatment success in 3 dimensions

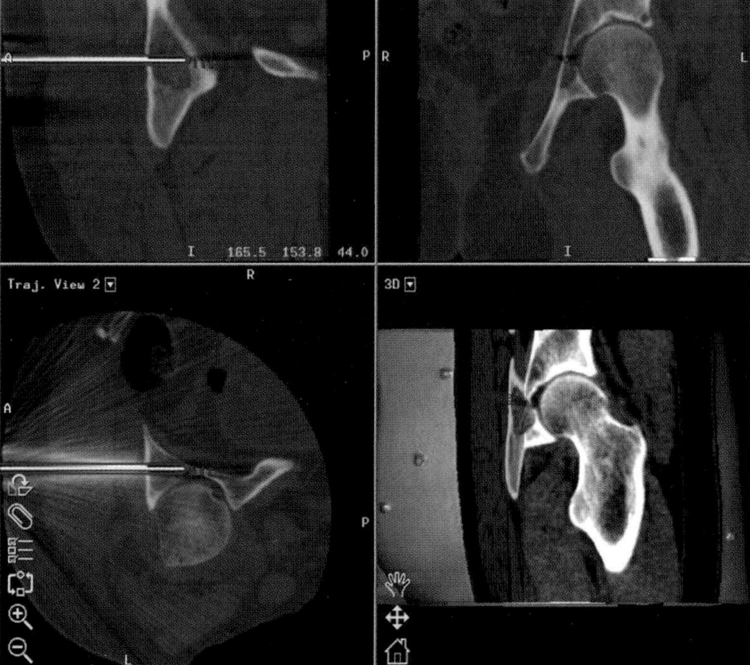

Fig. 20. Evaluating the accuracy of an image guided puncture for radiofrequency ablation of a hypernephroma metastasis in the right acetabulum: The intraoperative CT is fused with the pre-operative planning dataset and the actual position of the instrument is superimposed to the planned path

VBH mouthpiece, forming of individual mattresses, image acquisition, image fusion and diagnosis (WJ, PK).

I would like to thank the following doctors and physicists from the Department of Nuclear Medicine (Prof. Dr. I. Virgolini) for the exellent cooperation: Roy Moncayo, Eveline Donnemiller, Michael Gabriel, Dirk Heute, Dorota Kendler, Christian Uprimny, Peter Oberladstätter, Boris Warwitz.

In addition the following collaborators from other Departments are involved in the development and/or clinical applications of the SIP-Lab image fusion technology:

Department of Neurosurgery (Prof. Dr. K. Twerdy): Wilhelm Eisner, Johannes Burtscher, Thomas Fiegele, Michael Gabl, Martin Ortler

Department of Orthopaedics (Prof. Dr. W. Krismer): Franz Rachbauer

Department of Radiotherapy (Prof. Dr. P. Lukas): Reinhart Sweeney, Meinhard Nevinny, Karl Seydl

Department of Neurology (Prof. Dr. W. Poewe): Eugen Trinka, Günther Stockhammer, Iris Unterberger, Judith Dobesberger

Department of Surgery (Prof. Dr. E. Margreiter): Rupert Prommegger, Christoph Profanter

References

[1] Maintz JB, Viergever MA (1998) A survey of medical image registration. Med Image Anal 2: 1–36

[2] van den Elsen PA, Viergever MA (2004) Medical Image matching – a review with classification. IEEE Computer Graphics and Applications 12: 26–39

[3] Hanjal JH, Hawkes DJ, Hill D (2004) Medical Image Registration. [Series: Biomedical Engineering Series]. CRC Press, Boca Raton London New York, Washington D.C.

[4] Weese J, Penney GP, Desmedt P, et al (1997) Voxel-based 2-D/3-D registration of fluoroscopy images and CT scans for image-guided surgery. IEEE Trans Inf Technol Biomed 1: 284–93

[5] Maurer CR, Jr, Fitzpatrick JM, Wang MY, et al (1997) Registration of head volume images using implantable fiducial markers. IEEE Trans Med Imaging 16: 447–62

[6] Kremser C, Plangger C, Bosecke R, et al (1997) Image registration of MR and CT images using a frameless fiducial marker system. Magn Reson Imaging 15: 579–85

[7] Evans NT (1990) Combining imaging techniques. Clin Phys Physiol Meas 11 [Suppl A]: 97–102

[8] Zinreich SJ, Tebo SA, Long DM, et al (1993) Frameless stereotaxic integration of CT imaging data: accuracy and initial applications. Radiology 188: 735–42

[9] Hirschberg H, Kirkeby OJ (1996) Interactive image directed neurosurgery: patient registration employing the Laitinen stereo-adapter. Minim Invasive Neurosurg 39: 105–7

[10] Greitz T, Bergstrom M, Boethius J, et al (1980) Head fixation system for integration of radiodiagnostic and therapeutic procedures. Neuroradiology 19: 1–6

[11] Bergstrom M, Boethius J, Eriksson L, et al (1981) Head fixation device for reproducible position alignment in transmission CT and positron emission tomography. J Comput Assist Tomogr 5: 136–41

[12] Pilipuf MN, Goble JC, Kassell NF (1995) A noninvasive thermoplastic head immobilization system. Technical note. J Neurosurg 82: 1082–5

[13] Hauser R, Westermann B, Probst R (1997) Noninvasive tracking of patient's head movements during computer-assisted intranasal microscopic surgery. Laryngoscope 107: 491–9

[14] Gill SS, Thomas DG, Warrington AP, et al (1991) Relocatable frame for stereotactic external beam radiotherapy. Int J Radiat Oncol Biol Phys 20: 599–603

[15] Howard MA, III, Dobbs MB, Simonson TM, et al (1995) A noninvasive, reattachable skull fiducial marker system. Technical note. J Neurosurg 83: 372–6

[16] Martin A, Bale RJ, Vogele M, et al (1998) Vogele-Bale-Hohner mouthpiece: registration device for frameless stereotactic surgery. Radiology 208: 261–5

[17] Bale RJ, Vogele M, Freysinger W, et al (1997) Minimally invasive head holder to improve the performance of frameless stereotactic surgery. Laryngoscope 107: 373–7

[18] Bale RJ, Burtscher J, Eisner W, et al (2000) Computer-assisted neurosurgery by using a noninvasive vacuum-affixed dental cast that acts as a reference base: another step toward a unified approach in the treatment of brain tumors. J Neurosurg 93: 208–13

[19] Sweeney RA, Bale RJ, Moncayo R, et al (2003) Multimodality cranial image fusion using external markers applied via a vacuum mouthpiece and a case report. Strahlenther Onkol 179: 254–60

[20] Capek M, Wegenkittl R, Koenig A, Jaschke W, Sweeney RA, Bale RJ (2004) Multimodal Volume Registration based on spherical markers. Conference proceedings of the 9th International Conference in Central Europe on Computer Graphics, Visualization and Computer Vision 2001, WSCG'2001. 1, 17–24. University of West Bochemia, Pilsen, Czech Republic. Vaclav Skala

[21] Levin DN, Pelizzari CA, Chen GT, et al (1988) Retrospective geometric correlation of MR, CT, and PET images. Radiology 169: 817–23

[22] Pelizzari CA, Chen GT, Spelbring DR, et al (1989) Accurate three-dimensional registration of CT, PET, and/or MR images of the brain. J Comput Assist Tomogr 13: 20–6

[23] Wells WM, III, Viola P, Atsumi H, et al (1996) Multimodal volume registration by]maximization of mutual information. Med Image Anal 1: 35–51

[24] Studholme C, Hill DL, Hawkes DJ (1996) Automated 3-D registration of MR and CT images of the head. Med Image Anal 1: 163–75
[25] Lavallee S, Cinquin P, Szeliski R, et al (1995) Building a hybrid patient's model for augmented reality in surgery: a registration problem. Comput Biol Med 25: 149–64
[26] Bale RJ, Burtscher J, Eisner W, et al (2000) Computer-assisted neurosurgery by using a noninvasive vacuum-affixed dental cast that acts as a reference base: another step toward a unified approach in the treatment of brain tumors. J Neurosurg 93: 208–13
[27] Sweeney R, Bale R, Vogele M, et al (1998) Repositioning accuracy: comparison of a noninvasive head holder with thermoplastic mask for fractionated radiotherapy and a case report. Int J Radiat Oncol Biol Phys 41: 475–83
[28] Sweeney RA, Bale R, Auberger T, et al (2001) A simple and non-invasive vacuum mouthpiece-based head fixation system for high precision radiotherapy. Strahlenther Onkol 177: 43–7
[29] Bale RJ, Freysinger W, Gunkel AR, et al (2000) Head and neck tumors: fractionated frameless stereotactic interstitial brachytherapy-initial experience. Radiology 214: 591–5

Ten years experience with computer-assisted interventions from head to toe

R. Bale

Interdisciplinary Stereotactic Intervention- and Planning Laboratory (SIP-Lab), Department of Radiology (Chairman: Professor Werner Jaschke, MD), Medical University, Innsbruck, Austria

Computer-assisted navigation based on preoperative acquired 3D datasets gain increasing importance in various surgical disciplines, in particular in the cranial and in the musculoskeletal area. Especially in situations where the surgeon's orientation is irritated by destruction of normal anatomy (e.g. due to tumour or inflammation) navigation systems are helpful. Frameless stereotactic navigation systems allow for an interactive visualization of the actual position of the instrument with respect to the preoperative acquired image datasets. The surgeon can navigate on multiplanar reconstructed images in real-time. In contrast to conventional surgery the surgeon can identify, localize and access structures behind and in the vicinity of the surface. This is especially important if one deals with vital structures like vessels and nerves. Due to pre-operative planning and simulation standard surgical approaches can be adapted to the individual anatomic situation.

In spite of the apparent advantages such systems are currently confined to university clinics or other big centres. The reasons therefore are complex: In contrast to GPS navigation systems for the car a profound knowledge about the functionality of navigation systems is mandatory for a successful and safe application. The radiologist plays an important role in the whole procedure: He is responsible for the image acquisition, the diagnosis and the planning of the intervention. On one hand the acquired datasets should provide an accurate diagnosis, on the other hand they should serve as the basis for the image-guided surgery, thus special acquisition protocols are required. The selection of the respective protocols may affect the accuracy. It depends on the voxel size, which is influenced by the slice thickness and the field of view of the CT/MR data. MRI artefacts due to magnetic field inhomogenities and patient motion during image acquisition may also affect the accuracy. Most navigation systems require continuous slicing without gaps or overlaps. Acquisition with a tilted gantry leads to geometric distortions. Interdisciplinary cooperation is also necessary for data transfer from the scanner to the navigation systems via MOD, CD ROM or intranet.

Usually an additional planning CT is obtained the day before surgery with fiducial skin markers, invasive markers or reference frames. Additional procedures in the OR including system set-up, instrument calibration, registration, verification of accuracy, intraoperative application and dismantling of the navigation system may increase the operation time.

For the application of most navigation systems an additional person (technician) is still necessary. The costs for the purchase of the guidance system (approximately 100–300,000 €) and the additional costs for the man power are hardly affordable for small hospitals.

Ten years ago we started with the application of navigation systems for videoendoscopic ENT surgery. In 1995 we developed the worldwide first guidance devices for the application of navigation systems for precise percutaneous punctures. This was for the first time a symbiosis of navigation systems (frameless stereotaxy) with conventional frame-based stereotaxy. In the meantime many different devices and techniques were developed by our group in order to expand the use of image-guided surgery from the cranial area to the whole body.

In the following we present novel techniques and methods for percutaneous punctures of various structures in the whole body. In addition a novel unified concept for the application of the navigation system in the cranial area in order to safe surgery time, costs and effort is presented.

Basic principles of navigation systems

Computer-assisted surgery is based on preoperatively acquired Computed Tomographic (CT) or Magnetic Resonance (MR) images. Navigation systems consist of a workstation, a monitor, a three-dimensional digitizer (coordinate-detection or tracking system) and various pointers and instruments.

They show the actual position of the probe with respect to cross sectional images of the preoperative dataset. The software and the registration algorithms of most commercially available systems are similar. Standard tracking systems are based on electromechanic, optic or electromagnetic principles.

In 1995 we started with the use of the first commercially available navigation system, the ISG Viewing Wand System (ISG Technologies, Mississauga, Ontario, Canada) [7, 9, 19] using the FARO Surgicom (FARO Technologies, Inc., Lake Mary, Fla.) for computer-assisted videoendoscopic ENT surgeries. The mechanical articulated Faro arm is a six-jointed, six-degrees-of-freedom pointer.

It uses potentiometers to measure the angular position of each joint. The localization precision of the ISG viewing wand is 0.25 mm. Because its spatial system is entirely self-referential, rigid fixation of both the patient's head and the arm is an important prerequisite for successful implementation of the mechanical arm. In addition, due to its bulkiness the Viewing Wand was replaced by the following optical and electromagnetic systems.

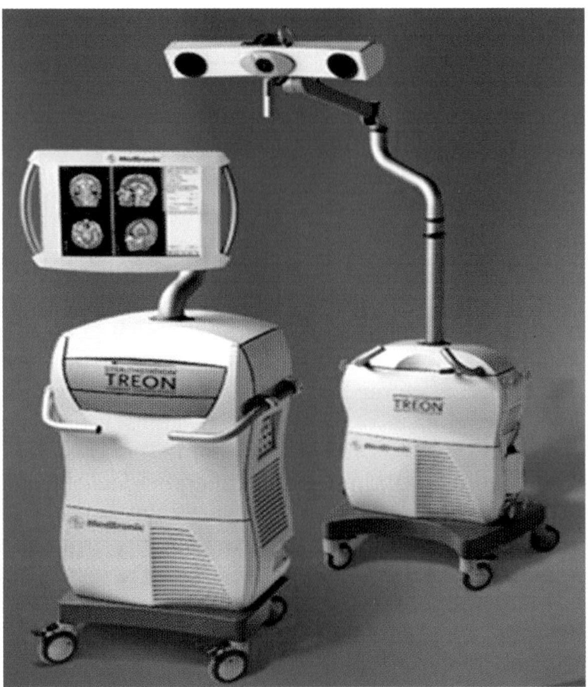

Fig. 1. Treon navigation system consisting of workstation, a camera and a monitor. The pointer is not displayed

Active optical systems (Medtronic, Brainlab, Stryker, Radionics, Robodent,...) [16] are equipped with a probe with infrared light-emitting diodes, two or three infrared position sensor cameras that are mounted on a trolley-stand (see Fig. 1) and a dynamic reference frame (DRF).

Instruments and anatomic structures are assumed as rigid bodies. DRFs, originally developed for spinal surgery, are used to track the actual position of the patient in space by providing a spatial coordinate system relative to the patient's anatomy. The DRF has to be rigidly attached to the patient. Once the patient is registered the rigid body (= patient with tracker or bone fragment with tracker) and the camera can be moved with respect to each other without loosing the spatial information. Due to the possible movements of the different vertebrae during spinal surgery the DRF has to be clamped to the spinal process of the vertebra that has to be treated.

In frameless stereotactic neurosurgery the tracker is usually attached to the head fixation device or the DRF may be screwed directly to the patient's head. Therefore, even if the patient's head moves, the system can compensate for such movement, thus avoiding the need to re-perform calibration. This may also be done by means of a plastic band. However the displacement of the DRF due to skin displacements may lead to serious inaccuracies, which might not be detected by the surgeon. Caversaccio et al. [8] and our group [1] mount the DRF to the patient by means of a non-invasive dental cast. Caversaccio uses his device for the attachment of the tracker only. Registration is performed using anatomical landmarks. The devices from our lab (VBH mouthpiece and SIP-Lab frame) are used for both, tracking of the patient and registration.

In contrast to active optical systems the instruments of passive systems (Medtronic, Brainlab) are equipped with reflective markers.

Infrared light signals that are emitted by two cameras are reflected by the markers and detected by the same cameras. The computer calculates the actual spatial position of the markers (instruments) on the basis of the angles of the incoming reflected light. The bench accuracy of active and passive instruments is in the range of 0.2 to 0.4 mm. DRFs may also be equipped with passive markers. In contrast to conventional active infrared systems the passive instruments are wireless which improves the surgeon's flexibility. As an alternative Stryker uses active wireless pointers which are equipped with batteries.

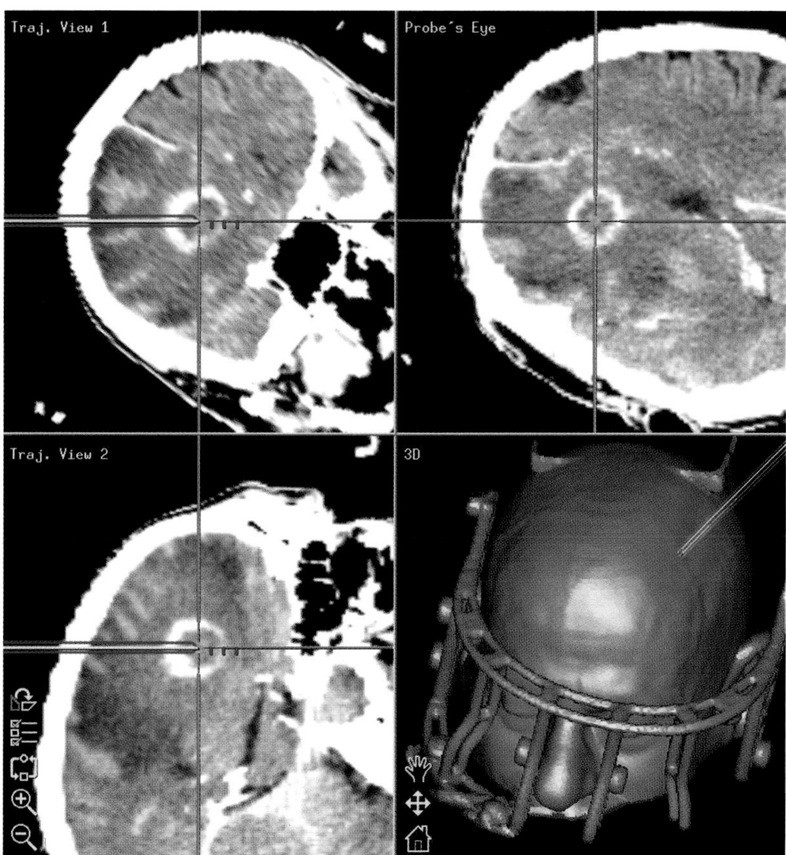

Fig. 2. The actual position of the probe is visualized with respect to the pre-operative acquired dataset in real time

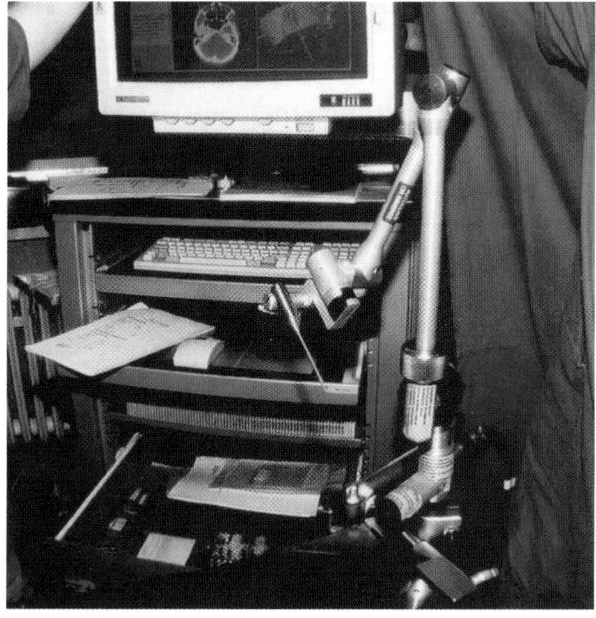

Fig. 3. The mechanical FARO arm is a six-jointed, six-degrees-of-freedom pointer

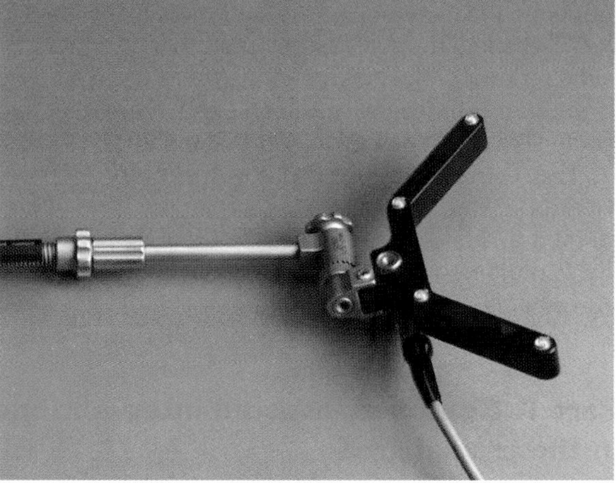

Fig. 4. Dynamic reference frame to be attached to the patient or the patient immobilization device

One major drawback of navigation systems based on optical technology is the requirement of a "line of sight" between the DRF, the instruments and the

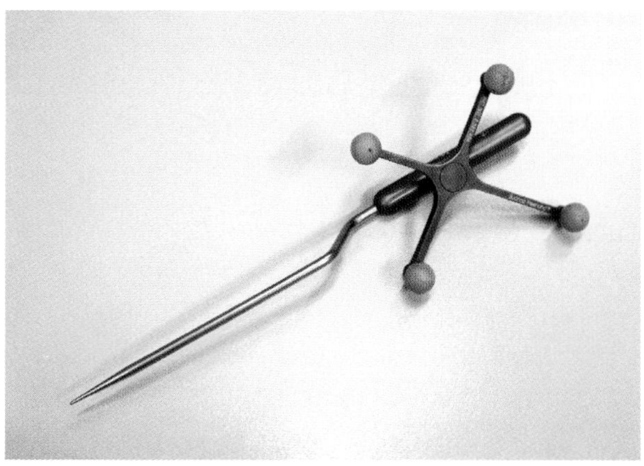

Fig. 5. Pointer equipped with passive reflective markers

camera. The navigation system InstaTrak (Visualization Technology, Inc., Boston, MA) [11] uses two electromagnetic sensors to provide positional information during surgery, not requiring a "line of sight". One sensor is incorporated into the instrument and the second is located on a headset that the patient wears during both the preoperative CT scan and the surgical procedure. The headset, which fits in the ear canals and on the bridge of the nose, serves two functions: it provides automated registration and compensates for head movements during surgery. Fried [11] reported a mean accuracy of the automatic registration of 2.28 mm, a 95th percentile of 2,5 mm and a maximum value of 5.08 mm. One major drawback of the system is that large metallic objects influence the accuracy of the system as is the case in the operating room. Another possible error source is the reproducible attachment of the reference frame to the skin. All devices and markers that are attached to the skin are sensitive to soft tissue shift.

The device we use in our institution (Treon, Medtronic Inc., Louisville, Colorado) has implemented a dual optical technology which allows for the simultaneous tracking of active and passive instruments.

Part I. Computer-assisted interventions in the cranial area

Preoperative steps

Usually 1 mm or 3 mm axial contiguous CT slices of the patient's head are obtained. Most authors use fiducials applied to the patient's skin during CT – or MR imaging. They must remain in place until surgery. The two dimensional CT data are transferred to the navigation system via optical disc/magnetic tape or network. Preoperatively the two-dimensional dataset is reconstructed to a 3D – dataset.

Intraoperative steps

After intubation the DRF has to be rigidly attached to the patient by means of an immobilization device. Various instruments including pointer, forceps, suction tube, endoscope are calibrated. The key step is the registration, during which the spatial configuration of the patient in the OR, is correlated with the pre-operative images of the patient. It is a correlation of the imaged space with the physical space. This is done by indicating the reference points (e.g. skin fiducials) on the patient with the probe of the navigation system and selecting the respective points on the dataset. It generally takes about 10 additional minutes to prepare the patient and complete the registration process. Using skin fiducials an accuracy of about 2–3 mm is usually achievable, inaccuracies of up to 8 mm may be observed due to soft tissue shift (personal experience in more than 100 ENT cases). Once the registration process has been completed, the tip of the probe is displayed in real time on the computer monitor. The position of the instrument's tip appears on the screen within various reconstructed images of the surgical area. Before the navigation system can be used during surgery the accuracy has to be checked by touching clearly identifiable landmarks. If the accuracy is not satisfactory the registration procedure may be repeated. Additional surface registration or landmark registration techniques may be added to improve the accuracy.

Alternative registration methods

The simplest registration method is the use of anatomical landmarks. Clearly defined external (nasion, spina nasalis, tragi, medial canthi) and/or internal landmarks are touched with the probe and correlated with their locations in the imaged CT- or MR-dataset. The advantage of using landmarks is that the diagnostic dataset can be used, thus necessitating an additional scan. Identification of the landmarks in both the patient and the imaged dataset is difficult, to a certain extent subjective and strongly depending on the experience of the operator (with a learning curve). Generally, these methods are inaccurate and they are time-consuming. Surface matching, which is done by touching about 40 points of the patient's skin or bone, can be used to refine anatomical registration. Pointing of the skin with the probe of the navigation system can also be replaced by a laser pointer. Such devices are commercially available from Medtronic and Brainlab. In most cases a sufficient accuracy can be obtained especially if the area of interest is close to the face whose contour is used for registration. However, all registration methods which are based on the skin surface are sensitive to skin shift which may lead to inaccuracies.

The most accurate registration can be achieved with markers implanted into the skull. Unfortunately they may cause major patient discomfort and should not left in place over an extended time.

Reproducible external reference frames [1, 12, 14] in combination with dynamic reference frames allow for registering the patient in his absence the day before surgery. In addition they allow for attaching DRFs non-invasively to the patient for tracking the patient's movement during surgery. The patient has to wear the frame during the CT scan.

The headset of the InstaTrak system, which fits in the ear canals and on the bridge of the nose, provides also external reference points and compensates for head movements during surgery. In addition the system automatically detects the markers in the headset. However, should the headset inadvertently shift in relation to the patient's skull, the surgeon does not get any feedback from the system, requiring an accuracy check before each application of the guidance tool.

The Vogele-Bale-Hohner (VBH) mouthpiece (Medical Intelligence, Schwabmünchen, Germany) is an individualized dental cast that is held against the upper jaw by negative pressure. The vacuum area is connected via a tube to the vacuum pump.

The Vogele-Bale-Hohner (VBH) mouthpiece in combination with registration rods or the SIP Lab Innsbruck frame (Medical Intelligence, Schwabmünchen, Germany) has successfully been used for immobilization and registration of the patient during more than 500 computer assisted surgeries in the cranial area. In contrast to the other external reference frames, repositioning can be controlled by the amount of negative pressure on the vacuum scale. Should the required negative pressure not be attained, the mouthpiece is not precisely repositioned. A volunteer study confirmed a repositioning accuracy of the VBH mouthpiece itself with respect to the patient's head with well under one millimetre, thus providing the most accurate non-invasive external reference points [14]. The mean localization accuracy of an optical navigation system using the VBH mouthpiece for registration with 3 mm axial CT slices was in the range of 0 and 2 mm [1]. One major drawback of the mouthpiece is its dependency on a minimum of two intact teeth.

CAS using the VBH mouthpiece

A VBH mouthpiece is fabricated prior to the scan taking about 10–15 minutes. The CT/MR scan is performed with the patient wearing the VBH mouthpiece and the SIP-Lab frame. In the SIP-Lab the DRF is mounted to the VBH mouthpiece. Due to the high repositioning accuracy of the VBH mouthpiece with respect to the skull and due to the application of the dynamic reference frame the registration can be performed in the laboratory in the absence of the patient. The registration protocol is stored on the navigation system. After oral or nasal intubation the VBH mouthpiece is introduced

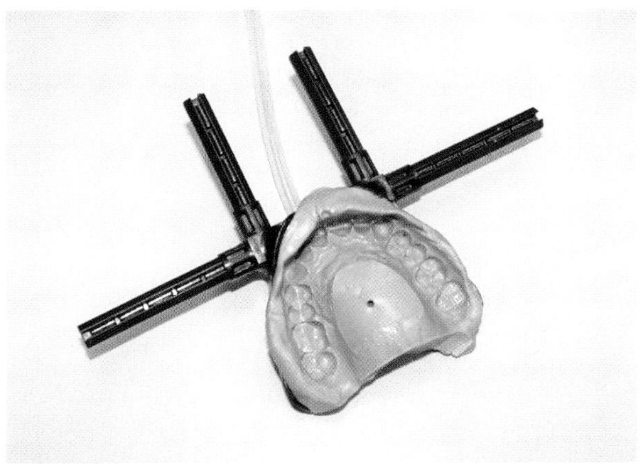

Fig. 6. The Vogele-Bale-Hohner (VBH) mouthpiece with the vacuum area in the centre. The anterior and lateral rods may be used for attachment of the reference frame and fixating arms

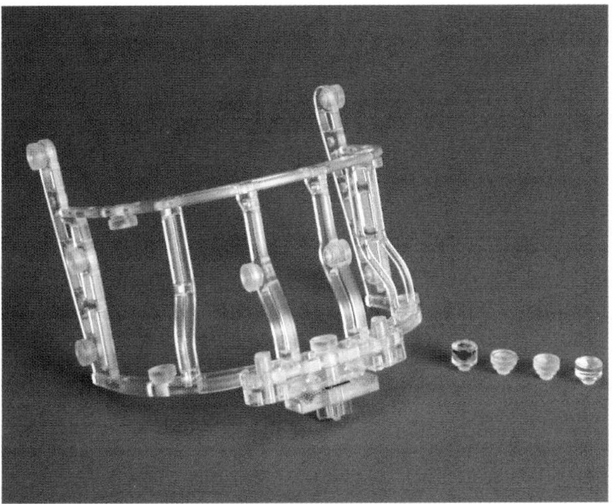

Fig. 7. The SIP-Lab Innsbruck frame is a universal registration device for CT-MR-SPECT-PET fusion and image-guided surgery

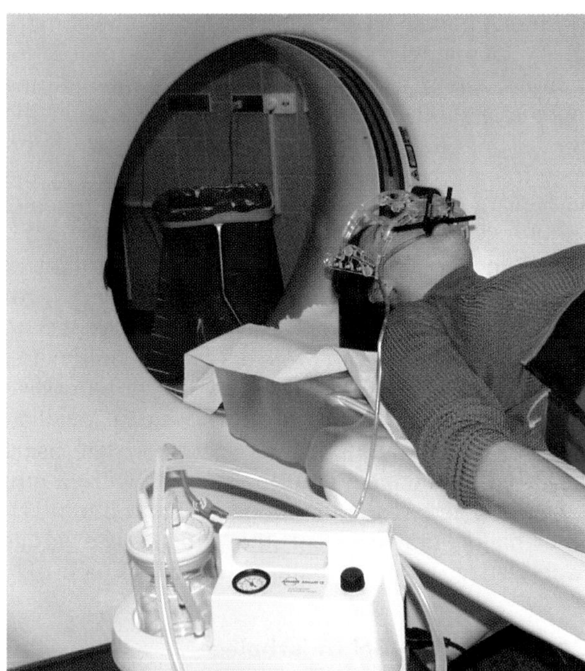

Fig. 8. Patient wearing the VBH mouthpiece and the SIP-Lab Innsbruck reference frame during a CT scan

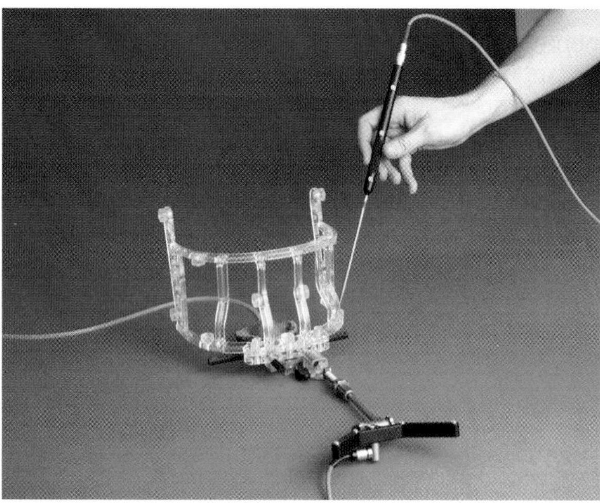

Fig. 9. Registration of the patient in his absence in the SIP-Lab. The DRF is mounted to the VBH mouthpiece. The reference points on the frame are indicated by the registration probe

into the patient's mouth and automatically registered by reloading the registration protocol. Due to the rigid attachment of the DRF on the mouthpiece the patient's head may be moved during surgery without loosing accuracy.

In phantom studies as well as in clinical studies an accuracy comparable to invasive markers could be achieved. This work is an important step towards a novel unified approach in the diagnosis and therapy of brain tumours.

Computer-assisted punctures in the cranial area

Besides the application of frameless stereotactic navigation systems for surgical procedures such systems may also be used for pre-planned image-guided punctures of different lesions or anatomical structures. Basically there are two ways to achieve that task: First, the CT/MR and the surgical intervention are performed in the same session. This is usually done with a conventional frame. It is invasively fixed to the skull and due to the lack of the possibility to reposition the frame with respect to the patient's skull the planning procedure and the intervention have to be performed in the same session, the patient being anaesthetized during the whole procedure in most cases.

The second option is the separation of image acquisition and therapy in time and location, necessitating precise markers for registration and rigid immobilization. Therefore the VBH mouthpiece/headholder is an ideal non-invasive registration and immobilization tool.

Before applying the VBH head holder the repositioning accuracy had to be evaluated. Due to the fact that precise repositioning of the patient is also an important prerequisite for fractionated radiotherapy our group decided to adapt the VBH

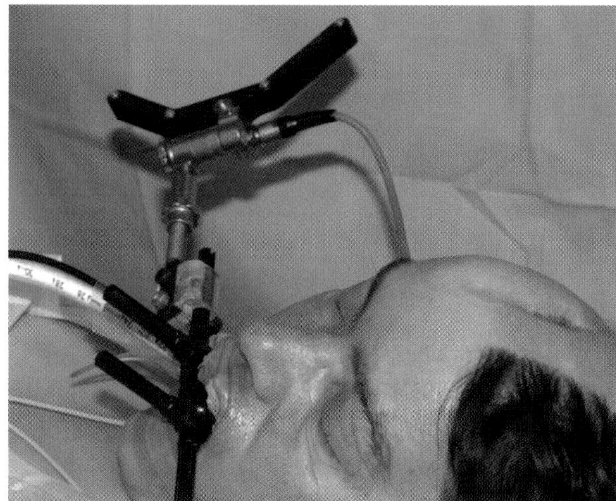

Fig. 10. For surgery the VBH mouthpiece with the DRF is repositioned in the patient's mouth necessitating intraoperative navigation

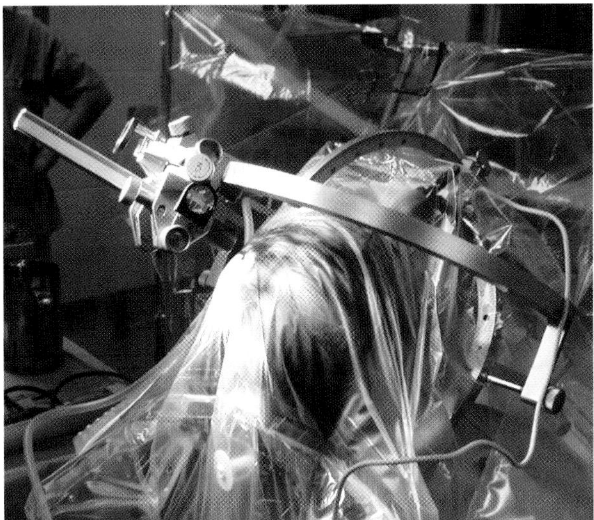

Fig. 11. Stereotactic frame that is rigidly attached to the patient's head by means of pins

head holder to the requirements of radiotherapy. In contrast to the studies performed by Martin et al. where only the repositioning accuracy of the VBH mouthpiece with respect to the patient's skull was determined the repositioning accuracy of the patient's head in the VBH head holder was evaluated. In 5 volunteers and in 250 measurements the mean repositioning accuracy was 1.02 mm, as compared to 3.05 mm using the conventional mask immobilization system [17].

Development of targeting devices for frameless stereotactic punctures

An important prerequisite for a precise linear targeting are not only a rigid patient (target) immobilization but also a rigid guidance of the instrument (endoscope, brachytherapy needle, biopsy needle, radiofrequency needle,...) that has to be advanced into the patient's body. In total four different aiming devices for computer-assisted punctures have been developed and patented by our group as early as 1995. Three of them have been commercialized in the meantime:

- Philips EasyTaxis™ Image-Guided Surgery System (Adams L., van den Brug W.P., Vogele M., Bale RJ: European Patent PHN 16.013/ alignment device)
- Medtronic VERTEK™ Targeting device (Vogele M., Bale R.J: European Patent 0871407).
- Medical Intelligence Atlas targeting device (Vogele M., Bale R.J: European Patent 0871407).

Using these targeting devices the worldwide first frameless stereotactic punctures with stabile guidance were performed by our group.

Computer-assisted interstitial brachytherapy of head and neck tumours

Brachytherapy is an established therapeutic option in selected patients with progressive inoperable ENT tumours (gr. brachy = short distance). Interstitial brachytherapy allows for the application of high radiation doses to the tumour via hollow needles.

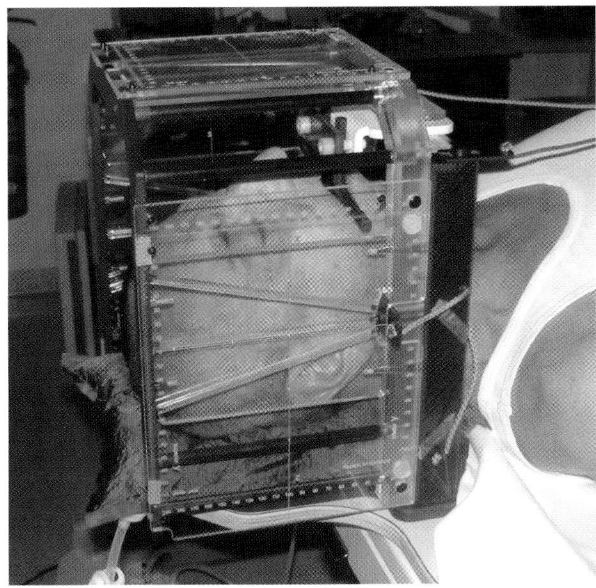

Fig. 12. VBH head holder for radiotherapy

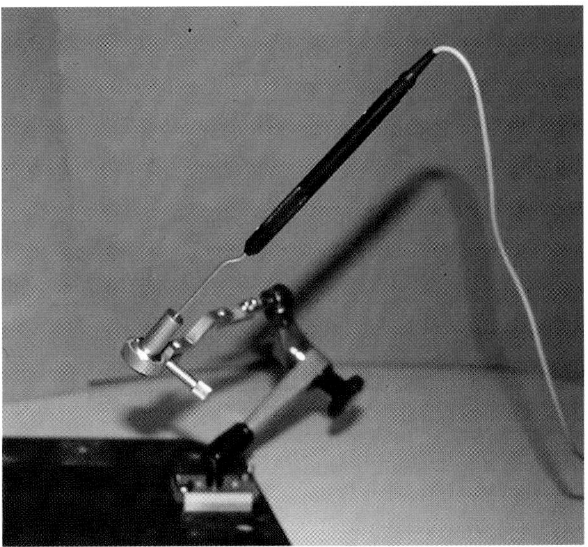

Fig. 13. Prototype of the EasyTaxis targeting device

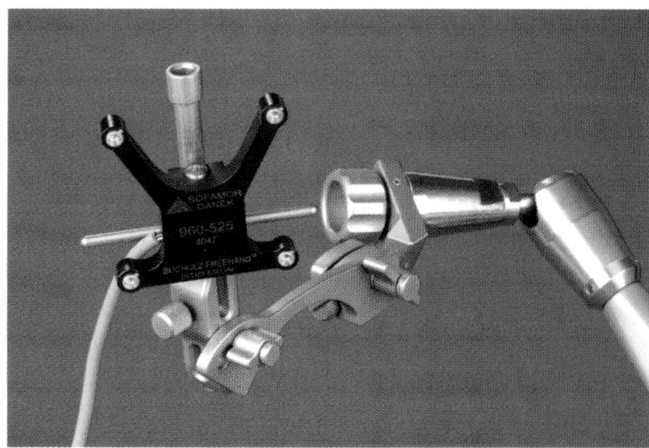

Fig. 14. Vertek targeting device

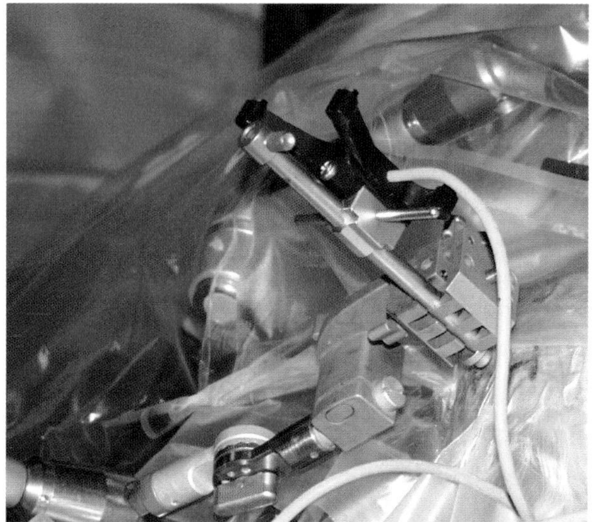

Fig. 15. Atlas targeting device

The short distance between the radiation source and the tumour allows for an optimal distribution within the tumour. However the precise placement of the needles in the centre of the tumour (if only one needle is used) or the optimal distribution of more than one needle is an important prerequisite. In 1995 we developed a novel technique for the reproducible placement of brachytherapy needles in the tumour for fractionated interstitial radiotherapy [3, 4].

The patient is immobilized in the VBH head holder during the CT- scan. The CT datasets are sent to the navigation system in the laboratory. The head holder is stored in the adjusted position which defines the position of the patient's head with respect to the base-plate of the head holder. The needle placement is planned according to the fused CT/MR/PET/SPECT data. The head holder is repositioned in the laboratory in the absence of the patient. The reference structure (e.g. SIP-Lab Innsbruck frame) on the VBH mouthpiece is used for registration of the virtual patient. In the laboratory the aiming device can be adjusted according to the planned pathway. For every needle one targeting device has to be adjusted. For brachytherapy the patient is repositioned in the VBH head holder and the needle is advanced through the adjusted targeting device to the pre-planned depth as given by the navigation system.

After verification of the real position of the needle in the CT the position may be adapted. Fractionated frameless stereotactic interstitial brachytherapy was performed in 12 patients. The accuracy of needle placement was depending on the localization of the tumour. In the cranial area high accuracies could be achieved (mean accuracy 1–3 mm, maximal deviation 4 mm), in the neck deviations of up to 20 mm occurred, mainly related to bad repositioning and movement of the soft tissue structures in this area. As a consequence image-guided punctures in the extracranial area have to be performed in one session the patient being immobilized during image acquisition, planning and intervention. One exception is the area of the ankle, where we developed a non-invasive reproducible fixation device (see below).

Computer-assisted punctures of brain tumours

The selection of the ideal slice thickness plays an important role for the intraoperative accuracy. In a phantom study Bale et al. [2] using the EasyGuide navigation system (Philips Medical Systems, Best, Netherlands) and our patented EasyTaxis aiming device a mean needle positioning error of 1.3 mm +/–

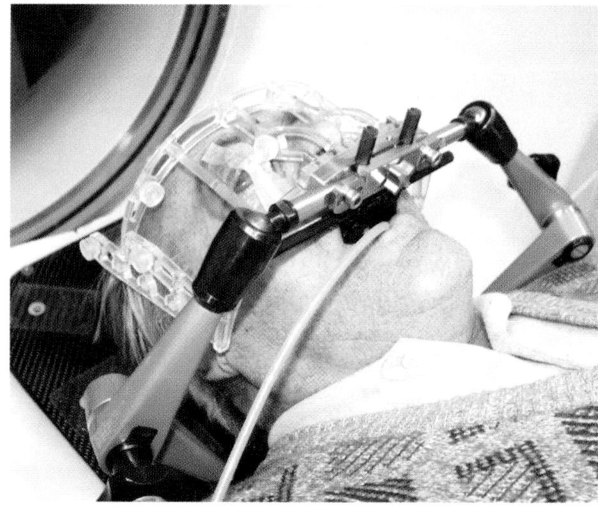

Fig. 16. The patient is immobilized in the VBH head holder during CT

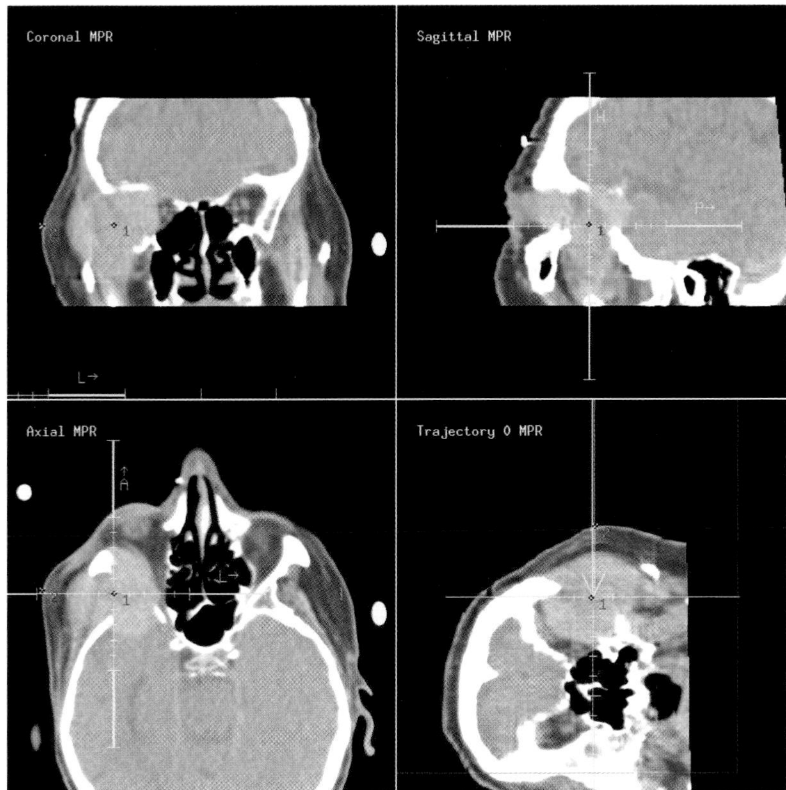

Fig. 17. Path planning for the placement of one brachytherapy needle in a large ENT tumour on various two-and three-dimensional reconstructions

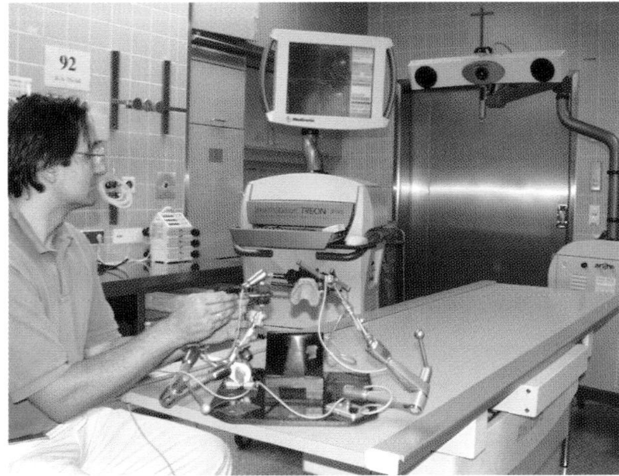

Fig. 18. Adjustment of the targeting device in the laboratory in the absence of the patient

0.7 mm was achieved using 1 mm CT slices. With increasing slice thickness the mean needle positioning error increases to 1.4 mm +/− 0.6 mm (3 mm slice thickness) and to 1.8 mm +/− 0.9 mm (5 mm slice thickness). For most stereotactic procedures in the cranial area a CT slice thickness of 3 mm is sufficient.

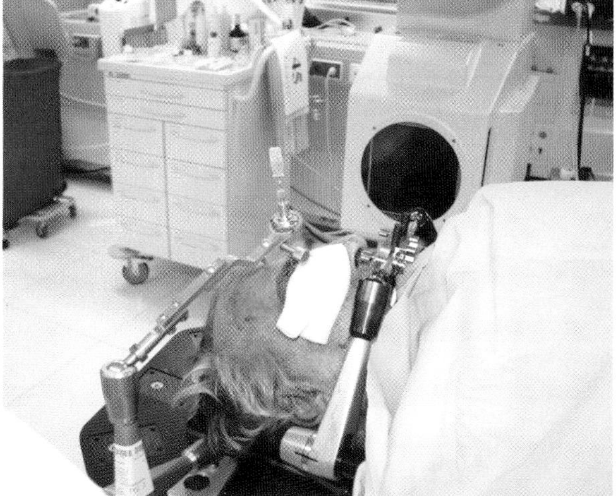

Fig. 19. For the intervention the patient is repositioned in the head holder. After sterile draping and local anaesthesia the needle is advanced through the pre-adjusted targeting device to the precalculated depth. In this case an intraorbital lymphoma was punctured

The same method as described above was also successfully used for thermal ablation of the trigeminal ganglion in 32 patients with trigeminal neuralgia.

The Gasserian Ganglion is reached via the oval foramen at the skull base, which has a diameter of 3.5 to 6 mm. In contrast to conventional fluoroscopy guided punctures the oval foramen can be reached at the first attempt. In four patients the control CT showed only a minimal deviation which could be successfully and easily be corrected manually. Using the similar procedure neurosurgical biopsies and computer-assisted neuroendoscopic procedures can be performed.

The precision can even be improved if the whole procedure is performed in one session directly in the CT room.

In such a setting the repositioning error of the patient in the head holder does not contribute to the overall application accuracy.

Improvement of accuracy

For the phantom study and for the initial clinical applications we used registration rods which were mounted bilaterally to the VBH mouthpiece. Markers with a diameter of only 1.5 mm (Beekley spots) served for registration. Using the SIP-Lab Innsbruck frame the accuracy can be improved. The localization error increases not only as a function of marker/fiducial localization error but also as the distance from the marker centroid to the point of interest increases [19]. Therefore the SIP-frame curves around the head with the most posterior markers located behind the ear. Since the markers are larger than the dimensions of a single voxel, defining their centre of mass in large magnification allows subvoxel registration accuracy.

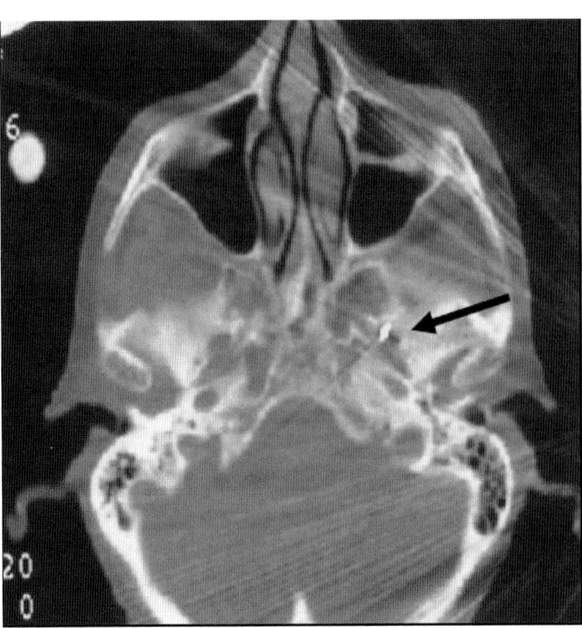

Fig. 20. Axial intraoperative CT scan showing the tip of the needle in the centre of the left foramen ovale (arrowhead)

The unified Innsbruck concept in the diagnosis and therapy of brain tumours

The application of the VBH mouthpiece for diagnostic, therapy and follow-up is currently evaluated at the University Clinic Innsbruck. An individualized

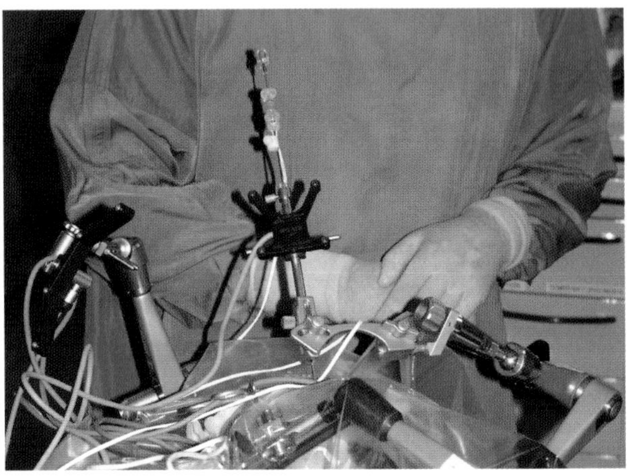

Fig. 21. Frameless stereotactic brain tumour biopsy using the Vertek aiming device. The patient is immobilized in the VBH head holder

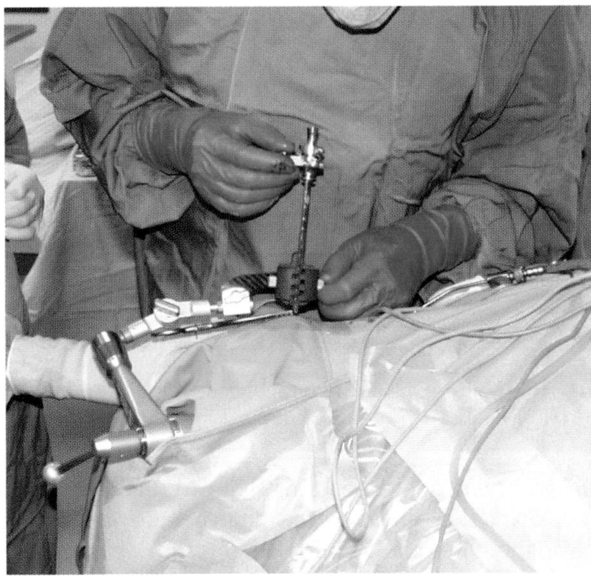

Fig. 22. The neuroendoscope is advanced through the preadjusted aiming device into an intraventricular cyst

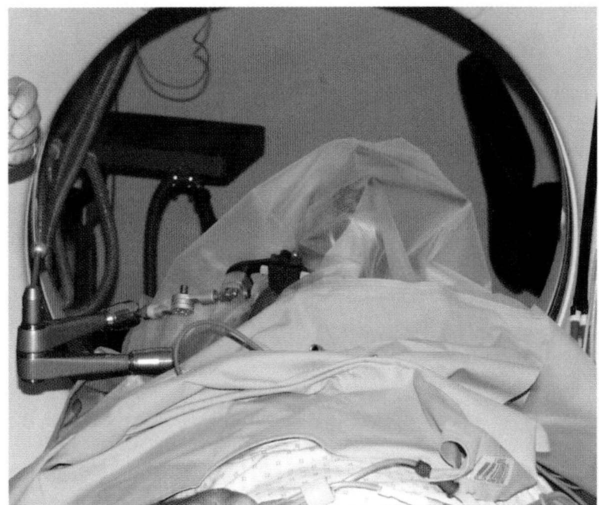

Fig. 23. Puncture of the Gasserian ganglion in the CT for radiofrequency ablation in an edentulous patient

VBH mouthpiece is fabricated in patients suspicious for having a brain tumour.

All the essential imaging modalities are obtained with the VBH mouthpiece and the SIP-Lab Innsbruck frame and the datasets are sent to the navigation system in the SIP-Lab. Image fusion of the different CT/MR/SPECT/PET datasets is performed on the basis of the external markers on the SIP-Lab Innsbruck frame. The fused datasets are the basis for diagnosis and therapy. In the case of therapeutic necessity the VBH vacuum mouthpiece can be used for non-invasive, precise and reproducible immobilization for biopsy, navigated surgery or radiotherapy, thus the VBH mouthpiece acts as a reference structure for all diagnostic and therapeutic steps.

Due to the lack of repositioning accuracy this concept cannot be applied in edentulous patients. In addition collaboration between the different departments is required.

Advantages of the unified approach:

1. **Image fusion**: The external markers allow for a precise image fusion of functional and anatomical data.

2. **Biopsy**: The gold standard for brain tumour biopsy is frame-based stereotaxy. A stereotactic frame is mounted to the patient's skull via invasive pins. The patient is scanned with the frame and – due to the lack of repositioning possibility – has to be treated in the same session. In contrast using the non-invasive reproducible VBH head holder image acquisition, planning and surgery can be separated in time and location resulting in a simplification of the procedure. In addition the anaesthesia time can be minimized because the patient is anaesthetized for the surgery only. The accuracy in the phantom study and in the first patients is comparable to conventional stereotaxy. There is no need for invasive immobilization of the patient.

2. **Computer-assisted surgery**: For computer-assisted surgery in most centres a planning CT or MRI with skin fiducials is performed the day surgery before surgery. On one hand the VBH mouthpiece improves the accuracy on the other hand all the diagnostic CT/MR/SPECT/PET datasets may be used for neuronavigation, thus an additional planning CT/MR the day before surgery is not required. In addition the dynamic reference frame may be mounted to the VBH mouthpiece during surgery allowing for intraoperative movement of the patient without decreasing accuracy [1].

3. **Radiotherapy**: Repositioning accuracy is crucial for fractionated external radiation therapy. The application of the VBH head holder allows for better repositioning accuracy of the patient compared to the conventional mask immobilization systems [6, 17]. Due to the use of the original VBH mouthpiece for reproducible immobilization during radiotherapy and the use of the diagnostic CT/MR/SPECT/PET datasets for radiotherapy planning costs may be reduced [18]. There is no need for the fabrication of a mask.

4. **Follow-up**: The original VBH mouthpiece may be used for CT/MR/SPECT/PET follow-up scans. Image fusion based on the external markers allows for a precise monitoring of tumour growth/regression and functional activity.

Part 2. Extracranial computer-assisted punctures

Retrograde computer-assisted drilling of osteochondral lesions of the talus for reperfusion

The principles for the therapeutic strategies of osteochondral lesions consist of debridement of the cartilaginous part and methods, which should revascularize necrotic bone. The latter is usually the intention for drilling of the sub-cartilaginous zone.

Due to the fact that an antegrade drilling of lesions located dorso-medial is technically difficult or even impossible and due to the invasiveness of the conventional approach with a medial tibial osteotomy retrograde drilling techniques were developed.

Our approach using computer-aided navigation technology is a further development of these already

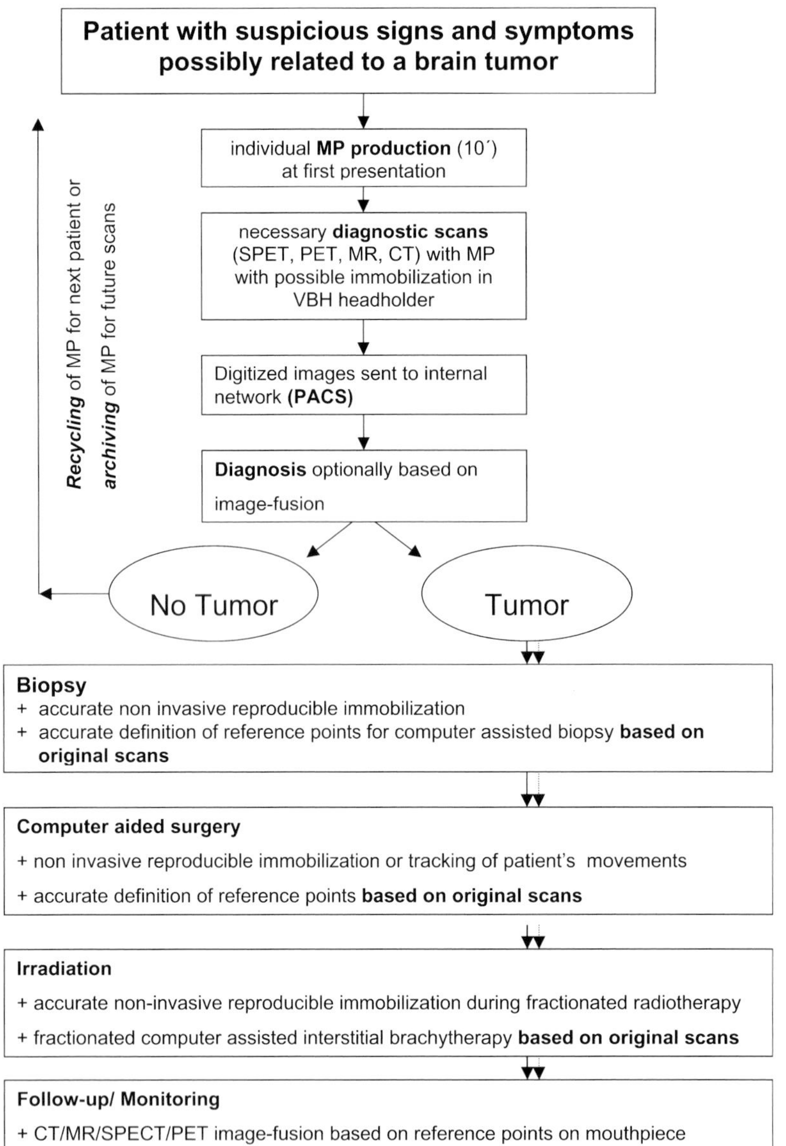

Fig. 24. Diagram showing the unified concept in the diagnosis and therapy of brain tumours (From: Bale R, Burtscher J, Eisner W, Obwegeser A, Rieger M, Sweeney RA, Dessl A, Giacomuzzi SM, Jaschke W (2000) Computer assisted neurosurgery with a non-invasive vacuum-dental cast acting as reference base – another step towards a unified approach in the treatment of brain tumors. J Neurosurg 93: 208–213)

existing techniques. An important prerequisite for precise computer-assisted targeting is a rigid fixation of the patient and a precise registration. Because osteochondritis dissecans stage 2 and 3 require additional arthroscopy and spongiosa plastic most of these procedures have to be performed in the OR. In addition we do currently not have a 3D image acquisiton tool (e.g. ISO C 3D, intraoperative CT) in the OR. Thus, a reproducible immobilization of the upper ankle is necessary in order to separate image acquisition, planning and therapy in time and location. This has been realized by the development of a special scotchcast fixation device (FiscoFix) [5, 10, 13, 15].

The steps of the procedure in this area are similar to those in the cranial area:

- The patient is immobilized during CT scan in the FiscoFix cast.
- The CT-data are sent to the navigation system in the SIP-Lab via network. After path-planning on the 3D- object the aiming device is adjusted in the laboratory in the absence of the patient.

- For the actual surgery the patient's leg is repositioned in the sterilized cast and the retrograde drilling is performed under fluoroscopic control by using the pre-adjusted targeting device.
- There is no need for a navigation system in the OR. Depending on the shape and size of the lesion the defect may be supplied with a spongiose bone autograft. In addition special guides allow for parallel drillings.
- The accuracy of pin placement in 10 cadavers was 1 to 3.5 mms. In the meantime more than 40 patients were treated with this method. The additional pre-operative efforts are compensated by the reduced operating time. Maybe this technology will be helpful in near future to guide complex retrograde cartilage-bone grafts surgery.

A novel immobilization method for computer-assisted extra-cranial interventions

In contrast to the cranial area and the ankle the remaining body parts may not be reproducibly immobilized due to the soft tissue shift. This is especially the case in adipose patients. Thus the concept had to be changed to an "all at once"-procedure. We developed and evaluated a novel fixation technique for immobilization during the time from the CT scan to the actual puncture. The so-called BodyFix (Medical Intelligence GesmbH, Schwabmünchen, Deutschland) is based on negative pressure technology.

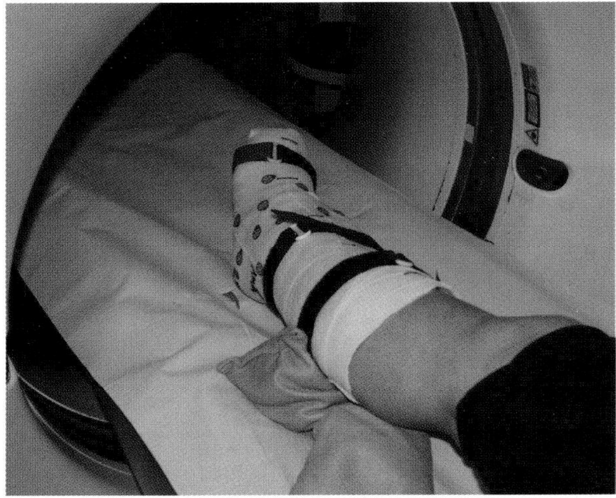

Fig. 25. During CT acquisition the patient is immobilized in the FiscoFix cast. Fiducials are attached to the fixation device

The BodyFix™ fixation device consists of a vacuum pump connected to different types of machine-washable pillows which are filled with tiny Styrofoam balls (similar to a vacuum splint) A thin plastic foil is used to cover the region of interest.

For hygienic reasons the patient is first covered by a thin cushion. Then, the patient's extremity is wrapped up with one of the pillows and covered with the plastic foil. The pillows are placed such that there is an area left for the surgical approach. When the vacuum pump is turned on, the air is evacuated from between the covering foil and the therapy couch, resulting in a hardening of the cushion, which is simultaneously sucked against the therapy couch together with the patient. The intensity of fixation can be selected by adjusting the degree of negative pressure built up by the vacuum pump.

Usually these interventions are performed directly in the CT room. Alternatively the patient can be brought from the CT to the OR/intervention room by a transfer-couch which is equipped with a battery for the BodyFix pump.

Procedure

The patient is immobilized in the BodyFix system on the CT table. Skin fiducials are attached to the patient and/or to the BodyFix.

A CT scan of the area of interest is obtained (1–3 mm slice thickness depending on the procedure). The CT datasets are sent directly to the navigation system in the CT room via intranet. The path is planned on the individual 2D and 3D reconstructed images.

After sterile washing and draping a sterile DRF is mounted to the frame of the BodyFix. Registration is performed by indicating the fiducials on the patient and selecting the corresponding markers on the 3D dataset.

The navigation system provides a value indicating the registration accuracy. In most systems it is the root mean square error (RMSE) which is defined as the mean of the distance of the paired points that were used for registration. If the markers are optimally distributed around the volume of interest this value is a very good indicator of the overall accuracy. Usually an RMSE in the range of 1 mm can be achieved. After an additional accuracy check by indicating the markers that were not used for registration the actual navigational procedure can start.

The sterile targeting device is mounted to the BodyFix frame and adjusted according to the preoperative plan.

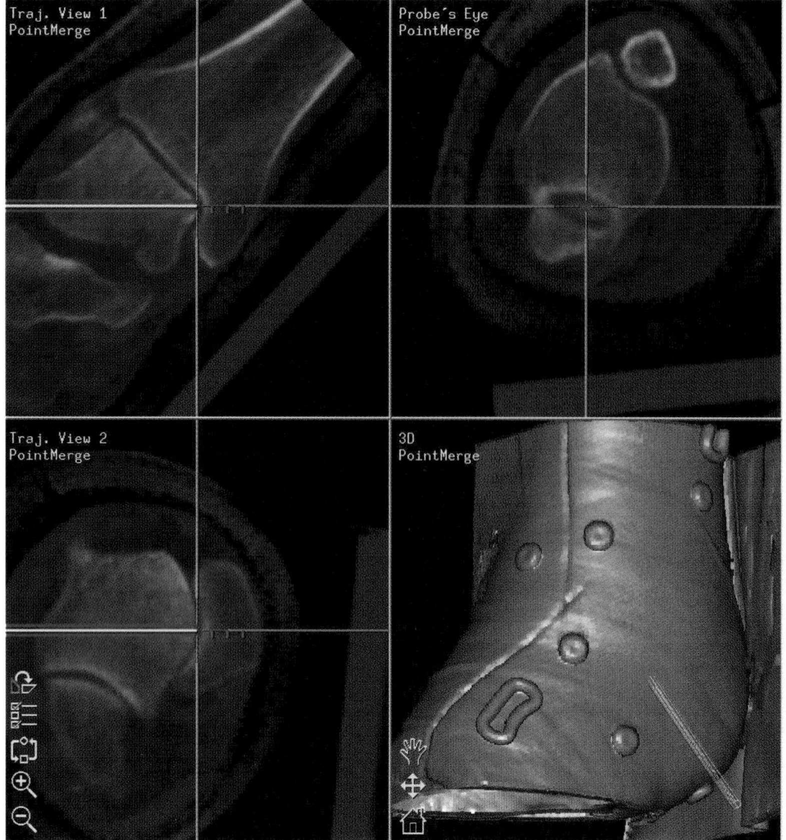

Fig. 26. Path planning for retrograde drilling of an osteochondral lesion in the medial talar dome on 2-and 3-dimensional reconstructed images

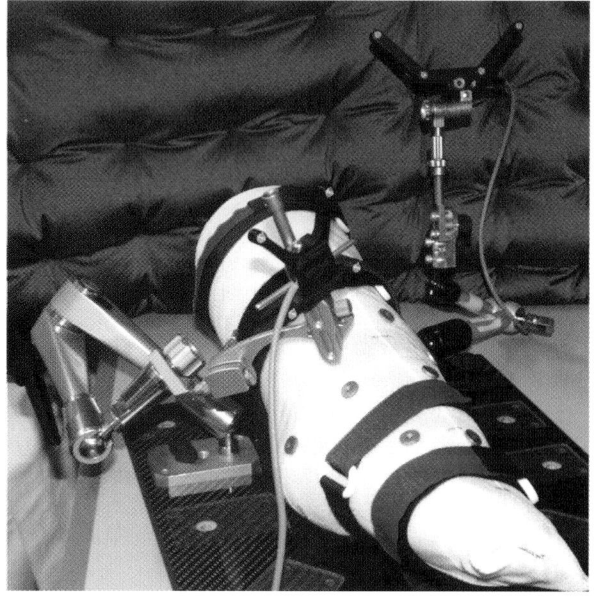

Fig. 27. The targeting device is adjusted in the laboratory in the absence of the patient

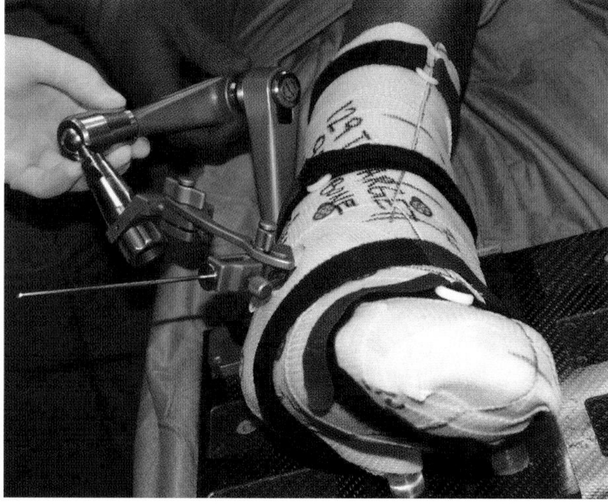

Fig. 28. Drilling of the osteochondral lesion through the pre-adjusted targeting device to the precalculated depth. There is no need for a navigation system in the OR

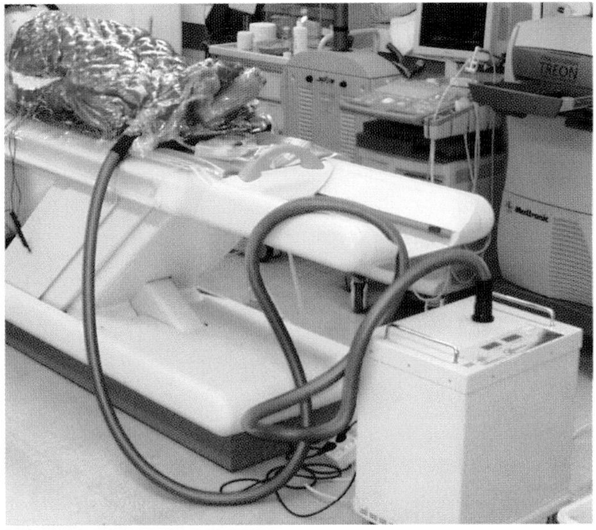

Fig. 29. BodyFix consisting of different pillows, a covering plastic foil and a tube leading to a vacuum pump

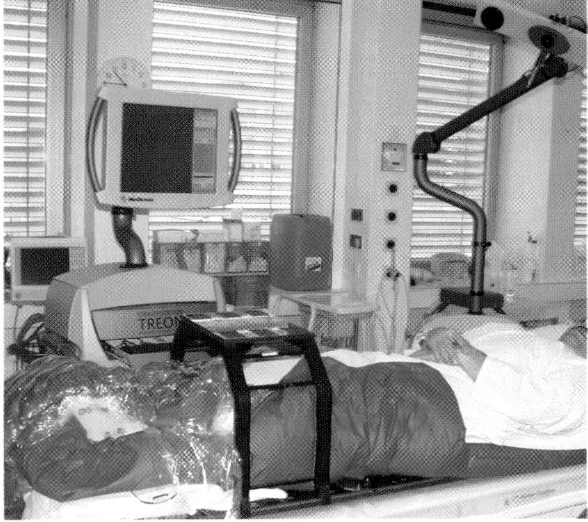

Fig. 31. Set-up for extracranial computer-assisted percutaneous interventions. The patient is immobilized in the BodyFix on the CT table. Markers are attached to the skin and the BodyFix

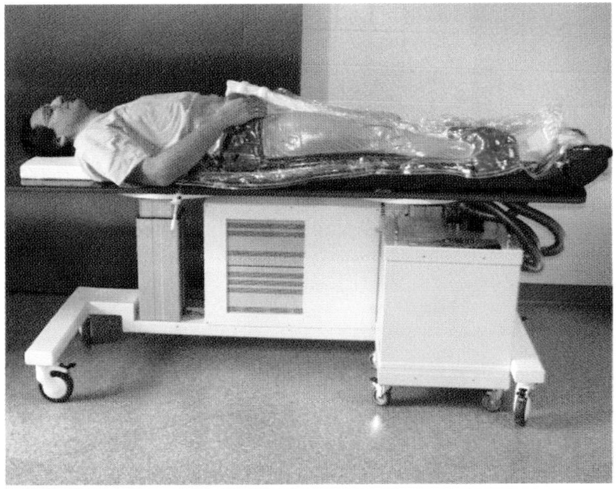

Fig. 30. Transfer couch

The needle or drill is advanced through the targeting device to the pre-planned depth.

A fusion of the intra-operative control CT (with the needle in place) with the planning CT (with the planned path) is performed allowing for a precise measurement of the accuracy of the puncture.

For interventions in organs that are sensitive to respiratory motion (the liver or the bases of the lungs) general anaesthesia is required in order to reposition the liver/lung with high precision. All the CT-scans, the registration procedure and the puncture are performed in maximal exspiration, which can be easily achieved by disconnection of the endotracheal tubus. Using this technique a repositioning accuracy of 1–3 mm can be achieved (unpublished data).

This technique is routinely performed at our institution for puncturing different lesions from head to toe e.g.:

- vertebral disc biopsy.
- vertebral discography.
- percutaneous fixation of pelvic fractures
- bone tumour biopsy.
- retrograde drilling of osteochondral lesions in the ankle, knee and hip.
- radiofrequency ablation of bone tumours (osteoidosteoma, metastasis).
- biopsy and radiofrequency ablation of liver, lung and kidney tumour (Computer assisted navigation allows for a precise 3D distribution of the needles around the tumour).

The time required for set-up is about 10–15 minutes. The time from the planning CT to the placement of the needle is about 30 minutes.

The application of navigation systems in combination with the BodyFix and the Vertek targeting device allows for a precise puncture in various regions of the body at the first attempt without the need for a correction of the position of the needle, thus even tiny lesions, which cannot be reached with conventional puncture techniques can be reached.

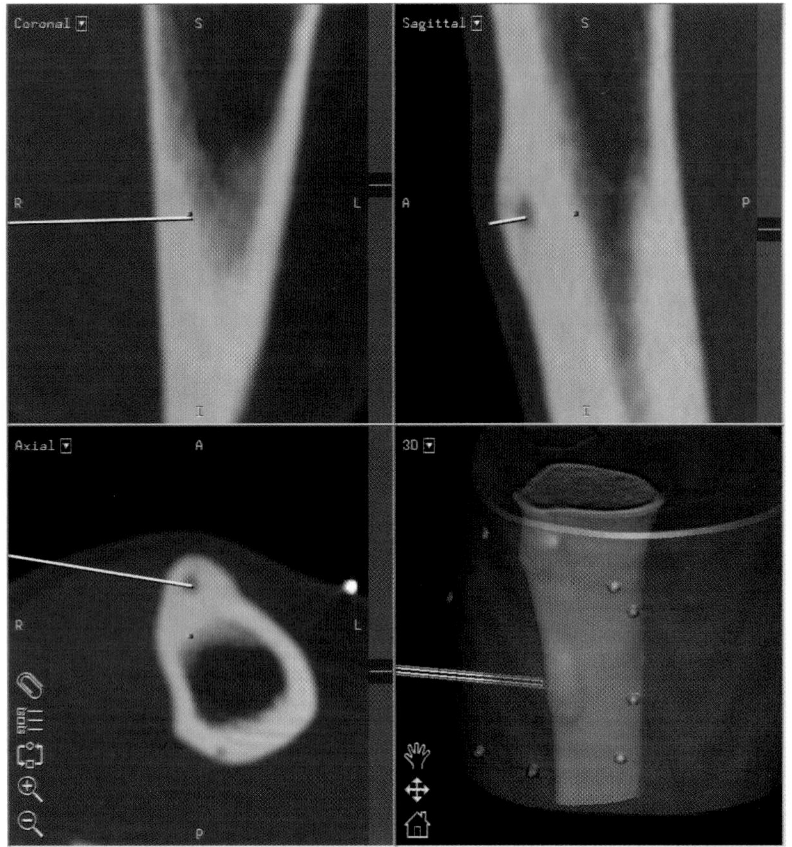

Fig. 32. Computer-assisted puncture of an osteoidosteoma in the right tibia. The path is planned on the individual 2D and 3D reconstructed images

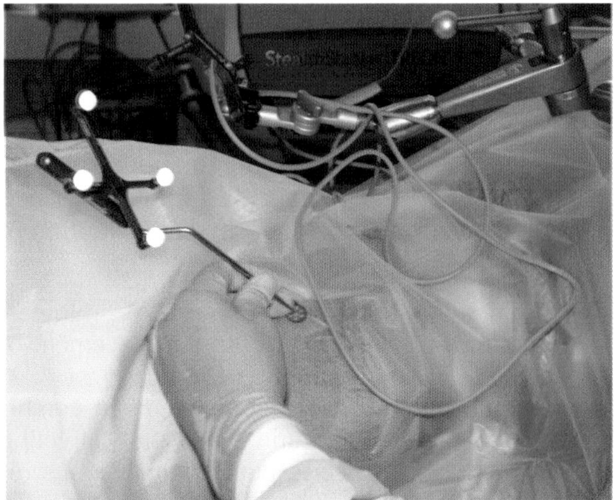

Fig. 33. Registration is performed by indicating the fiducials on the patient and selecting the corresponding markers on the 3D dataset

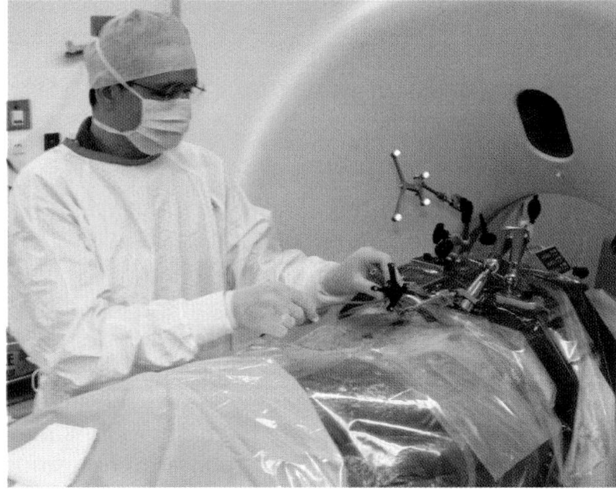

Fig. 34. Adjustment of Vertek targeting device for a puncture of a liver lesion for radiofrequency ablation

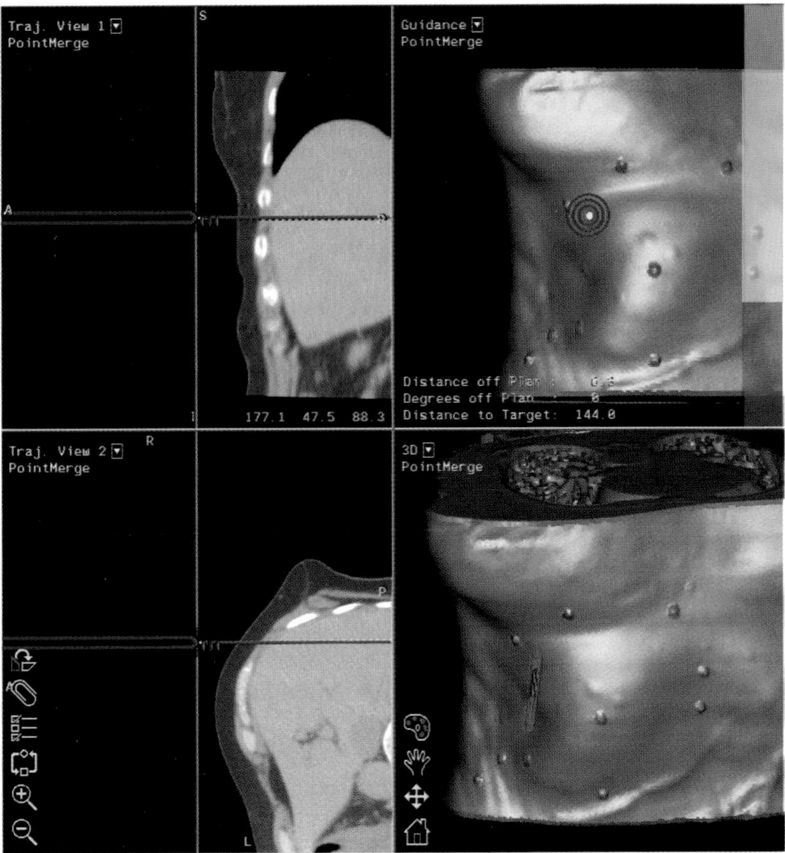

Fig. 35. The guidance view of the software of the navigation system allows for precise adjustment of the targeting device

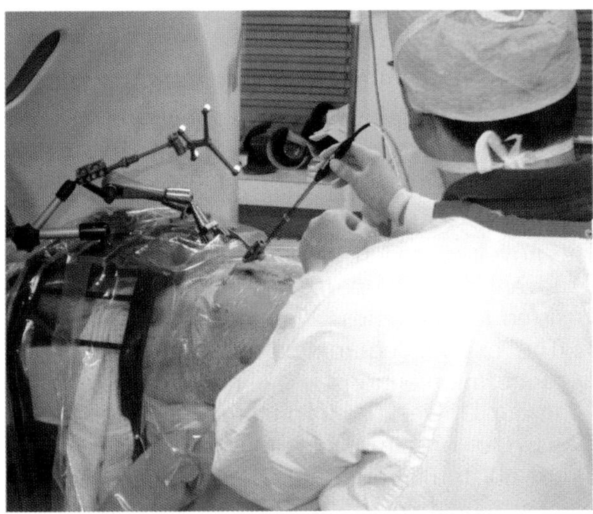

Fig. 36. The needle is advanced through the targeting device to the pre-planned depth

In contrast to conventional CT guided punctures double angulated approaches are feasible with high accuracy.

Image Guided Template Production in Oral Implant Surgery – the Innsbruck approach (Widmann G./Bale R.)

The introduction of computer-assisted diagnosis and therapy in the field of oral implant surgery shows significant advantages over conventional techniques:

1. Implant planning is based on 3-D CT-data, which overcomes all limits of 2-dimensional radiography.
2. The precise surgical realization is warranted through burr tracking or image guided template production (IGTP). Burr tracking navigation systems allow for an intra-operative real-time navigation of the dental drill along the predefined surgical plan, which is directly visualized on the CT-data of the patient. Alternatively, IGTP transfers the plan into a surgical template via positioning devices or CAD/CAM (computer aided design / computer aided manufacturing) stereolithographic, bone-, mucosa- or teeth supported templates.

Despite their challenging therapeutic advantages, costs and effort of existing systems remain still too

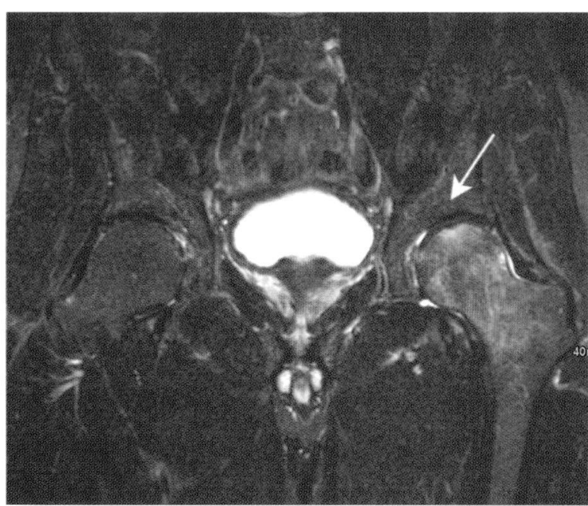

Fig. 37. Computer-assisted retrograde drilling of an osteochondral lesion in the left femoral head (arrowhead) – T2 weighted fat-saturated pre-operative image showing the osteochondral lesion and edema

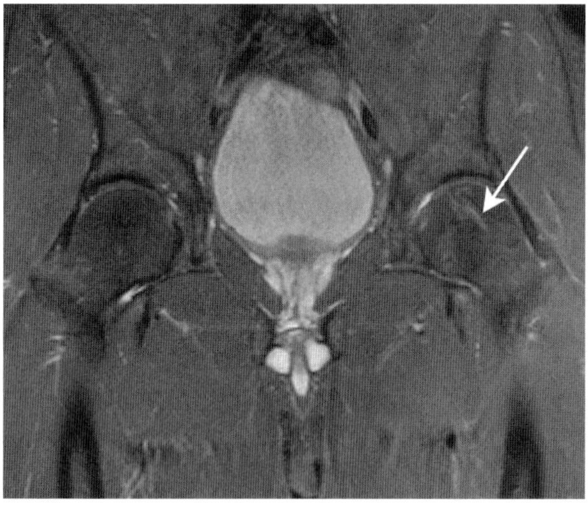

Fig. 38. Post-operative image 5 months after drilling reveals only minimal residual edema around the drill holes (arrowhead)

high for the routine application in private practice. We developed a novel concept of IGTP that may have the potential to overcome these drawbacks.

Preliminary in vitro studies of the obtained surgical templates show a mean accuracy in [xy] (normal deviation of the drill to a predefined target) of 0.49 +/– 0.34 mm (maximum 1.2 mm) and in [z] (accuracy of the introduction of the drill) of 0.25 +/– 0.12 mm (maximum 0.6 mm). The achieved accuracy lies within the top-range of existing developments and warrants its clinical application.

In our running clinical evaluation several patients were already successfully treated with excellent surgical, prosthetic, functional and aesthetic results. The present workflow consists of the following steps:

- The dentist takes dental impressions of the patient's jaws and an occlusal registration.
- The dental laboratory technician fabricates dental stone casts and mounts them on a dental articulator. A wax-reconstuction (wax-up) of the missing teeth is fabricated which will guide the position of the consecutive implants. A resin template is produced which is later completed to the final surgical template.
- The dental stone casts, the wax-up and the prefabricated template are sent to the SIP-Lab. A modified VBH-mouthpice is fabricated with maxillary and mandibular impressions under guidance of the dental articulator.
- A dental computed tomography of the patient is performed wearing the mouthpiece and the SIP-Lab Innsbruck dental reference frame. The DICOM-data is transferred to our 'Treon' navigation system.
- In the SIP-Lab the laboratory set-up holding the unmodified dental stone cast is registered to the CT-data. Together with the dentist, the wax-up is defined by the navigation probe and guides the implant planning on the 3D CT-data
- The surgical plan is transferred via the navigation system. A metal rod is guided through the Easy-Taxis or Vertek aiming device and positions a surgical burr tube which is glued into the prefabricated template by blue-light curing resin.
- The surgical template is delivered to the dentist and guides the surgical procedure.

The novel approach has the following additional advantages compared to other computer-assisted technologies

1. The existing equipment for frameless stereotactic interventions, which is already installed in our University Hospital, can additionally be used for oral implant surgery. Neither the dentist nor the laboratory technician needs to purchase any expensive products.
2. The work flow comes as close as possible to the standard procedure without image-guidance. Compared to burr tracking and existing IGTP-techniques there is no need for radiographic scan-templates, registration templates and modifications of the standard dental stone casts.

Instead a VBH-mouthpiece is needed for the initial registration.
3. Surgical templates with increasing diameter can be fabricated. Leaving the aiming device in the same position increasing burr tubes are positioned and glued into separately prefabricated templates. The following drillings of the implant drill-set are executed under precise template-guidance which may enhance the clinical accuracy and shorten the operative time.
4. Image-guidance is a successful basis for minimal invasive, flapless surgery which is generally a 'blind' surgical procedure. The treatment is less painful; it reduces the dental visits and enhances the acceptance of the patient. By means of immediate loading with the prefabricated prosthetic work the patient may immediately leave the office with the one-step integrated restoration.

In the near future the CT-scan of the patient may also be performed at a remote hospital. The DICOM CT-data may be sent to the SIP-Lab. We wish to introduce a different dental planning software that can be read by the software of our navigation system. By virtue of an interactive tele-conferencing network, the dentist may give his advises from his private practice or will be able to send his own computer-planning to the SIP-Lab.

The average dental office does not have the financial power and the necessary amount of implant patients to purchase an own burr tracking navigation system or a stereolithographic machine. Based on a interdisciplinary planning centre, our concept of IGTP may have the potential to provide high-tech implant planning and image-guided surgery to a broad number of patients with a minimum of effort and with affordable costs.

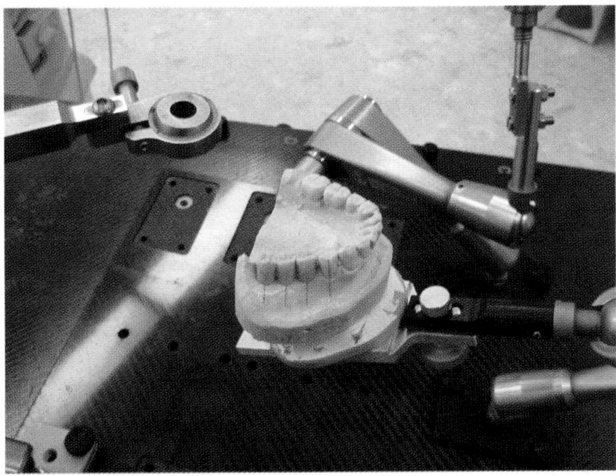

Fig. 39. Unmodified dental stone cast mounted on the laboratory set-up with the dental wax-up of the missing teeth

Current developments in cooperation with the SIP-Lab Innsbruck – a short overview

Current navigation systems were designed for the application in the OR. The use of navigation systems for percutaneous punctures in a CT suite is an additional application of these conventional navigation systems. In cooperation with CAS Erlangen and the Institute of Medical Physics we developed the CAPPA® IRAD, a novel navigation system which is adapted to the requirements for percutaneous punctures in the CT.

The reference frame that is scanned simultaneously with the patient is equipped with reflective markers that are automatically detected by the navigation system, thus allowing for an automatic registration. The interventional radiology can immediately start with the targeting procedure using our special targeting devices. This is an additional step towards a system which may also be used by radiologists who are not familiar with navigation technology. Another project focuses on the application of 3D – rotational angiography for percutaneous punctures of osseous lesions. Other projects deal with the development and/or evaluation of robots for an automatic adjustment of an aiming device along a given trajectory:

- A73 robot: cooperation with Medical Intelligence (Schwabmünchen, Germany), Medizinphysik Erlangen, ENT Department Erlangen and CAS Innovations (Erlangen, Germany)
- B-rob for CT-guided punctures: Cooperation with Seibersdorf, University Hospital Vienna and Medical Intelligence (Schwabmünchen, Germany)
- Innomotion robot for MR-guided punctures: Cooperation with Innomedic (Germany).

Part 3. The interdisciplinary Stereotactic Intervention-and Planning Laboratory (SIP Lab) Innsbruck – a novel concept

Many navigation systems have been sold in the last few years. Unfortunately most of these very expensive systems are rarely used. The reasons therefore are multifaceted, however, the main reason there-

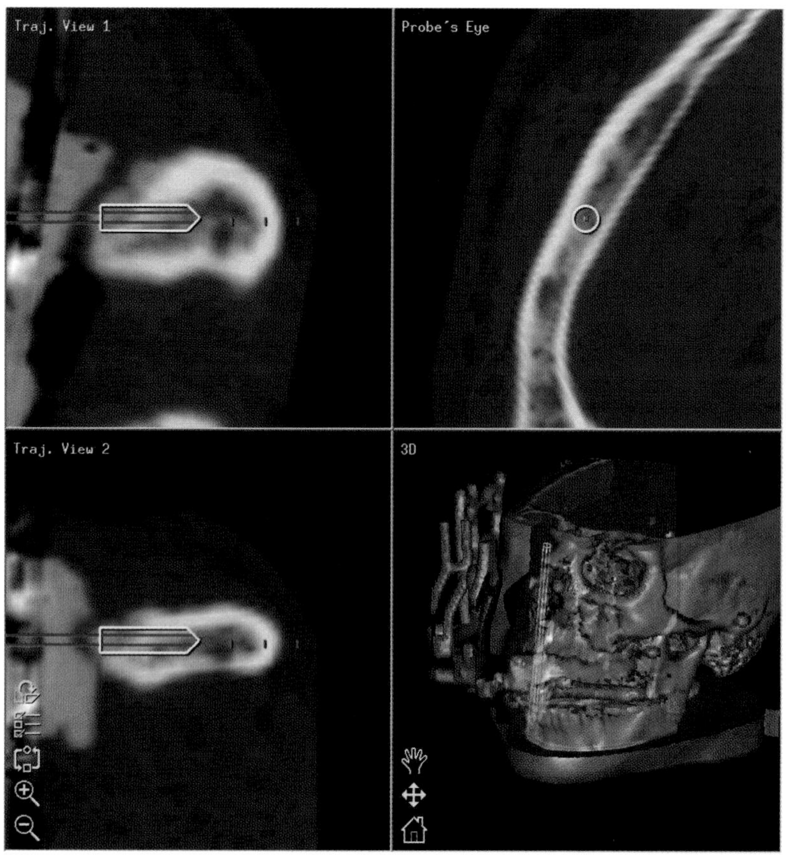

Fig. 40. Oral implant planning based on the 3D CT-data of the patient

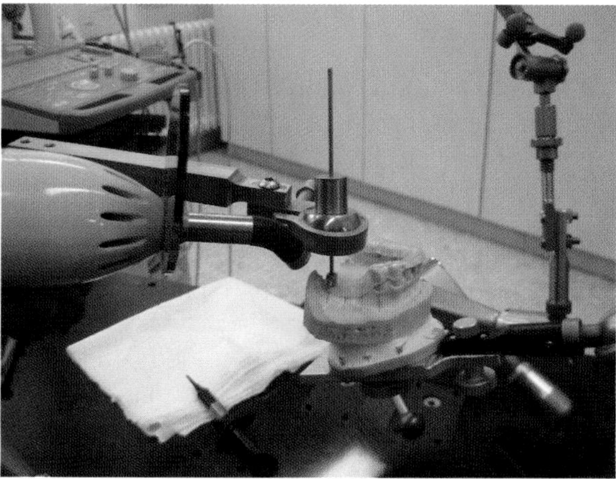

Fig. 41. Navigated positioning of the surgical burr tubes and fixation into the prefabricated template with blue light curing resin

fore is the challenge of the novel technology to medical doctors who do not have any knowledge in computer science or basics in navigation. Although

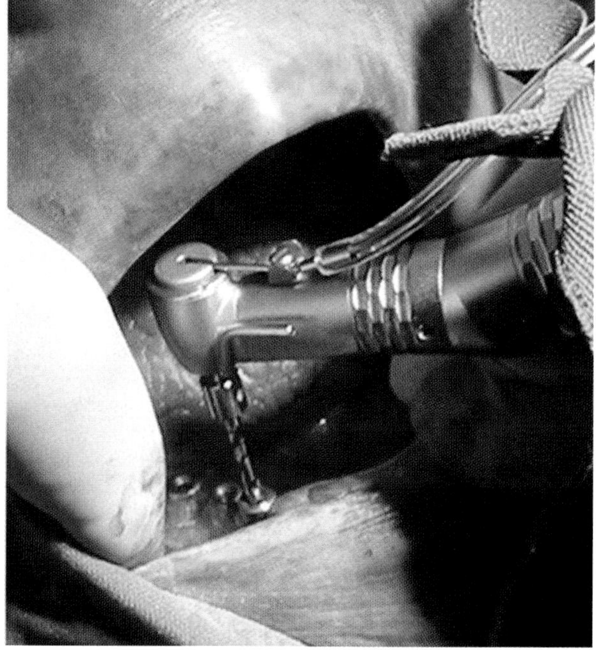

Fig. 42. Template-guided surgical procedure

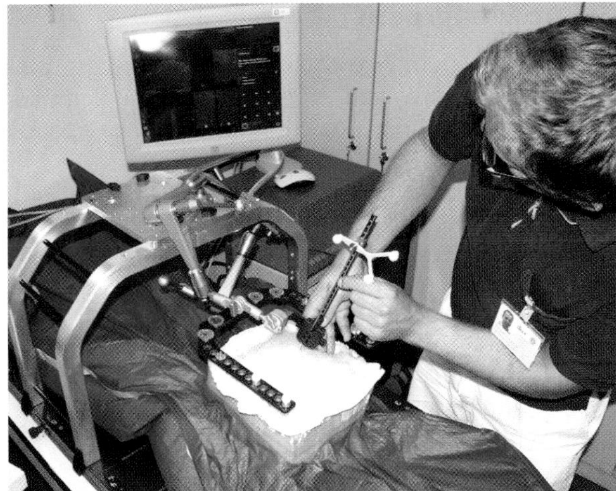

Fig. 43. Initial phantom study using the CAPPA® IRAD navigation system

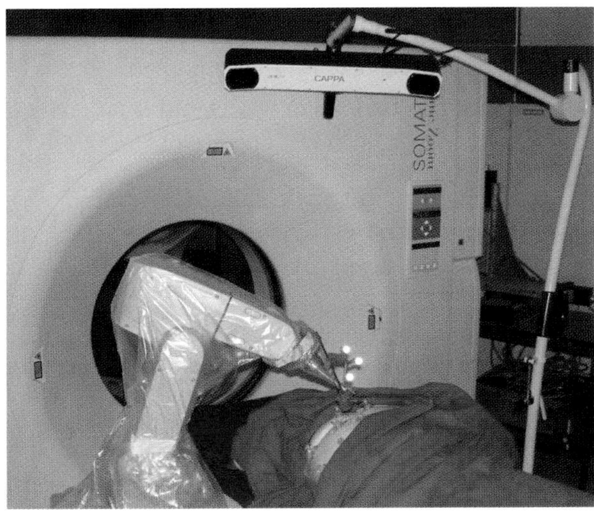

Fig. 44. The A 73 robot has 6DOFs and is tracked by an additional optical localization system

it is getting better most of the systems are still difficult to use. There is still a big learning curve adding additional stress to the surgeon. After a few bad experiences the system is placed somewhere in the corner....

The only way to overcome such a situation is to educate a group of medical doctors and support personnel (e.g. radiation technicians) to support the frustrated surgeons. Basically this could be done on every department (trauma surgery, orthopaedics, ENT, CMF,...). As radiologists we are used to collaborate with every department and it is just logical that this should be the place for a platform of navigation experts for the whole clinic. In addition only one or two navigated surgeries a week are performed in most departments. Thus it is much cheaper to buy one or two navigation system for a central well-trained team than to buy one system for every interested department.

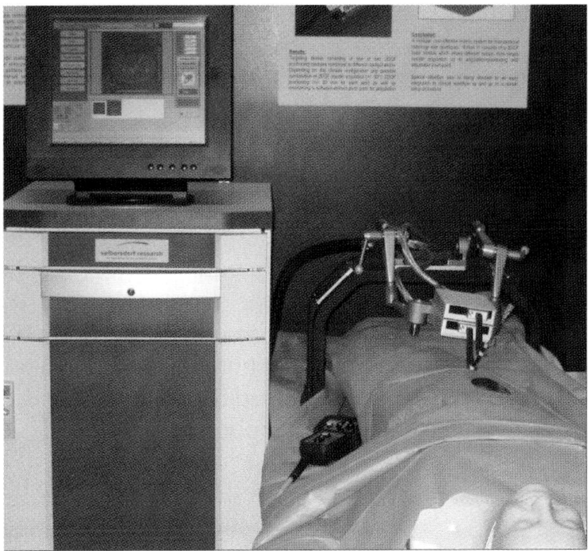

Fig. 45. The B-rob 2 is a smart robot, that is mounted to the mechanical arms of our navigation set-up instead of the manual aiming device

Two navigation systems, the Stealth Station and the Treon (Medtronic Inc., Louisville, Colorado, USA) represent the central technology in the SIP-Lab Innsbruck. Two radiologists and three radiation technicians with sophisticated knowledge about navigation techniques support different surgical disciplines during image guided procedures including brain tumour biopsy, neuroendoscopy and trauma surgery. The following work is done by the SIP-Lab team:

1. Support for the surgeon during computer-assisted navigation: image data acquisition and interpretation, image fusion, path planning, adjustment of the targeting device for computer-assisted punctures in the SIP-Lab or in the OR, and navigation in the OR. The navigation system, the registration devices, the immobilization devices and the targeting devices are provided by the SIP-Lab. One radiation technician and/or one radiologist operate the navigation system during surgery.
2. Precise computer-assisted punctures "from head to toe" in the CT as already described above.

3. Fabrication of the VBH vacuum mouthpiece which plays the central part for the unified concept in the diagnosis and therapy of brain tumours.
4. CT/MR/SPECT/PET and ultrasound image fusion in the whole body with the use of the image fusion software that is part of the navigation system.
5. For extra-cranial fusion the radiation technician from the SIP-Lab forms the vacuum mattresses and fixates the patient for the respective CT/MR/SPECT/PET image acquisition.
6. Development (targeting device, fixation devices, reference frames, robotic,....)

Conclusion

The progresses in the area of image-guided and minimal-invasive procedures lead to an increasing use of imaging data for planning, simulation and therapy. Many classical surgical approaches are replaced by less invasive methods. All these methods require pre-operative imaging data in order to allow for a safe navigation in the patient's body.

The spectrum of conventional CT-US-MR-guided punctures is enlarged by an additional computer-assisted puncture technique utilizing 3D image data. The 3D-guided puncture technique provides a better accuracy and a more sophisticated planning of the percutaneous path because the puncture plane can be selected individually. The pathway can be planned precisely thus sparing vital structures. In our opinion navigation system will be increasingly important for the radiologist. Besides data acquisition, data preparation and interpretation the radiologist of the near future should also use the 3D imaging data for percutaneous interventions.

By transfer of the planning phase and the adjustment of the targeting device out of the OR expensive OR time can be saved. Standardized surgical approaches can be adapted to the respective individual anatomical situation as visualized on the preoperative images.

However, computer-assisted navigation will never fully replace the surgeon. The novel technologies are only designed to assist the surgeon. The responsibility lies always in the hands of the surgeon/interventionalist. A fundamental knowledge of the basic principles and functionalities of the novel technologies is an important prerequisite for a reliable task in order to provide benefit for our patients.

Acknowledgment

The author would like to thank the following persons who are involved in the development and/or clinical applications of the SIP-Lab navigation technology:

SIP-Lab Team: P. Kovacs, T. Lang, M. Knoflach, C. Hinterleithner, G. Widmann

Department of Radiology Innsbruck (Prof. Dr. W. Jaschke): M. Freund, M. Rieger, W. Jaschke

Department of Neurosurgery (Prof. Dr. K. Twerdy): W. Eisner, J. Burtscher, T. Fiegele, I. Laimer, M. Ortler

Department of Traumatology (Prof. Dr. M. Blauth): R. Rosenberger, C. Fink, C. Hoser, B. Dolati

Department of Orthopaedics (Prof. Dr. W. Krismer): F. Rachbauer, R. Biedermann

Department of ENT (Prof. Dr. A. Gunkel): W. Freysinger, W. Thumfart

Department of Radiotherapy (Prof. Dr. P. Lukas): R. Sweeney, M. Nevinny, K. Seydl

Medical Intelligence GesmbH Schwabmünchen: M. Vogele

Medtronic Inc. USA: D. Legenstein

CAS Erlangen GesmbH.: R. Petzold

Institute of Medical Physics Erlengen-Nürnberg: M. Negel, W. Kalender

Forschungszentrum Seibersdorf: G. Kronreif

References

[1] Bale RJ, et al (2000) Computer-assisted neurosurgery by using a noninvasive vacuum-affixed dental cast that acts as a reference base: another step toward a unified approach in the treatment of brain tumors. J Neurosurg 93(2): 208–13

[2] Bale RJ, et al (1999) Application of the Vogele-Bale-Hohner (VBH) Head Holder in Computer-assisted Neurosurgery. In: Lemke HU, et al (eds) Computer assisted radiology and surgery. Elsevier, Amsterdam New York, pp 686–690

[3] Bale RJ, et al (2000) Head and neck tumors: fractionated frameless stereotactic interstitial brachytherapy-initial experience. Radiology 214(2): 591–95

[4] Bale RJ, et al (1998) First experiences with computer-assisted frameless stereotactic interstitial brachytherapy (CASIB). Strahlenther Onkol 174(9): 473–77

[5] Bale RJ, et al (2001) Osteochondral lesions of the talus: computer-assisted retrograde drilling–feasibility and accuracy in initial experiences. Radiology 218(1): 278–82

[6] Bale RJ, et al (1998) Noninvasive head fixation for external irradiation of tumors of the head-neck area. Strahlenther Onkol 174(7): 350–54

[7] Bale RJ, et al (1997) Minimally invasive head holder to improve the performance of frameless stereotactic surgery. Laryngoscope 107(3): 373–77

[8] Caversaccio M, et al (1999) The "Bernese" frameless optical computer aided surgery system. Comput Aided Surg 4(6): 328–34
[9] Drake JM, et al (1994) Frameless stereotaxy in children. Pediatr. Neurosurg. 20(2): 152–59
[10] Fink C, et al (2001) Computer-assisted retrograde drilling of osteochondral lesions of the talus. Orthopade 30(1): 59–65
[11] Fried MP, et al (1997) Image-guided endoscopic surgery: results of accuracy and performance in a multicenter clinical study using an electromagnetic tracking system. Laryngoscope 107(5): 594–601
[12] Hirschberg H, Kirkeby OJ (1996) Interactive image directed neurosurgery: patient registration employing the Laitinen stereo-adapter. Minim Invasive Neurosurg 39(4): 105–07
[13] Hoser C, et al (2004) A computer assisted surgical technique for retrograde autologous osteochondral grafting in talar osteochondritis dissecans (OCD): a cadaveric study. Knee Surg Sports Traumatol Arthrosc 12(1): 65–71
[14] Martin A, et al (1998) Vogele-Bale-Hohner mouthpiece: registration device for frameless stereotactic surgery. Radiology 208(1): 261–65
[15] Rosenberger RE, et al (2002) Computer-assisted drilling of the lower extremity. Technique and indications. Unfallchirurg 105(4): 353–58
[16] Smith KR, Frank KJ, Bucholz RD (1994) The NeuroStation–a highly accurate, minimally invasive solution to frameless stereotactic neurosurgery. Comput Med Imaging Graph 18(4): 247–56
[17] Sweeney R, et al (1998) Repositioning accuracy: comparison of a noninvasive head holder with thermoplastic mask for fractionated radiotherapy and a case report. Int J Radiat Oncol Biol Phys 41(2): 475–83
[18] Sweeney RA, et al (2003) Multimodality cranial image fusion using external markers applied via a vacuum mouthpiece and a case report. Strahlenther Onkol 179(4): 254–60
[19] Zinreich SJ, et al (1993) Frameless stereotaxic integration of CT imaging data: accuracy and initial applications. Radiology 188(3): 735–42

The therapeutic value of mapping and 3D modeling of cartilage lesions in the knee

K.-H. Kristen and A. Engel

Orthopedic Department, Danube Hospital, Vienna, Austria

To treat injuries and degenerative changes of strained cartilage of the knee joint is one of the chief problems in orthopedic surgery.

Knee injuries

Injuries and degenerative changes with subsequent osteoarthritis of the knee joint are becoming an increasing socioeconomic issue.

In the US almost 5 million people visit offices of orthopedic surgeons each year because of knee problems. More than 3 million of these visits are injury-related; the remaining are due to arthritis and other disorders. (Nat. Center of Health Statistics 1990–94). Another 1.4 million people go to a hospital emergency room because of knee problems. A biennial census by the American Academy of Orthopedic Surgeons of more than 14,000 orthopedic surgeons in the US disclosed the knee as the most often treated anatomical site. Orthopedists said that 26% of the total of their cases involved the knee. The sites of the injuries are the menisci and the collateral and cruciate ligaments. Chondral as well as osteochondral lesions occur, often injuries are combined. The injuries are satisfyingly resolved, except of the cartilage lesions. Once damaged, joint cartilage does not normally regenerate. Not only do such injuries cause pain and restrict mobility, chronic injuries to joint cartilage may finally lead to debilitating osteoarthritis. These manifestations can severely hinder a person's normal activities and occupation.

Cartilage injuries

Hyaline cartilage consists of chondrocytes (<5% total volume) and extracellular matrix (>95% total volume). The matrix contains a variety of macromolecules including type II collagen and proteoglycan. The structure of the matrix allows the cartilage to absorb shock and withstand shearing and compression forces. Healthy hyaline cartilage also has an extremely low coefficient of friction at the articular surface. Damage to articular cartilage caused by acute or repetitive trauma often results in pain and disability. Partly because hyaline cartilage is avascular, spontaneous healing of large defects is not possible. Osteoarthritis is associated with profound changes in articular cartilage. Cartilage is hyperhydrated and the proteoglycan concentration is decreased. The macromolecular matrix is disorganized and subsequently volumetric loss of cartilage occurs [22]. However, these observations can be made only after the onset of clinical symptoms and therefore reflect degenerative changes relatively late.

Imaging of cartilage injuries

Until recently, the earliest changes in articular cartilage could be assessed only by direct inspection using biomechanical and histological analyses [19]. Not invasive imaging modalities had been disappointing [2,3].

Plain radiographs are limited to detection of late manifestation of osteoarthritis such as narrowing of the cartilage space, sclerosis of subchondral bone and formation of osteophytes. Manifest structural alterations of the knee joint can be visualized in plaint radiographs. For the evaluation of axial deformities and malalignment of the joint, weightbearing radiographs still have an untouched indication and necessity for planning realignment operations.

CT scans provide excellent visualization of bone, but poor resolution of articular cartilage. Cartilage surface imaging can be achieved using CT with intraarticular contrast agent. Many reasons for acute or

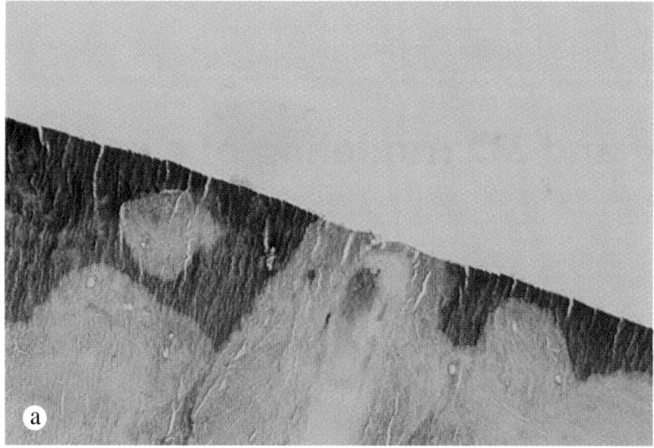

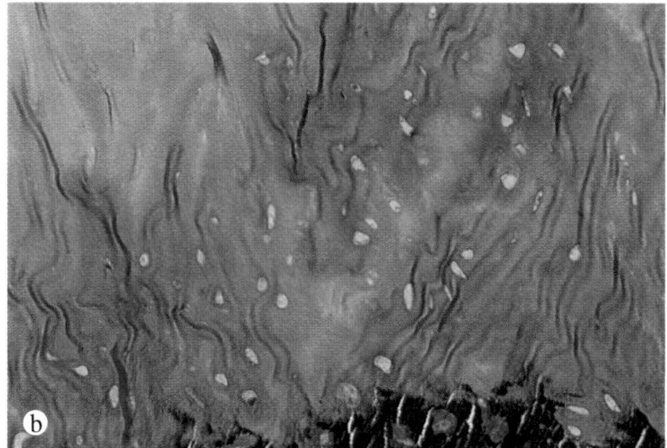

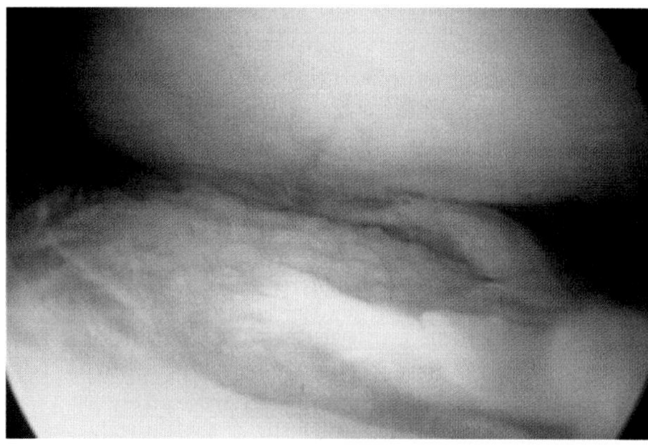

Fig. 1. Appearance of cartilage lesions. **a** Histologic section showing high grade degenerative changes with grade IV cartilage lesion, degenerative subchondral cysts and partial fibercartilage repair (undecalcified preparation). **b** Histologic section. Demasking of collagen fibers. HE. **c** Arthroscopic view of a grade III cartilage lesion/cartilage ulcer on the femoral condyle with central fibercartilage repair and cartilage delamination at the border. The corresponding patellar surface is on top

chronic knee pain cannot be detected using plain radiographs. Fortunately, the development of MRI has provided a non-invasive, non-irradiating technique that allows for high contrast resolution of soft tissue structures without adverse effects on tissue. The advantages of MRI have increased the interest in the application of this technology to the study of articular cartilage and osteoarthritis.

Purely cartilaginous lesions may heal spontaneously under partial repair with fibrocartilage. However, since fibrocartilage is known to be mechanically insufficient this repair often does not result in sufficient sports and working capacity. Therefore traumatic cartilage defects of the knee joint must be documented according to localization, surface involved and depth. Because the condition of the cartilage is increasingly accepted as a main factor in the whole osteoarthrosis issue visualization of cartilage compromising cartilage surface alterations, cartilage volume defects and cartilage 3D imaging will become a key point for future therapies and therapeutic decisions.

Therapy of cartilage injuries

Some people undergo arthroscopic surgery to smooth the surface of the damaged cartilage area. Other surgical procedures such as microfracture, drilling and abrasion, may provide symptomatic relief. The benefit, however, usually lasts only for a few years, especially if a person's pre-injury activity level is maintained [21].

These procedures are performed with the intent to allow bone marrow cells to infiltrate the defect,

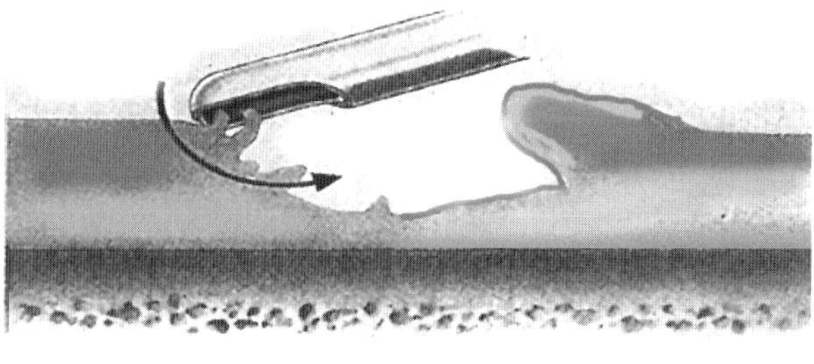

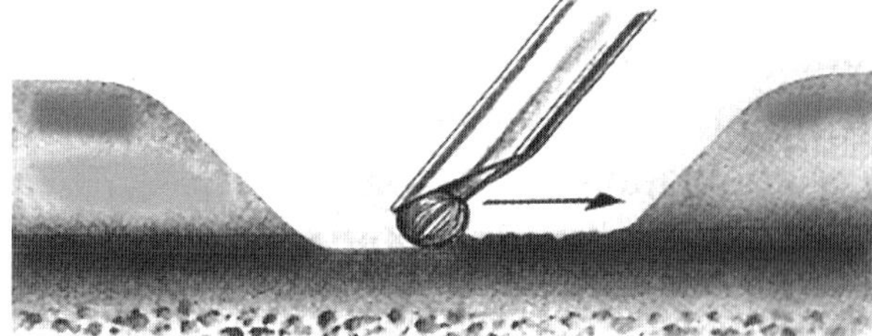

Fig. 2. The "old" arthroscopic operative debridement technique removing the degenerated cartilage tissue and loose cartilage flaps in grade II lesions. In grade III to grade IV lesions including the abrasion of subchondral bone to stimulate repair

resulting in the formation of a fibrous cartilage tissue, which is less durable and resilient than normal articular cartilage. Osteotomies with axial realignment may help to correct localized joint overpressure, especially in cases with related cartilage degeneration. More severe and chronic forms of knee cartilage damage can lead to greater deterioration of the joint cartilage and may eventually lead to some of the numerous total knee joint replacements performed each year. Approximately 200,000 total knee replacement operations are performed annually at a cost of about $25,000 each. The artificial joint generally has a life of 10 to 15 years and is considered a poor option for people younger than 50 years.

In order to avoid these late "complications" or cartilage lesion and cartilage degeneration ending up with total knee joint replacement as the ultimate solution, cartilage transplantation is a new and promising method. There are two technical options: One option is the autogenous transplantation of osteochondral plugs forming a mosaic. The advantage is that material is readily available for limited surface size [10,11].

A second option is the repair of hyaline-like cartilage using a chondrocyte suspension. It is used to treat larger surface defects, but two operations and cell culturing are needed [1,14].

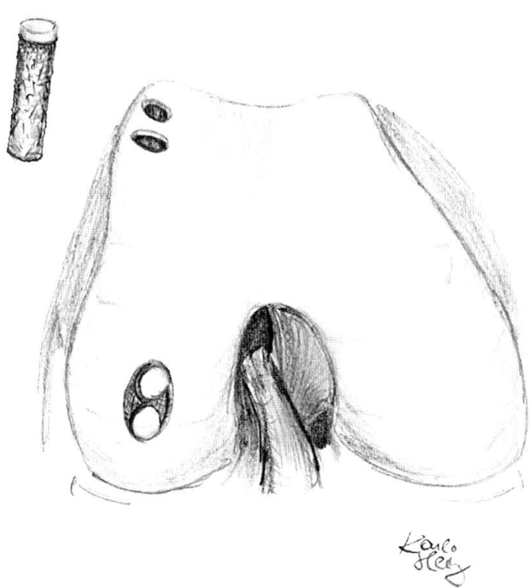

Fig. 3. Mosaicplasty technique (Hangody) harvesting cylindrical osteochondral plugs from non weightbearing areas of the knee and transplanting them into prepared holes in cartilage deficient areas in the weightbearing zone of the femoral condyle

These progressive surgical methods require a precise operation. It is a precondition that the basic disease – the injury of the cartilage – is detected in time. This in turn can only be achieved with the help of an excellent imaging diagnosis. To plan an operation two things are necessary: Objective imaging to chose the best operating technique for the individual patient, and a precise prognosis to inform the patient and to plan the rehabilitation. Excellent imaging and the presentation of cartilage are furthermore necessary to control the development of this disease in follow up studies.

The following is demanded of an objective imaging technique to present cartilage:

1. Quantitative imaging of cartilage in the joint
2. Optimized imaging of the surface to visualize local defects
3. Possibility of map-like imaging

The knee joint is especially suitable for such a procedure, due to its anatomic structure:

- The knee joint has the thickest cartilage
- Arthrosis and cartilage defects occur very frequently and carry high socio-economic consequences
- The knee joint is easily accessible in a MRI examination due to the relative absence of soft tissue

Ad I: Quantitative imaging of cartilage in the joint

To visualize articular cartilage in humans a variety of spin-echo and gradient-echo sequences have been used to acquire images. In most clinical studies of the human knee a slice acquisition of 3-mm range in thickness was used. The goal of these studies has been to identify focal defects and/or to measure cartilage thickness. Many of these studies have used knee arthroscopy as a "golden standard" for the evaluation of the efficacy of MRI in assessing articular cartilage. In an attempt to better delineate the interface between cartilage and synovial fluid, several authors have also used gadolinium as a contrast agent in conjunction with MRI [9]. Some authors prefer the use of a combination of two spin echo sequences – one for the cartilage-to-bone-interface and one for the cartilage-to-joint-fluid-interface visualization, thus minimizing the possibility of seeding errors during three dimensional reconstruction [15].

The use of fat suppressed flash sequences has currently proved to be the most successful and most

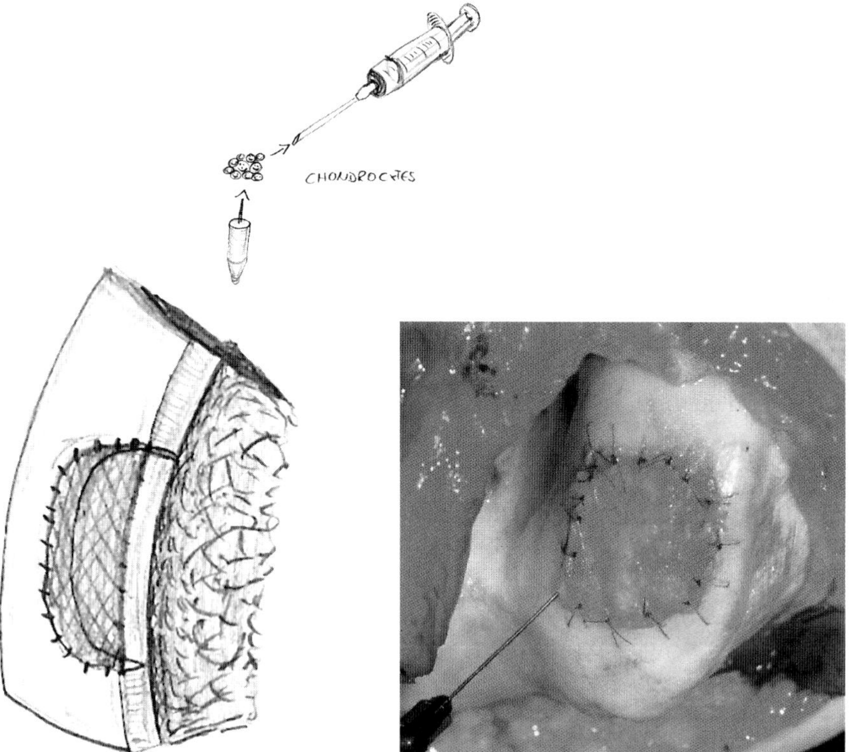

Fig. 4. Cartilage transplantation (Nehrer) suturing a periost flap in a focal cartilage defect area and filling the area between the periost and the subchondral bone with cultivated autologous chondrocyte cell suspension

efficient method in the native MR. Partly water excision flash sequences are used. The highest resolution of this sequence is 1.2 × 0.3 × 0.3 mm on a 1.5 Tesla instrument. However, this resolution may not be sufficient for the visualization of sharp structures. The subchondral plate, with an average bone density of 95–100% and a width of 0.2–0.6 mm (average 0.3 mm), is abruptly contiguous with a zone of low bone density.

The consequence in MRI is that the normal subchondral plate of 0.3 mm is not separately visualized, since its width lies below the pixel size. However, this zone and the subchondral bone component contribute jointly to the signal intensity of a pixel. The boundary between the cartilage and the subchondral bone as shown in a MR image therefore appears broader than the anatomical structure of the subchondral plate. The effect is reinforced by "smoothing programs" used to construct the image.

The imaging of cartilage with the gradient echo technique requires the presence of an intraarticular fluid, since this is the only way to achieve a sufficient contrast for the demarcation of the cartilage surface.

Cartilage volume

In studies investigating the total cartilage volume of the healthy human knee joint [5] using flash-3D-sequences with digital post processing and three-dimensional reconstruction, the conclusion was reached that the intra-individual total cartilage volume differs about ±19%. A correlation was found with the diameter of the tibial plateau, in which a standardization on the diameter of the tibial plateau resulted in an intra-individual variability of ±13%. These results appear logic in so far as that larger knee joints contain a larger volume of cartilage as smaller knee joints. A correlation with age, weight, height or bodymass-index was not significant. To qualify the results of mere volumetric analyses it must be said that already in young patients of almost the same age significant variations of cartilage volume are found retropatellar, however, without any signs of arthrosis. The volume of the patellar cartilage within 23–25 years old patients was 3.2 to 7.1 mm^3 (mean 4.8 to 28.6 mm^3) [23]. This reduces the possibility to judge an arthrosis by merely measuring cartilage volume.

MRI presents a clear picture of the decalcified cartilage. Calcification, especially in the area leading

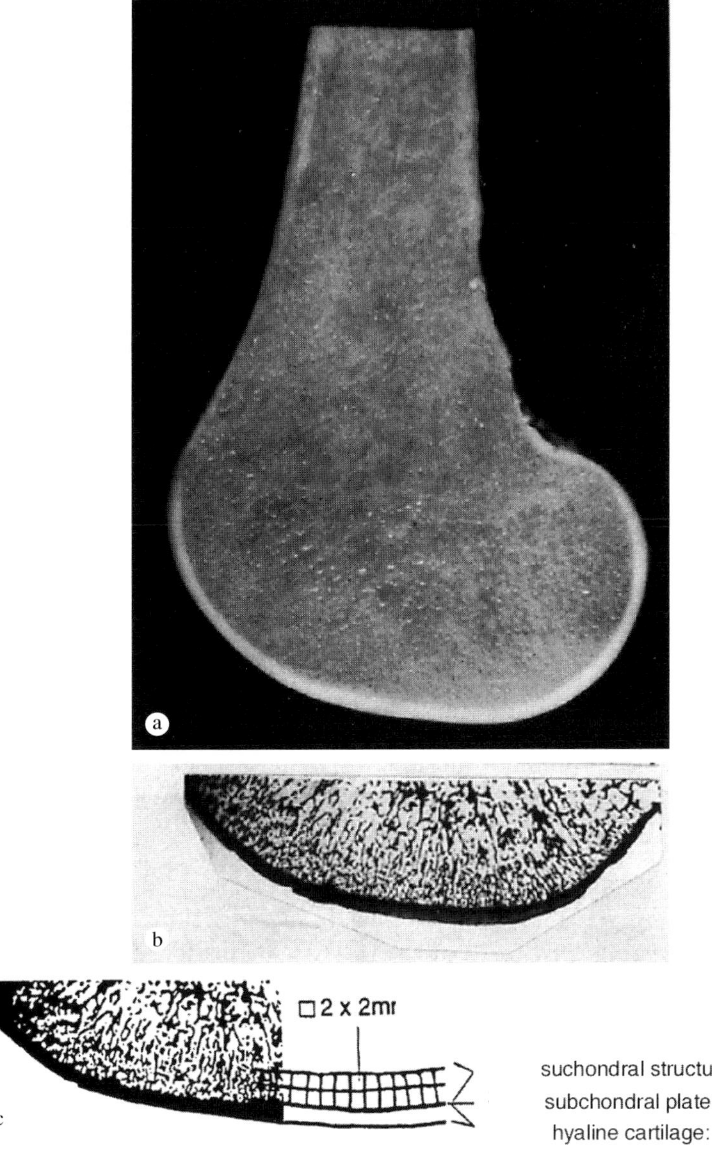

Fig. 5. Normal joint structures. **a** Sagittal section through the lateral condyle without signs of osteoarthritis. **b** Corresponding histological section for the measurement of the relative bone density of the subchondral cancellous bone (staining Kossa). **c** Graphic of the size of the cancellous subchondral bone structure (2.2 mm), the dimension of the subchondral plate (0.3 mm), and the hyaline cartilage

over to the subchondral area, however, cannot be demarcated clearly. This especially concerns degeneratively changed joint cartilage and transplanted cartilage. This presents one of the limits of this examination technique at the moment [8]. As studies have shown, the fat suppressed sequences used for cartilage imaging yield a high sensitivity for cartilage lesions. Concerning the assessement of arthrosis, it is only in the histological stages 2 and 3 that circumscribed superficial defects appear macroscopically as areas of roughness, uneveness or as deeper lesions.

The agreement between the histological, the macroscopic and the MRI findings is greatest in stages 3 and 4, since macroscopically extensive focal cartilage defects and areas with complete loss of the cartilage, which have been described as bare bone, are present [Fassbender 1985].

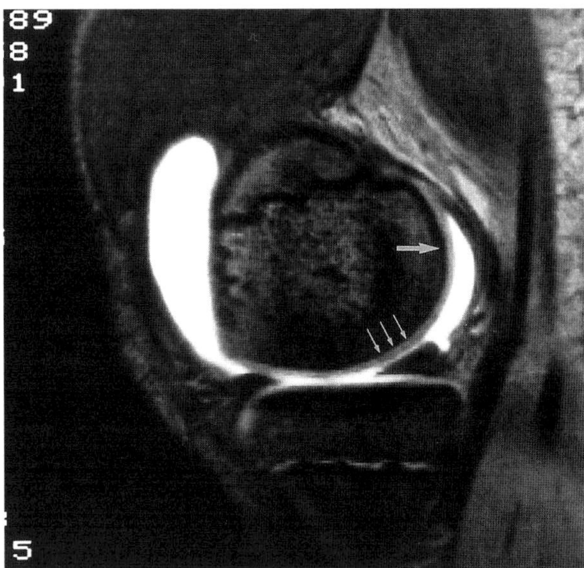

Fig. 6. MR arthrography (SE 700/15, sagittal plane, lateral condyle). Thin subchondral hypoindense zone in the anterior, central, and parts of the posterior section of the condyle. Broad subchondral hypoindense zone from the center of the posterior part of the condyle

Plain image vs	MRI	MR arthrography
T1	−0.41*	−0.35*
FLASH 3D	−0.08	−0.18*
*p = 0.05		

Fig. 7. Graph: difference of cartilage thickness (mm) between the plain image and MRI/MR-arthrography (Engel)

Possibility to reproduce cartilage volume examinations

Recent studies [20,23] have shown that the reproductivity of mean cartilage thickness in the area of the patella and the tibial cartilage lies within ±4% in the living test person.

To achieve a high contrast between the cartilage and the surrounding tissues, fat suppressed MRI sequences have been used. With these sequences, which require an imaging time of less than 5 minutes, the quantitative distribution of articular cartilage in the patella can be determined with high precision in vivo.

The cartilage volume measurement, also called chondro-crassometry, requires a framework for the examination techniques. The section plane should be orientated vertically towards the cartilage surface. This is especially easy to achieve for the patella and for the tibial plateau. Problems occur at the femoral condyles due to their 3D convex surface. These areas are therefore less precisely documented. To avoid the problem of different section planes in different examinations, three dimensional reconstruction techniques and digital data processing have been introduced. Thus the distribution of cartilage thickness can be determined independently of the original section plane. When longitudinal investigations of changes in cartilage thickness are envisaged, the position of the joint in the scanner will be different in each acquisition. Studies that investigate only the repeatability of thickness and volume measurements from the same data set, and examine the effect of repeated semiautomatic segmentation procedures are, therefore, of limited significance. It was shown that knee joints with arthrosis show a decrease of cartilage volume up to 58% [Hülig 1999].

Volume and strain

The question in how far mechanical strain can change cartilage volume was investigated by Eckstein et al. [5].

After the mechanical strain of 50 knee-bends healthy study patients showed a decrease in

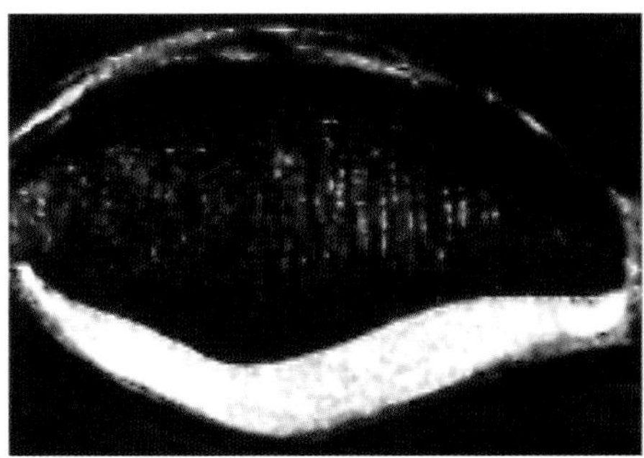

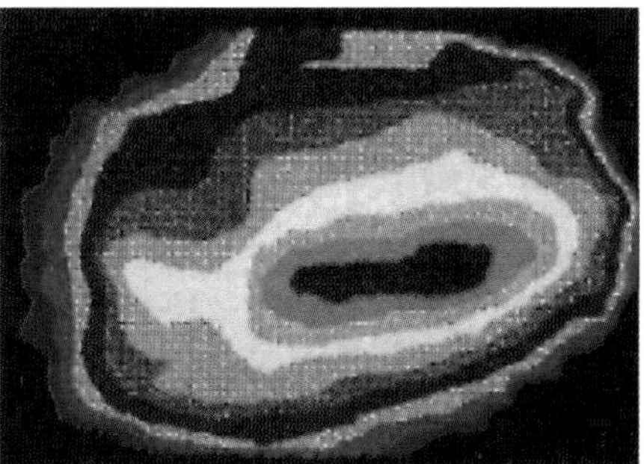

Fig. 8. 3D-MR-chondrocrassometrie (Lösch) visualizing the thickness distribution of cartilage on the patella by false colors onto the articular surface

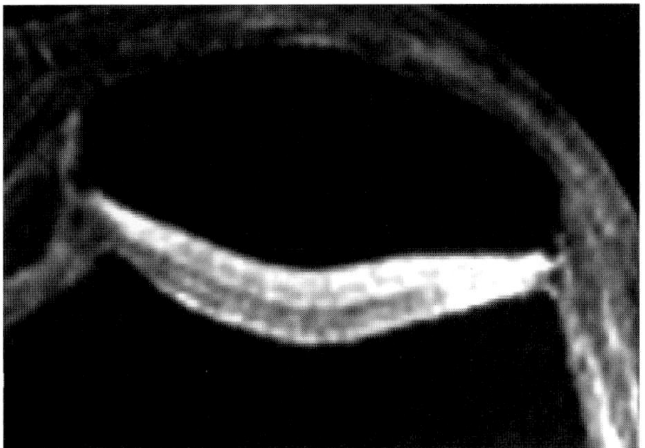

Fig. 9. Transverse fat suppressed MRI of the patellar region demonstrating good cartilage visualization but difficult cartilage surface visualization on areas with direct contact to corresponding cartilage surface

retropatellar cartilage volume of 6%. The fact that cartilage volume examinations must to be carried out on not strained cartilage, to require comparable results, was demonstrated in a study by Herberhold et al. (1999). It was shown that the strain of the knee joint with 150% of body weight for 32 hours meant a decrease in volume of 43% on average. After 1 minute strain under this weight the volume decreased around 3%.

Ad 2: Optimized imaging of the surface to visualize chaps and ulcers

The question to be asked is whether the measurement of cartilage volume is really the most relevant parameter for the control of the development, the prognosis and the planning of a therapy of a gonarthrosis. Other parameters of cartilage quality such as cartilage surface, the state of the cartilage and the localization of degenerations also appear to play a major role. To have a comparison: The measurement of the rubber volume of a tire is not sufficient to judge whether it is suitable for driving. Factors such as depth of tread, superficial chaps and possible deliminations have to be considered additionally. Similar criteria have to be considered in the evaluation of joint cartilage. At the moment arthroscopy is considered to be the "golden standard" in the evaluation of cartilage defects. The disadvantages, however, are the problems of standardization and the fact that it is an invasive method with all its possible complications.

The advantage of an arthroscopic examination lies in the optic imaging of cartilage surface with magnification and video resolution, which makes it possible to reach an excellent imaging and resolution. This cannot be achieved by a MRI examination at the moment. One examination technique that offers the best results for a surface imaging is the MR arthroscopy. Isotonar or, even better, Gardolinium are used as intraarticular contrast agents, with advantage that the contrast agent is presented in white color. Surface defects of the cartilage are presented more clearly in this way.

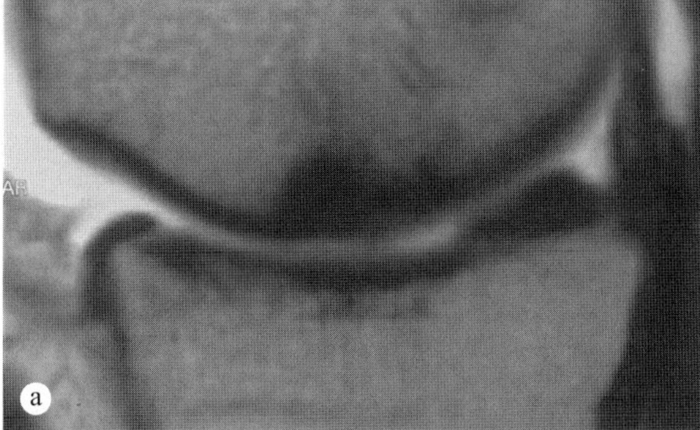

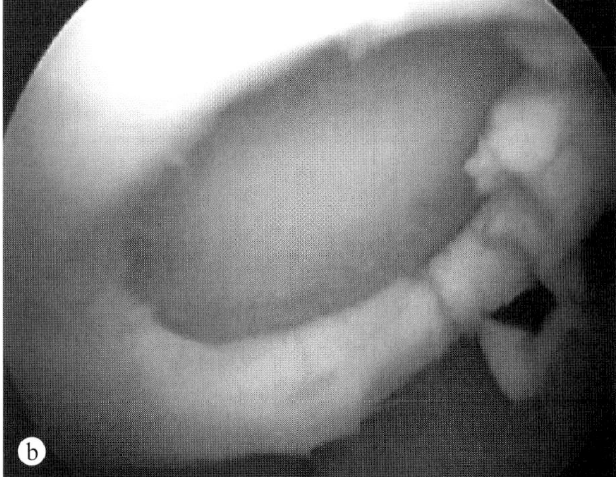

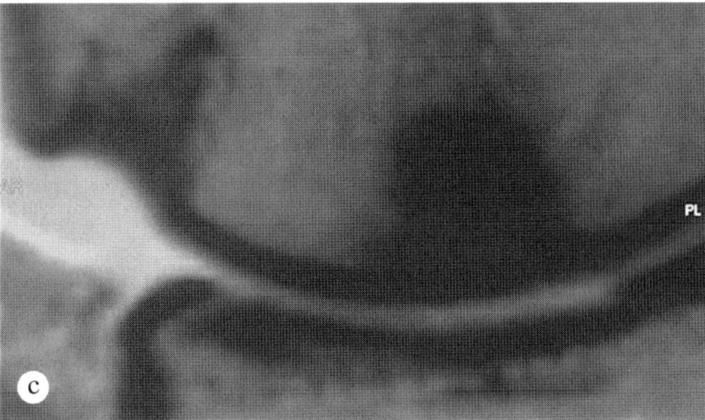

Fig. 10. Grade III (full thickness) focal cartilage lesion of the medial femoral condyle in the full weightbearing area in a 36 year old man. **a** Prae OP MR arthrography – T1 sagittal. **b** Intra OP arthroscopic view. **c** MR arthrography follow up after mosaic plasty

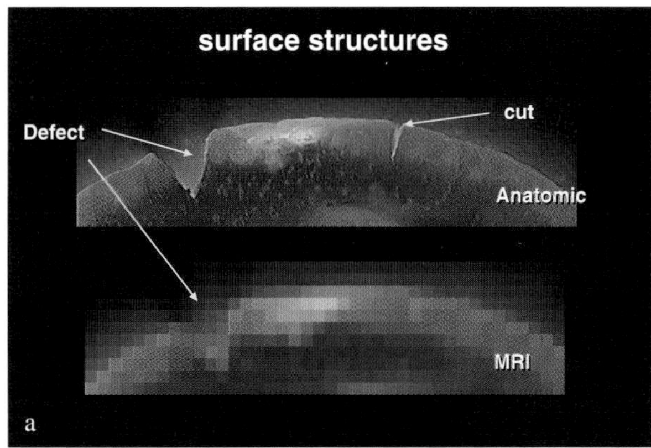

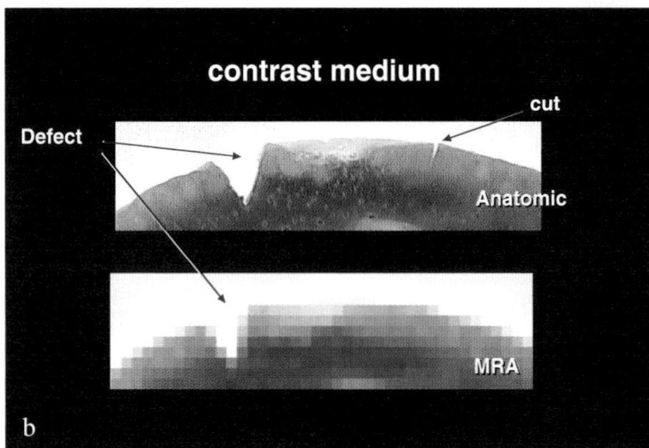

Fig. 11. Model showing the possibility of visualization of superficial defects, depending upon contrast agent and pixel resolution. The contrast is a black and white background, the resolution is optic/arthroscopic and the magnetic resonance pixel resolution. **a** Without contrast; **b** With contrast

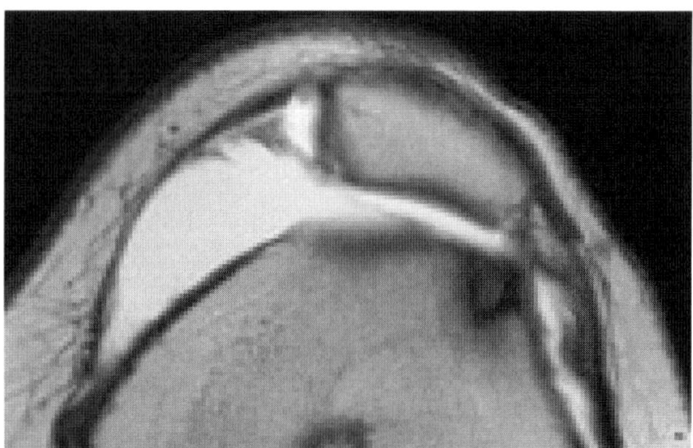

Fig. 12. Coronal MR arthrography of patella-femoral joint of a 36 year old woman with a osteochondral defect of the lateral femoral surface and a cartilage defect of the lateral patellar facet

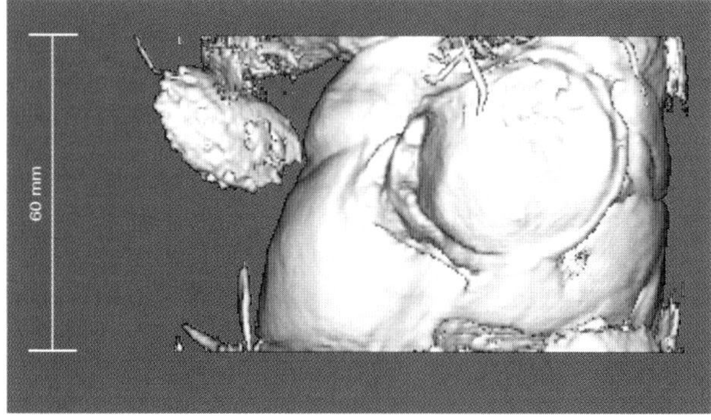

Fig. 13. Volume and surface reconstruction of a MR arthrography using the gradient of the Gadolinium to the surrounding structures – first steps to virtual arthroscopy

In opposition is the cartilage in the flash 3D imaging white itself and the danger exists that surface defects and delimination injuries are out-shined. The limits of surface imaging at the moment lie in the resolution, or in the size of pixel imaging respectively. However, in the future much more is to be expected due to faster processors. Another advantage of the arthrography is that because of the contrast agent the joint areas are separated, so that the problem of two inseparable, overlying cartilage areas is reduced but not solved. In any case does this method present a step towards virtual arthroscopy. The operator gets hold of a tool with which he is familiar in the way of visualization.

Possibility of map-like imaging

To visualize the cartilage as it presents itself in a standardized and reproducible MR examination, an image of a two-dimensional area similar to a map would be desirable. This provides the precondition for cartilage imaging of high quality and measurable and reproducible examinations. Similar to the technique used in cartography the cartilage coating of the knee joint has to be transferred onto a two-dimensional map. This cartographic imaging has the advantage that humans are used to the reading of maps, and that it is, therefore, easy for an experienced person to read three-dimensional information out of a two-dimensional map very quickly and without additional help. Similar to a map a raster divides the areas into the corresponding knee joint articulation areas, into medial and lateral part and into zones of main pressure. As the localization of a cartilage defect is far more important than the diagnosis of the defect itself, the defect has to be related to a defined area unambiguously. The third dimension, in cartography marked by the stratification of

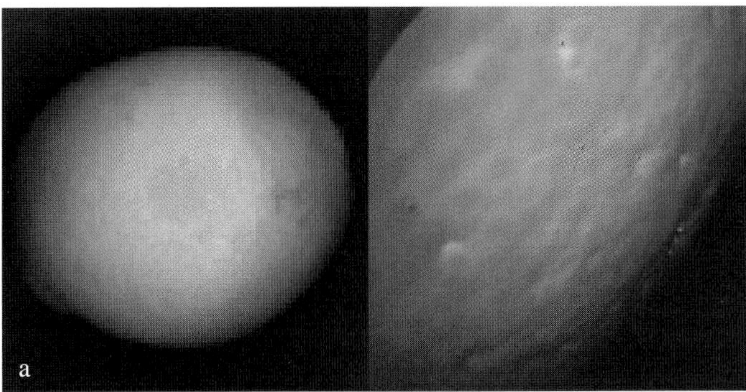

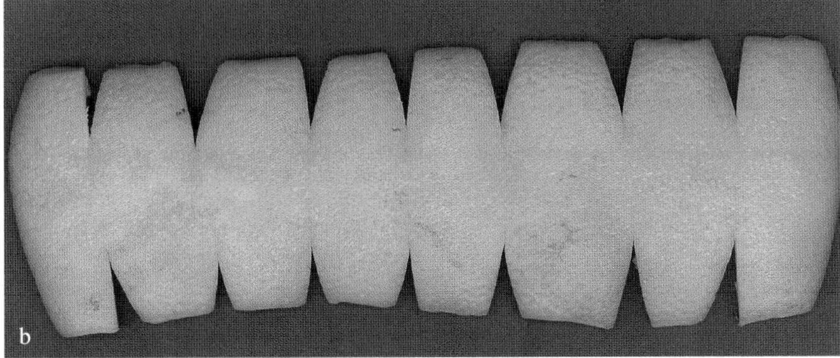

Fig. 14. An example for mapping of three dimensional curved surfaces using an orange. **a** Surface image; **b** Surface mapping

height with lines and the coloring of mountains and valley, has to be integrated into the cartilage imaging in an equivalent manner. In regard to the extension of cartilaginous defects, only lesions of grade III and IV are relevant for the therapy. The imaging can therefore be reduced to these kinds of cartilage lesions.

Recent problem: duration of the examination

The question of the duration of such cartilage volume examinations, which definitely presents an important factor in the practical use of such examinations, was raised in a study by Tieschky, Faber and Hauber (1997). The duration of the examination time needed for the reconstruction of the cartilage of the patella with fat suppressed 3D sequences resulted to last 4 minutes and 10 seconds. Marshall [15] described an examination time of only 11 minutes with an acceptable accuracy (96.5%) between measured and actual volume using combined SPGR and SFP sequences and a slice thickness of 1.5 mm.

The factor time does not only play a role in the taking of pictures but also in the postprocessing of the pictures. Here automated picture post processing applications have to reduce the time needed for the application.

The digital post processing to reduce the influence of positioning of the knee in follow up examinations was pointed out [23]. However, automated and integrated applications are necessary for routine use. procedures used that are necessary to convert the digital data and to transfer them to a graphic work station are time consuming and susceptible to interference. The segmentation of the cartilage is only semi automatic, meaning that areas of low contrast between the cartilage and the adjacent tissue, particularly the peripheral areas where the cartilage is in direct contact with the synovial folds have to be marked manually. The 3D reconstruction of the patellar cartilage including only the post processing carried our by an experienced technician required about 30 minutes. As the patella cartilage compromises only 1/7 of the knee joint area, a post processing time of 3–4 hours must be calculated for a whole knee cartilage 3D reconstruction.

Conclusion

It must be the aim to be able to judge the whole joint cartilage in an examination of the joint in the sense of a virtual arthroscopy. The examination must be possible in an acceptable time frame and with a satisfyingly high resolution. The cartilage should be visualized in a two-dimensional, map-like presentation in regard to localization and extension of the defect. This is the only way to include potential cartilage injuries, to localize them, to apply a standardized surgical procedure and to document the results in follow up studies. Therefore it is, on the one hand, the transplantation of cartilage and, on the other hand, the three-dimensional imaging of cartilage that can both lead to an optimization in the therapy of arthrosis. To construct cartilage models from MRI examinations presents a future possibility in the sense of biomechanic analysis and the calculation of finite elements (Vachum Project, http://www.ulb.ac.be/project/vakhum/index.html).

References

[1] Brittberg M, Lindahl A, Nilsson A (1994) Treatment of deep cartilage defects in the knee with autologous chondrocyte transplantation. NEJM 331: 889–894

[2] Chan WP, Lang P, Stephens MP (1991) Osteoarthritis of the knee: comparison of radiography, CT and MRI imaging to assess extent and severity. AJR 157: 799–806

[3] Daenen BR, Ferrara MA, Marcelis S, Dondelinger RF (1998) Evaluation of patellar cartilage surface lesions: comparison of CT, arthrography and fat-suppressed FLASH 3D MR imaging. Eur Radiol 8 (6): 981–985

[4] Eckstein F, Stammberger T, Priebsch J, Englmeier KH, Reiser M (2000) Effect of gradient and section orientation on quantitative analysis of knee joint cartilage. J Magn Reson Imaging Feb; 11 (2): 161–167

[5] Eckstein F, Tieschky M, Faber SC, Haubner M, Kolem H, Englmeier KH, Reiser M (1998) Effect of physical exercise on cartilage volume and thickness in vivo: MR imaging study. Radiology Apr; 07 (1): 243–248

[6] Eckstein F, Gavazzeni A, Sittek H, Haubner M, Losch A, Milz S, Engelmeier KH, Schulte E, Putz R, Reiser M (1996) Determination of knee joint cartilage thickness using three-dimensional magnetic resonance chondro-crassometry (3D MR-CCM). Magn Reson Med Aug; 36 (2): 256–265

[7] Eckstein F, Winzheimer M, Westhoff J, Schnier M, Haubner M, Englmeier KH, Reiser M, Putz R (1998) Quantitative relationships of normal cartilage volumes of the human knee joint – assessment by magnetic resonance imaging. Anat Embryol (Berl) May; 197 (5): 383–390

[8] Eckstein F, Sittek H, Gavazzeni A, Milz S, Kiefer B, Putz R, Reiser M (1995) Knee joint cartilage in magnetic resonance tomography. MR chondrovolumetry (MR-CVM) using fat-suppressed FLASH 3D sequence. Radiologe Feb; 35 (2): 87–93

[9] Engel A (1990) Magnetic resonance knee arthrography Acta Orthopaedica Scandinavica, suppl. No. 240, vol. 61. Munksgaard Copenhagen

[10] Hangody L, Sukosd L, Szigeti I (1996) Arthroscopic autogenous osteochondral mosaicplasty. Hungarian J Orthop Trauma 39: 49–54

[11] Herberhold C, Faber S, Stammberger T, Steinlechner M, Putz R, Engelmeier KH, Reiser M, Eckstein F (1999) In situ measurement of articular cartilage deformation in intact femoropatellar joints under static loading. J Biomech Dec; 32 (12): 1287–1295

[12] Jakob RP, Gautier E (1998) Complex knee trauma-cartilage injuries. Swiss Surg (6): 296–310

[13] Lösch A, Eckstein F, Hauner M (1995) 3D-MR-Chondrocrassometrie. Sportorthopädie – Sporttraumatologie, 11.3, 183–186

[14] Mankin H (1994) Chondrocyte transplantation – an answer to an old question. NEJM 331: 940–941

[15] Marshall KW, Mikulis DJ, Guthrie BM (1995) Quantitation of articular cartilage using magnetic resonance imaging and three-dimensional reconstruction. J Orthop Res Nov; 13 (6): 814–823

[16] Nagelberg A, Swason J, Oertel C, Christenson S (1997) 6 million a year seek medical care for knees. American Academy of Orthopaedic Surgeons, News Release

[17] Nehrer S, Minas T (2000) Moderne Behandlungsverfahren bei Knorpelschäden. Österr Journal für Sportmedizin 1: 6–11

[18] Potter HG, Linklater JM, Allen AA, Hannafin JA, Haas SB (1998) Magnetic resonance imaging of articular cartilage in the knee. An evaluation with use of fast-spin-echo imaging [see comments]. J Bone Joint Surg Am Sep; 80 (9): 1276–1284

[19] Radin EL, Ehrlich MG, Chernac R (1978) Effect of repetitive impulse loading on the knee joints in rabbits. Clin Orthop 131: 288–293

[20] Stammberger T, Eckstein F, Englmeier KH, Reiser M (1999) Determination of 3D cartilage thickness data from MR imaging: computational method and reproducibility in the living. Magn Reson Med Mar; 41 (3): 529–536

[21] Steadman J, Rodrigo J, Briggs K (1996) Long term results of full thickness articular cartilage defects of the knee treated with debridement and microfracture. Am J Sportsmed

[22] Thompson RC, Oegema TR (1979) Metabolic activity of articular cartilage in osteoarthritis: an in vitro study. J Bone Joint Surg (Am) 61: 407–416

[23] Tieschky M, Faber S, Haubner M, Kolem H, Schulte E, Englmeier KH, Reiser M, Eckstein F (1997) Repeatability of patellar cartilage thickness patterns in the living. J Orthop Res Nov; 15 (6): 808–813

Experiences and future aspects of neuronavigation

W. Pfisterer and M. Mühlbauer

Department of Neurosurgery, Donauspital SMZ-Ost, Vienna, Austria

Introduction

Ships have arrived at their destination harbours before GPS and intracranial lesions have been operated on before neuronavigation systems. The question is: Do we need navigation for intracranial procedures and did it have a major impact in the development of neurosurgical techniques? Technological advances in imaging and computerized systems have improved accuracy. The result is that for both – ships and patients – the journey is more safe.

The knowledge of the brain surface and neurological function allowed the first neurological surgeons to perform surgery on and in the brain just a century ago. In 1889, D.N. Zernov, a Russian surgeon, demonstrated the first brain navigator using a coordinate system: a device with an aluminium circular frame, which could be fixed to a patient's skull horizontally above the sagittal suture. For localization in the brain he used a polar coordinate system. The first stereotactic instrument for humans to be used clinically was invented by Spiegel and Wycis in Philadelphia in 1947 which is the beginning of the modern era of stereotactic neurosurgery [1].

Stereotactic methodology

Frame based systems

The construction of a stereotactic frame is based on a system of rectilinear coordinates along the x, y, z axes for determining a specific target point in the human brain. A second type of frame is based on a spherical or polar coordinate system. This requires trigonometric calculations based on geometric principles. One technique is to place the stereotactic frame directly on the skull and the target point is the centre of the arc. The more recent frame based techniques however have one ring fixed to the patient' s head with pins that impinge on the scalp and skull, and a second ring which is adjusted to the target coordinates at a phantom base and then transferred and attached to the frame on the patient's head.

Frameless systems

A new type of stereotactic instrumentation is the so-called "frameless instrument". These systems revolutionized the planning in neurosurgery and therefore altered the practice of neurosurgery as well. Instead of a frame screwed on the patient's head, simple adhesive markers are fixed on the scalp that give computer systems the necessary information to define the space within the head. These devices enable interactive image guided neurosurgery – the "Neuronavigation" was born. The navigator is the neurosurgeon who navigates the ships (instruments) through the sea (patient's brain) by support of the neuronavigation devices.

Neuronavigation requires three technological advances to make it useful and safe. Firstly precise imaging-methods of preparing thin slices of the brain to study the detailed neuroanatomy, secondly precise post-imaging processing allowing for reconstructed three-dimensional brain maps and thirdly the precise transfer of the coordinates of a specific target within the brain to a surgical instrument. The modern computed imaging techniques together with high speed computers and powerful graphic computer software now provide the technology to localize targets during brain surgery without a stereotactic frame and altered the practice of neurosurgery significantly.

Different localisation systems have been developed using either mechanical arms, magnetic arms, light emitting diodes (LED) or electromagnetic tracking systems. However all these devices need the supply of digitalized imaging technologies. The neuronavigation systems in the neurosurgical operating theatre are only one part of a technical revolution in the era of digital imaging of brain morphology and even of brain function.

Present application of a neuronavigation system in a fully digitalized hospital

Data acquisition – fiducial markers

In all patients with intracranial tumours, we perform a MRI or CT data set with fiducial markers as a slim mask for neuronavigation one to three days preoperatively. The fiducials used by us are adhesive ring markers with 1.5 cm diameter and a 1 mm defined centre (topographic Markers, EZ-AM Inc. Westbury, NY, USA). These markers are placed on the skin of the head. Stable scalp locations for marker placement are chosen: mastoid, frontal and parietal tuber and forehead. Additional fiducials are placed all around the visible contours of the head along an imaginary axis following the expected trajectory from the entry point to target point thus creating a stereotactic space for further volumetric calculation.

The imaging protocol for CT (Siemens Somatom Plus) defines a spiral scan mode with 3 mm thick slices/1 mm reconstruction index. For MRI-based navigation we usually use T1 weighted axial images after application of contrast medium with 1.3 mm slice thickness (Siemens Magnetom Expert).

Picture archive Communication System (PACS)

Due to the PACS, all radiological examinations are digital and are available within minutes on all peripheral workstations e.g. operating theatre, intensive care unit, planning workstation for 3-D-reconstruction and especially neuronavigation system. Imaging data can be immediately used for surgical planning, image-modality matching and neuronavigation. No data storage with tapes or CDs, for instance, is necessary for data transfer between the respective workstations.

Localization system

In 1995 we started frameless neuronavigation with the Aesculap SPOCS (Surgical Planning and Orientation Computer System), a first generation Interactive-Image-Guided Surgical (IIGS) planning and navigation device for surgery of space-occupying lesions in the head. Instrument tracking was based on a light emitting diode-based computer system.

Since 2003 we are using the TREON Stealth Station (Medtronic) which is also based on infrared instrument tracking. The TREON system includes several components: a mobile stand with the computer and the monitor, another mobile stand with two near infrared cameras fixed on a mobile arm allowing flexible positioning within the operating theatre, and a so called head follower equipped with several LEDs or with small reflecting balls in the visual field of the infrared cameras. As the head follower is attached to the patient fixation system, intraoperative repositioning of the patient is recognized by the computer and does not affect accuracy. A pointing device and also various surgical instruments are either equipped with LEDs or with reflecting markers and can therefore be tracked by the system. From the known geometry of the instrument, the computer calculates the position, direction and rotation of the instrument in space and shows its exact position in the patient's brain on the monitor.

3-D planning workstation

The TREON includes powerful graphic software. Using the thin-slice axial MR-data set it can display the MR images in the axial, coronal and sagittal plane and additionally in selectively defined trajectory views. 3-D reconstruction both of the surface of the head, but also of the brain surface for virtual visualisation of the gyri and sulci, the target, e.g. a tumour, and the blood vessels can easily be performed. An algorithm for automated multimodality image matching, for instance MRI with CT or MRI with PET, is also provided. All virtually created 3-D objects can be rotated and visualized from different angles for surgical trajectory planning. As this is an interactive procedure, the neurosurgeon can also improve his knowledge about the critical anatomical and pathological structures and he can use this device for teaching and even for some sort of virtual surgery.

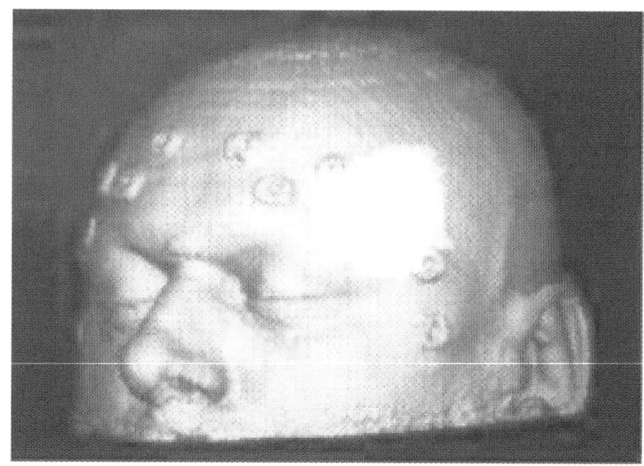

Fig. 1. 3D reconstruction of a patient's head with translucent skin and a tumour in the left perisylvian region (low grade glioma). Note the fiducials on the patient's forehead

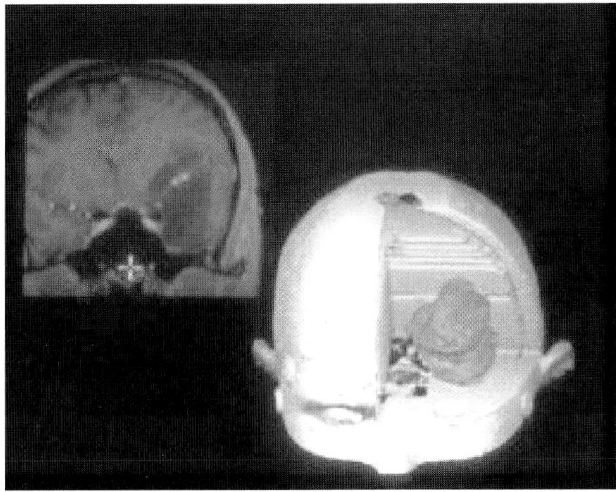

Fig. 2. Coronal T1-weighted MR and 3D reconstruction (cut planes) of a perisylvian tumour with vessels

Registration

In order to match the imaging data of the patient with the coordinates calculated for the position of the surgical instruments, the computer must first be provided with the information where the fiducial markers are regarding both the patient's CT- or MRI data set and regarding the patient's head after he has been positioned on the operating table in the theatre. For this registration procedure, the fiducials are identified and mouse-clicked on the 3-D reconstruction from the CT- or MRI data set. Then the fiducials on the patient's head are touched one by another with the infrared tracked pointer. This allows the computer for volumetric calculation of exact coordinates for any target point in the patient's brain

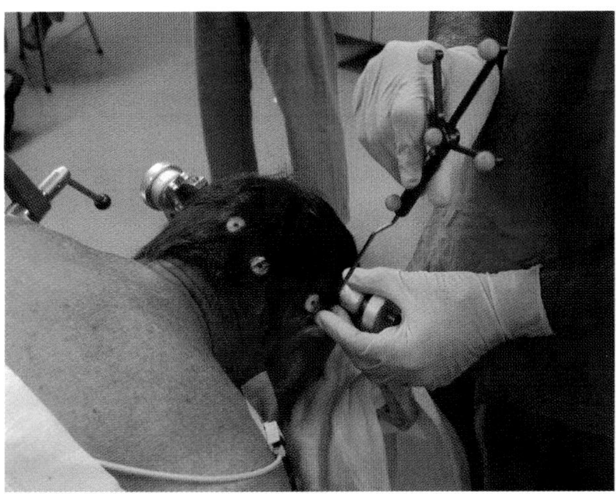

Fig. 3. Preoperative fiducial registration with pointer in a patient in prone position

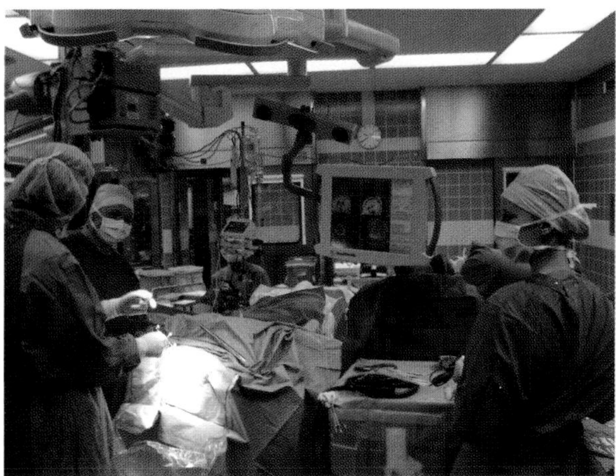

Fig. 4. Intraoperative TREON neuronavigation system set-up

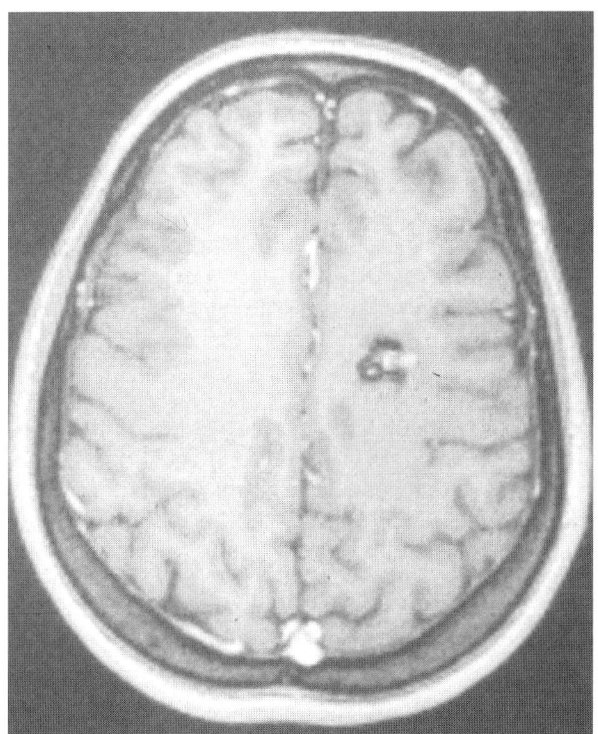

Fig. 5. MR (T1 weighted with contrast medium) of a deep seated cavernoma

and display it together with the MRI images or even inside the 3-D reconstructions on the monitor.

Registration accuracy

Registration accuracy is defined and measured as the root mean square error (RMS) in mm. This is calcu-

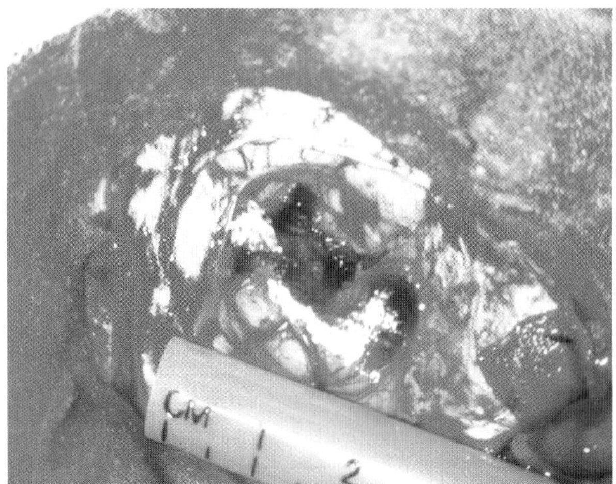

Fig. 6. Intraoperative situs after resection of the cavernoma

lated by the computer after the registration of all fiducial markers. It compares the relationship of the fiducial position on the patient's CT- or MRI images with the registered fiducial position on the patients head. It is dependant on skin movement between scanning and registration or fiducial displacement before or during registration and gives a rough orientation on how reliable the localization of target structures provided by the neuronavigation system will be in the respective procedure.

Application accuracy

Beside the calculated accuracy (RMS value), the application accuracy is useful to check the reliability of the respective procedure. It represents the totally achieved accuracy of the system in millimetres after successful registration by comparing the position of the skin (head surface) and of anatomical landmarks (e.g. glabella, external ear canal, eye bulb) on the CT- or MRI images with the real position on the patient' s head when these specific points are touched with a tracked instrument.

Intraoperative navigation tools

After registration is completed pathways may be defined from a chosen entrypoint towards the target deep inside the brain, and this trajectory is imposed either on the CT- or MRI pictures on the surgeon's monitor or even on the operating microscope's oculars. Any deviation from the chosen pathway can be visualized in realtime during surgery, and if necessary new pathways can be defined intraoperativly.

Frameless stereotactic biopsy

For a stereotactic biopsy of deep seated lesions there are instruments available that can be tracked by the system while they are introduced through the brain towards the target point. The application accuracy of the respective procedure defines the accuracy of the biopsy needles and forceps at the target point. Therefore lesions greater than 1 cm in diameter can effectively be reached with this timesaving procedure and without the need for mounting a stereotactic ring on the patient's head.

Framebased MRI stereotactic biopsy using CT data set

In rare cases, small deep seated lesions do not show up on CT but on contrast enhanced MRI only. If they require precise framebased stereotactic biopsy, a previously taken MRI can be used for defining the target point, but for the coordinate calculation a simple CT-scan taken with the stereotactic ring mounted on the patient's head is used. It is matched automatically with the MRI data set and then shows the target lesion also on the CT pictures. This spares the complicated procedure of taking an MRI with a mounted head ring in general anaesthesia.

Results (Tables 1–3)

The clinical applicability was proven for all standard patient positioning: prone-, side-, supine- and sitting position. To study the reliability and usefulness of neuronavigation we investigated the additional time effort, registration accuracy and application accuracy over a 4 year period (1996–1999).

Table 1. Diagnosis of 308 patients operated by assistance of neuronavigation

Diagnosis		Numbers
High grade gliomas		85
Low grade gliomas		25
Metastasis		60
Meningiomas:	Falx	13
	Skull base	27
	Convexity	26
Vascular malformation:	AVM	11
	Aneurysms	3
	Cavernomas	15
Pituitary adenomas		11
Cysts		8
Infectious diseases		6
Others		18

Table 2. Registration and application accuracy

Registration accuracy (RMS) mm:	1.0–2.75	154
	2.76–4.5	124
	>4.5	40
Application accuracy mm:	<2	126
	2–4	150
	>4	42

Table 3. Diameter of lesions and distance to the lesion from brain surface

Diameter lesion mm:	<20	60
	20–40	148
	>40	100
Distance to lesion mm:	0–15	140
	16–35	92
	<35	76

In 308 patients included in this study intracranial lesions were operated using a neuronavigation system (Table 1). In 283 patients MR, in 25 patients CT imaging studies were obtained before operation. The additional mean time effort for scanning, data transfer and registration was 30 minutes (range 20–60). Mean registration accuracy (root mean square error, RMS) was 2.9 mm (range 1.0–7.8 mm) (Table 2) and the mean application accuracy was 3.8 mm (range 1–7 mm).

The lesion diameters and the distances from the brain surface to the lesion were divided into three groups (Table 3). The provided application accuracy allowed an optimised planning both for skin incision and craniotomy, and for lesion localization and definition of its borders in all groups both for supra- and infratentorial brain tumour surgery. Trajectory guidance was especially helpful in approaching deep seated lesions.

Brain shift resulting from surgical intervention, from tumour debulking or from opening the ventricles led to progressive degradation in accuracy during the operation, with the greatest inaccuracy occurring when deep structures were manipulated.

An application accuracy of more than 4 mm, which was found in 42 cases in our study (13.8%), should not be accepted and the registration procedure should be repeated or completed with additional surface matching to achieve a better application accuracy for precise and reliable navigation.

Discussion and future aspects

Since the work of Roberts et al. in 1986, when he integrated an ultrasound based frameless stereotactic localization system into the operating microscope, many frameless stereotactic systems have been developed and a considerable number is nowadays commercially available [2–8]. At present mostly infrared based neuronavigation systems with tracking of a wide variety of neurosurgical instruments are used. Finally these systems have become very user-friendly, reliable, technically stable and most powerful for post-imaging processing and surgical planning [9–14].

Accuracy is the most important parameter for the usefulness of any neuronavigation system. In our study performed in 309 patients operated on with neuronavigation, a registration accuracy (RMS-value) of 2.9 mm mean was found. Higher RMS values derive from shift of fiducials in the time period between scanning and registration. Therefore, a short period between MR or CT scanning and surgery is essential for high registration accuracy. RMS-values smaller than 5 mm resulted in clinically useful application accuracy for lesion targeting, lesion border definition and identification of specific anatomical details.

Application accuracy is crucial to allow the surgeon relying on the neuronavigation system at all. In the literature application accuracy is correlated with the type of the system, the slice thickness of the CT- or MR images, the reported number of patients, the localization of the fiducials and the technique of head positioning [15–22]. This corresponds with the findings of our study.

We recommend 3 mm CT slices with 1 mm reconstruction index, and for MRI 1.3 mm images. Further to place the fiducials on less moveable skin areas, like mastoid, frontal and parietal bones. Any distortion of the scalp causing shift of the fiducials when fixing the head of the patient in the clamp should be avoided.

Clinical usefulness

When high registration and application accuracy allows the neurosurgeon to rely upon the information given by the computer of the navigation system, this results in considerable advantages for the patient. It both allows accurate approaching to the lesion, and it enables guidance for the borders of tumours. In glioma patients, the definition of their borders for resection guidance allows a more extensive surgical resection. This is particularly helpful in low-grad gliomas in eloquent areas. Whether this aids to complete tumour resection and lowering the risk of recurrence must still be proofed by further studies [23–25].

In meningeoma surgery, neuronavigation is helpful especially in cases of convexity and falx localization to better define the extent of the skin and bone flap and to securely localize the large venous sinuses and the surrounding vascular structures.

Small deep seated metastasis and cavernomas are challenging both for the neurosurgeon and the neuronavigation system. Neuronavigation allows us to approach such lesions by very small trepanations on a minimally invasive and less traumatic route through the brain and therefore reduce operative morbidity [4, 9, 23].

For stereotactic brain biopsy the use of frameless neuronavigation systems is save and offers advantages for time and cost of the procedure compared to frame-based stereotaxy. However application accuracy must be taken into account as limiting factor in very small lesions [13, 26].

In transsphenoidal resection of pituitary tumours neuronavigation helps us to localize critical anatomical structures such as the internal carotid artery covered from the sphenoid bone, for instance. Non visible areas ("dead angles") for the surgical microscope can be visualized with endoscopes. In such cases, as well as in neurosurgical procedures inside the ventricular system, we use navigated endoscopes. The combination of a navigation system with endoscopes allowing the use of small diameter instruments is a promising future aspect for "endonavigation" [27–29].

Virtual accuracy

Despite high accuracy and precise navigation at the beginning of the respective surgery, the clinical application of neuronavigation is impaired by the problem of brain shift. This is significant in large tumours with brain edema after opening the dura, further after manipulating such lesions during resection, and after opening the ventricles causing CSF loss. In such cases the previously defined target point moves, and therefore the calculated coordinates for this point do not represent its new position anymore. Even if accuracy is perfectly precise, it is "virtual accuracy", because it refers to a target point defined from a previously taken a radiological picture but not to the actual, real position of this point [9, 30, 31].

Promising methods for compensating this problem were recently introduced by the use of intraoperative ultrasound to redefine the target coordinates intraoperativly [32]. Further and already established techniques to overcome this problem are intraoperative CT or MRI [24, 33–36]. They either allow to perform an intraoperative update of the radiological data set while the operation is interrupted for a short time and the patient is put into an MRI-scanner next to the operating table. Using this intraoperative dataset new registration and definition of new target coordinates is performed together with the visualisation of the extent of tumour resection and the still remaining residual tumour portion [24, 25]. Other systems even allow real-time imaging during surgery while the operation is performed inside specially designed open MRI-scanners. This gives the surgeon real-time control both for the position of his instruments inside the brain and for the progress of the operation itself. However it still must be proved in further studies whether these complicated and expensive techniques really enable us to significantly improve survival and life quality after complex neurosurgical brain operations.

References

[1] Spiegel EA, Wycis HT (1950) Principles and applications of stereoencephalotomy. J Int Coll Surg 14: 394–402

[2] Roberts DW, Strohbehn JW, Hatch JF, Murray W, Kettenberger H (1986) A frameless stereotaxic integration of computerized tomographic imaging and the operating microscope. J Neurosurg 65: 545–9

[3] Watanabe E, Watanabe T, Manaka S, Mayanagi Y, Takakura K (1987) Three-dimensional digitizer (neuronavigator): new equipment for computed tomography-guided stereotaxic surgery. Surg Neurol 27: 543–7

[4] Golfinos JG, Fitzpatrick BC, Smith LR, Spetzler RF (1995) Clinical use of a frameless stereotactic arm: results of 325 cases. J Neurosurg 83: 197–205

[5] Wagner W, Tschiltschke W, Niendorf WR, Schroeder HW, Gaab MR (1997) Infrared-based neuronavigation and cortical motor stimulation in the management of central-region tumors. Stereotact Funct Neurosurg 68: 112–6

[6] Hata N, Dohi T, Iseki H, Takakura K (1997) Development of a frameless and armless stereotactic neuronavigation system with ultrasonographic registration. Neurosurgery 41: 608–13

[7] Tronnier VM, Wirtz CR, Knauth M, Bonsanto MM, Hassfeld S, Albert FK, Kunze S (1996) Intraoperative computer-assisted neuronavigation in functional neurosurgery. Stereotact Funct Neurosurg 66: 65–8

[8] Villalobos H, Germano IM (1999) Clinical evaluation of multimodality registration in frameless stereotaxy. Comput Aided Surg 4: 45–9

[9] Roessler K, Ungersboeck K, Dietrich W, Aichholzer M, Hittmeir K, Matula C, Czech T, Koos WT (1997) Frameless stereotactic guided neurosurgery: clinical experience with an infrared based pointer device navigation system. Acta Neurochir (Wien) 139: 551–9

[10] Roessler K, Ungersboeck K, Aichholzer M, Dietrich W, Czech T, Heimberger K, Matula C, Koos WT (1998) Image-guided neurosurgery comparing a pointer device system with a navigating microscope: a retrospective analysis of 208 cases. Minim Invasive Neurosurg 41: 53–7

[11] Wirtz CR, Tronnier VM, Bonsanto MM, Hassfeld S, Knauth M, Kunze S (1998) Neuronavigation. Methods and prospects. Nervenarzt 69: 1029–36

[12] Paleologos TS, Wadley JP, Kitchen ND, Thomas DG (2000) Clinical utility and cost-effectiveness of interactive image-guided craniotomy: clinical comparison between conventional and image-guided meningioma surgery. Neurosurgery 47: 40–7

[13] Alberti O, Dorward NL, Kitchen ND, Thomas DG (1997) Neuronavigation – impact on operating time. Stereotact Funct Neurosurg 68: 44–8

[14] Kleinpeter G, Lothaller C (2003) Frameless neuronavigation using the ISG-system in practice: from craniotomy to delineation of lesion. Minim Invasive Neurosurg 46: 257–64

[15] West JB, Fitzpatrick JM, Toms SA, Maurer CR, Jr, Maciunas RJ (2001) Fiducial point placement and the accuracy of point-based, rigid body registration. Neurosurgery 48: 810–6

[16] West J, Fitzpatrick JM, Wang MY, Dawant BM, Maurer CR, Jr, Kessler RM, Maciunas RJ, Barillot C, Lemoine D, Collignon A, Maes F, Suetens P, Vandermeulen D, van den Elsen PA, Napel S, Sumanaweera TS, Harkness B, Hemler PF, Hill DL, Hawkes DJ, Studholme C, Maintz JB, Viergever MA, Malandain G, Woods RP (1997) Comparison and evaluation of retrospective intermodality brain image registration techniques. J Comput Assist Tomogr 21: 554–66

[17] Sipos EP, Tebo SA, Zinreich SJ, Long DM, Brem H (1996) In vivo accuracy testing and clinical experience with the ISG Viewing Wand. Neurosurgery 39: 194–202

[18] Poggi S, Pallotta S, Russo S, Gallina P, Torresin A, Bucciolini M (2003) Neuronavigation accuracy dependence on CT and MR imaging parameters: a phantom-based study. Phys Med Biol 48: 2199–216

[19] Maurer CR, Jr, Fitzpatrick JM, Wang MY, Galloway RL, Jr, Maciunas RJ, Allen GS (1997) Registration of head volume images using implantable fiducial markers. IEEE Trans Med Imaging 16: 447–62

[20] Helm PA, Eckel TS (1998) Accuracy of registration methods in frameless stereotaxis. Comput Aided Surg 3: 51–6

[21] Barnett GH, Miller DW, Weisenberger J (1999) Frameless stereotaxy with scalp-applied fiducial markers for brain biopsy procedures: experience in 218 cases. J Neurosurg 91: 569–76

[22] Barnett GH (2001) Comment on "Fiducial point placement and the accuracy of point-based, rigid-body registration". Neurosurgery 48: 810–7

[23] Ganslandt O, Behari S, Gralla J, Fahlbusch R, Nimsky C (2002) Neuronavigation: concept, techniques and applications. Neurol India 50: 244–55

[24] Knauth M, Wirtz CR, Tronnier VM, Staubert A, Kunze S, Sartor K (1998) [Intraoperative magnetic resonance tomography for control of extent of neurosurgical operations]. Radiologe 38: 218–24

[25] Knauth M, Wirtz CR, Tronnier VM, Aras N, Kunze S, Sartor K (1999) Intraoperative MR imaging increases the extent of tumor resection in patients with high-grade gliomas. AJNR Am J Neuroradiol 20: 1642–6

[26] Dorward NL, Paleologos TS, Alberti O, Thomas DG (2002) The advantages of frameless stereotactic biopsy over frame-based biopsy. Br J Neurosurg 16: 110–8

[27] Scholz M, Deli M, Wildforster U, Wentz K, Recknagel A, Preuschoft H, Harders A (1996) MRI-guided endoscopy in the brain: a feasability study. Minim Invasive Neurosurg 39: 33–7

[28] Dorward NL, Alberti O, Zhao J, Dijkstra A, Buurman J, Palmer JD, Hawkes D, Thomas DG (1998) Interactive image-guided neuroendoscopy: development and early clinical experience. Minim Invasive Neurosurg 41: 31–4

[29] Schroeder HW, Wagner W, Tschiltschke W, Gaab MR (2001) Frameless neuronavigation in intracranial endoscopic neurosurgery. J Neurosurg 94: 72–9

[30] Dorward NL, Alberti O, Velani B, Gerritsen FA, Harkness WF, Kitchen ND, Thomas DG (1998) Postimaging brain distortion: magnitude, correlates, and impact on neuronavigation. J Neurosurg 88: 656–62

[31] Muhlbauer M, Pfisterer W, Haberler C, Knosp E (2002) Penetration failure and misdiagnosis of stereotactic biopsy caused by the uncommonly firm tissue of a gliomyosarcoma. Minim Invasive Neurosurg 45: 177–80

[32] Jodicke A, Deinsberger W, Erbe H, Kriete A, Boker DK (1998) Intraoperative three-dimensional ultrasonography: an approach to register brain shift using multidimensional image processing. Minim Invasive Neurosurg 41: 13–9

[33] Wirtz CR, Bonsanto MM, Knauth M, Tronnier VM, Albert FK, Staubert A, Kunze S (1997) Intraoperative magnetic resonance imaging to update interactive navigation in neurosurgery: method and preliminary experience. Comput Aided Surg 2: 172–9

[34] Wirtz CR, Knauth M, Staubert A, Bonsanto MM, Sartor K, Kunze S, Tronnier VM (2000) Clinical evaluation and follow-up results for intraoperative magnetic resonance imaging in neurosurgery. Neurosurgery 46: 1112–20

[35] Tronnier VM, Wirtz CR, Knauth M, Lenz G, Pastyr O, Bonsanto MM, Albert FK, Kuth R, Staubert A, Schlegel W, Sartor K, Kunze S (1997) Intraoperative diagnostic and interventional magnetic resonance imaging in neurosurgery. Neurosurgery 40: 891–900

[36] Oh DS, Black PM (2005) A low-field intraoperative MRI system for glioma surgery: is it worthwhile? Neurosurg Clin N Am 16: 135–41

F-18-FDG PET in oncology

P. Lind and D. Dapra

Department of Nuclear Medicine and Endocrinology, PET/CT Center, LKH Klagenfurt, Klagenfurt, Austria

Physical and technical principles of PET and PET/CT

Introduction

In tracing radioactively labeled isotopes within living organism, PET dominates the field of molecular imaging because of its undoubted sensitivity to even the smallest amount of tracer. PET is able to detect and reconstruct small radio-tracer concentrations in 3D space, thereby assessing biochemical and metabolic activity of organs and tissue in vivo.

Positron emission and annihilation

An unstable, neutron-poor, atomic nucleus usually decays by emitting a positron and a neutrino. The emitted positron is the antiparticle of the electron that means it has the same weight as the electron, but is conversely charged. Depending on the nuclide, a certain amount of kinetic energy is shared by the positron and neutrino. This positive particle travels a short distance within the surrounding matter. On its way through the matter, the positron loses almost the whole amount of its kinetic energy and finally recombines with an electron. The masses of both particles are converted into energy in accordance with Einstein's law of energy conservation. To conserve energy and linear momentum, the resulting electromagnetic radiation is in the form of two gamma-photons of 511 keV and emitted in opposite directions. This process is called annihilation and leads to a divergent emission of the two equal energy photons. The distance a positron covers before annihilation depends on the kind of isotope used (see Table 1).

Detection of annihilation radiation

The two divergently moving gamma-photons are detected simultaneously by two detectors in opposite locations. If the detection occurs within a certain short period of time, the photons are considered to originate from the same annihilation, and this is called a true coincidence event. These gamma rays simultaneously sensed by opposite detectors are presumed to come from an annihilation somewhere along the line between the detectors. This is the principle of the electronic collimation in Positron-Emission-Tomography (PET). Due to the fact that no mechanical collimation is needed, PET-cameras have a high sensitivity. A PET-scanner is assembled of many detectors packed tightly together and adjusted to a ring around the patient. Several of such rings build up a PET-camera. Each of the detectors accepts coincident events in combination with many opposite detectors, both in the same ring and in adjacent rings. The large number of potential coincident events in different directions allows collecting sufficient data to reconstruct the activity distribution in the examined patient.

Attenuation correction of PET-data

Unfortunately, not all coincident events are true events originating exclusively from the line of coincidence. Some of the 511 keV-photons interfere with the tissue and some are subject to scattering. Because of the interaction between photons and the surrounding matter the direction of the gamma-ray is altered and its energy decreases. Some of the photons are absorbed during collision with atoms in the tissue. The resulting attenuation is a function of the distance the photon has to travel in the tissue and of tissue density. Attenuation correction is absolutely necessary for quantitative tracer uptake calculations. Routine attenuation correction is usually performed by using transmission images or calculations based on the assumption of uniform tissue attenuation. Two other corrections to be taken into account are random coincident and scatter events. With an increasing number of photons some singles are detected with other photons originating

Table 1. Characteristics of common positron emitting Isotopes [79], radioactive half life, maximum positron energy and path length R_p in water within 50% (95%) of the positrons are stopped

Isotope	Half-life [min]	M_{max} [MeV]	Range R_p[mm]
^{15}O	2.05	1.72	0.7 (3.3)
^{13}N	9.9	1.19	0.5 (2.1)
^{11}C	20.4	0.97	0.3 (1.6)
^{18}F	109.7	0.64	0.2 (0.9)

from different annihilations, so-called random coincident events.

With a combination of PET and CT a new possibility emerges. It was originally shown by LaCroix and Tang that CT could be used for attenuation correction of PET images [76, 126]. They used a linear algorithm to transform the low energy CT data to the high energy of 511 keV. Today, bi-linear scaling methods [68] are widely accepted and used in daily routine [11]. The main advantage is the shortening of time needed for the acquisition of attenuation data. Time is reduced to less than one minute. On the other hand it must be considered that well known artifacts in the CT images, made for example by metal implants, affect the corrected PET image [44]. It is therefore recommended that PET images are read with care close to visible artifactual structures.

Spatial resolution

The physical limits of spatial resolution in PET are ultimately due to two factors. First the positron will travel a short distance between the site of emission and site of annihilation. This distance depends on the energy spectrum of the emitted positrons and the density of the tissue in which emission occurs. The other factor which can degrade spatial resolution is caused by the residual kinetic energy and momentum of the positron and electron at the moment they annihilate. This leads to an angle between the two resulting photons deviating slightly from 180 degree.

The non-colinearity and positron range effects restrict the absolute physical resolution of a PET system to approximately 2 mm [101]. Taking into consideration also technical limitations such as the crystal size, the current clinical systems are capable of 4–5 mm spatial resolution.

Production and synthesis of positron emitting tracers

Positron emitters are produced in a cyclotron, where stable nuclei are bombarded with protons or deuterons to generate the proton-rich atoms. Currently the most important isotope is fluorine-18, the master-element in drug design. There are also some generator-produced positron emitting isotopes including rubidium-82, copper-62 and gallium-68. Doses of these positron emitters can be eluted from the generator at regular intervals for the use in the PET centre. The parent isotopes are also produced by a cyclotron. Because of the short half-lives it is necessary to produce them as close to the positron tomography as possible. Therefore the synthesis of labeled products must be rapid. For this reason and because of radiation protection, it is very helpful to use automated devices for producing the labeled compounds.

Scintillation crystals for PET

A scintillator is a material with the ability to absorb ionizing radiation, such as g- or x-rays. It converts a fraction of the absorbed energy into visible or ultraviolet photons which are read out by photomultiplier tubes. The ideal detector for PET would have a combination of specific physical and scintillation properties. High atomic number is necessary for a large photoelectron cross section and high density for a large Compton-scattering cross section. High scintillation light yield usually results in good energy resolution. Good Energy resolution helps to reduce random events, because of filtering out radiation after a scatter interaction.

A short decay time of the scintillation light allows the use of a short coincidence timing window, reducing random events. BGO emerged in the early 1970s [134]. Its much higher detection efficiency has made it a popular choice for dedicated PET. More recently new crystals like LSO and GSO were characterized for the fast and efficient detection of radiation with 511 keV (see Table 2). Both have a short attenuation length for annihilation quanta and a short light decay. Although LSO emits much more light than GSO, their energy resolution is similar [98]. Currently the major companies of PET-CT favour different scintillation crystals: CTI and Siemens – LSO, GE – BGO and Philips – GSO. Currently, avalanche photodiodes as a semiconductor replacement for photomultiplier tubes are tested but are not yet available for clinical routine [136].

PET-CT

PET-CT is a combination of positron tomography and X-ray computed tomography. It combines functional and anatomical image techniques which allow the study of patients using both types of

Table 2. Scintillation crystals used for PET

	NaI(Tl)	LSO (Lu^2SiO^5:Ce)	GSO (Gd^2SiO^5: Ce)	BGO ($Bi^4Ge^3O^{12}$)
Wavelength	410	420	440	480
Light Yield (%NaI)	100	75	30	15
Decay constant (ns)	230	40	60	300
Attenuation length for 511 keV (mm)	30	12	15	11

techniques in close temporal relation. PET-CT is available from all major companies of PET imaging equipment: Siemens, CTI, GE, Philips. All these systems have in common that a commercial CT scanner is in conjunction with a commercial PET scanner. This construction creates the possibility to gather data from CT and PET and fuse them without having manually to register the images. For daily routine in clinical environment a standard acquisition protocol was generated. First a topogram is taken by CT. After defining the region of interest to scan a diagnostic- or low-dose- CT is recorded. Finally data from the PET are collected. The whole procedure takes from 20 to 40 minutes depending on the scanner, the activity injected and the crystal. The CT and PET images can be merged automatically. Because of the time difference between CT and PET movement artefacts can occur and must be taken into consideration. The construction of the PET-CT device implies also the possibility of reconstruction errors due to the low physical integration. Nevertheless the number of worldwide ordered PET-CT devices is highly increasing compared to the number of ordered PET stand alone solutions.

Clinical pharmacology of F-18-FDG

2-[F-18]-fluoro-2-deoxy-D-glucose (F-18-FDG) is a radiolabelled (positronen emitter) glucose analogue which allows the in-vivo investigation of glucose metabolism. Glucose is actively transported into the cell via membrane transport proteins. It was demonstrated that in malignant tumour cells there is an increase in glucose membrane transport proteins. The main membrane transporter of malignant tumour cells is called Glut-1 [59]. After intravenous injection F-18-FDG is transported into the cell similar to glucose with a half-live of less than one minute. Within the cell both are phosphorylated to glucose – or F-18-FDG-6-phosphate. However, the glycolytic enzyme glucose-6-isomerase does not recognise F-18-FDG. In contrast to glucose, F-18-FDG is trapped in the tumour cell [75]. Pharmakodynamic actions of F-18-FDG are not likely due to the minimal amount of deoxyglucose (<5 μg). 30% of the injected dose are eliminated via the kidney.

Indications and clinical trials of F-18-FDG PET in oncology

Results from far more than 100,000 applications of F-18-FDG in oncologic patients have been published up to now. F-18-FDG PET is indicated for tumour detection, staging of known tumours and therapy control.

Detection of primary tumours

For the detection of tumours, morphological methods such as x-ray, ultrasonography, computerized tomograpy (CT) or magnetic resonance imaging (MRI) are established methods in clinical routine. These non-invasive conventional methods detect lesions mostly on account of the different tissue densities of a tumour compared to normal tissue. However, a differentiation between benign and malignant tumours is not possible in most cases. It has been known for many years that malignant tumours demonstrate a higher glucose metabolism compared to benign lesions [132]. With the F-18 labelled glucose analogue deoxyglucose F-18-FDG) it is possible to image this elevated glucose metabolism using PET. For accurate therapeutic decisions there is a need for this kind of metabolic imaging.

Staging of known cancer

In case of known primary malignant tumour, therapy depends on the extent of the disease including lymph node involvement and the possible presence of distant metastases. Using CT for lymph node staging, lymph nodes larger than 1 cm in diameter (1.5 cm in the inguinal region) are considered to be pathologic in the sense of infiltration due to malignant cells. Histological work-up, however, has shown that while not all lymph nodes larger than 1cm (1.5 cm) demonstrate malignant infiltration, lymph nodes smaller than 1 cm are not always free of infiltration. Therefore in tumour staging, F-18-FDG PET imaging that represents glucose metabolism of viable tumour seems to be more accurate than morphological methods. A further advantage of F-18-FDG PET is the fact that this method can be performed as whole-body technique. Using whole body F-18-FDG PET, additional distant metastases, not known before, are often detected, which leads to a change of the therapeutic strategy.

Follow-up after therapy

One of the main problems in oncology is therapy control after chemotherapy or radiation therapy. These kinds of therapy may lead to a size reduction of the tumour, which is interpreted as therapy success. However, using morphological methods it is difficult or impossible to differentiate between scar and residual tumour tissue. Increasing data show that using F-18-FDG PET allows an accurate differentiation between scar or fibrosclerosis and residual tumour in most cases.

In the 3rd German Interdisciplinary Consensus Conference (GCC) Onko-PET III (July 21st and September 19th, 2000), guidelines for indication groups for F-18-FDG PET were defined [110].

Ia: Established clinical use
Ib: Clinical use probable
II: Useful in individual cases
III: Not yet assessable owing to missing or incomplete data
IV: Clinical use rare

According to the GCC on PET in oncology and more recent studies [42], F-18-FDG PET is of clinical relevance in the following tumour groups which will be described in detail:

3.1. Further evaluation of a solitary pulmonary nodule (SPN); staging of lung cancer
3.2. Follow up of differentiated thyroid carcinoma
3.3. Staging and therapy control of head and neck tumours including CUP
3.4. Restaging of malignant melanoma
3.5. Restaging of colorectal carcinoma
3.6. Staging of lymph nodes and distant metastases in oesophageal cancer
3.7. Staging and restaging of pancreatic carcinoma
3.8. Staging and therapy control of lymphoma
3.9. High grade glioma: differentiating recurrence from scar, localisation for tumor biopsy, detection of tumor dedifferentiation in relaps.

Protocol for FDG PET in oncology

+ Patient should be in a fasting state at least 6 (preferably 12) hours. Blood glucose should be less than 140 mg/dl.
+ Cold transmission scan using Ga-67 line or Cs-137 point sources
+ In case of PET/CT, CT will provide the best transmission images
+ Depending on the PET system and the acquisition mode (2D, 3D), intravenous injection of 200–500 MBq F-18 FDG.
+ Saline infusion containing 20 mg furosemide to lower background and renal activity since FDG is mainly excreted via the kidneys.
+ Uptake time from injection of FDG to emission scan: 60–90 minutes.
+ Emission scan with an acquisition time of 2–10 minutes per bed position depending on the crystal (LSO, GSO, BGO) and acquistion mode (2D, 3D) used.
+ 4–5 bed positions (partial body scan), preferably 7–9 bed positions (whole-body scan). In case that no cold transmission was performed, hot transmission during the emission scan using Cs-137 sources is possible.
+ Reconstruction using filtered back projection (preferably iterative reconstruction).
+ Visual interpretation of coronal, sagittal and transaxial slices,
+ Calculation of the standard uptake value (SUV)
+ Fusion and interpretation of fused images in case of PET/CT acquisition

Lung cancer

Introduction

Lung cancer is the most prevalent cause of death and accounts for 18% of all malignancies in men (incidence 75/100,000/year in men and 30/100,000/year in women). Lung cancer rate is five times higher in men than in women. However, whereas in men incidence has been stable over time, in women there is an increase of incidence of 3% per year. With a 5-year survival rate of 9% in men and 17% in women, lung cancer has the worst prognosis of most cancers. With respect to histopathological classification, 20% belong to small cell lung cancer (SCLC), whereas 80% are of NSCLC origin (squamous cell cancer, adeno-cancer, tall cell cancer). However, 5-year survival depends on histopathology and stage of cancer at the time of diagnosis. In general, SCLC is mainly diagnosed at an advanced stage and the 5-year survival rate is below 1%. In an early stage (pT1N0M0), the 5-year survival, especially in NSCLC, improves up to 50–85%.

Conventional diagnosis of lung cancer

Clinical signs of early-stage lung cancer are rare. Most of the tumours are diagnosed by chance on routine chest x-ray. Further conventional work up of a SPN includes CT and/or MRI and invasive methods such as CT guided transthoracic fine-needle aspiration biopsy (CT-TTFNA), bronchoscopy, mediastinoscopy and thoracoscopy [31, 91]. The specificity of non-invasive morphological methods ranges between 60% and 75% [32]. This means that up to 40% of nodules removed by surgery on the basis of morphological methods are benign [67]. Therefore invasive methods are necessary to improve the accuracy for malignancy. Bronchoscopy, an invasive method with low complication rate, is mainly the next step to detect malignancy. However, especially in SPN below a diameter of 2 cm, an accurate diagnosis is obtained in less than 40% of cases. CT-TTFNA is able to diagnose malignant tumours in up to 85%. However, complications such as pneumothorax (15–45%) or hemoptoe are frequent [25, 57]. In the light of the low specificity of morphological methods and the relative high complication rate of invasive diagnosis, non-invasive methods that use criteria other than morphological ones are needed for a better differentiation between malignant and benign disease. F-18 FDG PET images the elevated glucose metabolism of malignant tumours and therefore should be able to discriminate benign from malignant tumours in a non-invasive manner in most cases [88]. Similar problems as stated above exists with morphological methods for staging of lung cancer. Besides the tumour stage, the operability of lung cancer depends on the nodal stage. Nodal involvement of malignant cells up to stage N2 may be operated with curative outcome. However, nodal stage N3 (contralateral lymph node involvement) or distant metastases (M1) are contraindications for surgery. In this light, it is most crucial to know the correct nodal involvement before a therapeutic decision is made. Using CT for staging, a lymph node with a diameter above 1 cm is considered to be pathologic. However, it is evident that lymph nodes below 1 cm may also be infiltrated by malignant cells at an early stage of disease, and contrary lymph nodes above 1 cm may be enlarged due to non-neoplastic infiltration such as inflammation or other causes. Due to the fact that correct nodal staging by CT is achieved in only 75%, FDG PET may also play a major role in the pretherapeutic staging of lung cancer. This is true for nodal staging and the detection of distant metastases [4].

Role of FDG PET in the evaluation of solitary pulmonary nodule (SPN)

SPN is usually diagnosed by chest x-ray and CT. It is estimated that 50 to 60% of SPN are benign. Even if modern CT armamentarium is used, 20–40% of resected SPN are benign, which means unnecessary peri- and postoperative risk for the patient and unnecessary costs for assurance companies and the society.

In a multicenter trial, 89 patients with SPN had chest x-ray, CT, FDG PET and were scheduled for surgery [88]. Histopathology revealed that 60 SPN were malignant and 29 were benign. The calculated sensitivity for FDG PET was 92% (using only visual analysis 98%), the specificity 90%. This means that using FDG PET for decision making of surgery in this study would have reduced the number of unnecessary surgery from 30% to 10%. From a study in Belgium using FDG PET in patients with SPN, the positive predictive value (PPV) was 94%, the negative predictive value 100% [105]. According to literature overview the average sensitivity of FDG PET in SPN is 94%. The specificity ranges a slightly lower because granulomatous diseases, especially tuberculosis, demonstrates also an elevated glucose metabolism and therefore FDG uptake [52, 54, 63, 88, 103, 104, 107, 108]. Depending on the selection of patients the specificity ranges from 78%–93% with an average value of 85%. At our own department, in a period of 24 month, FDG PET was evaluated in 111 patients with SPN, resulting in a sensitivity of 96%, a specificity of 83%, PPV of 86% and NPV of 96%. Reviewing the current literature and our own experience FDG PET should be performed very early, immediately after CT, in the diagnostic work-up of SPN. This procedure reduces the need for invasive diagnostic approach and the rate of complications for the patients. Moreover the number of unnecessary surgery in case of benign nodules can also be reduced as well, which leads to an enormous decrease of costs and to a reduction of peri- and postoperative morbidity. From the economic point of view it could be demonstrated that, from among the different strategies in the work-up of lung cancer (wait and watch strategy, invasive surgical strategy, control CT strategy, CT and FDG PET strategy), the CT and FDG strategy is the most cost-effective one [43].

Role of FDG PET in staging of lung cancer

In case of suspected or known lung cancer, the therapeutic procedure depends on an accurate staging of the disease both within and outside the thorax. In case of ipsilateral lymph node involvement, surgery is the method of choice, because the node can be resected with the primary tumour (Fig. 1). Conversely, if contralateral nodes are involved or in case of extensive mediastinal involvement as well as pleural or distant metastases, surgery is contraindicated, because of morbidity and poor prognosis. Several studies have evaluated FDG PET for the staging of lung cancer [46, 50, 51, 74, 80, 93, 113, 118, 129, 130]. The reported sensitivities for staging lung cancer range from 82% to 100% (average: 91%), the specificity from 73 to

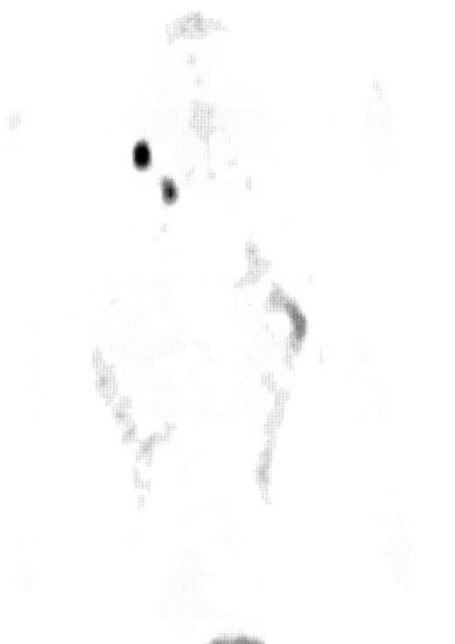

Fig. 1. 45 year old female with 1.5 cm large mass in the right upper lung lobe in the CT; no pathologically enlarged lymph node. FDG PET: hypermetabolic lesion in the right upper lobe and an additional FDG positive lesion in the right hilar region (coronal slice). Histopathology: well differentiated adeno-carcinoma pT1 N1 Mx

100% (average:87%). In a study by Steinert and co-workers, the PPV of CT in staging lung cancer was 76% compared to 96% for FDG PET [Steinert HC et al. 1998]. In a study from Belgium, the prevalence of nodal involvement was 58%. The values for sensitivity, specificity, PPV and NPV were calculated for FDG PET and CT as follows. FDG PET: 85%, 81%, 85%, 81%; CT: 64%, 68%, 67%, 65%. It is noteworthy that, in this study, CT both underestimated and overestimated the extent of disease compared to FDG PET. Not only the extent of nodal involvement but also the lack or presence of distant metastases changes the therapeutic strategy [19]. In a study by Werder an co-workers, FDG PET was performed in 94 patients with lung cancer and compared to conventional work-up. Thirteen out of 94 patients (14%) demonstrated distant extrathoracic metastases, which were not known before. Including lymph node involvement, 20% of patients were understaged by conventional work-up [135].

In a metaanalysis the sensitivity and specificity for F-18-FDG PET was 96% and 80% for the differentiation of benign and malignant pulmonary nodules, 88% and 92% for nodal staging and 94% and 97% for the detection of distant metastases [58].

Thyroid cancer

Introduction

Differentiated thyroid cancer is a relatively rare tumour. The incidence ranges from 4–9/100,000/year. The ratio between women and men is 3:1. 95% of thyroid cancer cases originate from epithelial cells. In iodine sufficient areas, papillary thyroid cancer is the most frequent one and accounts for about 60–70%; follicular thyroid cancer is less frequent (20–30%). Other malignant epithelial tumours of the thyroid gland such as medullary cancer (5–8%) or anaplastic cancer (2–4%) are very rare. The 10-year survival of differentiated thyroid cancer is high and ranges from 80–90% for papillary cancer and 60–70% for follicular cancer. Early diagnosis, adequate therapy and strict follow-up are most important for the prognosis and survival of the patients. As for other tumours, it is also true for thyroid cancer that the nodule is detected by chance mostly via palpation, ultrasonography or scintiscan. For further work-up of such nodules, ultrasonographically-guided fine-needle aspiration is most effective, especially for papillary thyroid cancer [95]. In case of follicular cancer, differentiation between benign adenoma and highly differentiated follicular carcinoma is very difficult or even impossible. Additional nuclear medicine methods such as Tl-201, Tc-99m Sestamibi or Tc-99m Tetrofosmin scintiscan were not able to provide a clear differentiation between follicular adenoma and carcinoma either [81]. Although only some reports with small patient numbers have been published on FDG PET in the preoperative assessment of thyroid nodule, this method seems to have no role for primary diagnosis of thyroid cancer [65]. Therapy of thyroid cancer includes near total or total thyroidectomy, radioiodine (I-131) remnant ablation and thyroid hormone suppressive therapy, in some special cases (pT4N1M0, R1) additional external radiotherapy. This is true for all TNM stages with the exception of papillary thyroid cancer pT1N0M0, in which I-131 remnant ablation is not performed. In case of malignant recurrence or distant metastases, several courses of high-dose I-131 therapy (up to a cumulative activity of 3,7–7,4 GBq) are performed as long as the metastases are well differentiated and store I-131. In case of less differentiated mostly iodine negative metastases, redifferentiation therapy using retinoic acid (before I-131 therapy) or new Y-90-labelled somatostatin receptor ligands are under investigation.

Conventional methods in the follow up of thyroid cancer

In the follow-up of differentiated thyroid cancer, the tumour marker serum thyroglobulin, ultrasonography and I-131 whole-body scintigraphy are well established methods [6, 69, 89]. Under T4-off conditions (bTSH >30 mU/l), serum thyroglobulin has a sensitivity of about 98%. Ultrasonography of the neck including ultrasonography guided fine-needle aspiration biopsy has a high sensitivity for the detection of local recurrences. In case of elevated serum thyroglobulin, I-131 whole-body scintigraphy (WBS) is performed in addition to sonography after 3–4 week withdrawal of thyroid hormone. The sensitivity of I-131 WBS depends on the administered activity. Whereas the diagnostic I-131 WBS (74–185 MbqI-131) has only a sensitivity of 56%, the post-therapeutic I-131 WBS (3700–7400 MBq I-131) has a higher sensitivity of 79%. However, since only 60–80% of cancer recurrences and distant metastases store I-131, additional methods are required to detect I-131-negative metastases in case of elevated serum thyroglobulin. Morphological methods such as CT or MRI play a minor role in the follow-up of thyroid cancer [116]. Non-specific radionuclides such as Tl-201 or newer kationic complexes (Tc-99m Tetrofosmin, Tc-99m Sestamibi) have demonstrated quite good a sensitivity in detecting I-131-negative metastases. The sensitivities for these non-specific tracers range from 45 to 90% [17, 61, 82, 83]. With the introduction of FDG PET in clinical oncology, the question arises: what is the role of FDG PET in the follow-up of differentiated thyroid cancer?

Role of FDG PET in the follow-up of thyroid cancer

FDG PET images the elevated glucose metabolism of malignant tumours. Comparative studies between I-131, Tc-99m Tetrofosmin, Tc-99m Sestamibi and FDG PET in the follow-up of thyroid cancer could demonstrate that the uptake of different tracers is correlated with the differentiation of the metastases. Whereas I-131 is mainly accumulated in well-differentiated metastases, FDG is stored in less differentiated metastases and mainly represents rapid tumour growth. The cationic complexes seem to be in between I-131 and FDG although the correlation to FDG is better than to I-131. Feine and co-workers investigated 41 patients using I-131 WBS and FDG PET in the follow-up of differentiated thyroid cancer. 34 of these patients had elevated serum thyroglobulin levels [37]. In 32/34 patients with elevated thyroglobulin, metastases could be demonstrated only by FDG PET (17 patients), only by I-131 (6 patients) or by both methods (5 patients). They found that most of the I-131-negative metastases demonstrated FDG uptake. In another study by Grünwald and co-workers, 54 patients with thyroid cancer were investigated comparing I-131, Tc-99m Sestamibi and FDG PET [49]. Similar to the above mentioned study, they found that 1) most of the I-131-negative metastases demonstrated FDG uptake; 2) FDG was better correlated to Tc-99m Sestamibi than to I-131; and 3) FDG was superior to Tc-99m Sestamibi in detecting metastases. Similar results were obtained by other authors using FDG PET in the follow-up of differentiated thyroid cancer [5, 26, 34, 131]. In a comparative study which was performed at our own department, 35 patients with elevated serum thyroglobulin had a posttherapeutic I-131 WBS, Tc-99m Tetrofosmin WBS and FDG PET [84, 85]. We found 5 different patterns of uptake within the metastases using these three tracers.

Table 3. Comparison of different methods to follow up differentiated thyroid cancer

Group	I-131	Tc-99m Tetro	F-18-FDG	Number
I	Positive	Positive	Positive	14
II	Negative	Positive	Positive	11
III	Negative	Negative	Positive	4
IV	Positive	Negative	Negative	5
V	Positive	Positive	Negative	1

Most of the I-131-negative metastases demonstrated FDG uptake, most I-131-positive ones failed to do so. In some cases there was I-131 and FDG uptake. Interestingly, FDG was much more sensitive than Tc-99m Tetrofosmin in detecting I-131 negative lesions (Fig. 2).

In contrast to preoperative diagnostics, where the role of FDG PET is not yet clearly evaluated [73, 81] FDG PET is of great value in the postoperative follow-up of differentiated thyroid cancer. In case of elevated serum thyroglobulin but negative I-131 WBS, FDG PET seems to be the method of choice to detect I-131-negative recurrences and metastases. FDG

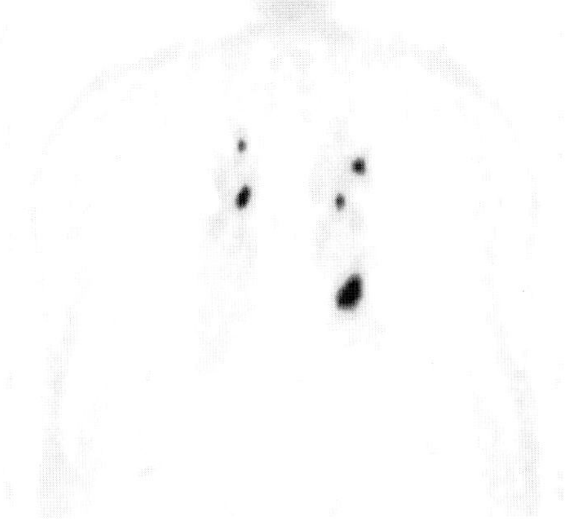

Fig. 2. 72 year old female with follicular thyroid cancer oxyphilic variant pT4 N1 M1 after several courses of radioiodine treatments and negative post-therapeutic I-131 whole-body scan after the last therapy with 5550 MBq I-131. FDG PET: several FDG positive lung metastases and a metastasis in the left adrenal gland (coronal slice)

uptake in metastases from differentiated thyroid cancer seems to be correlated with low differentiation and maybe bad prognosis.

Head and neck cancer including CUP

Introduction

Head and neck cancer is a heterogeneous group of cancers including salivary glands, nose, mouth, tonsillar region, epipharynx and hypopharynx. In men this tumour type is much more frequent than in women (3:1). The incidence is estimated to be 15–20 /100,000/year for men. In about 95% histopathology reveals squamous cell cancer; adeno-cancer, sarcoma or lymphomas are rare. Most cases of head and neck cancers are diagnosed by clinical investigation, especially inspection and palpation. While 60% of patients with head and neck cancer have enlarged lymph nodes at the time of diagnosis, only 40% do have lymph node metastases. The average five-year survival is >50% if no lymph nodes are involved, but only 30% in case of lymph node involvement. Correct staging therefore is important for the prognosis but also for an adequate therapy including surgery and/or radiotherapy or combined radiochemotherapy. For lymph node staging and especially in the follow up after chemo- or radiochemotherapy, morphological methods have difficulties to detect distinct malignant infiltration of the node or to differentiate between scar and viable tumour tissue.

Conventional diagnosis of head and neck cancer

Head and neck cancers are mostly diagnosed by clinical investigation including inspection and palpation. For further work-up, ultrasonography, CT, MRI and biopsies are established methods for pretherapeutic assessment and staging. There is evidence that especially for lymph node metastases, palpation may have a higher specificity than morphological methods [97]. Morphological methods yield information on the extent of the disease and allow also an interpretation of the tumour infiltration into adjacent normal tissue. Problems with morphological methods however, exist for lymph nodes that do not demonstrate morphological signs of malignant infiltration although metastases are present. For CT the sensitivity and specificity for lymph node staging in head and neck cancer range from 75%–82% and 78%–85% respectively [3, 55, 94, 120]. For restaging of head and neck cancer after chemo- or radiochemotherapy, using morphological methods, it is often impossible to differentiate between scar and viable residual tumour tissue. Another problem in the head and neck region is the fact that sometimes enlarged lymph nodes are detected. These lymph nodes are surgically removed. If histology reveals lymph node metastases of squamous cell or adeno-cancer, the question of the location of the primary tumour arises. However, despite intensive conventional work-up including multiple biopsies, no primary tumour can be detected in some cases.

Role of FDG PET in lymph node staging of head and neck cancer

Lymph node involvement is the most important prognostic factor in patients with head and neck cancer and influences also the therapeutic strategy. In this light, an accurate lymph node staging should be performed in all patients. For the interpretation of FDG images in head and neck cancer it is important to know that several structures, especially the muscles of the vocal cord and the tonsillae, demonstrate more or less intensive FDG uptake. Because most of the primaries are detected clinically and CT or MRI are accurate methods to demonstrate the extent of the tumour, FDG PET, with the exception of CUP, plays no major role for primary head and neck cancers. Most of the work up to now concerning FDG PET and head and neck cancers have concentrated on lymph node staging in case of known primary, therapy follow-up after radio- or combined radiochemotherapy and the detection of the primary tumour in case of CUP despite extensive conventional work up [1, 36, 90, 106]. It is well-known that morphological methods such as CT may under- or overestimate lymph node involvement. In a study published by Adams and co-workers, sensitivity and specificity of CT, MRI and FDG PET were compared in 1284 lymph nodes which were histologically investigated after resection [3]. Sensitivity and specificity for FDG PET were 90% and 94%, whereas the values for CT and MRI were 82% and 85% and 80% and 79% respectively. Similar results were published by other authors some years ago. Bailet and co-workers evaluated CT and FDG PET in 203 lymph nodes from 8 neck dissection specimens [7]. FDG PET accurately diagnosed 71% of involved nodes, whereas CT was correct in only 59%. In a study performed by Bender and co-workers, FDG PET was able to change the final staging in 25% of 150 patients investigated [10]. Based on 574 interpretable cases reported in the literature, sensitivity and specificity of FDG-PET alone in cervical lymph node staging are 85% and 91%, respectively, versus 76% and 78% for conventional imaging (CT/MRI/US). Similar values (82% and 100% for FDG-PET versus 81% and 81% for CT) have been confirmed recently [56]. All studies performed up to now have

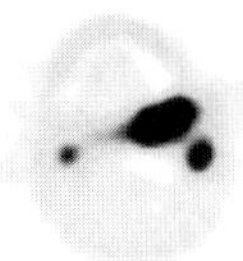

Fig. 3. 70 year old male with biopsy proven squamous cell carcinoma of the left tonsilla. FDG PET: a transaxial slice demonstrates a large hypermetabolic lesion in the left tonsillar region (primary tumour) and FDG positive spots on the right and left cervical region (lymph node metastases)

demonstrated that FDG PET has a major role in the correct staging of patients with head and neck cancer (Fig. 3).

Role of FDG PET in restaging after radio- or radiochemotherapy

In case of advanced tumour stage, radiotherapy or combined radiochemotherapy are the therapeutic options of choice. In these patients is often difficult to differentiate between scar and viable residual tumour tissue. Several studies were performed to evaluate the role of FDG PET in the follow-up of these patients. Greven and co-workers investigated 18 patients 4 months after radiotherapy using FDG PET [47]. Eleven out of 18 patients had a negative FDG PET at the primary site and non of them developed recurrent disease. From the remaining 7 patients with positive FDG PET, 6 had a biopsy-proven residual or recurrent tumour. Concerning the lymph nodes, all 15 patients with negative FDG PET were negative in the follow- up, however, in 2 out of 3 patients with positive FDG PET biopsy-proven residual nodal disease could be demonstrated. In a study by Lowe and co-workers, FDG PET was evaluated in 28 patients before and after chemotherapy because of head and neck cancer [87]. Sensitivity of FDG PET in this study was 90%, specificity 83%. From the same group the results were published recently with the additional statement that there was positive correlation between percent reduction in tumour volume by CT and SUV by FDG PET ($p < 0.04$, $r = 0.60$). The authors conclude that FDG PET and CT imaging are at least equivalent in correctly assessing tumour response to chemotherapy with a trend towards better performance by PET [28]. Several studies are in progress to evaluate the role of FDG PET in patients after combined radiochemotherapy. FDG PET therefore may have a role in the future in the re-evaluation of patients after radio- or radiochemotherapy (Fig. 4). However, it is important to bear in mind that the time of FDG PET imaging after the last chemotherapy or radiochemotherapy should not be less than 6 weeks and 4 months respectively. Whether an early FDG PET during chemo- or radiochemotherapy may predict the outcome of therapy or lead to a change of the therapeutic strategy is under investigation but is not yet clear.

Role of FDG PET in carcinoma of unknown primary (CUP)

It is a known problem that in some cases with histologically proven lymph node metastases the primary tumour is unknown despite intensive work-up including biopsies in the head and neck area. The sensitivities for FDG PET in detecting the primary in case of CUP after conventional work up range from 25–53%. In a study by Braams and co-workers, FDG PET was able to detect the primary in 4 out of 13 patients with CUP [15]. In study by Aassar and co-workers, the sensitivity for FDG PET to detect the primary in case of CUP was

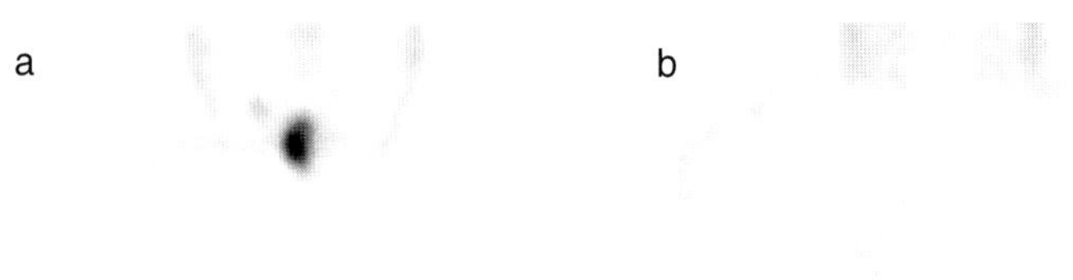

Fig. 4a. 56 year old male with biopsy proven sqamous cell carcinoma of the larynyx. FDG PET: hypermetabolic lesion in the right larynx and a FDG positive lymph node metastasis nod demonstrated by CT (coronal slice); the patient underwent radiochemotherapy. **b.** Same patient 3 months after radiochemotherapy; FDG PET: no hypermetabolic lesion indicating viable tumour tissue

53% [1]. Similar results were obtained in recent studies [14, 66, 109]. According to our own experience FDG PET was able to detect 9 out of 15 primaries with CUP [72] (Fig. 5).

Malignant melanoma

Introduction

Malignant melanoma (MM) belongs to the most aggressive tumours of the skin and mucosa. The incidence of MM has been increasing over the last decades and ranges, depending on geography, from 10/100,000/year (Europe) to 40/100,000/year (Queensland). The key factor influencing prognosis is the thickness of the primary tumour [16]. Whereas the 5-year survival is high in clinical stages Ia (97%) and Ib (90%), it decreases in stages IIa (73%) and IIb (53%). Lymph node metastases decrease the 5-year survival to 37% (stage III), distant metastases to below 10% (stage IV). Detection at an early stage is most important for the survival of the patient because surgery and radiotherapy in lower stages may be curative. On the other hand, an accurate staging of patients, especially in case of higher suspicion of metastases (stage III), is necessary. Due to a very high glycolytic metabolism of MM, FDG PET should be able to detect metastases of MM in the staging of high-risk patients as well as in the follow-up.

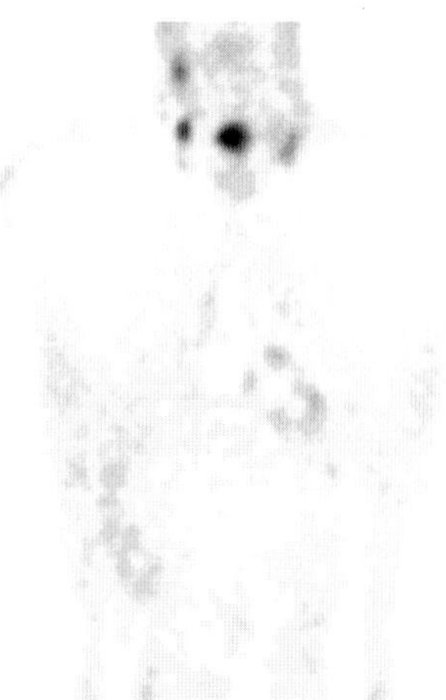

Fig. 5. 45 year old male with lymph node enlargement on both cervical sides and histologically proven metastases of squamous cell carcinoma; no primary found; only MRI demonstrated suspicion of an abnormality on the base of the tongue on the left side. FDG PET: clear uptake in several lymph nodes on both cervical sides but also a hypermetabolic lesion on the base of the tongue according to the primary carcinoma

Conventional diagnosis in malignant melanoma

As most of the MMs are located on the skin, the diagnosis of the primary tumour is made by inspection and excision biopsy. In case of non-palpable nodes, ultrasonography may detect changes in the lymph node suspicious for metastatic infiltration in up to 30% [12]. However, for non-palpable lymph nodes, the sentinel node concept with the identification and removal of the sentinel node is the most accurate method to detect lymph node metastases [112]. In case of palpable lymph nodes, ultrasonography and fine-needle aspiration biopsy are performed. Ultrasonography has a high sensitivity (94%) and a rather good specificity in those cases (87%). For the detection of systemic metastases, a variety of methods with different sensitivities and specificities including abdominal sonography, CT, MRI and nuclear medicine methods such as Ga-67 scintigraphy and scintigraphy with monoclonal antibodies are performed. However, not all modalities are effective in all areas. Whereas MRI is the method of choice for metastases in the brain and liver, CT has an advantage over MRI in the lung. In addition to the possibility of whole-body imaging using FDG PET, this modality may have a role in the early detection of distant metastases due to the elevated glucose metabolism.

Role of FDG PET in malignant melanoma

There is consensus today that high-resolution FDG PET using a ring scanner is the best method to detect metastases from MM in most regions of the body with the exception of brain and liver (Fig. 6). In a study by Gritters and co-workers an overall sensitivity of 91% for detecting metastases and a sensitivity of 97% for metastases > 5 mm was achieved [48]. In another study by Steinert and co-workers, 33 patients were investigated using FDG PET [119]. While 10 patients had newly diagnosed MM stage IIa with a higher risk for metastases, metastases were already known in 23 patients. From a total of 53 lesions, 40 were proven to be metastases. FDG PET correctly identified 37 out of 40 metastases (93%). Three small metastases below 3 mm in diameter were missed by FDG PET. In a study by Nguyen and co-workers involving 45 patients, FDG PET was performed due to high-risk (n = 15) or recurrent (n = 30) melanoma. FDG PET facilitated clinical decision-making in 33% mostly due to detection of distant metastases, rendering a surgical procedure inappropriate [99]. In 6% FDG PET was false positive, in 14% false negative. False negative scans were noticed in very small lung metastases and in brain metastases, the false positive in benign liver lesions

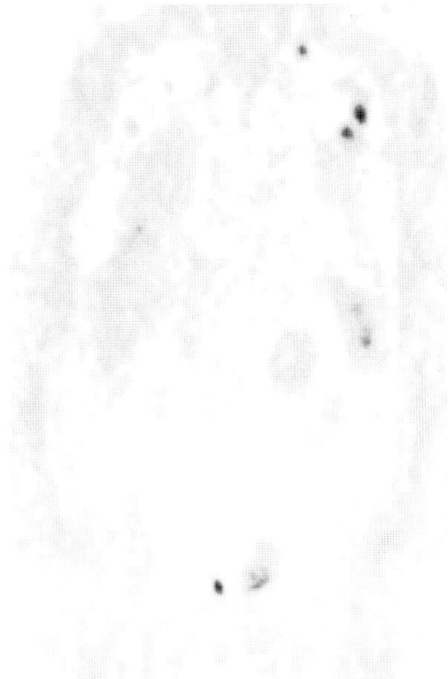

Fig. 6. 58 year old male with malignant melanoma level IV in the left shoulder. Surgical removal of axillary lymph node metastases, chemotherapy and external radiation therapy. FDG PET: restaging of this patient revealed several FDG positive hot spots spread all over the body including both axillae, mediastinum, liver, adrenal gland and spleen (only partially shown on this 7 mm coronal slice)

and sarcoidosis. Prospectively, Tyler and co-workers investigated 106 whole body PET scans obtained after injection of 2-[^{18}F]fluorine-2-fluoro-2-deoxy-D-glucose (FDG) in 95 patients with clinically evident stage III lymph node and/or in-transit melanoma metastases [128]. 13/39 false-positive areas were due to recent surgery, 3 to arthritis, 3 to infection, 2 to superficial phlebitis, 1 to a benign skin naevus and 1 to a colonic polyp. The sensitivity, specificity was 87.3% (144/165 areas), 43.5%, respectively. FDG PET changed management in 16/106 patients (15.1%). In contrast to the role of FDG PET in the detection distant metastases, recurrent disease and follow-up staging, its value is not yet clear in primary lymph node staging. However, it is likely that in a study comparing the SLN concept with FDG PET, which has yet to be undertaken, FDG PET would miss micrometastases.

Colorectal cancer

Introduction

Colorectal cancer is one of the most frequent cancers in western countries. With an incidence of 43/100,000/year in men, it is the third most frequent cancer after prostate and lung cancer. In women, colorectal cancer ranges behind breast and lung cancer with an incidence of 28/100,000/year. Twenty years ago, about 25% of colorectal cancer were inoperable at the time of diagnosis [21]. Due to screening programs, this situation has changed over time. Prognosis of colorectal cancer depends on stage and radical resection. Whereas the 5-year survival in stage I is 100%, it decreases to 87% for colon and 69% for rectal cancer and is below 50% in stage III. For the diagnosis of colorectal cancer, feces blood investigation, rectal palpation, rectosigmoideoscopy or coloscopy including biopsy are established methods. Surgery is the only curative treatment whether for primary or for recurrent disease. In the follow-up of patients with colorectal cancer it important to detect malignant recurrence at an early stage and to detect distant metastases when they are not wide-spread. As in other cancer types, morphological methods such as CT have the problem in the postoperative follow-up that a differentiation between scar and recurrence is difficult or impossible at an early stage. It could also be demonstrated that serum CEA has only a marginal role in the early detection of recurrences. Especially in early extraluminal recurrence detection and early detection of distant metastases, FDG PET should have advantages over morphological methods.

Conventional diagnosis in the follow-up of colorectal cancer

Locoregional recurrences appear in 75% within 2 years after surgery. They may occur at the site of the anastomosis, locoregionally, as lymph node or distant metastases. The results of therapy are greatly influenced by the time of diagnosis. The postoperative follow-up of colorectal cancer includes determination of serum CEA, coloscopy, CT, MRI and sometimes anti-CEA IS [86]. Although the overall sensitivity for serum CEA is high, for the special group of early recurrence serum CEA may be negative. For the detection of intraluminal recurrences, coloscopy and intraluminal ultrasonography (especially in the rectosigmoidal area) are suitable methods, in case of suspicious extraluminal recurrences, lymph node and distant metastases ultrasonography, CT and MRI are established. However, sometimes it is very difficult to differentiate postoperative scar from early recurrence using CT or MRI [41]. A second problem with morphological methods is the early detection of distant metastases, especially of liver metastases. Only 20% of liver metastases with a diameter below 1 cm are diagnose by ultrasonography. Immunoscintigraphy using Tc-99m labelled monoclonal antibodies against CEA could demonstrate that early detection of locoregional recurrence is possible despite normal serum CEA and unsuspicious CT. As regards the detection of liver metastases, anti CEA-IS is able to detect metastases earlier than other methods in some cases, however, the physiological uptake of the antibody in the liver makes the diagnosis much more difficult compared to other regions. The sensitivity of anti- CEA IS for detecting local recurrences or distant metastases ranges between 38% and 91% the specificity between 67% and 100%.

Role of FDG PET in the restaging of colorectal cancer

While the role of FDG PET in the preoperative evaluation has not yet been established, several studies have been able to demonstrate that FDG PET is an important method to follow up patients with colorectal cancer. The early detection of recurrent disease is desirable because about 30% of recurrences are resectable. In addition, single metastases or metastases of limited extent in liver and lung are resectable. In a very early study conducted in 1989, Strauss and co-workers investigated 29 patients after rectum resection who had equivocal CT mass [123]. Histology revealed malignant recurrence in 21 and scar tissue in 8 cases. FDG PET demonstrated elevated FDG uptake in 20 out of 21 patients with malignant recurrence. In one false negative case, FDG uptake was only moderate. All 8 patients with scar tissue did not demonstrate FDG uptake. In a comparative study between CT and FDG PET in patients with suspicion of recurrent or metastasizing colorectal cancer, Ogunbiyi and co-workers found a much higher sensitivity and specificity for FDG PET (91% and 100%) compared to CT (52% and 80%) [100]. Debelke and co-workers compared FDG PET with CT and CT portography in 52 patients with suspicion of liver metastases [29]. The diagnostic accuracy for FDG PET was 92% compared to 78% for CT and 80% CT portography. In a study by Lai and co-workers in 34 patients with suspicion of recurrent colorectal cancer, FDG PET detected extrahepatic metastases in 11 patients (32%) not known before, which resulted in a change of therapy in 10 patients (29%) [77]. Some data exist also on the therapy control after radiotherapy and chemotherapy. In a study performed by Haberkorn and co-workers, 20 patients with inoperable colorectal cancer were investigated before and after radiotherapy. In 11 patients there was a decrease, in 2 patients an increase and in 7 patients no change in FDG uptake [53]. This underlines that FDG PET performed immediately after radiotherapy cannot predict the therapeutic effect. It is therefore recommended that the time interval between radiation therapy and therapy control using FDG PET should be 4–6 months. Similar studies were performed using FDG PET before and after chemotherapy. Findley and co-workers investigated 20 patients before, 1–2 and 4–5 weeks after combined 5-FU/INF alpha chemotherapy using FDG PET [39]. Response to chemotherapy did not correlate with the initial tumour /liver ratio. Metastases with response after chemotherapy demonstrated a marked reduction of FDG ratio tumour/liver. This was predictive for therapy response 4–5 weeks after chemotherapy.

Pancreatic cancer

Introduction

Among the gastrointestinal malignancies, pancreatic cancer has the worst prognosis. In a small number of patients pancreatic cancer is diagnosed at an early stage. The incidence ranges from 3–5/100,000/year. Pancreatic cancer is more frequent in men than in women. Clinical signs are non-specific and do not allow early diagnosis. If a tumour in the pancreatic region is diagnosed, mostly during routine investigation by ultrasonograpghy, the question arises whether this tumour is benign or malignant. It is also important to know whether the tumour is resectable or not and whether there are distant metastases, which means inoperability for the patient. To answer these questions several modalities like endosonography, CT or MRI and ERCP should be performed.

Conventional diagnosis of pancreatic cancer

Pancreatic tumours are often diagnosed by chance during routine investigations. If clinical symptoms or laboratory changes occur, the disease is in advanced stage in most cases. Spiral CT is considered to be the most sensitive method for staging pancreatic tumours and to answer the question whether the tumour is resectable [13, 33]. However, inflammatory pseudotumours may also produce results similar to pancreatic cancer with infiltration and lymph node enlargement and lead to false positive results. Endosonography has a similar sensitivity for pancreatic tumours, however, it is extremely dependent on the experience of the investigator. The results of MRI are comparable with spiral CT. Despite the high sensitivity of morphological methods between 85–92%, there is a role for metabolic imaging in selected cases.

Role of FDG PET in the staging of pancreatic cancer

Most pancreatic cancers demonstrate an elevated FDG uptake. If a standard uptake value (SUV) is calculated, the best cut-off between cancer and chronic inflammation or benign disease is 2. If no SUV is calculated, the uptake should be higher than in normal liver tissue. In a study by Ho and co-workers, 12 patients with intermediate pancreatic mass on CT and 2 with typical malignancy signs were investigated using FDG PET [60]. Eight out of 14 patients had pancreatic cancer. FDG PET was able to identify cancer in all 8 patients using an SUV cut-off of 2.5. Two out of the 6 benign lesions were false positive on FDG PET. In another study published by Stollfuss and co-workers, CT and FDG PET was compared in 73 patients with suspicious pancreatic cancer [122]. Using a SUV above 1.53 for malignancy, the sensitivity for FDG PET was 93% with a specificity of 93%. Visual interpretation gave a sensitivity of 95% and a specificity of 90%. Abdominal CT in contrast had much lower values (sensitivity: 80%, specificity 74%). Bares and co-workers investigated 40 patients with suspicious pancreatic cancer and compared FDG PET, CT and sonography not only for the primary tumour but also for lymph node involvement [9]. FDG PET in this study had a sensitivity of 92% and a slightly lower specificity of 84%. Concerning lymph node involvement, the sensitivity of FDG PET was much higher (76%) compared to CT (17%) and ultrasonography (6%). In another study in 106 patients with pancreatic mass the sensitivity was 85%, the specificity 84% [137]. Although only few studies have been performed on FDG PET in pancreatic cancer compared to other tumour types, it seems that FDG PET plays a role in the non-invasive evaluation of pancreatic tumours and the detection of metastatic disease. The role for lymph node staging has to be investigated in larger series.

Lymphoma

Introduction

Lymphomas originate from lymphoid tissue and account for about 8–10% of malignancies. They are divided into Hodgkins lymphoma (HL) and Non-Hodgkins lymphoma (NHL). According to Ann Arbor classification there are 4 stages of disease extent. The extent of involvement is the most important factor for failure-free survival and survival of patients. The incidence of HL is 3/100 000/year with a peak between 15–35 years. From the 4 histological types of HL, nodular sclerosis is the most common type (65%) and it is usually located in the mediastinum. Accurate staging and appropriate therapy has led to remission rates of 80–90%. The incidence of NHL is 4–5 /100,000/year with a peak beyond the age of 50. 70% of NHL are B-cell, 30% T-cell, 30% high-grade (untreated survival: weeks), 70% low-grade (untreated survival: years) lymphomas. Most patients have stage III or IV at presentation and up to 40% have bone marrow involvement. Appropriate staging and treatment leads to 50–70% remission in NHL. Correct staging of the patients appropriate treatment and correct restaging after treatment are most important for a good outcome. With the general use of CT and MRI in recent years, staging of patients for lymphoma has improved.

Conventional diagnosis and staging of lymphoma

For the diagnosis of HL and NHL, clinical and laboratory investigations as well as morphological methods such as CT are performed, but finally histology is necessary. If HL or NHL has been histologically proven staging of disease is most important for appropriate therapy [22, 38]. CT is a useful method to define the sites and the extent of nodal and extranodal disease [Castellino RA et al. 1998]. A lymph node larger than 1 cm is considered to be pathologic. The same is true for MRI. Neither CT nor MRI are able to detect structural abnormalities within involved lymph nodes. This means that morphological method do not provide any direct information on the infiltration of the lymph node with malignant cells. It is evident that CT and MRI may therefore under- as well as overestimate the extent of disease. However, this problem of morphology-based definition of the extent of disease, plays a more pronounced role in the restaging after chemo- and/or radiotherapy. In case of bulky disease, a CT mass of several centimeters in diameter often remains. It is very difficult or even impossible to differentiate fibrosclerosis from residual tumour using CT in those patients. Yet this differentiation is most important for the further therapeutic strategy and, in the end, for the survival of the patient. On the other hand, a reduction of enlarged lymph nodes below 1 cm after therapy is usually interpreted as therapy response and remission. However, every recurrence after remission means that, despite normal CT or MRI at the time of restaging the patient was not disease-free. It is therefore evident that also lymph nodes below 1cm after therapy may still be infiltrated with malignant cells. This is the reason why we need methods that are based on other criteria than morphological ones.

Role of FDG PET in staging and restaging of lymphoma

Due to the high glucose metabolism of HL and NHL, FDG PET should lead to a further improvement in the staging and especially restaging of lymphoma patients (Fig. 7). Moog and co-workers investigated 60 patients (33 HL, 27 NHL) comparing FDG PET and CT for initial staging [96]. Discordant results between the two methods were verified by biopsy or clinical follow-up. 160 out of 740 lymph nodes evaluated were interpreted as being involved via both methods. PET detected 25 additional regions with elevated FDG uptake (7 true positive, 2 false positive, 16 unresolved). CT demonstrated 6 lesions not imaged by FDG PET (3 false positive, 3 unresolved). Hoh and co-workers compared FDG PET and conventional staging in 18 patients with lymphoma (7HL, 11NHL). FDG PET demonstrated accurate staging in 17 of 18, conventional staging in 15 of 18 patients. FDG PET showed additional lesions in 5, conventional staging in 4 patients [62]. In a study by Bangerter and co-workers 44 newly diagnosed patients with HL underwent FDG PET. PET findings were compared with findings of conventional staging including CT, US, BS (bone scintigraphy), bone marrow biopsy, liver biopsy and laparatomy. Different results between FDG PET and conventional work up were seen when re-evaluated by biopsy, if possible, or MRI. FDG PET was positive in 38 out of 44 (86%) patients at the site of documented disease. FDG PET led to an upstaging in 5 patients and a downstaging in one patient. A change in therapeutic strategy due to FDG PET results was necessary in 14% of patients [8]. Similar results, demonstrating the superiority of FDG PET over other methods were reported by Talbot and others in several additional studies in recent years [70, 125]. Clear data on the advantage of FDG PET compared to CT are given in the study by Stumpe and co-workers [124]. They investigated 50 patients with lymphoma (35 HL, 15 NHL). There was no major difference for sensitivity and specificity of FDG PET between HL and NHL. Also sensitivity for FDG PET and CT were similar. However, FDG PET showed much better specificity compared to CT in HL as well as NHL (see Table 2).

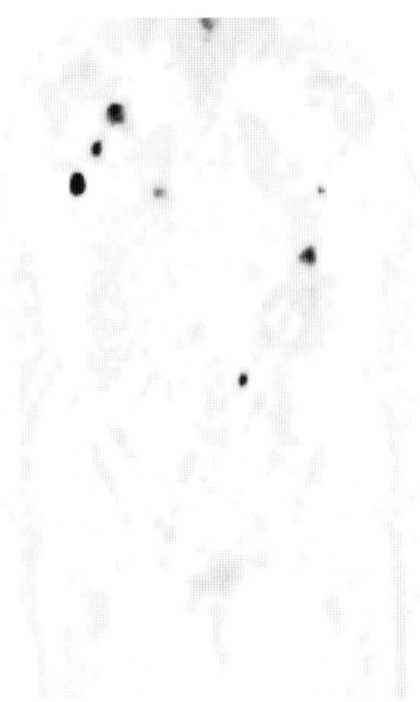

Fig. 7. 59 year old female with NHL CSIII. PET demonstrates on a whole body scan multiple FDG positive lesions in the right axilla, left axilla (not shown on this coronal slice), right hilus, splee, paraaortal region (not shown on this coronal slice) and right iliacal region

Thill and co-workers pointed out in 27 lymphoma patients that FDG and CT was equal in the cervical region, but FDG PET was much more sensitive in all other regions, especially in the abdomen, compared to CT [127].

One of the most interesting indications for FDG PET is the therapy control after chemo- or radiotherapy. In a study by Mainolfi and co-workers, 32 patients were investigated using FDG PET and CT before and after chemotherapy [92]. In 78% of lesions there was agreement between FDG PET and CT, 30 in complete remission, 15 in partial regression and 17 in progression. In the remaining 22% there was disagreement between the 2 methods. No FDG uptake was found by FDG PET in 9 patients with fibrosclerosis despite CT abnormalities. Slight FDG uptake was found by PET in 8 patients with residual disease despite normal CT. FDG PET is highly sensitive and specific to evaluated residual tumour tissue or remission in the follow-up of lymphoma patients after chemotherapy. Gambhir reported changes in patient management in 10% of cases investigated for recurrence work-up (n = 158). Higher rates (up to 60%) were reported in a recent study by Schroeder and coworkers [42, 115]. Römer and co-workers pointed out that FDG PET 6 weeks after chemotherapy was superior in the prediction of long term outcome over FDG PET 1 week after chemotherapy

Table 4. Sensitivity and specificity of PET and CT in HD and NHL according to Stumpe et al. 1998 [124]

	FDG PET(HL)	CT(HL)	FDG PET(NHL)	CT(NHL)
Sensitivity	86	81	89	86
Specificity	96	41	100	67

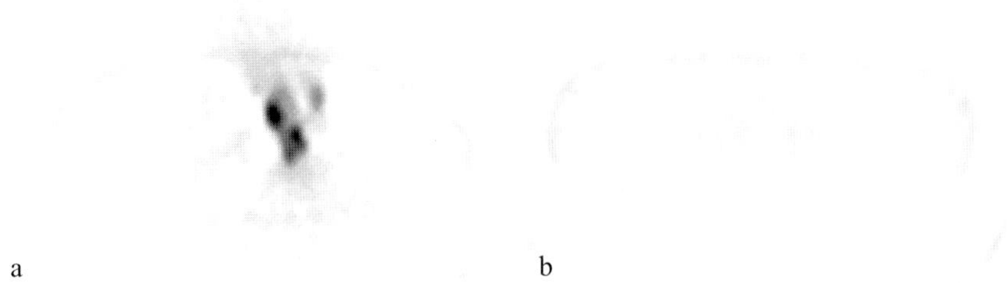

Fig. 8a. 34 year old male with HL with bulky disease in the mediastinum (CT:9 × 8 × 7 cm mass in diameter). FDG PET: hypermetabolic FDG positive lesion in the mass described by CT; this patient underwent chemotherapy. **b.** Same patient 3 months after chemotherapy, CT yet demonstrated a mass of 4 cm in diameter. FDG PET: no pathologic FDG uptake in the mediastinum indicating that viable tumor tissue is not likely

[111]. Today it seems to be accepted that in the therapy control of tumour patients, especially of lymphoma patients, FDG PET should be performed not earlier than 6 weeks after chemotherapy and 3 months after radiotherapy.

Cost – effectiveness of FDG PET in oncology

There are several studies that demonstrate that using FDG PET at an early stage of cancer diagnosis is cost effective in most cancer types described above. For SPN and lung cancer cost effectiveness was described by Ghambir and others [35, 43]. The cost-effectiveness of FDG-PET in the management of NSCLC has also been evaluated in Japan by Kosuda, who conducted a decision-tree analysis to assess whether comparable results may be obtained in Japan where different management strategies are in use (e.g. less frequent mediastinoscopy and more frequent bronchoscopy) and costs of medical interventions differ markedly compared to western countries (e.g. very low cost of bronchoscopy). A simulation of a cohort of 1000 patients with suspected NSCLC indicated that the chest CT + chest FDG-PET strategy would reduce the number of bronchoscopies (−50%) and of unnecessary exploratory thoracotomies, while the number of medastinoscopies and curative thoracotomies would increase. Life expectancy would increase by 0.6 year, as would do the costs by 1.730 €/life-year saved/patient [71]. These results are in contrast with the European and American studies and indicate that cost-effectiveness studies are closely related to the social and economical context. Also for head and neck cancer FDG-PET is likely to be cost-effective in staging, due to the possibility, in FDG conclusive patients, to avoid other expensive examinations such as repeated panendoscopy and invasive procedures the cost of a neck dissection being considerably higher than that of a PET examination. There is also a cost associated with random biopsies of potential sites of residual/recurrent disease, and its potential patient morbidity because of the risk of biopsy-associated soft-tissue necrosis or infection [120, 121]. A lower morbidity for the patient is expected from FDG PET, consequence of an earlier and more correct diagnosis, leading to a better adapted management. Furthermore, a positive PET examination can direct the clinician to the most likely biopsy site to yield tumour, and intervention can be accomplished early, when the likelihood of successful salvage therapy is the greatest. In some cases, a false-positive scan may be associated with the additional cost of what proves to be an unnecessary biopsy if the clinician feels a biopsy is warranted. These costs, however, are more than balanced by the savings and the lower morbidity, resulting from the high negative predictive value of the technique [40]. A cost-effectiveness analysis of FDG-PET *versus* CT for the

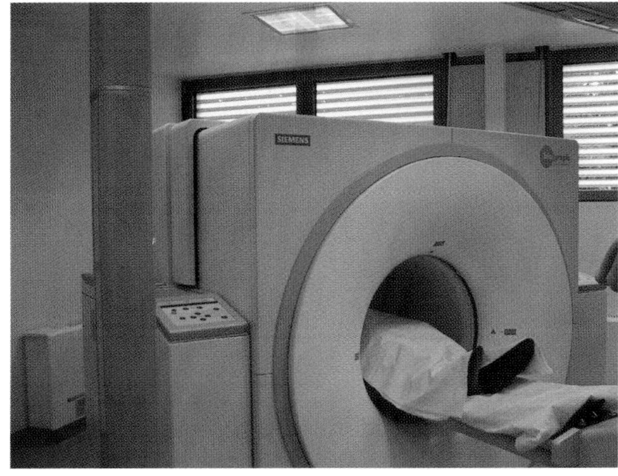

Fig. 9. Combined PET/CT Scanner: Biograph ® Siemens/CTI with a dual slice CT and full ring LSO PET scanner

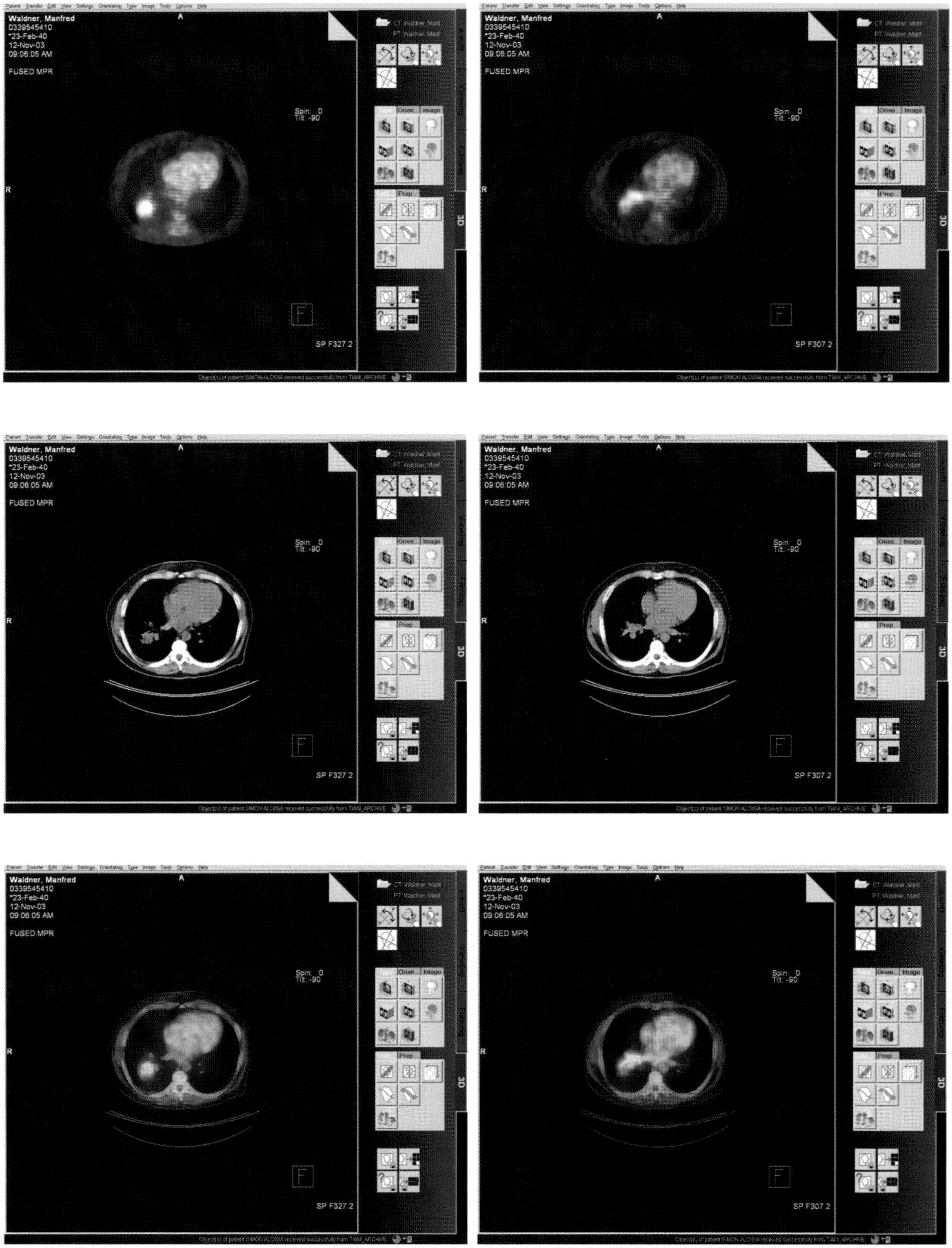

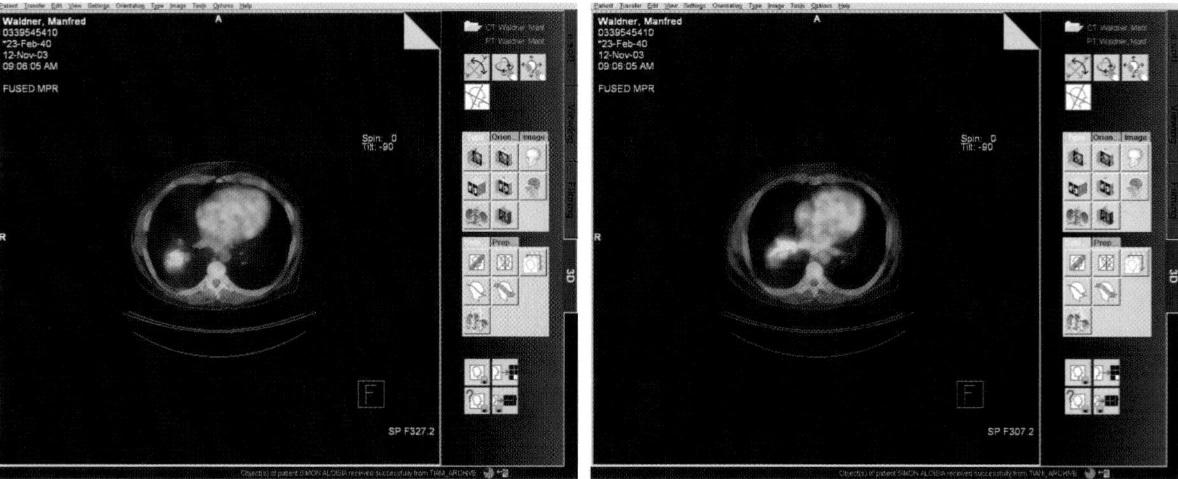

Fig. 10. PET/CT in a 63 year old male with SPN in the right lower lobe. FDG PET demonstrates elevated FDG uptake in the SPN; in addition lymph node metastases in the right hilus were detected. PET (**a**), CT (**b**) and PET/CT (**c**) is shown for the primary tumor (left row) and for the hilar lymph node metastases (right row)

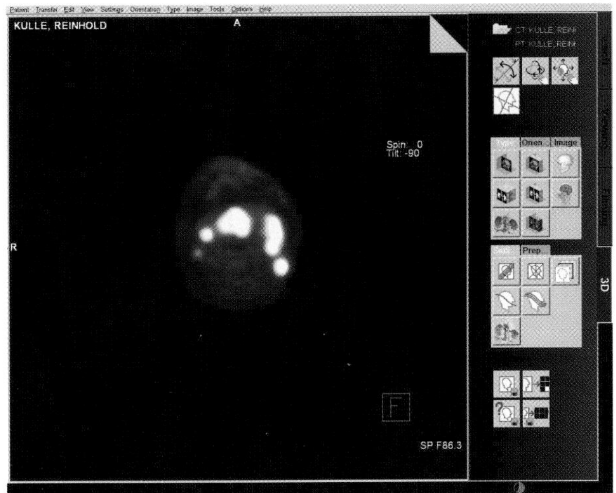

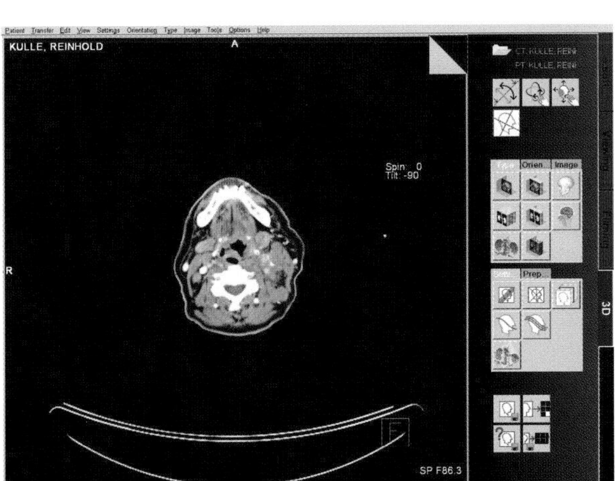

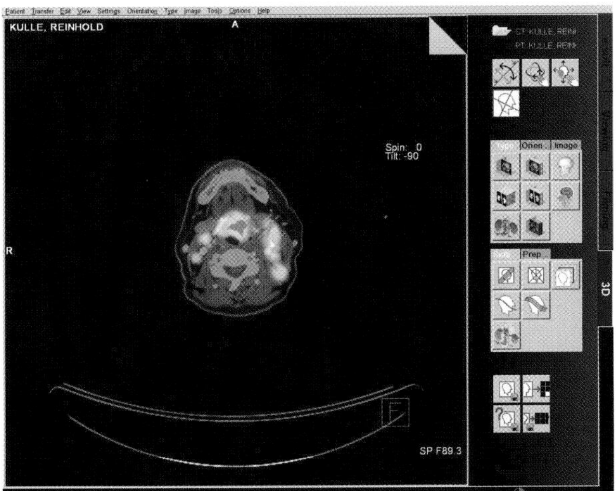

Fig. 11. PET/CT in a 73 year old male with suspicion of cancer in dorsal area of the tongue. PET (**a**), CT (**b**) and PET/CT(**c**) demonstrates pathologic FDG uptake in the primary tumor and in lymph nodes on both sides of the cervical region

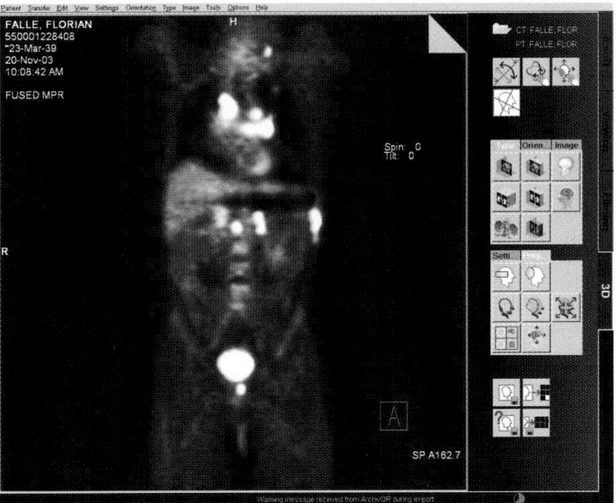

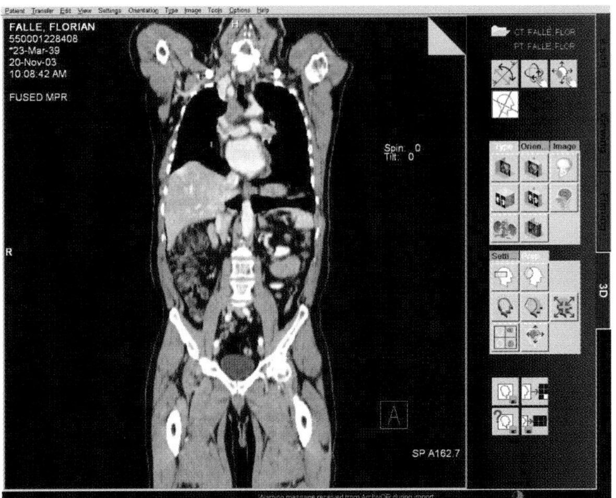

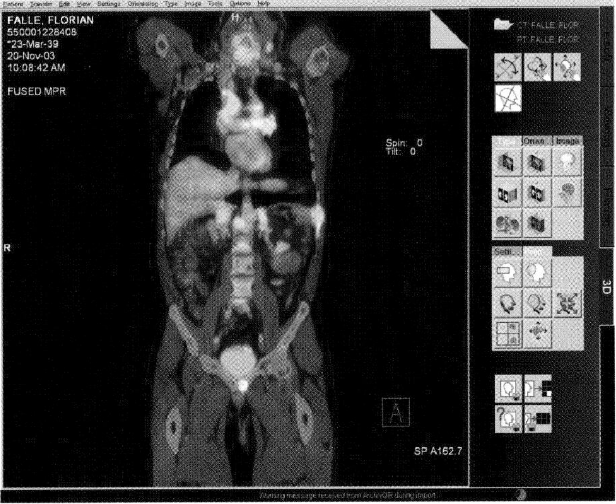

Fig. 12. PET/CT in a 64 year old male after surgery of a malignant melanoma of the right thumb (pT4a N0 Mx), Clark level IV, Breslow 4.5 mm in June 2001. FDG PET/CT was performed for restaging due to an elevated

primary staging of lymphomas, was carried out in 22 patients by Klose and co-workers [69]. Incremental cost-effectiveness ratios (i.e. the additional costs of a more effective diagnostic strategy per additional correctly staged patient) were 478 € for CT *versus* the "no diagnostics" strategy, and 3133 € for FDG-PET *versus* CT. If extra-cost can be estimated to be in the neighbouring of 500 € per patient as compared to CT alone (961 € for PET and 391 € for CT) for the initial staging of lymphoma, FDG-PET additional costs must be put in parallel with the clinical impact (4 patients were upstaged), the costs of unnecessary treatments, that the method allows to avoid, and with the treatment costs of HD (up to 135,000 €) and NHL (up to 75,000 €). Cost-effectiveness in malignant melanoma is difficult to appreciate, since there is no well-established work-up pattern for the metastasized disease, due to the small size and the highly variable metastatic spread. For this reason, whole-body scanning with FDG-PET seems very useful and can be used instead of the battery of usual screening tests (chest X-rays, CT of the brain, chest and abdomen, ultrasonography of the abdomen and LN) that are generally necessary for extensive exploration. Several cost-effectiveness studies attempted to estimate the savings that might result from preoperative PET in recurrent colorectal cancer patients: Without taking into account the costs for (avoided) surgical interventions, Staib and co-workers evaluated retrospectively that US$39.735 could have been saved for 100 patients simply by omitting the procedures which could have been replaced by PET, i.e. ~ US$400 per patient, a value similar to US$445 found by Abdel-Nabi [2]. Valk estimated, from data obtained in 134 colorectal cancer patients explored for preoperative evaluation of recurrence, that the reduction of surgery for non-resectable tumour from the usual ~40% rate to less than 20% could result in savings of US$3000 per patient, after subtraction of PET costs [117]. Park used a rigorous decision tree analysis based on theoretical models (and current prices of CT and FDG-PET in the USA), to assess the cost-effectiveness of a strategy in which FDG-PET is performed after CT for the diagnosis and management of recurrent colorectal cancer, compared to a CT-alone strategy. They found that the

Fig. 12 (Continued)
supraclavicula lymph node on the left side. PET (**a**), CT (**b**) and PET/CT (**c**) demostrates multiple lymph node metastases cervical, supraclavicular, in the left axilla, in the mediastinum, in the abdominal and retroperitoneal region (not all shown on this slice); in addition multiple lung and bone metastases were detected

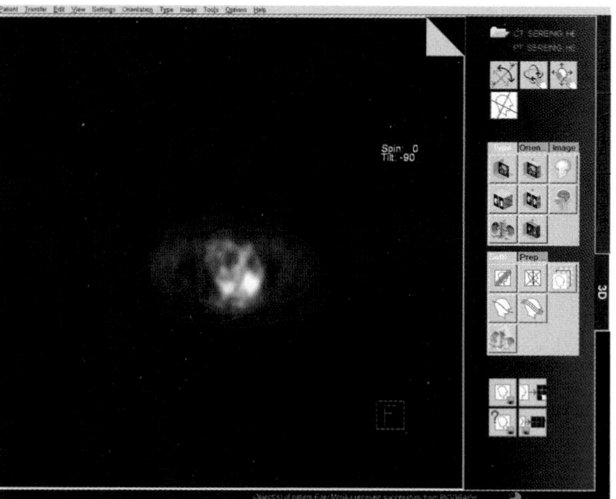

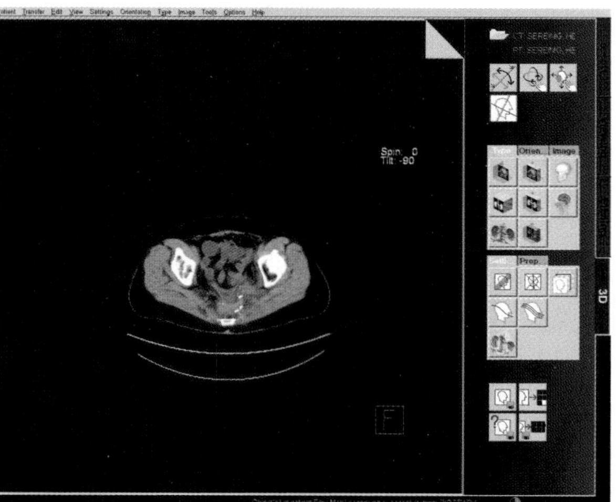

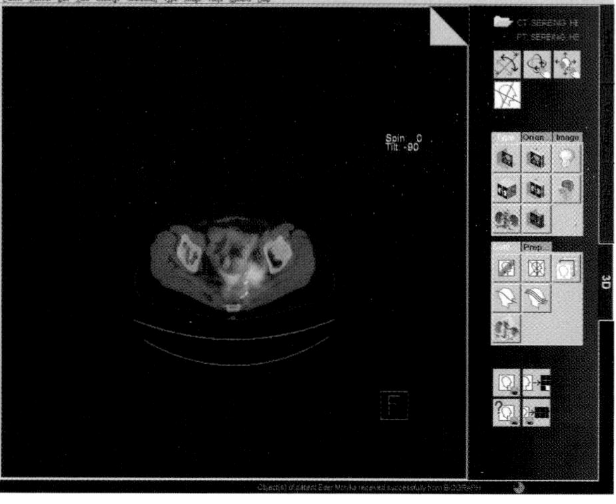

Fig. 13. PET/CT in a 70 year old female after operated rectal cancer (pT3 N1 G2 Mx). PET (**a**), CT (**b**), and PET/CT (**c**) demonstrates local recurrence (soft tissue metastasis) in the left pelvic region

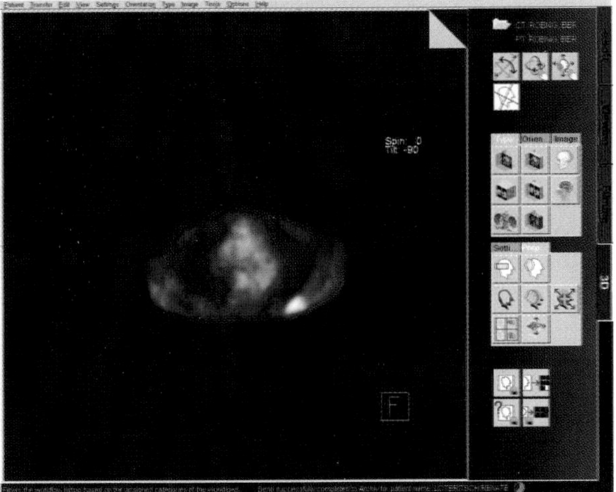

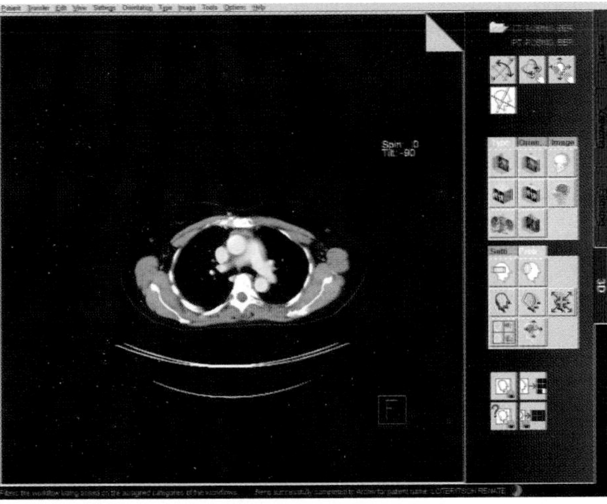

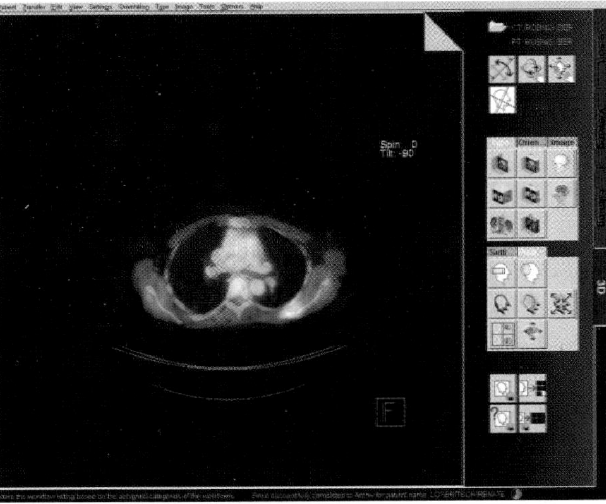

Fig. 14. PET/CT in a 53 year old female after thyroidectomy and 2 times radioiodine therapy due to follicular thyroid cancer (insular variant) with increasing thyroglobulin. PET (**a**), CT (**b**) and PET/CT (**c**) demonstrates a FDG positive metastasis originating from the left medial scapula infiltrating the soft tissue

CT+PET strategy had a higher mean cost of only US$ 429 per patient, but may result in an increase in mean life expectancy of 9.5 days per patient [102].

PET/CT

Since 2001 dedicated PET/CT (full ring PET scanner and spiral CT), as a combined metabolic/morphologic imaging modality, is available (Fig. 9). With the introduction of this new modality of imaging in oncology the question arises whether PET/CT is superior to PET and CT alone and if so, can PET/CT affect patients management better than both modalities alone. PET can assess for example metabolism, protein synthesis, gene expression and tissue hypoxia depending on the tracer used, whereas CT mainly reflects anatomy and to some degree perfusion [114]. In the combined modality CT data are used for calculation of attenuation correction as well as for anatomic information. The question whether CT should be performed as contrast enhanced diagnostic CT or only as "low dose CT" for anatomic correlation is not yet answered. There is also some debate on the use of oral contrast media for PET/CT imaging. First clinical results of PET/CT in oncology reveal that in general there is much better reliability of the results and higher diagnostic confidence using PET/CT compared to each modality alone [18, 78, 114]. Due to the fusion of anatomy and metabolism, exact localisation of hypermetabolic spots (e.g. osseous versus soft tissue lesions) on the one hand and metabolic evaluation of anatomic lesions on the other hand can be achieved. For NSCLC for example it could be demonstrated that PET/CT provided additional information in 20 out of 49 patients. With the combination of PET/CT T-staging was correct in 88% compared to 58% for CT and 40% for FDG PET alone [78]. For recurrent and metastatic colorectal cancer PET/CT is more accurate that PET or CT alone [Burger I et al. 2003]. The combination of PET and CT is most helpful in the cervical and abdominal region. Our own experience in the first 200 patients using PET/CT for staging and restaging of various tumors confirm that there is additional information in about 45% of patients and change of management in 15% of patients (Figs. 10–14). In addition it could be demonstrated that pitfalls of PET (e.g. normal structures in the head and neck region that are positive on FDG PET, bowel activity, muscle activity, excretion via the kidneys and subsequent sometimes circumscribed ureter activity, brown fat tissue etc.) can be reduced using PET/CT (Fig. 15). In conclusion, first results on PET/CT in oncology provide increased diagnostic confidence, reduction of equivocal results

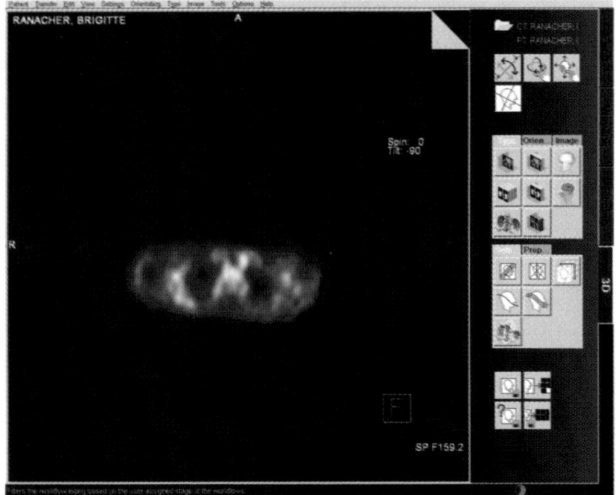

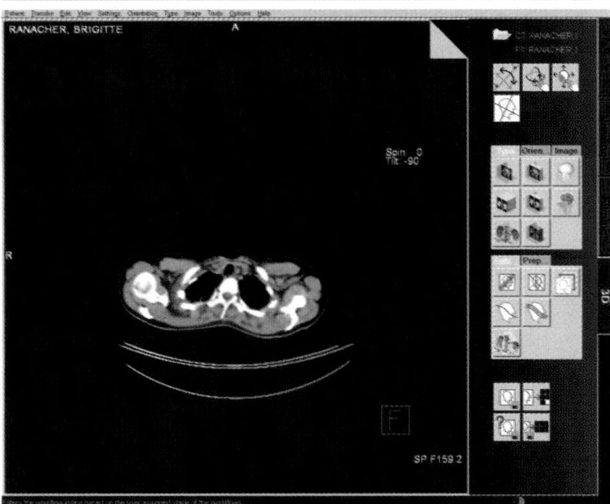

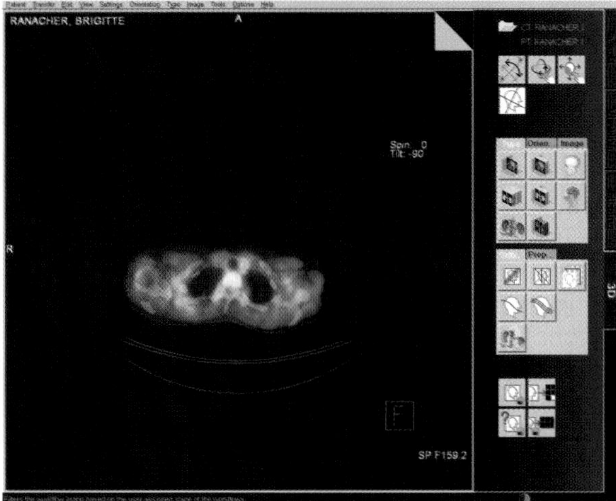

Fig. 15. PET/CT in a 29 year old female with distinct elevation of thyroglobulin (2.4 ng/ml) but negative I-131 WBS. The multiple areas with FDG uptake in the cervical region however corresponded to fat tissue in the CT (pitfall brown fat tissue). PET (**a**), CT (**b**) and PET/CT (**c**) is demonstrated. The fused images were able to exactly localise the areas with FDG uptake

in PET and CT alone, additional information in about 45% and change of therapeutic management in about 10–15% of patients.

The authors want to thank all the coworkers at the Nuclear Medicine department and the colleagues from the Radiologic Department for their assistance: H.J. Gallowitsch, MD; P. Mikosch MD; E. Kresnik, MD; I. Gomez, MD; Gerhild Kumnig, MD; Isabel Igerc MD, Sabine Matschnig, MD, P. Reinprecht, MD, K. Hausegger MD.

References

[1] Aassar OS, Fishbein NJ, Caputo GR, et al (1999) Metastatic head and neck cancer: role and usefulness of FDG PET in locating occult primary tumors. Radiology 210: 177–181

[2] Abdel-Nabi H, Doerr RJ, Lamonica DM, et al (1998) Staging of primary colorectal carcinomas with fluorine-18 fluorodeoxyglucose whole-body PET: correlation with histopathologic and CT findings. Radiology 206 (3): 755–760

[3] Adams S, Baum RP, Stukkensen T, et al (1998) Prospective comparison of 18F-FDG PET with conventional imaging modalities (CT,MRI, US) in lymph node staging of head and neck cancer. Eur J Nucl Med 25: 1255–1260

[4] Al-Sugair A, Coleman RE (1998) Application of PET in lung cancer. Semin Nucl Med 28: 303–319

[5] Altenvoerde G, Lerch H, Kuwert T, et al (1998) Positron emission tomography with F-18-deoxyglucose in patients with differentiated thyroid carcinoma, elevated thyroglobulin levels and negative iodine scans. Langenbecks Arch Surg 383: 160–163

[6] Antonelli A, Miccoli P, Ferdeghini M, et al (1995) Role of neck ultrasonography in the follow up of patients operated on for thyroid cancer. Thyroid 5: 25–28

[7] Bailet JW, Abemayor E, Jabour BA, et al (1992) Positron emission tomography: a new precise modality for detection of primary head and neck tumors and assessment of cervical adenopathy. Laryngoscope 102: 281–288

[8] Bangerter M, Moog F, Buchmann I, et al (1998) Whole-body 2-(18F)-fluoro-2-deoxy-D-glucose positron emission tomography (FDG PET) for accurate staging of Hodgkins disease. Ann Oncol 9: 117–1122

[9] Bares R, Klever P, Hauptmann S et al (1994) F-18 fluorodeoxyglucose PET in vivo evaluation of pancreatic glucose metabolism for detection of pancreatic cancer. Radiology 192: 79–86

[10] Bender H, Straehler-Pohl HJ, Schomburg A, et al (1998) Value of F-18-FDG PET in the assessment of head and neck tumors. J Nucl Med 38: 153

[11] Beyer T, Townsend D, Blodgett T, et al (2002) Dual-Modality PET/CT tomography for clinical oncology. Quart J Nucl Med 46: 24–34

[12] Blessing C, Feine U, Geiger L, et al (1995) Positron emission tomography and ultrasonography – a comparative retrospective study assessing the diagnostic validity in lymph node metastases of malignant melanoma. Arch Dermatol 131: 1394–1398
[13] Bluemke DA, Fishman EK (1998) CT and MR evaluation in pancreatic cancer. Surg Oncol Clin N Am 7: 103–124
[14] Bohuslavizki KH, Klutmann S, Kroger S, et al (2000) FDG PET detection of unknown primary tumors. J Nucl Med 41 (5): 816–822
[15] Braams JW, Pruim J, Kole AC, et al (1997) Detection of unknown primary head and neck tumors by positron emissions tomography. Int J Oral Maxillofac Surg 26: 112–115
[16] Breslow A (1970) Thickness, cross sectional areas and depth of invasion in the prognosis of cutaneous melanoma. Ann Surg 172: 902–908
[17] Briele B, Hotze A, Kropp J, et al (1991) Vergleich von Tl-201 und Tc-99m MIBI in der Nachsorge des differenzierten Schilddrüsencarcinoms. Nuklearmedizin 30: 115–124
[18] Burger I, Görres G, von Shulthess G, et al (2002) PET/CT: diagnostic improvement in recurrent colorectal carcinoma compared to PET alone. Radiology 225: 424 (p)
[19] Burry T, Paulus P, Dowlati A, et al (1996) Staging of the mediastinum: value of positron emission tomography imaging in non-small cell lung cancer. Eur Resp J 9: 2560–2564
[20] Bury T, Dowlati A, Paulus P, et al (1996) Evaluation of solitary pulmonary nodule by positron emission tomography imaging. Eur Expir J 9: 410–414
[21] Cappel I, Blum U, Ungeheuer E (1983) Bedeutung der Vorsorgeuntersuchung für die Prognose des Dickdarmkarzinoms. Schweiz Med Wochenschr 113: 550–552
[22] Castellino RA, Hoppe R, Blank N, et al (1984) Computed tomography, lymphography and staging laparatomy: correlation in initial staging of Hodgkins disease. AJR 143: 37–41
[23] Castellino RA, Hoppe R, Blank N, et al (1986) Hodgkins disease: contribution of chest CT in the initial staging evaluation. Radiology 160: 603–605
[24] Cherry SR, Phelps ME (1996) Positron emission tomography: methods and instrumentation, Diagnostic nuclear medicine. Williams & Wilkins, ISBN 0–683–07503–9
[25] Conces DJ, Tarver RD, Gray WC, et al (1988) Treatment of pneumothoraces utilizing small caliber chest tubes. Chest 94: 55–57
[26] Conti PS, Durski JM, Bacqai F, et al (1999) Imaging of locally recurrent and metastatic thyroid cancer with positron emission tomograpgy. Thyroid 9: 797–804
[27] Dadparvar S, Krischna L, Brady LW, et al (1993) The role of I-131, thallium-201 imaging and serum thyroglobulin in the management of differentiated thyroid carcinoma. Cancer 71: 3767–3773
[28] Dalsaso TA, Lowe VJ, Dunphy FR, et al (2000) FDG PET and CT in evaluation of chemotherapy in advanced head and neck cancer. Clin Pos Imag 3: 1–5
[29] Debelke D, Vitola JV, Sandler MP, et al (1997) Staging recurrent metastatic colorectal carcinoma with PET. J Nucl Med 38: 1196–1201
[30] Dehdashti F, Griffith LK, McGuire AH, et al (1992) FDG-PET evaluation of suspicious pulmonary and mediastinal masses. J Nucl Med 32: 961 P
[31] Dewan NA, Reeb SD, Gupta NC, et al (1995) PET FDG imaging and transthoracic needle lung aspiration biopsy in evaluation of pulmonary lesions. Chest 108: 441–446
[32] Dewan NA, Shehan CJ, Reeb SD, et al (1997) Likelihood of malignancy in a solitary pulmonary nodule. Comparison of Bayesian analysis and results of FDG PET scan. Chest 112: 416–422
[33] Diel SJ, Lehmann KJ, Sadick M, et al (1998) Pancreatic cancer: value of dual-phase helical CT in assessing resectability. Radiology 206: 373–378
[34] Dietlein M, Scheidhauer K, Voth E, et al (1997) Fluorine-18 fluorodeoxyglucose positron emission tomography and iodine-131 whole body scintigraphy in the follow up of differentiated thyroid cancer. Eur J Nucl Med 24: 1342–1348
[35] Dietlein M, Weber K, Gandjour A, et al (2000) Cost-effectiveness of FDG-PET for the management of solitary pulmonary nodules: a decision analysis based on cost reimbursement in Germany. Eur J Nucl Med 27 (10): 1441–1456
[36] Farber LA, Bernard F, Machtay M, et al (1999) Detection of recurrent head and neck squamous cell carcinoma after radiation therapy with 2–18F-fluoro-2-deoxy-D-glucose positron emission tomography. Laryngoscope 109: 970–975
[37] Feine U, Lizenmayer R, Hanke JP, et al (1996) Fluorine-18 FDG and iodine-131 uptake in thyroid cancer. J Nucl Med 37: 1468–1472
[38] Fishman EK, Kuhlman LE, Jones RJ, et al (1991) CT of lymphoma: spectrum of disease. RadioGraphics 11: 647–669
[39] Findley M, Young H, Cunninham D, et al (1996) Noninvasive monitoring of tumor metabolism using fluorodeoxyglucose and positron emission tomography in colorectal cancer liver metastases: correlation with tumor response to fluorouracil. J Clin Oncol 14: 700–708
[40] Fischbein NJ, OS AA, Caputo GR, et al (1998) Clinical utility of positron emission tomography with 18F-fluorodeoxyglucose in detecting residual/recurrent squamous cell carcinoma of the head and neck. Am J Neuroradiol 19 (7): 1189–1196
[41] Freeny PC, Marks WM, Ryan JA, et al (1986) Colorectal carcinoma evaluation with CT: preoperative staging and detection of postoperative recurrences. Radiology 158: 347–353
[42] Ghambir SS, Czernin J, Schwimmer J, et al (2001) A tabulated summary of FDG PET Literature. J Nucl Med 42: 1S–93S
[43] Gambhir SS, Shepherd JE, Shah BD, et al (1998) An analytical decision model for the cost effective

management of solitary pulmonary nodules. J Clin Oncol 16: 2113–2125

[44] Goerres GW, HAny TF, Kamel E, et al (2002) Head and neck imaging with PET and PET/CT: artifacts from dental metallic implants. Eur J Nucl Med 29: 367–370

[45] Gould MK, Lillington GA (1998) Strategy and cost in solitary pulmonary nodule. Thorax 53: 32–35

[46] Graeber GM, Gupta NC, Murray GF (1999) Positron emission tomography imaging with fluorodeoxyglucose is efficacious in evaluating malignant pulmonary diesease. J Thorac Cardiovasc Surg 117: 719–727

[47] Greven KM, Williams DW, Keyes JW, et al (1994) Positron emission tomography of patients with head and neck carcinoma before and after high dose irradiation. Cancer 74: 1355–1359

[48] Gritters LS, Francis IR, Zasadny KR, Wahl RL (1993) Initial assessment of positron emission tomography using 2-fluorine-18-fluoro-2-deoxy-D-glucose in the imaging of malignant melanoma. J Nucl Med 34: 1420–1427

[49] Grünwald F, Menzel C, Bender H, et al (1997) Comparison of 18FDG-PET with 131iodine and 99m Tc-sestamibi scintigraphy in differentiated thyroid cancer. Thyroid 7: 327–335

[50] Guhlmann A, Storck M, Kotzerke J, et al (1997) Lymph node staging in non-small cell lung cancer: evaluation by [18F FDG positron emission tomography (PET). Thorax 52: 438–441

[51] Gupta NC, Graeber GM, Rogers SJ, Bishop HA (1999) Comparative efficacy of positron emission tomography with FDG and computed tomographic scanning in preoperative staging of non small cell lung cancer. Ann Surg 229: 286–291

[52] Gupta NC, Malof J, Gunel E (1996) Probability of malignancy in solitary pulmonary nodules using F-18 FDG and PET. J Nucl Med 37: 943–948

[53] Haberkorn U, Strauss LG, Dimitrakopopoulou A, et al (1991) PET studies of fluoro-deoxyglucose metabolism in patients with recurrent tumors receiving radiotherapy. J Nucl Med 32: 1485–1490

[54] Hain SF, Curran KM, Beggs AD, et al (2001) FDG-PET as a "metabolic biopsy" tool in thoracic lesions with indeterminate biopsy. Eur J Nucl Med 28: 1336–1340

[55] Hanasono MM, Kunda LD, Segall GM, et al (1999) Uses and limitations of FDG positron emission tomography in patients with head and neck cancer. Laryngoscope 109: 880–885

[56] Hannah A, Scott AM, Tochon-Danguy H, et al (2002) Evaluation of 18F-fluorodeoxyglucose positron emisison tomography and computed tomography with histopathological correlation in the initial staging of head and neck cancer. Ann Surg 236 (2): 208–217

[57] Haramati LB, Austin JHM (1991) Complications of CT guided needle biopsy through aerated versus non-aerated lung. Radiology 181: 778

[58] Hellwig D, Ukena D, Paulsen F, et al (2001) Meta-analyse zum Stellenwert der Positronen-Emissions-Tomographie mit F-18-Fluorodeoxyglucose (FDG PET) bei Lungentumoren. Pneumologie 55: 367–377

[59] Hiraki Y, Rosen OM, Birnbaum MJ (1988) Growth factors rapidly induce expression of the glucose transporter gene. J Biol Chem 27: 13655–13662

[60] Ho CL, Dehdashti F, Griffeth LH, et al (1996) FDG-PET evaluation of intermediate pancreatic masses. J Comput Assist Tomogr 20: 363–369

[61] Hoefnagel CA, Delprat CC, Marcuse HR, de Vijlder JJM (1986) Role of thallium-201 total body scintigraphy in follow up of thyroid carcinoma. J Nucl Med 27: 1854–1857

[62] Hoh CK, Glaspy J, Rosen P, et al (1997) Whole-body FDG PET imaging for staging Hodgkins disease and lymphoma. J Nucl Med 38: 343–348

[63] Hubner KF, Buonocore E, Singh SK, et al (1995) Characterisation of chest masses by FDG Positron Emmission Tomography. Clin Nucl Med 20: 293–298

[64] Hüfner M, Stumpf HP, Grussendorf M, et al (1983) A comparison of the effectiveness of I-131 whole body scans and plasma Tg determination in a diagnosis for metastatic differentiated carcinoma of the thyroid: a retrospective study. Acta Endocrinol 104: 32–332

[65] Joensuu H, Ahonen A, Klemi PJ (1998) F-18-fluorodeoxyglucose imaging in preoperative diagnosis of thyroid malignancy. Eur J Nucl Med 13: 502–506

[66] Jungehulsing M, Scheidhauer K, Damm M, et al (2000) 2[F]-fluoro-2-deoxy-D-glucose positron emission tomography is a sensitive tool for the detection of occult primary cancer (carcinoma of unknown primary syndrome) with head and neck lymph node manifestation. Otolaryngol Head Neck Surg 123 (3): 294–301

[67] Khouri NF, Mezziane MA, Zerhouni MA, et al (1987) The solitary pulmonary nodule – assessment, diagnosis and management. Chest 91: 128–133

[68] Kinahan PE, Townsend DW, Beyer T, et al (1998) Attenuation correction for a combined 3D PET/CT scanner. Med Phys 25: 2046–2053

[69] Klose T, Leidl R, Buchmann I, Brambs HJ, Reske SN (2000) Primary staging of lymphomas: cost-effectiveness of FDG-PET versus computed tomography. Eur J Nucl Med 27 (10): 1457–1464

[70] Kostakoglu L, Leonard JP, Kuji I, et al (2002) Comparison of fluorine-18 fluoro-deoxyglucose positron emission tomography and Ga-67 scintigraphy in evaluation of lymphoma. Cancer 94 (4): 879–888

[71] Kosuda S, Ichihara K, Watanabe M, et al (eds) (1998) Decision-tree sensitivity analysis for cost-effectiveness of chest 2-fluoro-2-D-[(18)F]fluorodeoxyglucose positron emission tomography in patients with pulmonary nodules (non-small cell lung carcinoma) in Japan. In: Fischbein NJ, OS AA, Caputo GR, et al (eds) Clinical utility of positron emission tomography with 18F-fluorodeoxyglucose in detecting residual/recurrent squamous cell carcinoma of the head and neck. Am J Neuroradiol 19 (7): 1189–1196

[72] Kresnik E, Mikosch P, Gallowitsch HJ, et al (2001) Evaluation of head and neck cancer with F-18-FDG PET: a comparison with conventional methods. Eur J Nucl Med 28: 816–821
[73] Kresnik E, Gallowitsch HJ, Mikosch P, et al (2003) F-18-FDG PET in the preoperative assessment of thyroid nodules in an endemic goiter area. Surgery 133: 294–299
[74] Kutlu CA, Pastorino U, Maisy M, Goldstraw P (1998) Selective use of PET scan in the preoperative staging of NSCLC. Lung Cancer 21: 177–184
[75] Kuwabara H, Gjedde A (1991) Measurements of glucose phosphorylation with FDG and PET are not reduced by dephosphorylation of FDG-6-phosphate. J Nucl Med 23: 918–922
[76] LaCroix KJ, Tsu BMW, Hasegawa BH, et al (1994) Investigation of the use of X-ray CT images for attenuation correction in SPECT. IEEE Trans Nucl Sci 41: 2793–2799
[77] Lai DT, Fulham M, Stephen MS, et al (1996) The role of whole-body positron emission tomography with 18F-fluorodeoxyglucose in identifying operable colorectal cancer metastases to the liver. Arch Surg 131: 703–707
[78] Lardinois D, Weder W, Hany TF, et al (2003) Staging of non-small-cell lung-cancer wirth integrated positron emissiontomography and computed tomography. N Engl J Med 348: 2500–2507
[79] Levin CS, Hoffmann EJ (1999) Calculation of positron range and its effect on the fundamental limit of positron emission tomography system spatial resolution. Phys Med Biol 44: 781–799
[80] Lewis P, Griffin S, Marsden P, et al (1994) Whole-body FDG positron emission tomography in preoperative evaluation of lung cancer. Lancet 344: 1255–1266
[81] Lind P (1999) Multi-tracer imaging of thyroid nodules: is there a role in the preoperative assessment of nodular goiter. Eur J Nucl Med 26: 795–797
[82] Lind P, Gallowitsch HJ (1996) The use of non specific tracers in the follow up of differentiated thyroid cancer: Results with Tc-99m Tetrofosmin whole body scintigraphy. AMA 23: 69–75
[83] Lind P, Gallowitsch HJ, Langsteger W, et al (1997) Technetium-99m Tetrofosmin whole body scintigraphy in the follow up of differentiated thyroid carcinoma. J Nucl Med 38: 348–352
[84] Lind P, Gallowitsch HJ, Unterweger O, et al (1998) FDG PET in the follow up of thyroid cancer: comparison with Tc-99m tetrofosmin and I-131 whole body scintigraphy. Eur J Nucl Med 25: 974
[85] Lind P, Kresnik E, Kumnig G, et al (2003) F-18-FDG PET in the follow up of thyroid cancer. AMA 30: 17–21
[86] Lind P, Lechner P, Arian-Schad K, et al (1991) Anti-carcinoembryonic antigen immunoscintigraphy (Tc-99m monoclonal antibody BW 431/26) and serum CEA levels in patients with suspected primary and recurrent colorectal carcinoma. J Nucl Med 32: 1319–1325
[87] Lowe VJ, Dunphy RS, Varvares M, et al (1997) Evaluation of chemotherapy response in patients with advanced head and neck cancer using F-18 fluorodeoxyglucose positron emission tomography. Head Neck 19: 666–674
[88] Lowe VJ, Fletcher JW, Gobar L, et al (1998) Prospective investigation of Positron Emmission Tomography in lung nodules. J Clin Oncol 16: 1075–1084
[89] Lubin E, Mechlis-Frish S, Zatz S, et al (1994) Serum thyroglobulin and I-131 whole body scan in the diagnosis and assessment of treatment for metastatic differentiated thyroid carcinoma. J Nucl Med 35: 257–262
[90] Macapinlac HA, Yeung HWD, Larson S (1999). Defining the role of FDG PET in head and neck cancer. Clin Pos Imag 2: 311–31
[91] Mack MJ, Hazelrigg SR, Landreneau RJ, Acuft TE (1993) Thoracoscopy for the diagnosis of intermediate solitary pulmonary nodule. Ann Thorac Surg 56: 825–832
[92] Mainolfi C, Maurea S, Varella P, et al (1998) Positron emission tomography with fluorine-18-deoxyglucose in the staging and control of patients with lymphoma. Comparison with clinico-radiologic assessment. Radiol Med 95: 98–104
[93] Marom EM, McAdams HP, Erasmus JJ, et al (1999) Staging non-small cell lung cancer with whole body PET. Radiology 212: 803–809
[94] McGuirt WF, Greven K, Williams D, et al (1998) PET scanning in head and neck oncology: a review. Head Neck 20: 208–215
[95] Mikosch P, Gallowitsch HJ, Kresnik E, et al (1999) Value of ultrasound guided fine-needle aspiration biopsy of thyroid nodules in an endemic goiter area. Eur J Nucl Med (in press)
[96] Moog F, Bangerter M, Diederichs CG, et al (1997) Lymphoma: role of whole body 2-deoxy-2-[F-18]fluoro-D-glucose (FDG) in nodal staging. Radiology 203: 795–800
[97] Moreau P, Goffart J, Collignon J (1990) Computed tomography of metastatic cervical lymph nodes. A clinical computed tomographic, pathologic correlative study. Arch Otolaryngol Head Neck Surg 116: 1190–1193
[98] Moszynsky M, Kapusta M, Wolski D, et al (1998) Energy resolution of scintillation detectors readout with large area avalanche photodiodes and photomultipliers. IEEE Trans Nucl Sci 45: 472–477
[99] Nguyen AT, Akhurst T, Larson SM, et al (1999) PET scanning with 18F- 2- fluoro-2-deoxyD-glucose (FDG) in patients with Melanoma: benefits and limitations. Clinical Positron Imaging 2: 93–98
[100] Ogunbiyi OA, Flanagan FL, Dehdashti F, et al (1997) Detection of recurrent and metastatic colorectal cancer: comparison of positron emission tomography and computed tomography. Ann Surg Oncol 4: 613–620
[101] Ostertag H (1992) Positronen Emissions Tomographie (PET): Ein diagnostisches Verfahren zur in vivo-

Stoffwechseluntersuchung mit Positronenstrahlern. Physikalische Blätter 48(2): 77–83

[102] Park KC, Schwimmer J, Shepherd JE, et al (2001) Decision analysis for the cost-effective management of recurrent colorectal cancer. Ann Surg 233 (3): 310–319

[103] Patz EF, Lowe VJ, Goodman PC, Herrndon J (1995) Thoracic nodule staging with PET imaging with 18FDG in patients with bronchogenic carcinoma. Chest 108: 1617–1621

[104] Patz EF, Laue VJ, Hofmann, et al (1993) Focal pulmonary abnormalities: Evaluation with FDG-PET scanning. Radiology 188: 487–490

[105] Paulus P, Benoit TH, Bury TH, et al (1995) Positron Emmission Tomography with F-18 FDG in the assessment of solitary pulmonary nodules. Eur J Nucl Med 22: 775

[106] Paulus P, Sambon A, Vivegnis D, et al (1998) 18FDG-PET for the assessment of primary head and neck tumors: clinical, computed tomography and histopathological correlation in 38 patients. Laryngoscope 108: 1578–1583

[107] Prauer HW, Weber WA, Römer W, et al (1998) Controlled prospective study of positron emission tomography using the glucose analogue [18f] fluorodeoxy-glucose in the evaluation of pulmonary nodules. Br J Surg 85: 1506–1511

[108] Rege SD, Hoh CK, Glaspy JA, et al (1993) Imaging of pulmonary mass lesions with whole-body positron emission tomography and fluorodeoxyglucose. Cancer 72: 82–90

[109] Regelink G, Brouwer J, De Bree R, et al (2002) Detection of unknown primary tumours and distant metastases in patient with cervical metastases: value of FDG-PET versus conventional modalities. Eur J Nucl Med 29 (8): 1024–1030

[110] Reske SN, Kotzerke J (2001) FDG PET for clinical use. Eur J Nucl Med 28: 1707–1723

[111] Römer W, Hanauske AR, Ziegler S, et al (1998) PET in Non-Hodgkins lymphoma: Assessment of chemotherapy with FDG. Blood 91: 4464–4471

[112] Rettenbacher L, Koller J, Kässmann H, Galvan G (1997) Selective regional lymphadenectomy in malignant melanoma using a gamma probe. AMA 24: 79–80

[113] Sasaki M, Ichiya Y, Kuwabara Y, et al (1996) The usefulness of FDG positron emission tomography for the detection of mediastinal lymph node metastases in patients with non-small cell lung cancer: comparative study with x-ray computed tomography. Eur J Nucl Med 23: 741–747

[114] Schöder H, Erdi YE, Larson SM, Yeung HWD (2003) PET/CT: a new imaging technology in nuclear medicine. Eur J Nucl Med Mol Imaging 30: 1419–1437

[115] Schröder H, Meta J, Yap C, et al (2001) Effect of whole-body 18F-FDG PET imaging on clinical staging and management of patients with malignant lymphoma. J Nucl Med 42 (8): 1139–1143

[116] Schlumberger M, Challeton C, De Vathaire F, et al (1996) Radioactive Iodine treatment and external radiotherapy for lung and bone metastases from thyroid carcinoma. J Nucl Med 37: 598–605

[117] Staib L, Schirrmeister H, Reske SN, Beger HG (2000) Is (18)F-fluorodeoxyglucose positron emission tomography in recurrent colorectal cancer a contribution to surgical decision making? Am J Surg 180 (1): 1–5

[118] Steinert HC, Hauser M, Allemann F, et al (1997) Non-small cell lung cancer: Nodal staging with FDG PET versus CT with correlative lymph node mapping and sampling. Radiology 202: 441–446

[119] Steinert HC, Huch-Böni RA, Buck A, et al (1995) Malignant melanoma: staging with whole-body positron emission tomography and 2-[F-18]-fluoro-2-deoxy-D-glucose. Radiology 195: 705–709

[120] Stokkel MP, ten Broek FW, van Rijk PP (1999) Preoperative assessment of cervical lymph nodes in head and neck cancer with fluorine –18 fluorodeoxyglucose using a dual head coincidence camera: a pilot study. Eur J Nucl Med 26: 499–503

[121] Stokkel MP, Ten Broek FW, Hordjik GJ, et al (2000) Preoperative evaluation of patients with primary head and neck cancer using dual-head 18fluorodeoxyglucose positron emission tomography. Ann Surg 231 (2): 229–234

[122] Stollfuß JC, Glatting G, Friess H, et al (1995) 2-(fluorine-18)-fluoro-2-deoxy-D-glucose PET in detection of pancreatic cancer: value of quantitative image interpretation. Radiology 195: 339–344

[123] Strauss LG, Clorius JH, Schlag P, et al (1989) Recurrence of colorectal tumors. PET evaluation. Radiology 170: 329–332

[124] Stumpe KDM, Urbinelli M, Steínert HC, et al (1998) Whole-body positron emission tomography using fluorodeoxyglucose for staging of lymphoma: effectiveness and comparison with computed tomography. Eur J Nucl Med 25: 721–728

[125] Talbot JN, Haioun C, Rain JD, et al (2001) F-18-FDG positron imaging in clinical management of lymphoma patients. Crit Rev Oncol Hematol 38: 193–221

[126] Tang HR, Schreck CE, Hasegawa BH, et al (1999) ECT attenuation maps from X-ray CT images. J Nukl Med 40: 113P

[127] Thill R, Neuerburg J, Fabry U, et al (1997) Comparison of 18-FDG PET and CT for pretherapeutic staging of malignant lymphoma. NuclearMedicine 36: 234–239

[128] Tyler DS, Onaitis M, Kherani A, et al (2000) Positron emission tomography scanning in malignant melanoma – clinical utility in patients with stage III disease. Cancer 89: 1019–1025

[129] Valk PE, Pounds DR, Hopkins DM, et al (1995) Staging lung cancer by PET imaging. Ann Thor Surg 60: 1573–1582

[130] Vansteenkiste JF, Stroobants SG, DeLeyr PR (1998) Lymph-node staging in non-small cell lung cancer with FDG PET scan: a prospective study on 690 lymph node stations from 68 patients. J Clin Oncol 16: 2142–2149

[131] Wang W, Macapinlac H Larson SM, et al (1999) [18F]-2-fluoro-deoxy-D-glucose positron emission tomograpgy localizes residual thyroid cancer in patients with negative diagnostic (131)I whole body scans and elevated serum thyroglobulin levels. J Clin Endocrinol Metab 84: 2291–2302

[132] Warburg O (1993) The metabolism of tumours. Smith RR Inc, New York, pp 129–169

[133] Weber W, Römer W, Ziegler S, et al (1995) Clinical value of F-18 FDG PET in solitary pulmonary nodules. Eur J Nucl Med 22: 775

[134] Weber MJ, Monchamp RR (1973) Luminescence of $Bi^4Ge^3O^{12}$: spectral and decay properties. J Appl Phys 44: 5495–5499

[135] Weder W, Schmid RA, Bruchhaus H, et al (1998) Detection of extrathoracic metastases by Positron Emmission Tomography in lung cancer. Ann Thorac Surg 66: 886–892

[136] Ziegler SI, Pichler BJ, Boening G, et al (2001) A prototype high resolution animal positron tomograph with avalanche photodiode arrays and LSO crystal Eur J Nucl Med 28: 136–143

[137] Zimny M, Bares R, Fass J, et al (1997) Fluorine-18 fluorodeoxyglucose positron emission tomography in the differential diagnosis of pancreatic carcinoma: a report of 106 cases. Eur J Nucl Med 24: 678–682

Perfusion and spectroscopy in cerebral magnetic resonance tomography (MRT)

F. A. Fellner

Institute of Radiology, Landes-Nervenklinik Wagner-Jauregg, Linz, Austria

Introduction

Perfusion magnetic resonance tomography (MRT) has been discussed in scientific papers for some 10 years but has been integrated into clinical routine only slowly. Modern evaluation programmes that enable colour-coded evaluation of the parameters according to Østergaard have made it possible to perform the procedure within an acceptable time limit (5–10 minutes) so that it can now be incorporated into routine diagnostic procedures.

How the measurement is performed

For a perfusion MRT scan we use an echo-planar imaging (EPI) sequence with a high temporal resolution of about 150 ms per image. In order to achieve a sufficiently high perfusion curve a high flow rate is needed (for example, 5 ml/second) and the flow needs to be homogenous. For this purpose an automated injector of contrast medium is required. Perfusion investigations can be done by using "simply" relaxant contrast mediums (such as Magnetivist, Omniscan, Dotarem, etc) but also by using more highly relaxant mediums (such as Gadovist, Multihance). For the perfusion, the generation of a significant signal drop during first pass of the contrast medium through the tissue is of vital importance. Our current preference is therefore more highly effective contrast mediums as these can achieve an excellent bolus curve. The measurement parameters are given at the end of the chapter.

Evaluation of the measurement

Evaluation according to Østergaard includes measuring the following variables: regional cerebral blood volume (rCBV), regional cerebral blood flow (rCBF), mean transit time (MTT), and time to peak (TTP). The measurements are currently relative values as reliable quantitative measurements using MRT in clinical practice are currently not within the realm of the possible. Of importance is the colour-coded display of the perfusion results, which enables easier interpretation of the images than monochrome images.

Areas of clinical use

Diagnostics of acute stroke

Whether MRT is of use in diagnosing acute strokes is still being evaluated scientifically and is the subject of controversy. MRT certainly has the advantage that in a short time of investigation (measurement time less than 10 minutes), it provides a large amount of information from the different sequences: rapid FLAIR sequence, time-of-flight-MR-angiography, diffusion and perfusion. Although the predictive value or use of the mismatch between diffusion and perfusion has thus far not been sufficiently clarified, in clinical practice it can be useful in reaching decisions concerning acute treatment of borderline clinical cases (Fig. 1).

When MRT is used to diagnose an acute stroke, perfusion measurement should therefore be performed in any case. Clinical practice has shown that in cases of insufficient clinical information (patient may not be conscious or able to communicate, history incomplete even when taken with the help of others), MRT with optimised stroke protocol and performed after an normal CT scan has often be found to be helpful in establishing a diagnosis of stroke or not. This helps to avoid the problem that patients in whom acute ischaemia is suspected are subjected to thrombolysis as a result of an normal CT scan, although no infarction is present but their symptoms are due to another cause (e.g. post-ictal status).

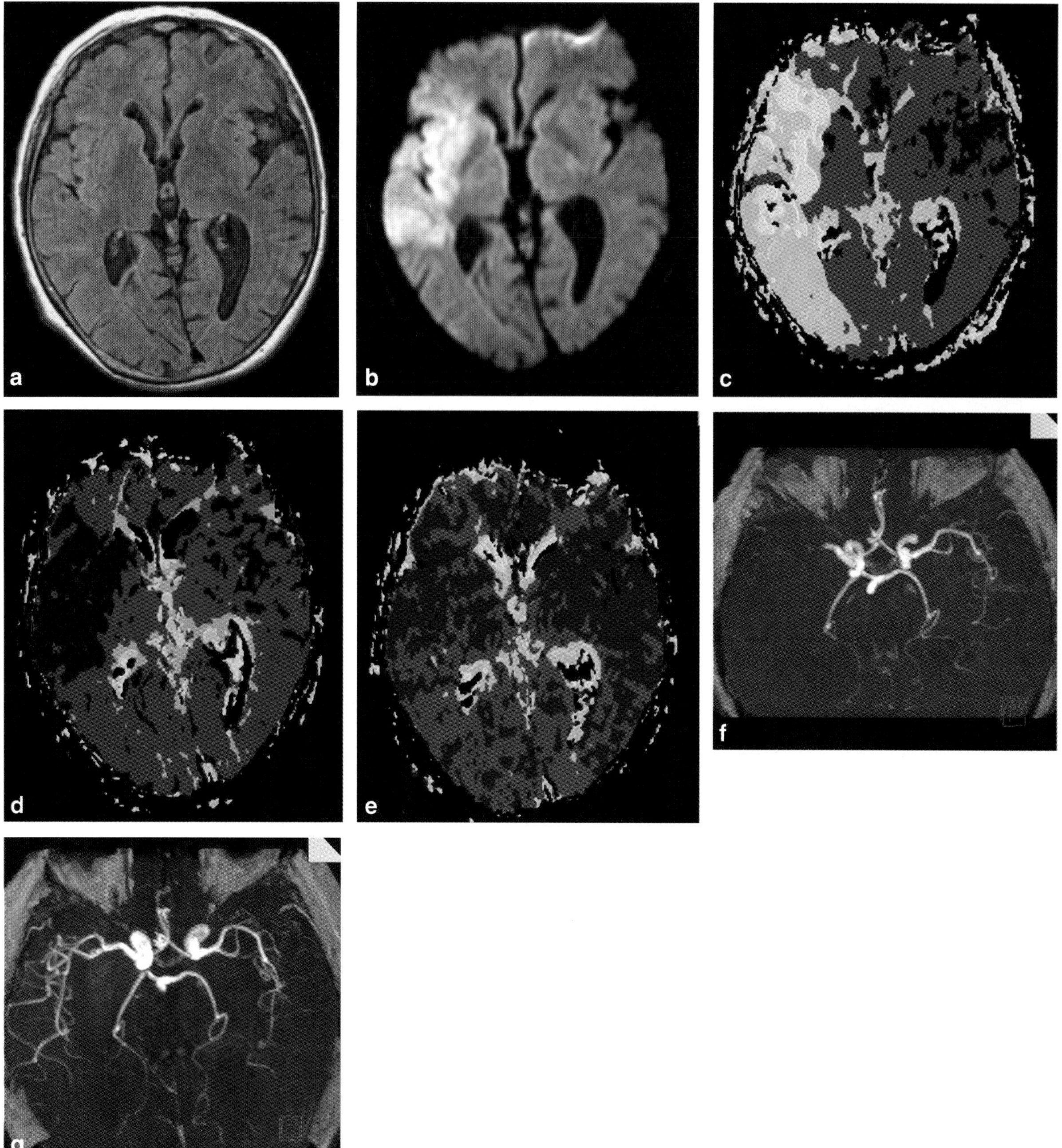

Fig. 1. Acute stroke. A 79 year old patient with acute left hemiplegia, central facial paresis, and eye deviation to the right side. The event started about 3 1/2 hours before the patient was admitted. The FLAIR sequence (**a**) is not showing a significant signal change. On diffusion MRT (**b** value = 1000 s/mm^2) a restricted diffusion is visible in wide areas of the arteria cerebri media. The perfusion (time to peak map) (**c**) shows a complete lack of perfusion in this area. The clear mismatch between diffusion and perfusion influenced the decision to start thrombolysis in spite of the time delay. After intravenous thrombolysis with rTPA the patient achieved restitutio ad integrum. MR control scans after three days (**d**) and 15 days (**e**) show increasingly normal perfusion. The MR scan before thrombolysis (**f**) shows an occlusion of the proximal parts of the arteria cerebri media, which showed complete reperfusion after thrombolysis (**g**)

Further uses in investigating vascular changes

Vascular pathologies such as vasculites, moya-moya disease, or intracranial or extracranial atherosclerotic stenoses, for which invasive therapeutic measures are planned, are further disease entities where we use perfusion MRT (Fig. 2).

Diagnosis of intracranial tumour

Pretherapeutic diagnosis

Perfusion MRT has been of some use in the preoperative diagnosis and classification of intracranial tumours. Highly malignant astrocytomas (WHO grade III-IV) mostly show an increased blood volume compared with normal white matter; astrocytomas of lesser malignancy show a lower blood volume. Very rarely such tumours have been misdiagnosed, as apparently only a very low number of astrocytomas WHO III can have a low blood volume. The view to date has been that WHO III-IV astrocytomas could not be diagnosed through perfusion MRT, but according to a more recently reported study, differentiation can be made with the help of semi-quantitative evaluations.

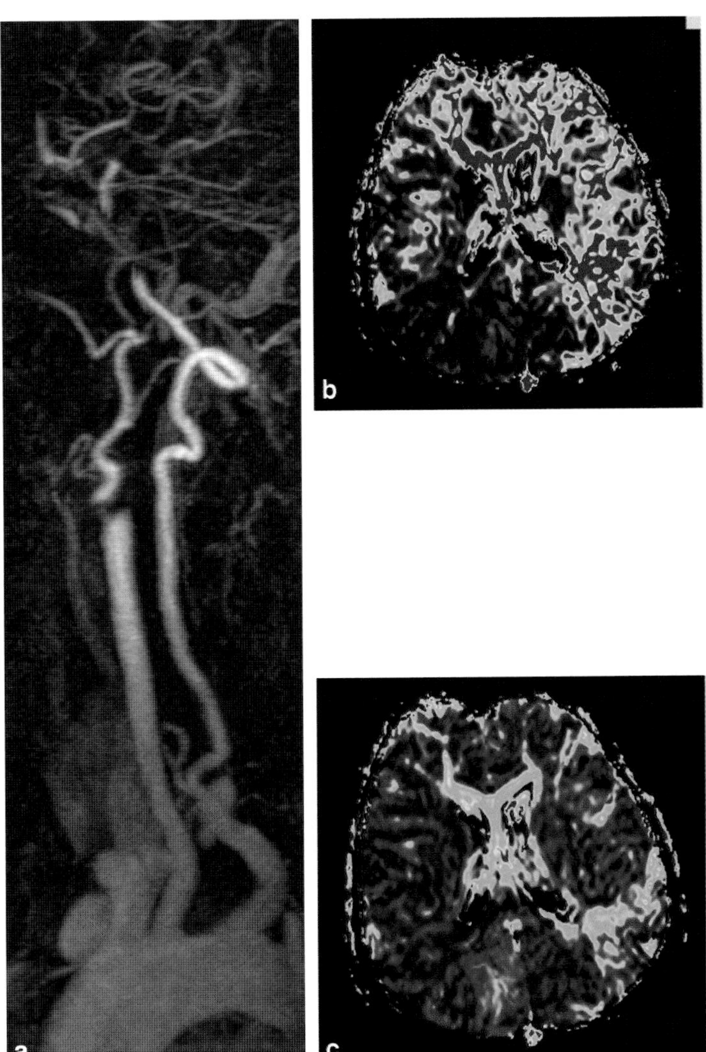

Fig. 2. Perfusion changes in stenoses and occlusions of the carotid arteries. A woman aged 64 presented with recurring syncope. The patient's internal carotid artery was occluded on both sides and the external carotid artery was stenosed (to the left more than to the right). The contrast-enhanced MR angiogram shows a high grade stenosis of the external carotid artery on the left hand side (**a**). The perfusion scan shows a clearly delayed perfusion of the arteria cerebri media on the left compared with that on the right (**b**). After the patient received a stent to help the stenosis in the left external carotid artery, perfusion of the left hemisphere shows to have normalised compared with that on the right (**c**)

We use perfusion MRT routinely in pretherapeutic diagnoses as it can be used without any major expense in terms of time, but always in combination with MR spectroscopy measurements. In our experience to date, MR spectroscopy (MRS) is, from a clinical perspective, by far the most valuable method in this context. The extent of the choline peak is known to be directly proportional to the grade of malignancy. As a rule of thumb, the clearer the choline peak the higher the grade of malignancy (Fig. 3).

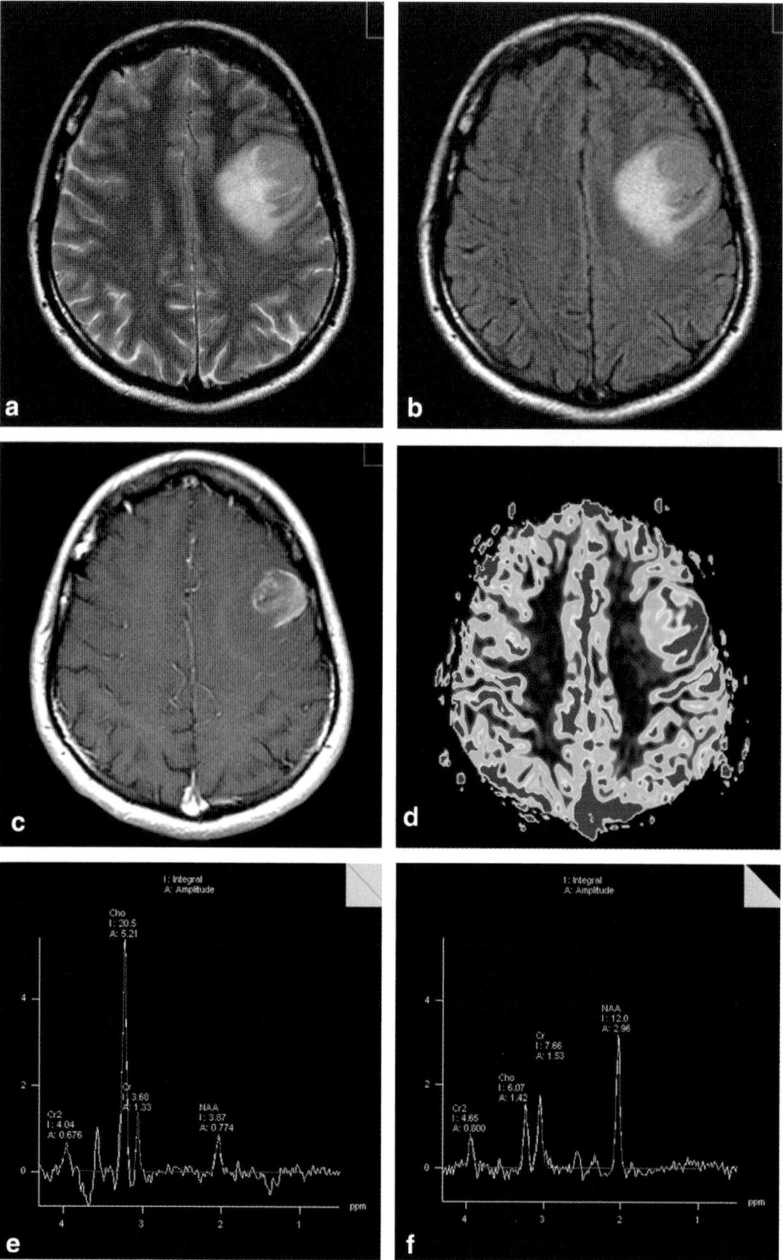

Fig. 3. Glioblastoma multiforme. Conventional MRT including T2-weighted turbo spinecho (**a**), FLAIR (**b**), and T1-weighted spinecho sequences after contrast medium (Gadovist) (**c**) shows a partially strong enhancing mass lesion in the left frontal lobe. In perfusion MRT the relative blood volume is shown to be significantly raised (**d**), which is consistent with a highly malignant tumour. MR spectroscopy with an echo time of 135 ms shows a massively raised choline peak in the tumour (**e**) – such as occurs, for example, in glioblastomas or primitive neuroectodermal tumours (PNET). By way of comparison, the normal spectrum is shown as measured in the normal parenchyma of the opposite side (**f**)

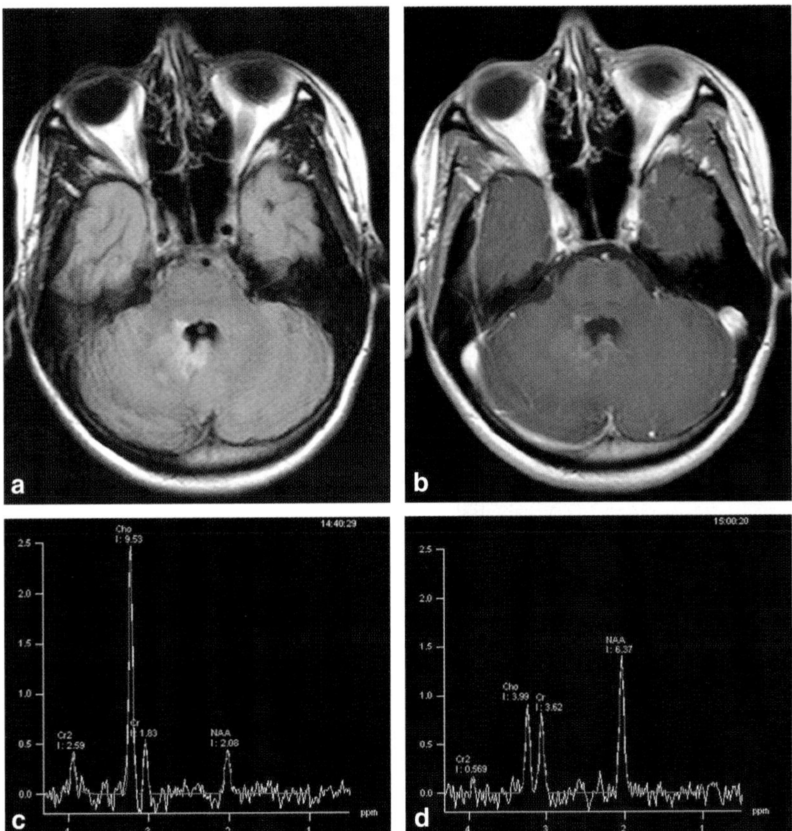

Fig. 4. Primitive, neuroectodermal tumour/medulloblastoma of the posterior fossa (PNET-MB). Conventional MRI, FLAIR (**a**) and contrast enhanced T1-weighted spinecho sequence (**b**) shows a formation of unclear aetiology in the environment of the fourth ventricle (dorsal and right lateral). As there were no signs of expansive growth it is not clear that this finding indicates a tumorous lesion. The differential diagnosis may be an inflammatory lesion. MR spectroscopy (**c**) shows a substantial reduction of NAA and Cr as well as an exorbitantly raised choline peak compared with the healthy opposite side (**d**). This implies the presence of a highly malignant tumour. We have not observed such high choline peak in MS. The histological finding was PNET-MB

The combination of MRS and perfusion MRT is especially helpful in establishing differential diagnoses – for example, whether the lesion is actually a tumour. Differential diagnosis is often difficult, especially when trying to distinguish between tumorous lesions and inflammatory conditions (Fig. 4 and Fig. 5). Differential diagnosis between tumour and multiple sclerosis (MS) is, however, to be undertaken with care and attention: according to the stage of the plaque, the resulting spectra can be diverse and in rare cases MS plaques can simulate a tumour spectrum. In such cases additional information – such as clinical presentation, CSF diagnostics, etc – is essential to minimise further misdiagnosis (Fig. 6).

As far as tumorous lesions are concerned, perfusion MRT and especially MRS are helpful in differentiating types. Necrotising glioblastomas often have a lactate peak. Ependyomas normally have a myoinositol peak and meningeomas a choline monopeak. These are only a few examples of how much pretherapeutic MRT differential diagnostics of intracranial tumours have improved. More insights are expected for the future.

Monitoring the clinical course of intracranial tumours

Perfusion MRT is of particular importance in monitoring the clinical course of more highly malignant intracranial tumours after treatment. During pretherapeutic diagnosis, the advantages are unequivocally with MRS, but perfusion MRT is superior in monitoring the development of more highly malignant tumours. Owing to the high blood volume of highly malignant astroctyomas perfusion MRT enables a much better differentiation between treatment-induced necroses and recurrent tumours than conventional gadolinium MRT (Fig. 7). A high blood

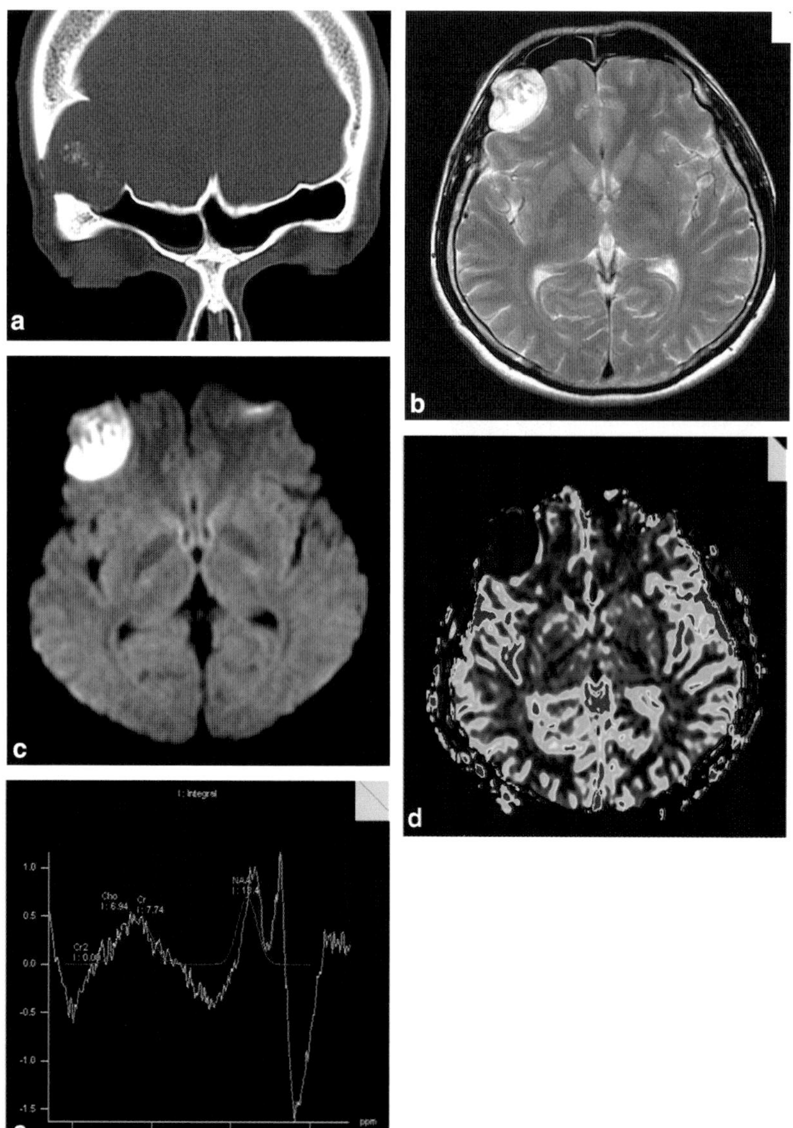

Fig. 5. Chronic actinomycosis abscess. A 33 year old patient presented with chronic sinusitis of the frontal sinus, for which he had received unsuccessful treatment for a year. A CT scan that was performed in another institution (**a**) raised the suspicion that the lesion was in fact a slow-growing, benign, tumour in extra-axial location. The patient had a preoperative MRI scan: T2-weighted turbo spinecho sequence (**b**), diffusion with a b-value of 100 s/mm^2 (**c**), and MR perfusion (rCBV) (**d**). The significantly high signal in the diffusion may imply at a differential diagnosis of an inflammatory process such as in an abscess. MR perfusion shows a complete lack of perfusion, which would be unusual in a tumour. MR spectroscopy (**e**) shows neither an absolute nor a relative rise in choline, but a clear lactate peak is obvious. This supported the idea of an inflammatory genesis. The diagnosis, obtained by histology, was a chronic actinomycosis abscess

volume in perfusion seems to indicate a recurrence reliably whereas lower blood volumes mostly indicate necroses. In our clinical experience of more than 200 cases, however, two patients incorrectly had a recurring tumour diagnosed, which turned out to be actinic neovascularisation within radiation necroses. Since these also necessitate surgery because of the danger of serious bleeds, this currently does not seem to present a substantial clinical problem.

Perfusion MRT also seems useful in monitoring the development of moderately malignant tumours since it may help to diagnose a potential malignisation more easily.

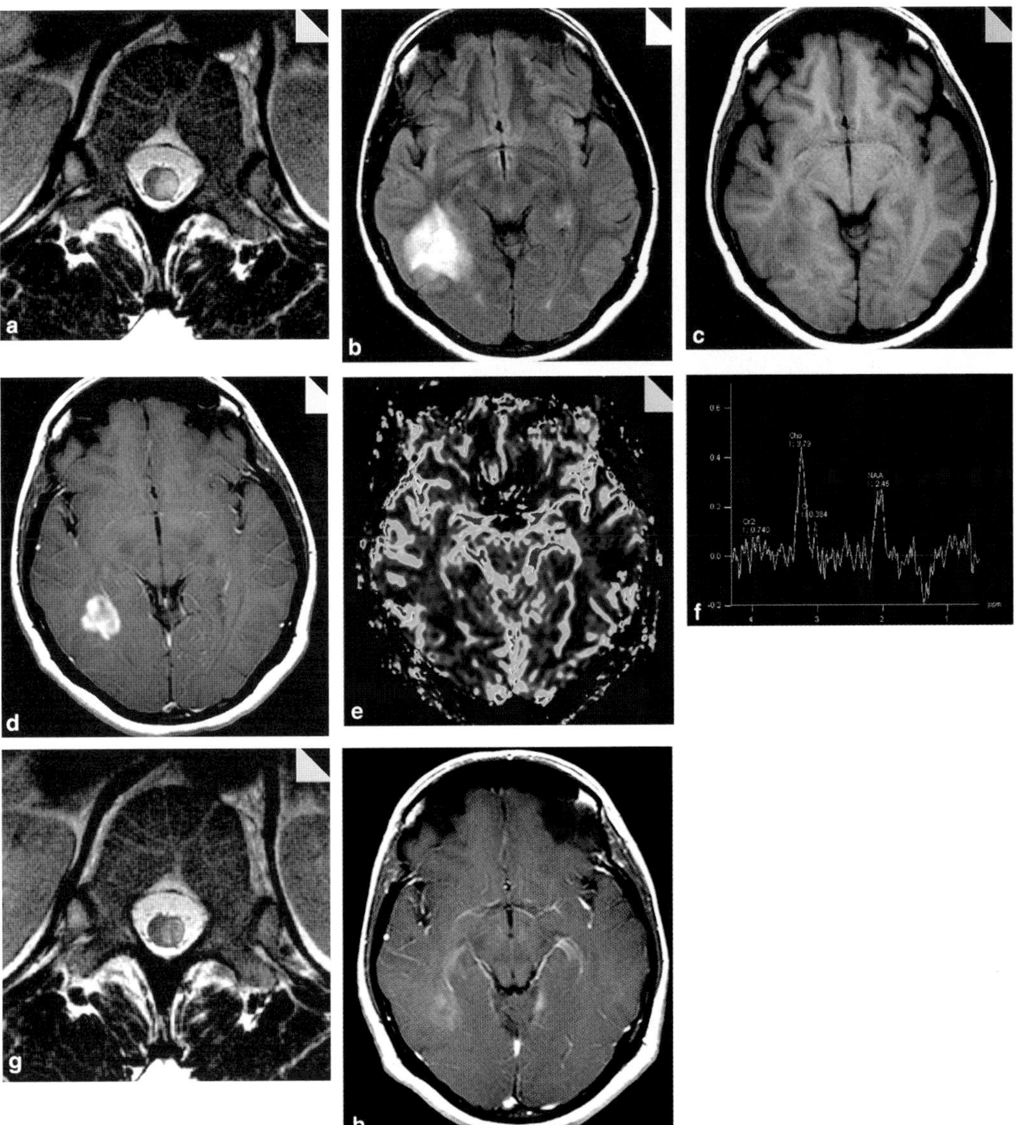

Fig. 6. Suspected multiple sclerosis. A 40 year old woman presented with paraesthesias in both lower arms and hands, hypaesthesias and motor deficits of the left lower limb. An MR scan of the thoracic and lumbar spine shows an extended focus in the myelon in the T2-weighted image (**a**). The primary thought was that of an inflammatory focus, such as in MS, for example. MR investigations of the brain show an extended tumour with significant contrast enhancement in the right temporal lobe: FLAIR (**b**), T1-weighted spinecho sequence before (**c**) and after (**d**) administration of contrast medium (Gadovist). It is of note that this lesion shows a low blood volume on the perfusion scan (**e**), which is not consistent with a highly malignant tumour. MR spectroscopy with an echo time of 135 ms (**f**) shows lowered NAA and creatine and an absolute raise in choline and presence of lactate (peak inversion at 1.3 ppm). This spectrum, in contrast to the perfusion result, implies a more highly malignant tumour. The undulating clinical course with disseminated symptoms pointed in the right direction, although CSF tested negative for MS. No invasive methods were undertaken to confirm the diagnosis; instead the patient was monitored for four weeks. No drug treatment was initiated (for example, with cortisone). The examination after four weeks without treatment showed significant remission of the focus in the myelon (**g**) and the cerebral lesion (**h**) and clear clinical improvement. This confirmed the suspicion of a chronic inflammatory pathology, such as MS. The patient is being monitored regularly

Perfusion MRT is less useful in differentiating moderately malignant parts of the tumour from radiation necrosis since both have a low blood volume. In such cases MRS is the imaging technique of choice.

From a practical point of view perfusion MRT is highly superior to MRS. Data acquisition and evaluation for MRS also take considerably longer than for perfusion MRT.

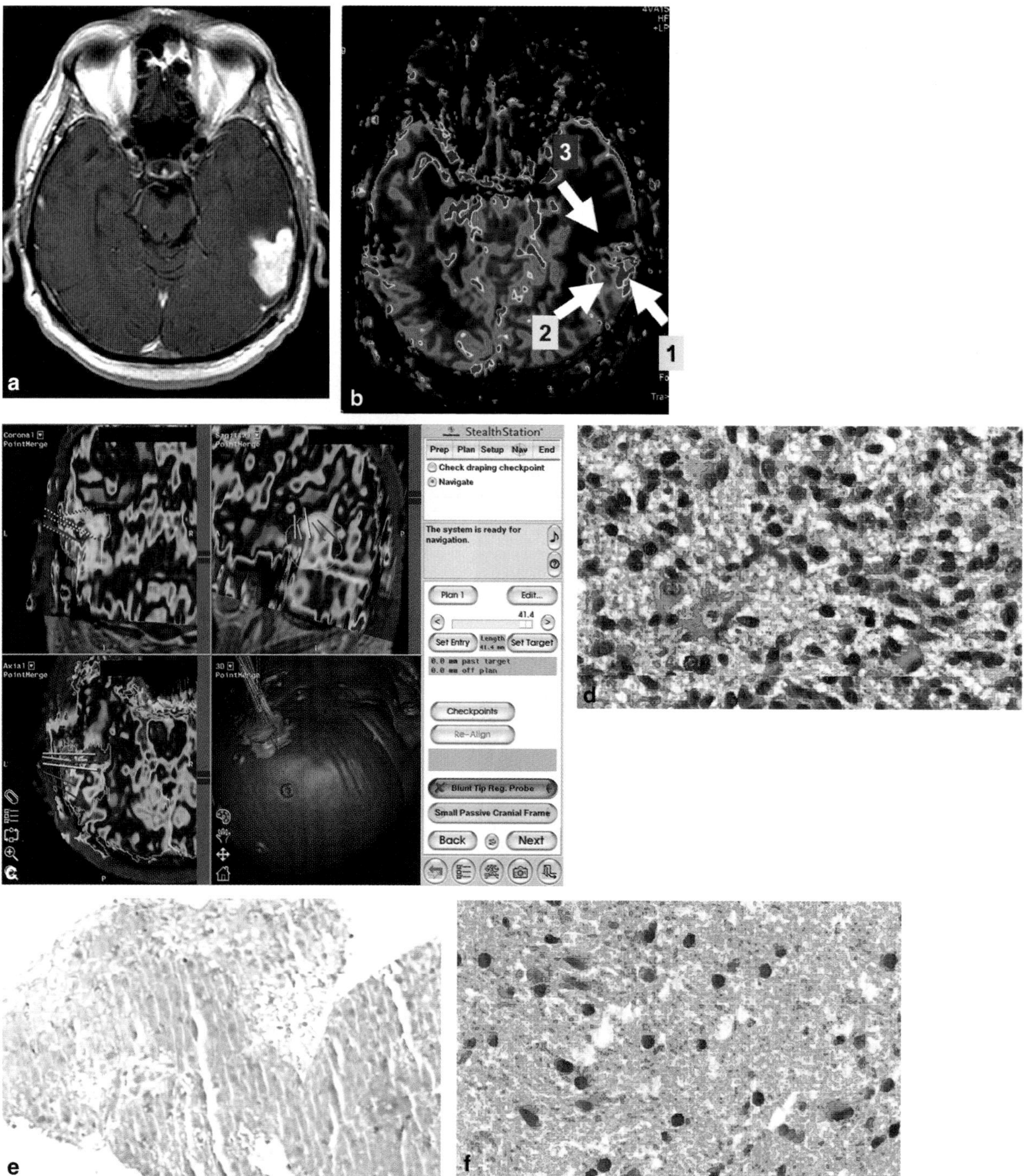

Fig. 7. Recurring glioblastoma multiforme with necrosis. A 54 year old male patient had undergone resection of a glioblastoma multiforme of the left temporal lobe. After surgery he had radiation treatment and chemotherapy. Four weeks after the radiation treatment had ended, the patient presented with a grand mal seizure. External MRI raised clinicians' suspicion of a recurrence. After contrast medium had been administered, a mainly homogenous formation is visible in the former location of the tumour (**a**) in the T1-weighted image. Perfusion MRT (**b**) shows raised rCBV in the lateral part of the lesion, which may indicate a recurrence of the tumour (1). Within the lesion, an area with lower CBV is visible, indicating a pathology of non-tumorous origin, such as necrosis (2). The surrounding parenchyma also showed low rCBV, which may be due to a reaction to the treatment (3). Before the entire lesion was resected, the neurosurgeon took guided biopsies, among others in areas 1, 2, and 3. (**c**) Shows how the biopsies and surgery were planned from the neuronavigation point. The

Fig. 7. (continued)
coloured lines mark the conducted biopsies. Histology produced the following results: **d**) area 1 shows spindle-shaped, partly small-cell, very polymorphous-cell sections on a fibrous background, necroses and atypical vascular proliferations in the sense of a recurrence of a glioblastoma. High rate of mitosis. **e**) Area 2 shows necrosis – adjacent to the tumour recurrence – which may be due to radiation. No vital tissue. **f**) Area 3 consists of reactively changed brain parenchyma without any trace of glioma parts (HE, 100x). The histological findings were confirmed by a reference centre

MR equipment

MR system	**SIEMENS Magnetom Symphony**
Gradients	Quantum gradients Maximum field strength: 30 mT/m Minimum rise time: 240 μs
Software version	Syngo 2002b (VA 21)
Sequence parameter perfusion	
Sequence	EPI
TR	2310 ms
TE	47 ms
FOV	220×220 mm^2
Orientation	transverse
Flip angle	60°
slice thickness	6 mm
slice gap	1.2 mm
Number of slices	19
Number of measurements	40
Measuring time	1 min 37 s
Voxel size	$1.7 \times 1.7 \times 6.0$ mm^3
Matrix size	128×128
Injection parameters perfusion	
Contrast medium	Gadobutrol 0.2 ml/kg body weight flow rate: 5 ml/s
Saline flush	20 ml flow rate: 5 ml/s

Acknowledgements

The experiences that are briefly summarised in this chapter are the result of an excellent interdisciplinary and friendly collaboration between the **Department of Neurology** (head: Prof. Dr F T Aichner) and the **Department of Neurosurgery** (head: Prof. Dr J Fischer), Dr J Pichler (**internal medicine**, special subject neuro-oncology), and the **Institute of Pathology** (head: Prof. Dr R Silye). I cannot thank my collaborators enough for all their help and input.

I also want to thank my colleagues who were actively involved in the cases described in this chapter:

Institute of Neurosurgery: Prof. Dr K Holl, Dr G Wurm, Dr B Tomancok

Institute of Neurology: Dr H-P Haring, Dr F Gruber, Dr Staudacher

Institute of Pathology: Dr R Silye

I also thank my colleagues in the Institute of Radiology for their valuable support, especially Dr S Wimmer and Dr J Trenkler, as well as Dr C Fellner for their constructive suggestion during revision of the manuscript.

Dr. med. Franz A. Fellner
Institute for Radiology
Landes-Nervenklinik Wagner-Jauregg
Wagner-Jauregg-Weg 15
A-4020 Linz
and
Zentrales Radiologie Institut
Allgemeines Krankenhaus (AKH)
Krankenhausstraße 9
A-4021 Linz, Austria
(Correspondence address)

References

[1] Cha S (2003) Perfusion MR imaging: basic principles and clinical applications. Magn Reson Imaging Clin N Am 11:403–413

[2] De Crespigny A (2003) Editorial comment–mismatch or misconception? Stroke 34:1683–1685

[3] Fountas KN, Kapsalaki EZ, Vogel RL, Fezoulidis I, Robinson JS, Gotsis ED (2004) Noninvasive Histologic grading of solid astrocytomas using proton magnetic resonance spectroscopy. Stereotact Funct Neurosurg 82:90–97

[4] Kwong KK, Chesler DA, Weisskoff RM, Donahue KM, Davis TL, Østergaard L, Campbell TA, Rosen BR (1995) MR perfusion studies with T1-weighted echo planar imaging. Magn Reson Med 34:878–887

[5] Latchaw RE (2004) Cerebral perfusion imaging in acute stroke. J Vasc Interv Radiol 15(1 Pt 2):S29–46

[6] Latchaw RE, Yonas H, Hunter GJ, Yuh WTC, Ueda T, Sorensen AG, Sunshine JL, Biller J, Wechsler L, Higashida R, Hademenos T (2003) Guidelines and recommendations for perfusion imaging in cerebral ischemia: a scientific statement for healthcare professionals by the Writing Group on Perfusion Imaging, From the Council on Cardiovascular Radiology of the American Heart Association. Stroke 34:1084–1104

[7] Law M, Yang S, Wang H, Babb JS, Johnson G, Cha S, Knopp EA, Zagzag D (2003) Glioma grading: sensitivity, specificity, and predictive values of perfusion MR imaging and proton MR spectroscopic imaging

compared with conventional MR imaging. AJNR Am J Neuroradiol 24:1989–1998

[8] Østergaard L, Weisskoff RM, Chesler DA, Gyldensted C, Rosen BR (1996) High resolution measurement of cerebral blood flow using intravascular tracer bolus passages. I. Mathematical approach and statistical analysis. Magn Reson Med 36:715–725

[9] Østergaard L, Sorensen AG, Kwong KK, et al (1996) High resolution measurement of cerebral blood flow using intravascular tracer bolus passages. II. Experimental comparison and preliminary results. Magn Reson Med 36:726–736

[10] Preul C, Kuhn B, Lang EW, Mehdorn HM, Heller M, Link J (2003) Differentiation of cerebral tumors using multi-section echo planar MR perfusion imaging. Eur J Radiol 48:244–251

[11] Smith JK, Castillo M, Kwock L (2003) MR spectroscopy of brain tumors. Magn Reson Imaging Clin N Am 11:415–429, v-vi

[12] Sorensen AG, Copen WA, Østergaard L, Buonanno FS, Gonzalez RG, Rordorf G, Rosen BR, Schwamm LH, Weisskoff RM, Koroshetz WJ (1999) Hyperacute stroke: simultaneous measurement of relative cerebral blood volume, relative cerebral blood flow, and mean tissue transit time. Radiology 210:519–527

[13] Sugahara T, Korogi Y, Torniguchi S, Shigematsu Y, Ikushima I, Kira T, Liang L, Ushio Y, Takahashi M (2000) Posttherapeutic intraaxial brain tumor: the value of perfusion-sensitive contrast-enhanced MR imaging for differentiating tumor recurrence from nonneoplastic contrast-enhancing tissue. AJNR Am J Neuroradiol 21:901–909

[14] Tugnoli V, Tosi MR, Barbarella G, Ricci R, Leonardi M, Calbucci F, Bertoluzza A (1998) Magnetic resonance spectroscopy study of low grade extra and intracerebral human neoplasms. Oncol Rep 5:1199–1203

[15] Tzika AA, Cheng LL, Goumnerova L, Madsen JR, Zurakowski D, Astrakas LG, Zarifi MK, Scott RM, Anthony DC, Gonzalez RG, Black PM (2002) Biochemical characterization of pediatric brain tumors by using in vivo and ex vivo magnetic resonance spectroscopy. J Neurosurg 96:1023–1031

[16] Vuori K, Kankaanranta L, Hakkinen AM, Gaily E, Valanne L, Granstrom ML, Joensuu H, Blomstedt G, Paetau A, Lundbom N (2004) Low-grade gliomas and focal cortical developmental malformations: differentiation with proton MR spectroscopy. Radiology 230:703–708

[17] Wegener S, Gottschalk B, Jovanovic V, Knab R, Fiebach JB, Schellinger PD, Kucinski T, Jungehulsing GJ, Brunecker P, Muller B, Banasik A, Amberger N, Wernecke K, Siebler M, Rother J, Villringer A, Weih M, and for the MRI in Acute Stroke Study Group of the German Competence Network Stroke (2004) Transient ischemic attacks before ischemic stroke: preconditioning the human brain?: a multicenter magnetic resonance imaging study. Stroke 35:616–621

Digital mammography

R. Schulz-Wendtland[1], K.-P. Hermann[2], and W. Bautz[1]

[1]University Erlangen-Nürnberg, Institute for Diagnostic Radiology (Director: Professor W. Bautz MD)
[2]Georg-August-University Göttingen, Faculty of Medicine, Division for Diagnostic Radiology
(Director: Professor E. Grabbe MD)

Introduction

For many years, almost all types of diagnostic radiology have had digital imaging technology at their disposal, but no adequate digital alternative was available for traditional screen film mammography (SFM) [1–5]. Even in "filmless" hospitals, mammographies were therefore performed in the traditional manner. The reason is that mammography has special requirements vis-à-vis the quality of images, and digital imaging methods are not capable of meeting these requirements just like that. Traditional screen film mammography is thus far the only imaging technique that helped to achieve a reduction in breast cancer mortality when used as a regular screening tool [6]. Its advantages include its comparatively low costs, a high resolution in the high contrast area (up to 20 lp/mm), and easy viewing on a viewbox. In addition to having to find a compromise between definition and exposure, the disadvantages of the imaging system include its low effective quantum efficiency (DQE). Owing to the sigmoid gradation curve of conventional screen film systems, each system can be usefully employed only when radiation dosages are clearly defined.

The information conveyed by a radiograph is best described with the so-called signal to noise ratio (SNR). This ratio depends on the radiation dose and the quantum flow that was used to obtain the image, but also on the structural attributes of the imaging systems. The DQE is a further important measure to gauge the capacity of a mammography system, by indicating how effectively the SNR or the information contained in the radiograph – produced by X-rays that have passed through the chest – is transferred on to the mammogram. The ideal is a transfer ratio of 1:1, i.e. a DQE of 100%. Real equipment, however, is not capable of such high quality, owing to noise and other processes that reduce the contrast. The resulting quality of the image is therefore always reduced, and the DQE falls to less than 100%. The reduction in the SNR results in an inferior reproduction of small details in the breast, such as microcalcifications. The DQE is dependent on the radiation dose and the local frequency. With the same dose, a system with a high DQE produces images with less noise, or it produces images of equal quality with a smaller radiation dose than a system with a lower DQE. The DQE enables objective comparison between different radiographical imaging systems on the basis of the image quality and dose efficiency. Currently no standardised procedures exist to help determine the DQE for mammography imaging systems, and especially not for complete mammography workstations with a complete set of components, including image viewers. The DQE values provided by manufacturers of digital mammography systems can therefore not be compared and can be used only as approximate guidelines.

In digital mammography, conventional screen film mammography is replaced by an electronic detector that absorbs the incoming X-rays and produces an electric signal. This signal is digitalised in an analogue-to-digital converter and can therefore be processed, exposed, and stored on a computer. In conventional film screen mammography, the entire imaging process is linked to the radiograph, whereas in digital radiography, the actual imaging is split into three steps: recording, processing, and reproduction. This means that each individual step can be optimised, and in addition an opportunity arises for electronic image transfer in the sense of tele-radiography. A digital mammogram consists of a finite number of pixels, which are arranged in a two-dimensional image matrix. The distance between two adjacent pixels is known as the sampling frequency or, more generally, as the pixel size. The grey value of each individual pixel is quantified

– i.e., represented by a finite number of signals. These values range from 0 to $2^n - 1$, with n equalling the number of bits that are used to digitalise the variation of the analogue signal in the detector. Systems than can be used for mammography capture the data with a depth of up to 16 bit/pixel, equalling $2^{16} = 65536$ shades of grey. The greater the number of pixels and shades of grey, the greater the storage requirement of an individual mammogram.

The digital mammography systems that are currently licensed by the US Food and Drug Administration achieve a resolution of 5–12.5 lp/mm (max). To reach the very high resolution of conventional film screen mammography (of up to 20 lp/mm), digital detectors would have to have a maximum pixel size of 25 μm, which would mean an image matrix of $7200 \times 9600 = 69.1$ million pixels for a detector area of 18×24 cm^2. Nishikawa et al. [7], however, found in 1987 that the detection of critical structures is limited more by an SNR that is too low and has too little contrast than by the resolution of the digital imaging system. In spite of this finding, the quality of resolution and its importance in assessing a digital mammography system were at the centre of technical discussions for a long time. In Germany, the requirements for resolution are now different for conventional film screen mammography ($\geq$ 10 lp/mm) and digital mammography ($\geq$ 5 lp/mm). At a European level, work is being done on an addendum to the section covering "digital mammography" in the European protocol for quality control of the physical and technical aspects of mammography screening, to introduce the threshold contrast visibility as the crucial measure of image quality. The lower requirements vis-à-vis local contrast visibility for digital mammography systems are being justified with the fact that lesions are detected because of their contrast to their background and that contrast visibility or other functions of transmission that use contrast are a more appropriate measure than the modulation transfer function used by film screen systems or the threshold frequency of visual perception that is derived from it [8]. The contrast resolution is determined as the smallest radiological contrast that produces a visible difference in the image for an image detail of a particular size.

Two types of digital mammography systems have to be distinguished: tape-based (off-line) and integrated (online) imaging systems. Off-line systems include storage devices (plates, etc) that can be used with any conventional mammography equipment if the exposure variable is selected accordingly. Integrated imaging systems are installed into each individual mammography system and cannot be moved. Further distinction has to be made between full-field systems and scanning systems. Full-field detectors are exposed like a film screen system, whereas in the case of scanning systems, an array of detectors is moved very slowly across the area that is to be imaged, and the X-rays are sent through a slot and therefore limited to the width of the row of detectors.

Digital mammography systems with FDA licence

1. Senographe 2000 D (GE Medical Systems, Waukesha, USA)

The digital mammography system Senographe 2000 D by manufacturer GE Medical Systems uses a flat panel digital detector of 19×23 cm^2. The detector is based on a semiconductor layer from amorphous silicium, which has been vapourised on to a glass mount as the sensor matrix. Each individual element of the matrix contains thin-film diodes or transistors, which allow the selection, pixel by pixel, of a charge profile produced on the detector by radiation. The silicium in the sensor matrix is not sufficiently sensitive to the radiation quality used in mammography, so that the matrix is combined with a scintillator layer of CsI:Tl. In this layer, X-rays are converted into visible light. The needle shape of the caesium iodine crystals focuses the light on to the detector elements, so that loss through scattering can be mostly prevented [9, 10, 11] (Table 1).

2. SenoScan (Fischer Imaging, Denver, USA)

The digital mammography system SenoScan by manufacturer Fischer Imaging uses a "slot scan" detector measuring 1×22 cm^2 and consisting of four charge coupled devices (CCDs), using a default pixel size of 54 μm. CCD technology uses a particular attribute of silicium – namely, it converts incoming light photons into mobile charge carriers. As the CCD sensors are not very sensitive to X-rays, incoming radiation first has to be converted by the scintillators into visible light. The intensity of light behind the scintillator is then adopted as the charge profile, in a multitude of spatially arranged individual elements and converted into digital imaging information [9, 10, 11]. The size of the CCD sensor is limited to about 5×5 cm^2 as single crystal silicium discs have to be used. Digital full-field mammography is possible only by arranging four small CCD receptors in an array and in combination with scanning technology. Scanning systems have the advantage that "stray" radiation from the breast can be efficiently kept from the detector even without a filter, which helps to

Table 1. Digital mammography-systems

	Senographe 2000D	SenoScan	LDBI	Selenia	FCR 5000MA
Manufacturer	GE Medical Systems	Fischer Imaging	Hologic/Lorad	Hologic/Lorad	Fujifilm
Conversion Material	Scintillator CsI:Tl	Scintillator CsI:Tl	Scintillator CsI:Tl	Photoconductor aSe	Phosphor Storage Screen
Detector Material	aSi	4 CCDs (slot detector)	12 CCDs (mosaic detector)	aSi	
Pixel Size	100 μm	50 μm	40 μm	70 μm	50 μm (laser width)
Field of View	19×23 cm^2	21×29 cm^2 (scan system)	19×25 cm^2	24×29 cm^2	24×30 cm^2
DQE	42	50	55	65	45
Spatial Resolution[1]	5 lp/mm	10 lp/mm	12.5 lp/mm	7.1 lp/mm	10 lp/mm
Memory Depth	14 Bit	12 Bit	14 Bit	12 Bit	10 Bit
FDA Approval	January 2000	September 2001	March 2002	October 2002	2004 (4)

[1]The designated spatial resolution is the resulting Nyquist frequency from the given pixel size.

improves contrast visibility and SNR. Another advantage is that the detector at any time has to capture only the radiation that has passed behind part of the breast and therefore, with a given pixel size, fewer detector elements are required than with full-field systems. For scanning systems, the acquisition time for a complete mammogram is 3–6 seconds. As each part of the breast is exposed only for a very short moment, this does not result in movement related blurring, which is a familiar outcome of film screen mammography. Imaging artefacts may, however, arise if the breast is being moved during the scanning process (Table 1).

3. LDBI (Hologic/Lorad, Bedford, USA)

The Lorad Digital Breast Imager (LDBI) works with a digital image acquisition system, which consists of 12 CCDs that are arranged in the form of a mosaic, and that are coupled with a large scintillator plate that is thallium doped caesium iodide. This receptor covers an area of 18.6×24.8 cm^2. Hologic is, however, not planning further marketing of the CCD-based units but is concentrating its activities on the flat panel digital detector consisting of amorphous selenium (Table 1).

4. Selenia (Hologic/Lorad, Bedford, USA)

Lorad's digital mammography system Selenia uses a 24×29 cm^2 flat panel detector, which, instead of a scintillator, has a semiconductor layer of amorphous selenium. Selenium enables the direct conversion of X-rays into electrical charge. This technology uses a voltage of about 2.5 kV, applied to a layer of selenium of about 250 μm thickness. Behind the selenium layer is a pixel matrix consisting of electrodes to receive the charge, storage condensers, and field effect transistors. The charge produced in the selenium layer by X-rays is passed along the field lines to the charge electrode underneath and stored in the condenser. If a particular transistor is aimed at the charge is passed on to an analogue to digital converter [9, 10, 11]. When selenium technology is used, the incoming radiation is converted directly into electrons. Since every step of the conversion makes additional disturbances possible, direct conversion should result in an improved noise characteristic. The detector has a pixel size of 70 μm and thus reaches a maximum local resolution of 7.1 lp/mm (Table 1).

5. FCR 5000MA (Fujifilm, Tokyo, Japan)

Fuji's full-field mammography system FCR 5000MA includes an image plate reader with a resolution of 50 μm for all mammography formats, with dual-sided reading technology. Computed radiography (CR) technology is currently the most widely used procedure for digital projection radiography in clinical practice. Digital mammography using photo-stimulated phosphor imaging plates has been used in clinical practice for some 20 years now. This technology uses X-rays that elevate electrons in a crystal structure to a higher energy level. The number and distribution of these electrons correspond to the intensity of the radiation. In a separate reading unit, a laser beam scans the imaging plate. During this process, electrons revert back to their original state while emitting light. A photomultiplier registers the amount of light at the site. After the analogue signals have been converted into digital signals, each pixel in the image is allocated an intensity value. The concluding, homogeneous incidence of light deletes the remaining imaging information [9, 10, 11]. For use in mammography, high resolution imaging plates with a sampling rate of 10 Pixel/mm were selected. Since March 2001 a new imaging plate with a thicker emulsion layer and a transparent support layer has become available, which in the FCR 5000MA is selected simultaneously, on both sides, with an sampling rate of 20 Pixel/mm. In this way, the local resolution of 5 lp/mm, which has theoretically been possible so far, was increased to 10 lp/mm, and through the dual-sided selection process, the DQE was also raised. The CR system can be used in combination with any conventional mammography system if the automatic exposure is adjusted accordingly (Table 1).

Results from clinical studies

Ad I.

Obenauer et al. [12, 13] and Fischer et al. [14] compared digital mammography (GE-System) and conventional screen film mammography in clinical and control investigations and found comparable results or slight superiority (not significant) of the digital technique. Grebe et al. [15] and Schulz-Wendtland et al. [16], however, found no significant differences between the two systems. In a comparative study of 692 female patients, Venta, Hendrick et al. [17] found agreement between conventional film screen mammography and digital mammography in 82%, part-agreement in 14%, and no agreement in 4% of results, which they explained this with interobserver variability. Another study by Lewin, Hendrick et al. [18] that included 4945 female patients found on comparing conventional and digital mammography a total of 35 cases of breast cancer – the conventional system detected 22 cases and the digital system 21 cases. The authors found no significant difference in the detection rate, but a lower recall rate in digital mammography than in conventional mammography (11.5% *v* 13.8%, respectively). They did not find a significant difference in the rate of positive biopsies (19% *v* 30%). Lewin and Hendrick, in a study in 2002 [19] with 6736 patients whose condition was generally diagnosed through both imaging modalities, found 42 malignancies in 181 biopsies, of which 15 were detected exclusively though conventional mammography and only 9 through digital mammography. They did not find a significant difference in the detection rate for malignancy, but a lower recall rate for digital mammography. The study by Skaane et al. [20] included 1832 women who were examined with both techniques (additionally generally double reading). The authors did not find significant differences in the detection rate but a higher rate of air ingress and average parenchymal dosis for the digital system than for the conventional system. This study has met with substantial criticism with regard to different variables, and in addition the results are diametrically opposed to those of Hermann et al. [21, 22], who found a dose reduction of 25% for digital mammography compared with conventional mammography.

Ad 2. and 3.

There are no clinical studies. Only studies with small field detectors, such as the one by Undrill et al. [23], found, in a phantom study, significantly better results in clarity of detail for the CCD technique than for film screen mammography, without significant interobserver variability.

Ad 4.

There is no literature reporting clinical studies investigating amorphous selenium used in digital mammography.

Ad 5.

The available studies, among others by Schulz-Wendtland et al. [24, 25], show equivalence of luminescence radiography and conventional film screen mammography.

Currently, two large, prospective, randomised clinical trials including a total of 49 000 women, are under way [26, 27]. The US Department of Defense (DOD) is sponsoring a study that compares the systems manufactured by Lorad, Fischer, und GE. This study investigates digital full-field mammography as well as conventional film screen mammography in all patients and analyses the findings them independently of each other. A minimum follow up of 18 months is planned. Eight centres are participating in the study by the International Digital Mammography Development Group (IDMDG), which assesses the digital systems manufactured by Lorad, Fischer, und GE. Results from either study can be expected for 2005 at the earliest. It remains to be seen whether the two studies prove a significant superiority of one of the two systems as interobserver variability tends to be substantial.

Discussion

The literature overview shows that few clinical studies to date have compared conventional and digital mammography. Tendentially, on the basis of phantom and clinical studies, luminescence radiography with high resolution imaging plates (CR-M) (Fuji/Siemens) and digital full-field mammography (GE) (using a digital amorphous silicium detector) has been found to be of equal value or slightly superior to conventional film screen systems [12–25]. The validity of the available studies meets the criteria only for classification II B-C (prospective, non-randomised studies) of the ASCO (American Society of Clinical Oncology) [28]. No studies that meet classification I criteria (prospective, randomised studies) are currently available. Notably, however both digital mammography devices manufactured by Lorad (detector from amorphous selenium, and CCD basis), the digital full-field mammography device manufactured by Fischer (digital CCD detector), and the device manufactured by General Electric (digital amorphous silicium detector) have been licensed by the US FDA, which for digital mammography with high resolution imaging plates is not expected before 2004. Along with others we think that digital mammography is a promising future technology for the diagnostics of the breast. Whether Pisano et al. [26, 27] are correct in assuming that, that owing to theoretical considerations, our hopes for the future lie in full-field systems on the basis of CCD detectors and the advantages of digital systems in view of high local resolution (threshold visibility more than 10 lp/mm) and DQE >0.6, has to be questioned critically.

On this background, the results from the studies of the US Defense Department and the International Digital Mammography Development Group, are of particular importance. Additionally, opportunities may open up for computer assisted diagnosis (CAD), tomosynthesis, and tele-radiography on the basis of primarily digitally composed images.

References

[1] Bick U (2000) Digitale Vollfeldmammographie. RöFo 173: 957–964

[2] Grabbe E, Fischer U, Funke M, Hermann KP, Obenauer S, Baum F (2001) Wert und Bedeutung der digitalen Vollfeldmammographie im Rahmen eines Mammographie – Screenings. Radiologe 41: 359–365

[3] Herman KP, Funke, M, Grabbe E (2002) Physikalisch-technische Aspekte der digitalen Mammographie. Radiologe 42: 256–260

[4] Säbel M, Aichinger U, Schulz-Wendtland R, Bautz W (1999) Digitale Vollfeld-Mammographie: Physikalische Grundlagen und klinische Aspekte. Röntgenpraxis 52: 171–177

[5] Feig SA, Yaffe MJ (1998) Digital mammography. Radio Graphics 18: 893–901

[6] Schreer I (2001) Auswertung der bisherigen Mammographie – Screening – Studien in Europa und in Nordamerika. Radiologe 41: 344–351

[7] Nishikawa RM, Mawdsley GE, Fenster A, Yaffe MJ (1987) Scanned projection digital mammography. Med Phys 14: 717–727

[8] European Commission (2001) European guidelines for quality assurance in mammography screening, 3rd. edn. Office for Official Publications of the European Communities, Luxemburg

[9] Busch HP (1999) Digitale Projektionsradiographie. Technische Grundlagen, Abbildungseigenschaften und Anwendungsmöglichkeiten. Radiologe 39: 710–724

[10] Neitzel U (2000) Systeme für die digitale Bildgebung. In: Ewen K (Hrsg) Moderne Bildgebung. Thieme, Stuttgart, S 127–136

[11] Schulz RF (2001) Digitale Vollfeld – Mammographie: Physikalische Grundlagen und klinische Aspekte. Fortschr Röntgenstr 173: 1137–1146

[12] Obenauer S, Hermann KP, Schorn C, Funke M, Fischer U, Grabbe E (2000) Digitale Vollfeldmammographie: Phantomstudie zur Detektion von Mikrokalk. RöFo 172: 646–650

[13] Obenauer S, Hermann KP, Schorn C, Fischer U, Grabbe E (2000) Digitale Vollfeldmammographie: Dosisabhängige Detektion von simulierten Herdbefunden und Mikrokalzifikationen. RöFo 172: 1052–1056

[14] Fischer U, Baum F, Obenauer, S, Luftner-Nagel, S, Von Heyden D, Vosshenrich R, Grabbe E (2002) Comparative study in patients with microcalcifications: full – field digital mammography vs. screen-film mammography. Eur Radiol 12: 2679–2683

[15] Grebe S, Dieckmann F, Bick U, Paepke S, Winzer KJ, Hamm B (2000) Initial clinical experiences with digital full-field mammography. Zentralbl Gynäkol 122: 589–594

[16] Schulz-Wendtland R, Aichinger U, Lell U, Kuchar I, Tartsch M, Bautz W (2002) Erfahrungen mit Phantommessungen an verschiedenen Mammographiesystemen. RöFo 174: 1243–1246

[17] Venta LA, Hendrick RE, Adler YT, De leon P, Mengoni PM, Scharl AM, Comstock CE, Hansen L, Kay N, Coveler A, Cutter G (2001) Rates and causes of disagreement in interpretation of full-field digital mammography and film-screen mammography in a diagnostic setting. AJR 176: 1241–1248

[18] Lewin JM, Hendrick RE, D' Orsi CJ, Isaacs PK, Moss LJ, Karellas A, Sisney GA, Kuni CC, Cutter GR (2001) Comparison of full-field digital mammography with screen-film mammography for cancer detection: results of 4,945 paired examinations. Radiology 218: 873–880

[19] Lewin JM, D' Orsi CJ, Hendrick RE, Moss LJ, Isaacs PK, Karellas A, Cutter GR (2002) Clinical comparison of full-field digital mammography and screen-film mammography for detection of breast cancer. AJR 179(3): 671–677

[20] Skaane P, Skjennald A, Gangeskar L, Pedersen K (2001) Population-based Full Field Direct Digital Mammography (FFDDM) Screening: The Oslo Project. Digital Mammography 2001, Toronto

[21] Hermann KP, Obenauer S, Grabbe E (2000) Die Strahlenexposition bei der digitalen Vollfeldmammographie mit einem Flachdetektor aus amorphem Silizium im Vergleich zur konventionellen Film-Folien-Mammographie. RöFo 172: 1052–1056

[22] Hermann KP, Obenauer S, Marten K, Kehbel S, Fischer U, Grabbe E (2002) Mittlere Parenchymdosis bei der digitalen Vollfeldmammographie mit einem Detektor aus amorphem Silizium – Klinische Ergebnisse. RöFo 174: 696–699

[23] Undrill PE, O'Kane AD, Gillbert FJ (2000) A comparison of digital and screen-film mammography using quality control phantoms. Clin Radiol 55: 782–790

[24] Schulz-Wendtland R, Aichinger U, Säbel M, Böhner C, Dobritz M, Bautz W (2002) Experimentelle Untersuchungen zur Bildgüte konventioneller Film-Folien-Mammographie, digitaler Mammographie mit Speicherfolien in Vergrößerungstechnik und voll digitaler Mammographie in CCD-Technik. RöFo 172: 965–968

[25] Schulz-Wendtland R, Aichinger U, Säbel M, Böhner C, Dobritz M, Wenkel E, Bautz W (2002) Expermental investigations of image quality in X-ray mammography with conventional screen film system (SFS), digital phosphor storage plate in/without magnification technique (CR) and digital CCD-technique (CCD). Röntgenpraxis 54: 53–55

[26] Pisano ED, Cole EB, Major S, Zong S, Hemminger BM, Muller KE, Johnston RE, Walsh R, Conant E, Fajardo LL, Feig SA, Nishikawa RM, Yaffe MJ, Williams MB, Aylward SR (2000) Radiologistś preferences for digital mammographic display. The International Digital Mammography Development Group. Radiology 216: 820–830

[27] Pisano E, Yaffe M, Hemminger B, Hendrick R, Niklason L (2000) Current status of full-field digital mammography. Acad Radiol 7: 266–280

[28] ASCO (American Society of Clinical Oncology) (1999) Guidelines. J Clin Oncol 17: 1312

New advances for imaging laryngo / trachealstenosis by post processing of spiral-CT data

E. Sorantin[1], D. Mohadjer[1], L. G. Nyúl[2], K. Palágyi[2], F. Lindbichler[1], and B. Geiger[3]

[1]Division of Digital Information and Image Processing, Department of Radiology, University Hospital Graz, Graz, Austria
[2]Department of Applied Informatics, Josef Attila University Szeged, Szeged, Hungary
[3]Siemens Corporate Research Princeton Inc., Josef Attila University Szeged, New Jersey, USA

Endotracheal intubation is the most common cause of laryngo-tracheal stenoses (LTS), followed by trauma and prior airway surgery [1, 2, 3]. In rare cases LTS may have resulted also from inhalation injuries, gastro-esophageal reflux disease, neoplasia and autoimmune diseases like Wegeners granulomatosis or relapsing polychondritis [1, 4]. In pediatric patients vascular compression of the trachea is a common cause of tracheal indentations [5]. Clinical management of these conditions requires information on localization, grade, length and dynamics of the stenosis. Exact LTS information is necessary, since stenoses with a length less than 1.0 cm can be treated by an endoscopic surgery [6, 7]. Besides fiberoptic endoscopy (FE), which represents the gold standard for airway evaluation, imaging modalities like conventional radiography, fluoroscopy, tracheal tomograms, Magnetic Resonance Imaging and above all Spiral Computed Tomography (S-CT) are an essential part of the clinical work up [1, 8]. S-CT and the recent introduction of multislice imaging allows volumetric data acquisition of the laryngo-tracheal tract (LTT) during a short time span. Decreased motion artifacts and increased spatial resolution form the basis for high quality post processing [9, 10].

The improved performance of today's workstations permits the use of sophisticated post processing algorithms even on standard hardware like personal computers. Thus real time 3D display and virtual endoscopic views (virtual endoscopy) are just one mouse click away. Other algorithms compute the medial axis of tubular structures like airways or vessels in 3D, which can be used for the calculation of 3D cross sectional profiles for better demonstration of caliber changes [11]. Thus display of S-CT axial source images is moving rapidly to 3D display. Moreover, established network connections within and between institutions allows telemedical cooperation. Web technologies offer an easy to use way for information exchange.

The objective of this book contribution is to give an overview about 3D display and quantification of LTS as well as to provide information how these results can be presented and shared with the referring physicians on the hospital's computer network. This contribution is structured in 7 parts:

- S-CT data acquisition for LTS imaging
- Airway Segmentation
- 3D Display
- Virtual Endoscopy
- Objective LTS degree and length estimation using LTT 3D – cross – sectional profiles
- Intranet Applications
- Conclusion

S-CT data acquisition for Imaging of LTS

Positioning

All CT studies should be performed in helical mode. The patient is scanned supine and special care has to taken for head positioning in order to faciliate comparable results for follow-up studies. In our institution we prefer a head position, where the vertical beam of the CT machine laser positioning tool targets the lateral orbital angle and the tragus cartilage. This procedure puts the head in a neutral position and is easy to reproduce.

Scan range

Helical scanning is performed from the caudal mastoid border to the tracheal bifurcation.

Scan parameters

Modern multislice scanners allow a beam collimation of about 0.75 mm to 1.25 mm and the highest pitch levels as recommended by the manufacturer. In order to keep the radiation as low as possible a low tube current should be used. At reconstruction an overlap of 50% to 70% should be used. Thus a whole study ends up with about 200 to 300 axial source images.

Intravenous contrast medium injection

For LTT evaluation usually there is no need for intravenous (i.v.) contrast medium injection. Exceptions are oncologic staging investigations, especially laryngeal cancers, and the suspicion of vascular anomalies in children. Whenever i.v. contrast injection is necessary an power injector should be used, the flow rate should be set to 3 ml/s and bolus tracking systems used.

Airway segmentation

Segmentation can be defined as procedure to define the boundaries of the "Organ of Desire" or more general speaking "Regions of Interest" (ROI's). An ideal algorithm should be as much as possible free from the operators influence and fast. Several algorithms can be used – from simple manual tracing and region growing to more sophisticated ones like the "Fuzzy Connectedness" algorithm – the later ones will be presented in more detail below.

Region growing

Due to the air content of the upper respiratory tract the attenuation coefficients are well below −150 Hounsfield Units [12]. Axial S-CT slices are displayed at lung window settings (center/width -600/1200 Hounsfield Units). By starting from a seed point inside the trachea, neighboring voxels are added if their attenuation coefficients are below a specified threshold (usually less than −150 Hounsfield Units) [12]. Due to the partial volume effects boundary pixels, respective voxels, exhibit a variation of the attenuation coefficients. Thus organ boundaries are frequently not closed on axial source images. Therefore, by choosing a fixed threshold value keeps the segmented contour either to "close" or "bleeding" occurs (meaning the extension of the segmented region to unwarranted dimensions). As workaround, the chosen threshold can be adapted on slice to slice basis to the individual S-CT patient data [13]. Next, the middle of the segmented region is determined and projected to the next slice, where it serves as a new seed point. The entire process is repeated until the whole upper respiratory tract has been defined and each step is performed under the control of the operator. This approach inherits the disadvantage of being highly operator dependent.

Fuzzy connectedness

"Fuzzy Connectedness" captures the image inherent fuzziness as well as the spatial-coherence of the voxels in a well defined manner [14, 15]. In case of LTT, air has a well defined range of Hounsfield units. Therefore the parameters, needed for the definition of the fuzzy affinities, can be set once and used for all studies without a per-study training. On one or more axial slices the operator selects by a mouse click a "seed point" within the LTT center for seeding the fuzzy connected objects.

Since absolute "Fuzzy Connectedness" is used and a single object is segmented, the uncertain boundary regions (due to partial volume effects) are not captured by the fuzzy objects. Thus the resulting segmented LTT was uniformly smaller than the physicians expectations. Hence a 3D dilation using a $3 \times 3 \times 3$ structuring element was applied to the segmented fuzzy connected object. Finally the operator controlled at fixed window settings (center −600 Hounsfield units, width 1200 Hounsfield units) the results of segmentation on the computer screen, where the segmented LTT boundaries were outlined on original axial slices (Fig. 1). In an own investigation the "Fuzzy Connectedness" algorithm was applied for LTS segmentation in 26 patients and 18 normal controls. On average 3.9 slices had to be edited in patients and 2.4 in the normal controls – this difference was found to be statistically insignificant ($p = 0.06$). In 90% of all cases only less than five slices had to be corrected manually [11]. In another study the accuracy and precision of three different approaches for LTS segmentation were investigated, namely: free hand tracing, manual tracing augmented by splines and the "Fuzzy Connectedness" algorithm [16]. Segmentation results revealed no statistically significant differences regarding accuracy and precision, but the "Fuzzy Connectedness" algorithm proved to be the fastest, just lasting 15–20 seconds for a complete run of LTT segmentation. Therefore the conclusion can be drawn, that the "Fuzzy Connectedness" algorithm represents a fast and robust tool for LTT segmentation.

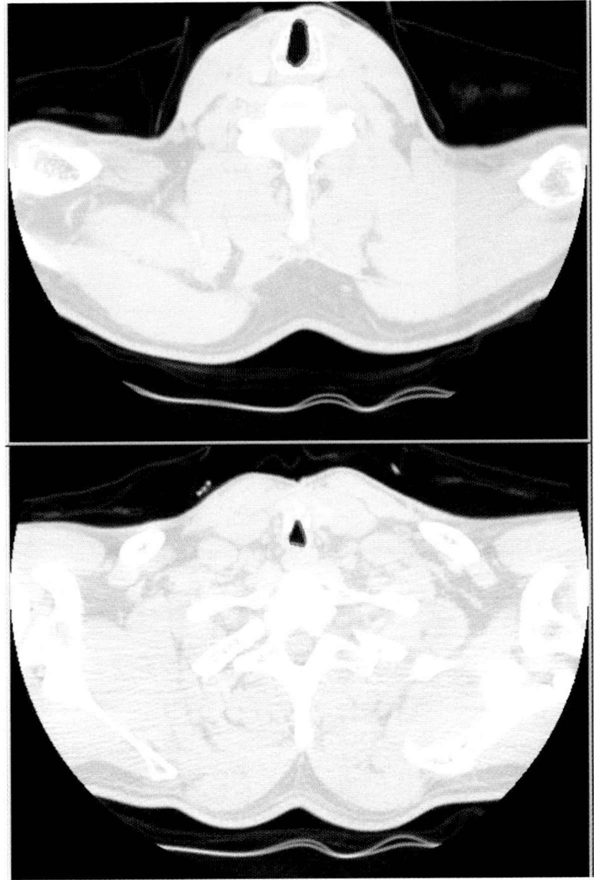

Fig. 1. S-CT, LTT segmentation based on fuzzy connectedness: the red line, superimposed on the original axial S-CT image outlines the results of segmentation for the laryngeal region (upper part) and for a tracheal stenosis (lower part)

3D-display

It is well known in medical literature that the mental reconstruction process of multiple, transaxial sections may fail in patients with tracheobronchial deformities [12, 17]. On axial CT the shape of tubular structures like airways depends on the angle between the structure itself and the slice plane: If this angle is 90 degrees to the longitudinal axis of the tubular structure the true cross section, e.g. a circle, is displayed. If this angle is oblique or approaches zero the displayed shape will change e.g. will get more elliptic. Therefore the true caliber and shape in 3D are hard to determine on axial slices alone. 3D reconstructions help to avoid this problem. So for example Remy-Jardin published a paper regarding the comparison between reading axial slices alone and volume rendered transparent bronchographic images. It was found, that the volume rendered bronchographic 3D reconstructions were superior to reading axial slices alone [17]. 3D-display allows to demonstrate clinical colleagues CT findings in an easy and impressive way. It addition, they are useful for follow-up investigation, since the underlying patho-anatomy is displayed on just a few views.

In medical image processing mainly "Multiplanar Reformation", "Surface Rendering" and "Volume Rendering" are used – these techniques will be described in the following.

Multiplanar reformation (MPR)

For computing MPR's all images are stacked in order to built up a volume. Care has to be taken in order to keep the correct aspect ratio – either interpolation is used or the volume is stretched according the ratio between the x,y- and z-voxel-size. MPR's are known for assessment of spinal CT investigations. Similar, sagittal and coronal MPR enable additional LTS view. In case of a buckled LTT it is not possible to display the LTT in one view, but this can be achieved using curved MPR's. In addition, thick MPR's (MPR with a thickness of more than one pixel) can be used for better overview (see Fig. 2).

Surface rendering (Synomina: Shaded surface display, isocontour rendering)

After segmentation the contours of the ROI's can be extracted easily. Using the morphological operation of erosion, one layer of the segmented surface voxels can be "peeled off" [18]. The difference between the resulting data volume and the original volume are just the surface voxels. Therefore once the data volume has been subtracted from the original volume only the contours will remain. In order to obtain polyhedral surface models these contours are converted into 3D models using the Delaunay triangulation method [19]. Figure 3 displays the contours of a segmented trachea. Figure 4 shows the result after triangulation.

These surface models can be rendered at interactive speed at a workstation. Properties such as color and transparency may be manipulated. A 3D model after color mapping can be seen in Fig. 5, demonstrating a patient suffering from a subglottic stenosis. In addition, real time rotation, panning and zooming are possible. By conversion of such 3D models according the standards of the Virtual Reality Modeling Language 2.0 (VRML) they can even be visualized on a Personal Computer using a standard web browser [20].

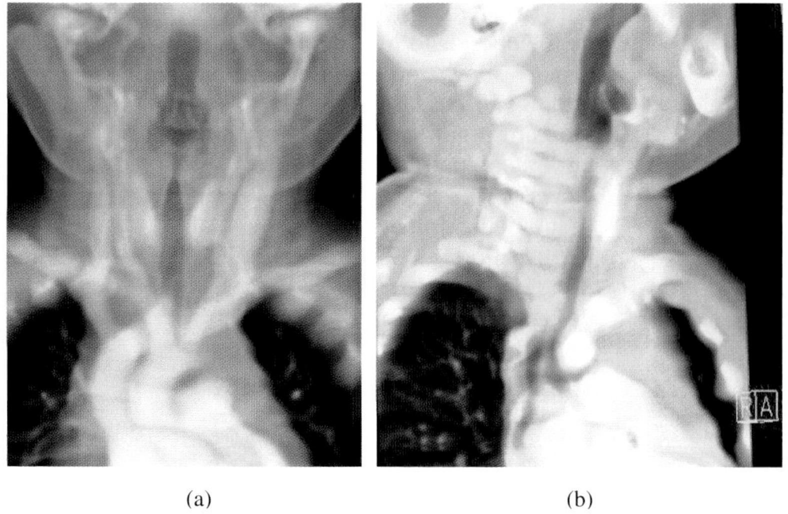

(a) (b)

Fig. 2. S-CT, thick MPR reconstruction: tracheal compression caused by the brachiocephalic artery. **a** Shows an ap – view and **b** a lateral view. On both views the tracheal compression can be percepted

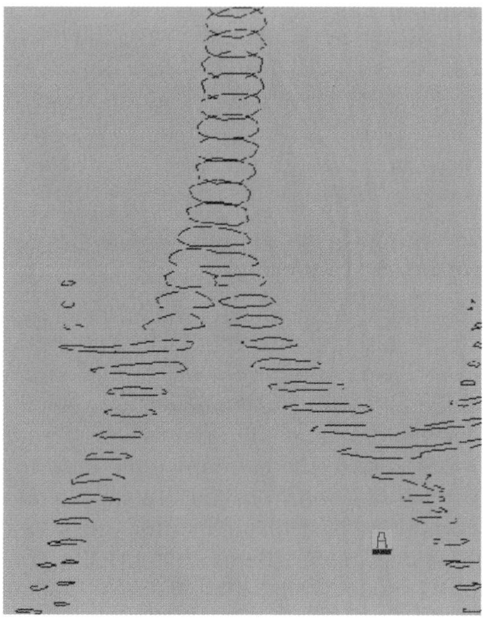

Fig. 3. The extracted LTT contours after segmentation are displayed

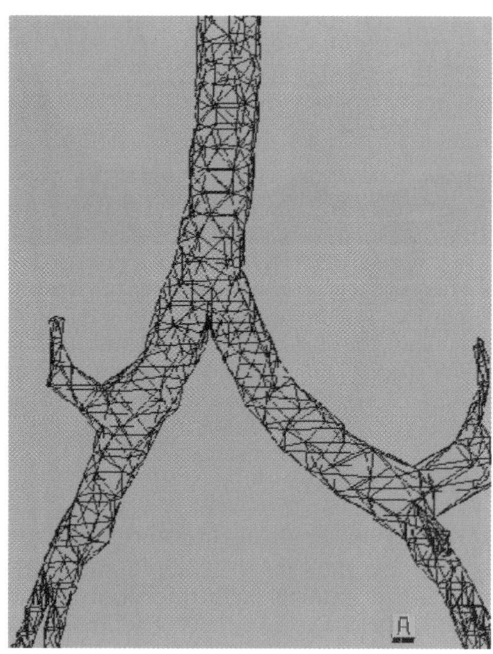

Fig. 4. LTT contours after triangulation – the contours of the individual slices are connected in order to form a wireframe

The main disadvantage of "Surface Rendering" is the necessity of segmentation. The procedure works only well in areas of high contrast – e.g. 3D-display of bones based on native CT scans, or air filled organs like the LTT. As already mentioned in section "Region growing", due to partial volume effects the boundaries of biological structures like the LTT are often not closed, thus leading to "bleeding". Consecutively, (sometimes exhausting) editing of the segmented boundaries are necessary. Moreover, only the prior segmented organ boundaries can be displayed in 3D. Thus for display just about 10% of all available source data are used. Therefore anatomical information is limited to the boundaries of the segmented organs.

Due to it's undemanding computational needs "Surface Rendering" was on of the earliest techniques for 3D-display.

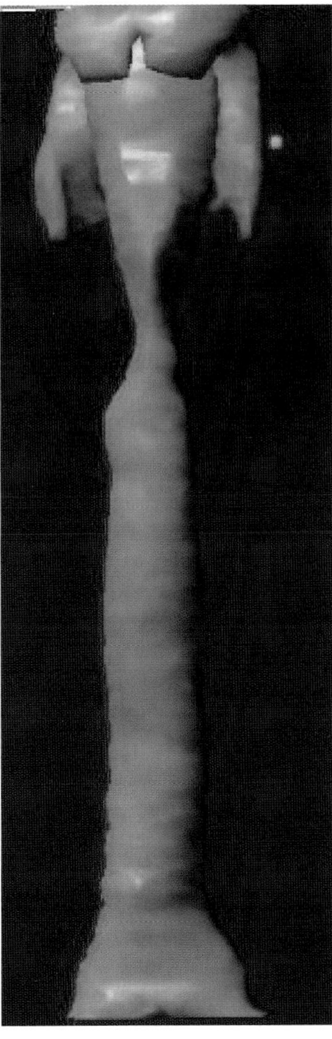

Fig. 5. "Surface Rendering": the colored LTT model of a patient suffering from a subglottic stenosis is shown and the site of the stenosis clearly depicted

Volume rendering (Synonym: Percentage rendering)

A completely different approach is used by the volume rendering algorithm. No segmentation is needed using this 3D reconstruction method. Basically, an "opacity curve" is constructed for a given data volume. This curve assigns every Hounsfield Unit a particular opacity, ranging from 0% (= completely transparent) to 100% (= completely opaque). By manipulating the opacity curve different anatomical structures can be displayed. A virtual ray is sent through the data volume. All grey values along the ray are collected and their opacity is changed according the chosen shape of the opacity curve. Details of the algorithm have been published elsewhere [9].

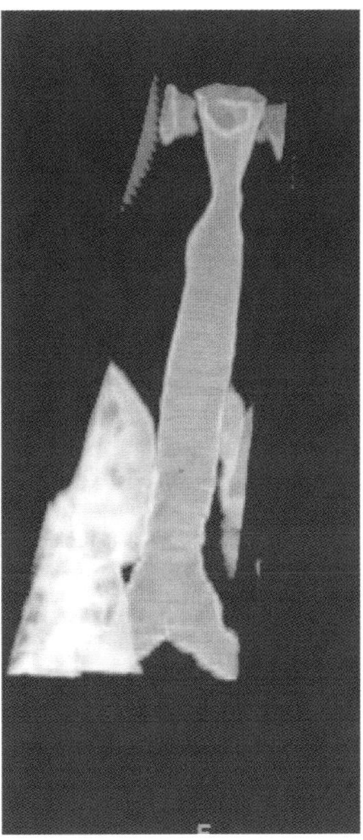

Fig. 6. "Volume Rendered" 3D reconstruction of the airways similar to bronchography. The opacity curve was adjusted in order to make the airways semitransparent

Figure 6 demonstrates the result after adjusting the opacity curve in order to display the airways semitransparent similar to bronchography. In order to achieve high quality 3D reconstructions with multiorgan display the desired organ systems need good contrast to the surrounding anatomy. As mentioned above, whenever vessels are of interest, intravenous contrast administration by a power injector is mandatory.

Volume rendering offers several challenges for the radiologist in presentation of S-CT findings. The most important step is the adjustment of the opacity curve. This can be tricky sometimes especially at low contrast states.

By using different colors for the airways and displayed surrounding anatomy, topographic relationsships can be displayed clearly (Fig. 7). The LTT as well as the surrounding anatomy can be shown in a comprehensive way.

Hybrid rendering

The combination of "Surface Rendering" and "Volume Rendering' is called "Hybrid Rendering". This

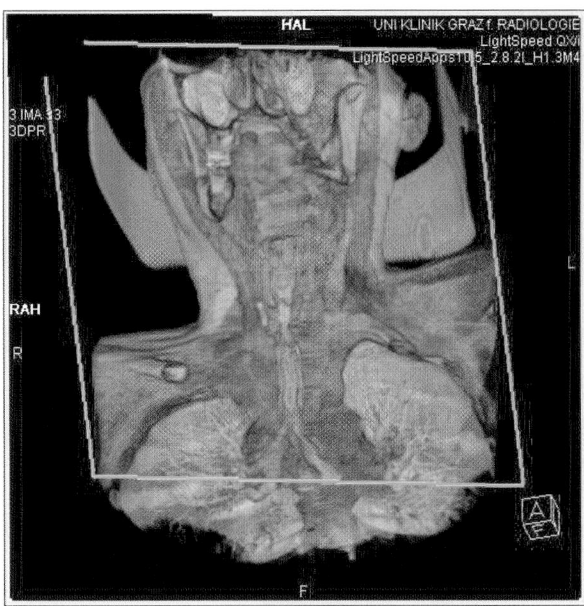

Fig. 7. S-CT after iv. contrast injection, multiorgan display: "Volume Rendered" 3D reconstruction of the neck and upper chest in a patient suffering from a tracheal carcinoma. The blue rectangle indicates the oblique frontal cutting plane. Skin, subcutaneous tissue, opacified vessels and the airways including the tracheal stent are shown

makes sense, if in low contrast situations (e.g. tumors) the patho-anatomy cannot be displayed by "Volume Rendering" alone. Prior segmentation (even using manual tracing) allows to define the boundaries of low contrast structures. By displaying both, the segmented boundaries by "Surface Rendering" and the surrounding anatomy by "Volume Rendering", usually a sufficient 3D representation can be achieved.

Virtual endoscopy

Virtual endoscopy (VE) was defined as a method that creates visualizations from 3D medical image scans similar to those produced by fiberoptic endoscopy [21]. There are many synonyms of VE especially concerning the gastro-intestinal tract: CT based virtual endoscopy, virtual colonoscopy, CT colography, three dimensional Spiral-CT pneumocolon, 3D colonography, to name but a few [22]. Rogers has suggested a new policy in naming VE images, mainly attaching the suffix -graphy to the organ system rendered. In order to indicate which imaging modality was used, a prefix is formed from that modality e.g. CT-tracheabronchography (CT-TB), CT-colonography [22].

The generation of these virtual views from inner body surfaces is based on surface and volume rendering algorithms as described above. By using perspective, i.e. objects closer to the virtual camera will appear larger than objects of the same size farther away from the virtual camera. It is the same effect as looking down from a skyscraper: a person just beneath us appears properly sized whereas people down in the street appear tiny.

Fiberoptic tracheoscopy (FTB) enables the inspection of the airway surface including mucosal changes as well as the dynamics. Information regarding the surrounding anatomy is limited to the perception of abnormal shapes or vessel pulsations. S-CT on the other hand, due to its excellent spatial and contrast resolution, provides information on intra- and extraluminal anatomy, but visualization of mucosal changes is not possible. As mentioned above, the shape of the trachea or bronchus depends on the angle between the axis of the trachea or bronchus and the CT slice plane. In a normal individual, where the trachea is just a little bent to the right and slightly angulated from superior anterior to caudal posterior, it can be expected that the axial S-CT slice will characterize the shape of the airways properly. But this may not be assumed in pathological cases, where the trachea can be buckled in any direction. Therefore LTS characterization on axial slices can be a troublesome topic. But CT-TB enables the radiologist to navigate through the airways in any direction interactively, to inspect every part from different views and to assess changes in diameter and shape directly, similar to FTB. In addition, findings of CT-TB can easily be compared to those of FTB. This is supported by a study of McAdams, who compared findings on axial CT slices and those of CT-TB in lung transplant recipients regarding the length and degree of airway stenosis [23]. They concluded, that CT-TB was more accurate than axial CT for diagnosis of clinical relevant stenosis. By comparing findings of axial CT slices (including MPR) with axial CT slice, MPR and virtual endoscopy, there was a clear advantage of using all three display modes and a reduction of false negative findings [13].

At FTB, the film documentation of a patient's CT will be on the lightbox and the endoscopist tries to match the information from FTB with that of CT in his/her mind. Computer simulations can help in this situation.

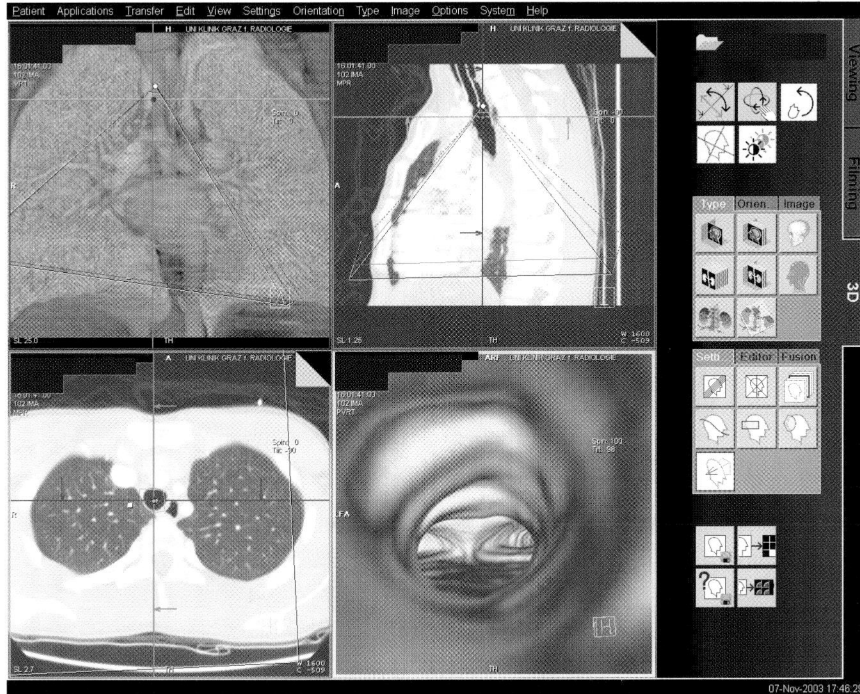

Fig. 8. "Virtual Endoscopy" – composition of the workstation screen, which is divided into four parts: left upper part displays a "Volume Rendered" semitranparent 3D reconstruction of the chest, the right upper part a sagittal MPR, whereas in the left lower part the axial slice in lung window settings is shown. On all three parts there is superimposed the position and opening angle of the virtual camera. On the right lower quadrant the virtual endoscopic view using "Volume Rendering" is shown

Since the underlying S-CT slices of CT-TB contain information about the surrounding anatomy too, this can be exploited by displaying additional views. As shown in Fig. 8 the global view of the airways, the axial S-CT slice and the virtual endoscopic view can be displayed simultaneously. The position of the virtual camera is marked on all views in order to establish anatomical cross reference. This display allows to study the topographic relationships of a patient's anatomy in a comprehensive way. In addition, this kind of display is a promising tool for teaching students and residents.

There are even more advantages of CT-TB. In planning for a transbronchial biopsy the best suited place for sampling can be chosen interactively [24]. Potential hazards of injuring vessels or other vital structures can be simulated without any danger to the patient. If transparent rendering of the tracheal wall is used, the extraluminal anatomy can be inspected within the 3D shape. Airways that cannot be explored by FTB, can be passed with the virtual endoscope and virtual, retrograde endoscopic views can be computed as well (Fig. 9). This is far beyond the possibilities of FTB.

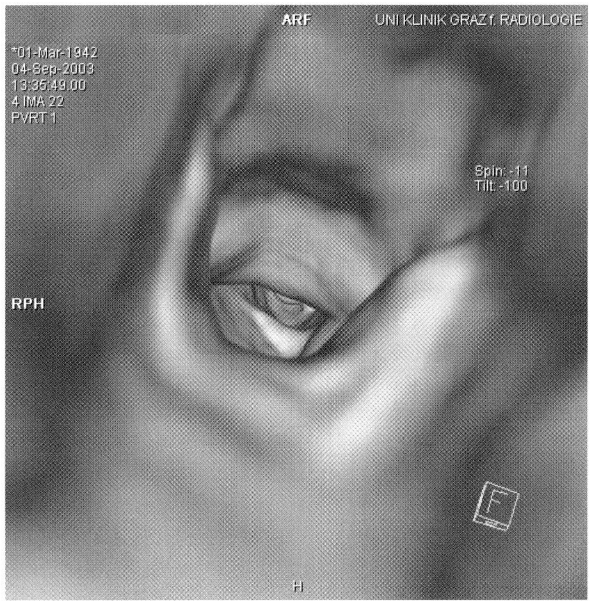

Fig. 9. Virtual retrograde, endoscopic view of a tracheal stenosis – this kind of view cannot be obtained by FTB

Moreover, for imaging of caliber changes during the respiratory cylce dynamic CT has to be performed, which is not undertaken routinely at every institution. Therefore both, FTB and S-CT including CT-TB, are not competitive but complementary.

Objective LTS degree and length estimation using LTT 3D-tracheal cross sectional profiles

Clinical management of patients suffering from LTS is based on FTB and imaging modalities [1]. Based on FTB there are several classifications for LTS, but they are either not practicable or do not predict the clinical course [1, 25]. Moreover, at FTB the estimation of the length and degree in LTS is regarded to be operator dependent [26].

Unfortunately imaging modalities have their inherent weak points too. Conventional radiographs allow to estimate the sagittal and transverse diameter of the airways. For assessment of LTS, where the trachea may be shaped asymmetrically, sagittal and transversal diameters do not characterize the shape of the airways properly. This was confirmed by Huber et al. who investigated different methods including radiographs of the neck, tracheoscopy, direct surgical measurements as well as necropsy measurements for assessment of tracheal stenosis [27]. They concluded that accurate measurements of tracheal stenosis cannot be done by radiographs and tracheoscopy.

Using conventional CT or electron beam CT, changes in the cross sectional area of the upper respiratory tract had been reported for healthy volunteers and for the evaluation of chronic airway obstruction in children [28, 29]. In both studies the cross sectional area was determined on axial slices alone. As mentioned already, in the case of a LTS, where the trachea may not be straight but buckled in any direction, the measured cross sectional area on axial slices will not be a reliable characterisation of the lumen as it will for healthy individuals. Own investigations yielded, that estimating LTS degree on axial S-CT slices and MPR alone are burdened by a high interobserver error – on average 43.3%, up to a maximum of 141.2% [30]. For the same reason the length of a stenosis cannot be estimated by just calculating the difference of slice positions. Curved multiplanar reformation could be used for length measurements, thus making it necessary to draw the medial axis on sagittal or coronal reconstructions. In case of LTS with a buckled trachea, this is a difficult task and the resulting medial axis will be again operator dependent. In addition, not all vendors of medical workstations are capable of obtaining length measurements from curved multiplanar reformations. 3D reconstructions, as described in section 3, helps to display the 3D shape and extension of the airways but the length and degree of LTS have to been estimated visually and semiquantitative by the reporting radiologist. Although the authors has no scientific evidence, it is their belief, that this visual assessements will suffer from an similar interoperator error as FTB.

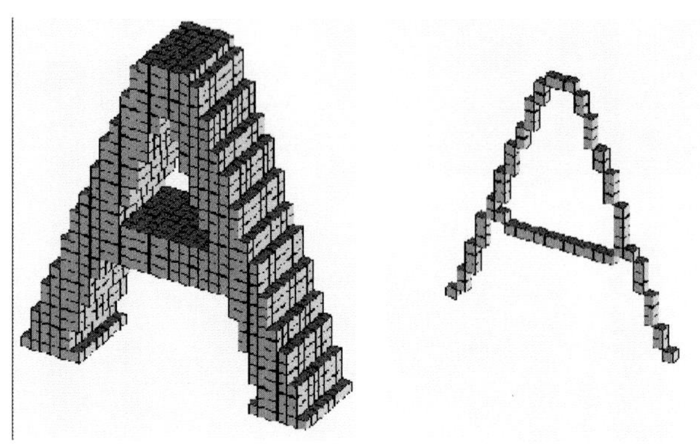

Fig. 10. Subfigure A) displays a 3D model of character A, whereas subfigure B) shows the result after skeletonization: the basic shape is preserved and the character A is still recognizeable

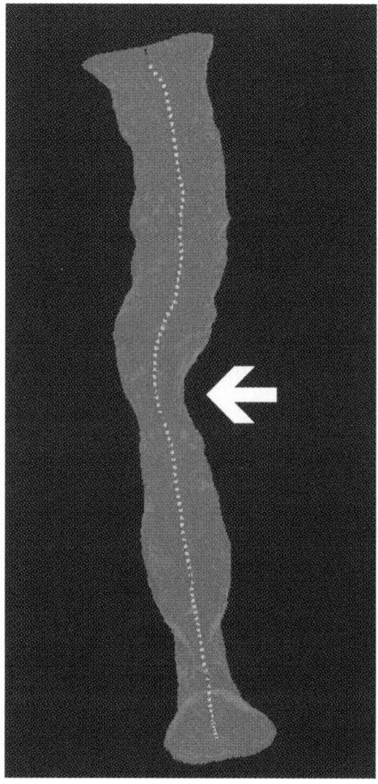

Fig. 11. 3D tracheal model form a patient suffering from a trachealstenosis. Site of the stenosis is indicated by the white arrow. The tracheal medial axis is shown as bright line in the center

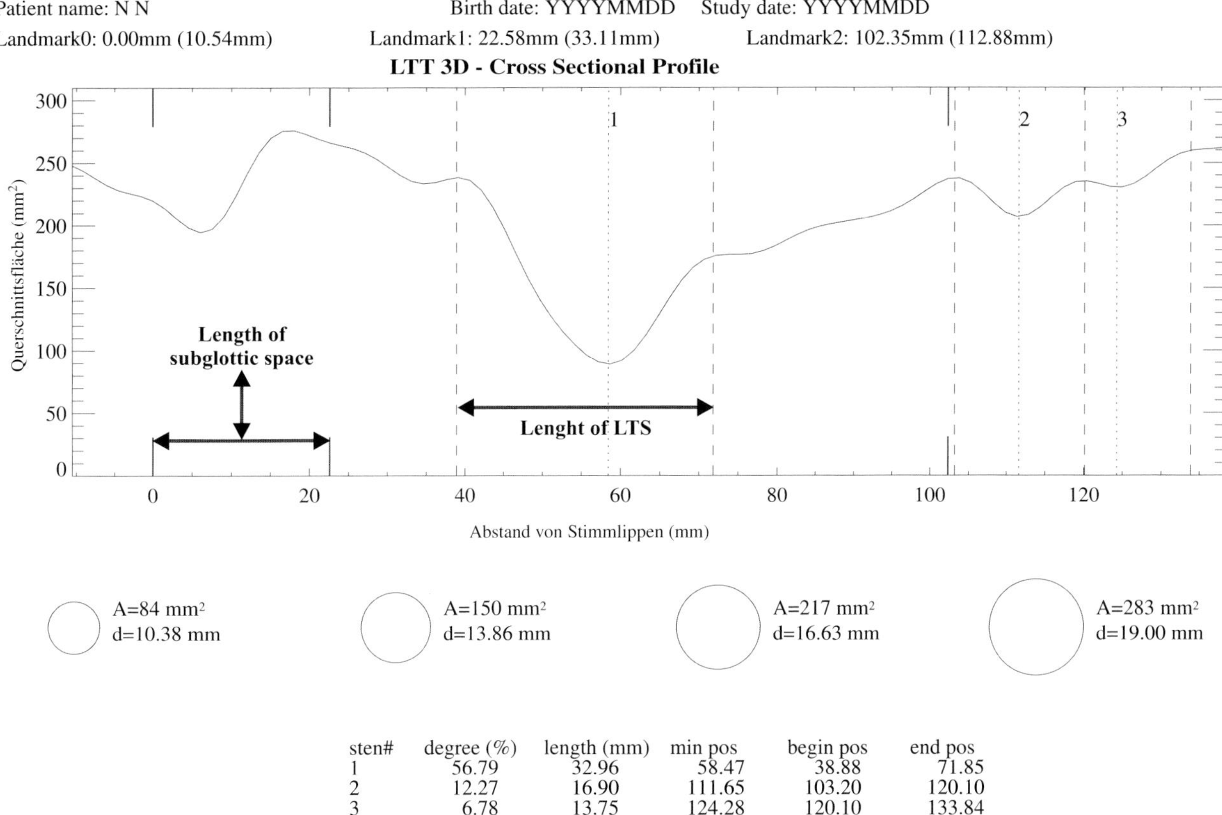

sten#	degree (%)	length (mm)	min pos	begin pos	end pos
1	56.79	32.96	58.47	38.88	71.85
2	12.27	16.90	111.65	103.20	120.10
3	6.78	13.75	124.28	120.10	133.84

Fig. 12. LTT 3D cross sectional chart from a patient suffering from tracheal stenosis. The short vertical bars represent the three chosen anatomic landmarks. Distal the caudal border of the cricoid cartilage three drops of of the cross sectional area can be seen: one major one ⇒ representing the stenotic segment, and two non pathologic areas of LTT minor caliber changes. For better correlation between caliber changes on 3D-cross sectional chart and the "Real World" there are four circles drawn in real size below the chart, covering the range of the plotted cross sectional areas. In addition the table with the quantification results is shown. The following abbreviations were used: degree ⇒ degree of LTT minor caliber changes, ⇒ length of the LTT minor caliber changes

A potential solution for these problems is the calculation of the S-CT based LTT 3D-cross sectional profile using a skeletonization algorithm [11]. A very illustrative definition of skeletonization is provided by the prairie-fire analogy: the boundary of a structure is set on fire and the skeleton is formed by the loci where the fire fronts meet and quench each others [31]. The skeleton of an object provides shape features that are extracted from binary data e.g. the segmented LTT (segmentation already described in section "Airway segmentation"). It's objective is to reduce the volume of elongated objects to their skeletons, which represent the abstraction of the object's shape. Figure 10a displays the capital letter "A" as a 3D object. After skeletonisation the basic shape is still recognizable (Fig. 10b). Different algorithms for computation of the skeleton of an object exist already [31]. One method used at our institution is a recently published 3D extension of a thinning algorithm, which computes the object's skeleton including its medial axis [31]. Thinning may be compared to peeling onions. It is an iterative method which removes the superficial layer of the segmented airways and repeats this process until the "skeleton" is left. After the skeletonization the extracted LTT medial axis is used afterwards for calculation of the 3D-cross sectional along that axis. Finally, the results of the 3D cross sectional profile are presented as a line chart. Values on the x-axes represent positions on the medial axis, and are normalized to the position of the vocal chords, which represent the zero position. Added anatomic landmarks help to establish cross reference with 3D reconstructions and FTB. Figure 11 shows a 3D model of a trachea in a patient suffering from a tracheal stenosis. At Fig. 12 the corresponding cross sectional profile is depicted. The vertical bars mark the position of the vocal chords, caudal border of the cricoid cartilage and that of the jugular fossa. The (marked) drop of

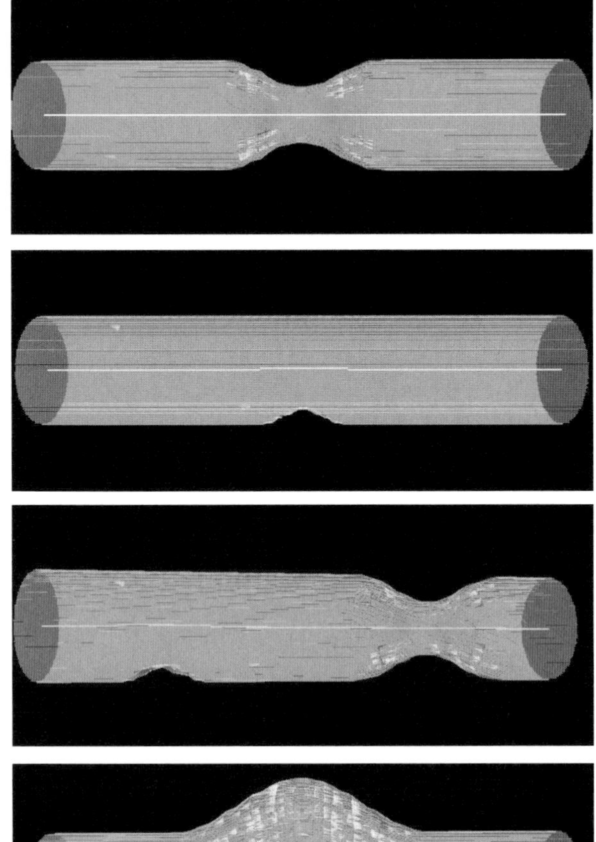

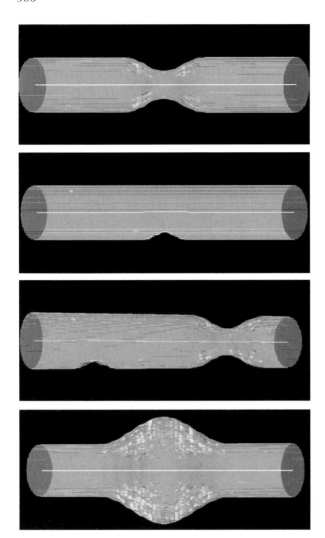

Fig. 13. VGB's for assessing accuracy and precision of the 3D-cross sectional profile. They consisted of tubes with symmetric and asymmetric narrowings (upper three) and an intersection of a sphere with a tube

the cross sectional area outlines the stenosis. By subtraction of the end position from the start one the true length in 3D can be calculated along the LTT medial axis. Therefore, the tracheal caliber changes can be displayed on this charts in a quantitative way and length and degree of LTS can be determined.

Accuracy and precision of the 3D cross sectional profiles where evaluated using virtual geometric bodies (VGB) containing narrowed and expanded areas (Fig. 13). These VGB's were generated mathematically in 3D as binary data volumes and for symmetrical caliber changes the true3D cross sectional profile was known as well as the degree and length of caliber changes. Furthermore, in order to simulate (the always existing) noise in the CT slices, VGB's with a "rough" surface were computed too

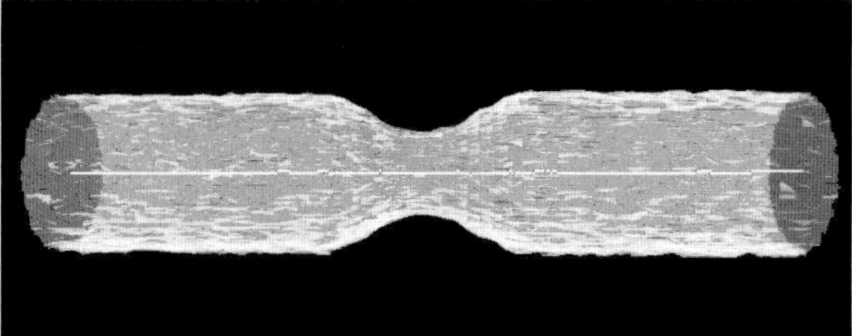

Fig. 14. VGB with added surface noise

(Fig. 14) [11]. Comparison of the true and the computed 3D cross sectional profile by linear regression yielded excellent results (Fig. 15).

Intranet applications

As described in the preceding sections there are several possibilities for imaging of LTS. Unfortunately, the above described techniques for LTS imaging and assessment involve different computer platforms, operating systems and software, not all being embedded in an existing Picture Archiving and Communications System (PACS). At the Department of Radiology Graz/Austria an intranet application was developed, which allows to collect all images and data of a particular patient using standard network computer interfaces (e.g. ftp, network drives, samba clients). Using the scripting language PHP, the application is fully operating system independent [32]. Since the software runs in a web browser window, it can be started from any computer connected to the hospitals network by just using a webbrowser. Of course, attention has to be payed to security items. The collected data are processed automatically and displayed as web pages on the hospitals intranet. Multimedia content, like digital videos from virtual endoscopy, can be viewed by using free software like media players, which can be downloaded from the internet for almost all operating systems. Therefore the referring physicians can observe these videos even on his/her desktop computer at no extra costs.

On the internet web server software is free available for almost all computer- and operating systems, the most utilized being the Apache software [33]. Therefore, as long as a hospital's network exists, almost every computer can be turned in a web server without spending additional money for infrastructure.

Moreover, by using a SQL database (e.g. MySQL) for patient data administration, automated web server administration systems can be programmed [34]. At our institution such software takes care in order to keep the list of accessible patient data as low as reasonable, which more or less means, not to

VBG#1 - Comparison between the theoretical 3D cross sectional profile and that one obtained by skeletonisation: overplot (upper) and linear regression (lower)

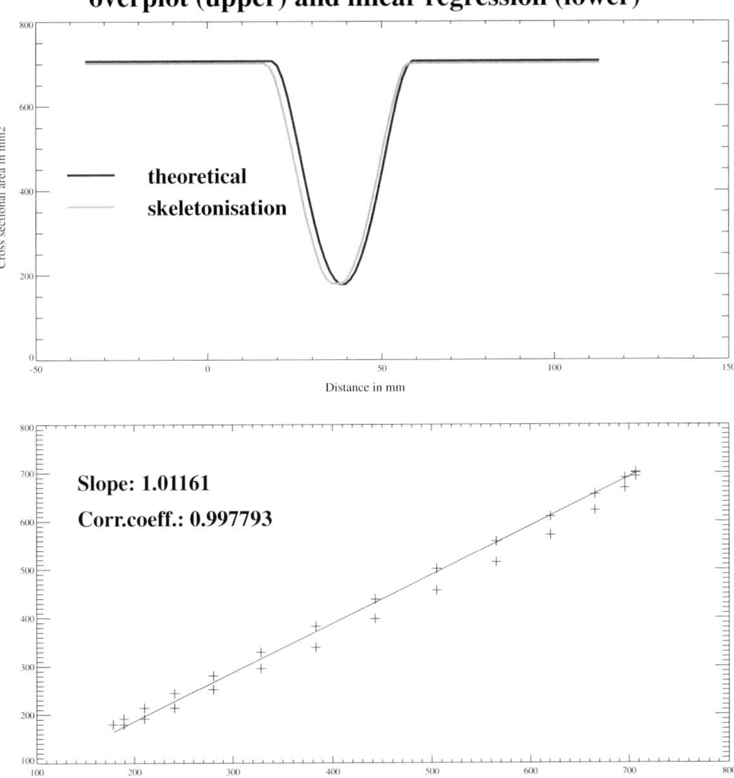

Fig. 15. Correlation between the theoretical cross sectional profile (black line) and that obtained by skeletonization (gray line) of the VGB as displayed in Fig. 13, upper row. Linear regression revealed an an excellent correlated between both ($p << 0.005$)

show up not any more needed patients. Algorithms like "First in first out" will prevent the display of a particular patient at a prior chosen watermark – e.g. all patients data, generated more than three months ago will be shown. Cash algorithms represent a better solution. The software will check the date of the patient's data last assessment, and remove those, who were not opened for a previously fixated time span. Therefore, only the needed patients are kept dynamically. Of course, all patient data, not saved to the PACS System, have to be archived according the national laws.

Conclusion

As described in the previous sections, post processing of S-CT offers challenging possibilities for Radiology including LTS imaging and assessment. The inherent information of S-CT can be displayed in different ways to the referring clinician in order to facilitate optimal patient management. Modern information technology and affordable computer hardware allow for new ways of data exchange and interaction between hospital departments. By using internet technology, asynchronous, interactive access to results of imaging and post processing can be provided. For imaging of LTS many facettes of the anatomy can be shown in order to provide a road map for therapeutical decisions. Looking at all these possibilities together, it is safe to say that a digital revolution is taking place in Radiology.

Acknowledgments

Surface -and volume rendered 3D reconstructions including CT-TB were done with the Siemens Virtuoso3D or Leonardo workstation (Siemens MED, Erlangen, Germany). Skeletonization and Intranet applications were developed within the CEEPUS (Central European Exchange Program for University Studies [35]) framework as interuniversitary cooperation. Special thanks to Ms. Irene Stradner for typographical assistance and to Ms.Eveline Therisch for support in image management.

References

[1] Couray M, Ossoff R (1998) Laryngeal stenosis: A review of staging, treatment, and current research. Current Opinion in Otolaryngology, Head and Neck Surgery 6: 407–410

[2] Grillo H, Dnonahue D, Mathiesen D, Wain J, Wright C (1995) Postintubation tracheal stenosis: Treatment and results. J Thorax Cardiovasc Surg 109: 486–492

[3] Lano C, Duncavage J, Reinisch L, Ossoff R, Couray M, Netterville J (1998) Laryngotracheal reconstruction in the adult: A ten year experience. Ann Otol Rhinol Laryngol 107: 92–96

[4] Spraggs H, Tostevin P (1997) Management of laryngotracheobronchial sequelae and complications of relapsing polychondritis. Laryngoscope 107: 936–941

[5] Berdon W, Condon V, Currarino G, Fitz C, Leonidas J, Parker B, Slovis T, Wood B (1993) Caffey's Pediatric X-Ray Diagnosis. Mosby, Chicago

[6] Coleman J, VanDuyne J, Ossoff R (1995) Laser treatment of lower airway stenosis. Otolaryngol Clin North Am 28: 771–783

[7] Ossof R, Tucker G, Duncavage J, Toohill R (1985) Efficacy of bronchoscopic carbon dioxide laser surgery for benign strictures of the trachea. Laryngoscope 95: 1220–1223

[8] Czaja J, McCaffrey T (1996) Acoustic measurement of subglottic stenosis. Ann Otol Rhinol Laryngol 105: 504–509

[9] Kuszyk B, Heath D, Bliss D, Fishman E (1996) Skeletal 3D-CT: Advantages of volume rendering over surface rendering. Skeletal Radiol 25: 207–214

[10] Zeiberg A, Silverman P, Sessions R, Troost T, Davros W, Zeman R (1996) Helical (spiral) CT of the upper airway with three-dimensional imaging: Technique and clinicalassessment. AJR 166: 293–299

[11] Sorantin E, Halmai C, Erdöhelyi B, Palágyi K, Nyúl L G, Ollé K, Geiger B, Lindbichler F, Friedrich G, Kiesler K (2002) Spiral-CT based assessment of tracheal stenoses using 3d-Skeletonisation. IEEE TMI 21: 263–273

[12] Lacrosse M, Trigaux J, van Beers B, Weynants P (1995) 3d sprial CT of the tacheobronchial tree. J Comput Assist Tomogr 19(3): 341–347

[13] Sorantin E, Geiger B, Lindbichler F, Eber E, Schimpl G (2002) CT-based virtual tracheobronchoscopy in children – comparison with axial CT and multiplanar reconstruction: preliminary results. Pediatric Radiol 32: 8–15

[14] Udupa J, Samarasekera S (1996) Fuzzy connectedness and object definition:theory, algorithms, and applications in image segmentation. Graphical Models and Image Processing 58(3): 246–261

[15] Udupa J, Odhner D, Samarasekera S, Goncalves R, Lyer K (1994) 3DVIEWNIX: An open, transportable, multidimensional, multimodality, multiparametric imaging software system. SPIE Proceedings 2164: 58–73

[16] Mohadjer D (2001) Analyse der Einflußfaktoren und Reproduzierbarkeit von Querschnittsprofilen zur Charakterisierung von Tracheallumina. Ph.D. thesis, Univ. Hospital Graz, Karl Franzens University, Austria

[17] Remy-Jardin M, Remy J, Artaud D, Fribourg M, Duhamel A (1998) Volume rendering of tracheobronchial tree: Clinical evaluation of bronchographic images. Radiology 208: 761–770

[18] Gonzalez C, Woods R (1993) Morphology. Addison-Wesley, New York

[19] Boissonnat J, Geiger B (1993) Three dimensional reconstruction of complex shapes based on the (delaunay) triangulation. In: Acharya R, Goldgof D (eds) Biomedical image processing and biomedical visualization. SPIE Proceedings, San Jose, CA, pp. 964–975

[20] Carey R, Bell G (1996) The Annotated VRML 2.0 Reference Manual. Addison-Wesely Developers Press, New York

[21] Blezek D, Robb R (1997) Evaluating virtual endoscopy for clinical use. J Digit Imaging 3 [Suppl 1]: 51–55

[22] Rogers L (1998) A day in the court of lexicon: Virtual endoscopy. AJR 171: 1185

[23] McAdams H, Palmer S, Erasmus J, Patz E, Connolly J, Goodman P, Delong D, Tapson V (1998) Bronchial anastomotic complications in lung transplant recipients: Virtual bronchoscopy for noninvasive assessment. Radiology 209: 689–695

[24] Rubin G, Beaulieu C, Argiro V (1996) Perspective volume rendering of CT and MR images: Applications for endoscopic imaging. Radiology 199: 321–330

[25] McCaffrey T, Czaja J (1992) Classification of laryngeal stenosis. Laryngoscope 102: 1335–1340

[26] Jewett B, Cook R, Johnson K, Logan T, Rosbe K, Mukherji S, Shockley W (1999) Subglottic stenosis: Correlation between computed tomography and bronchoscopy. Ann Otol Rhinol Laryngol 108: 837–841

[27] Huber M, Henderson R, Finn-Bodner S, Macinitre D, Wrigh J, Hankes G (1997) Assessment of current techniques for determining tracheal luminal stenosis in dogs. AJVR 10: 1051–1054

[28] Stern E, Graham C, Webb R, Gamsu G (1993) Normal trachea during forced exspiration: Dynamic CT measurements. Radiology 187: 27–31

[29] Frey E, Smith W, Grandgeorge S, McCray P, Wagener J, Jr, F E, Y S (1987) Chronic airway obstruction in children: Evaluation with cine-CT. AJR 148: 347–352

[30] Sorantin E: unpublished data

[31] Palágyi K, Kuba A (1998) A 3d 6-subiteration thinning algorithm for extracting medial lines. Pattern Recognition Letters 19: 613–627

[32] http://www.php.net.

[33] http://www.apache.com.

[34] http://www.mysql.com.

[35] Sorantin E: http://www.kfunigraz.ac.at/radwww/ceepus.

Current development and economic issues

Flat panel detectors – closing the (digital) gap in chest and skeletal radiology

K.J. Reiff

Siemens AG, Malvern, USA

Abstract

In the radiological department today the majority of all X-ray procedures on chest and skeletal radiography is performed with classical film-screen-systems.

Using digital luminescence radiography (DLR or CR, which stands for computed radiography) as a technique has shown a way to replace this 100 year old procedure of doing general radiography work by acquiring the X-rays digitally via phosphor screens. But this approach has faced criticism from lots of radiologists world wide and therefore hasn't been overall implemented except in the intensive care environment.

A new technology is rising based on the use of so called flat panel X-ray (FD) detectors. Semi-conducting material detects the X-rays in digital form directly and creates an instantaneous image for display, distribution and diagnosis. This ability combined with a large field of view and – compared to existing methods – excellent detective quantum efficiency represents a revolutionary step for chest and skeletal radiography and will put basic X-ray-work back into the focus of radiological solutions.

This paper will explain the basic technology of flat panel detectors, possible system solutions based on this technology, aspects of the user interface influencing the system utilization and versatility as well as the possibility to redefine the patient examination process for chest and skeletal radiography.

Furthermore the author discusses limitations of the first systems, upgrades for the installed base and possible scenarios for the future, e.g. fluoroscopy or angiography application.

History vs. introduction

More than 100 years after the discovery of X-rays radiological exams of chest and skeleton still have not stepped into the digital age. For fluoroscopy and angiography the development of large image intensifiers combined with digital imaging systems was a major step, but – depending on the department – the majority of all X-ray procedures still remain to be either chest or skeletal radiography. Percentages range from 50 to 80 depending on the department and the spectrum of diagnostic systems.

A first step to overcome conventional work was made in 1982 by introducing a system that uses storage phosphor plates instead of conventional film-screens. This method uses the possibility of storage phosphor plates to grab and release energy. However, a special reader to evaluate the cassettes where the stored analog image was transferred into a digital data file is still required. The whole handling is equivalent to film, and the method itself hasn't been a major breakthrough (excluding Japan) within the medical community [1]. Also using it in intensive care, where performing radiography always is most difficult in terms of patient positioning and the correct exposure data, can be cumbersome.

Another more recent solution has been the development of systems based on charged coupled devices (CCD) which are optically communicating to a scintillator. This approach shortens the total examination time today but has the disadvantage of an extreme optical reduction factor caused by the small CCD surface area.

Another approach for radiography is based on amorphous selenium where X-ray is directly converted into an electrical charge with the sampling of information inside an electrical field. This solution appears to be very well accepted for chest and genrad work, but – due to the obtainable signal-to-noise-ratio – it is questionable, whether this technology is capable of performing fluoro work [2].

The latest and most promising approach to cover single exposure as well as fluoro imaging is a flat

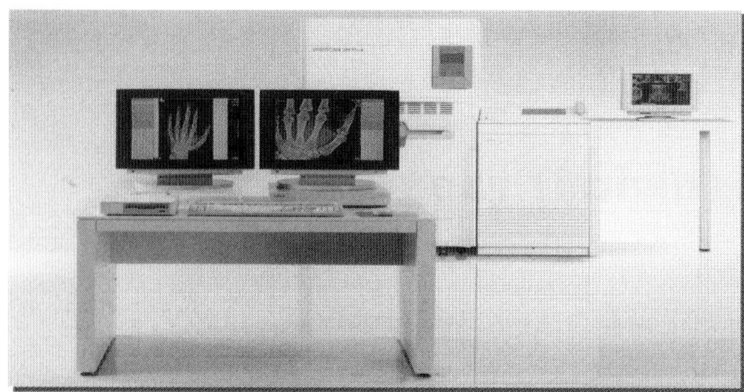

Fig. 1. Typical storage phosphor system with patient registration console, storage phosphor reader and diagnostic reporting console

detector based on a combination of a cesium iodide scintillator and an active read-out-matrix of amorphous silicon [3–5].

Technology (FD-principle)

The flat panel detector technology can be described as follows:

A layer of 450 μm thallium-doped cesium iodide is used to convert X-ray into light [6]. The benefits of this material are an excellent absorption of X-ray radiation, a high conversion factor as well as a very good geometrical resolution due to its needle shaped crystalline structure. This leads to a zero-frequency detective quantum efficiency of approximately 65% at a tube voltage of 70 kV and a MTF (modulation transfer function) value of more than 30% at 2.5 Lp/mm. These values are considerable higher than any conventional film-screen or storage phosphor system [4].

The light (visible range photons) is then converted into an electrical charge in the photodiodes of the amorphous silicon matrix. There the charge is read out with dedicated electronics and converted to a digital signal with 14-bit resolution (16384 gray levels). The most significant 12 bits are used to generate the digital image, which is processed by special hardware, displayed on a monitor and transferred into a network.

Detector technical data:

Pixel size	143 μm^2
Pixel matrix	2981 × 3021
Active area	42.6 cm × 43.2 cm
Spatial resolution	~3.5 Lp/mm
DQE	>60%
X-ray generator voltage range	40–150 kV
Overall dimensions	~56 × 49 × 4.5 cm
Weight	20 kg

Potential of the detector

Film-screen-systems have been developed and designed to a nearly perfect combination of patient positioning capabilities, X-ray procedure and developing of images. So there must be more in that technology for it to match today's state of the art systems.

This leads automatically to the question, why one wants to spend a substantial amount of money to purchase this new technology.

The technology of flat panel detectors described above has the potential of direct digital imaging with no need of additional read out devices. Detectors have been constructed and tested by various companies throughout the world using plates of smaller sizes at the beginning and fully sized detectors later [3,4,7,8]. Many papers have been published on those tests and clinical results and – even in the early phase of that new development – the authors have been very positive in judging the potential [9–14]. A few quotations are listed in the following:

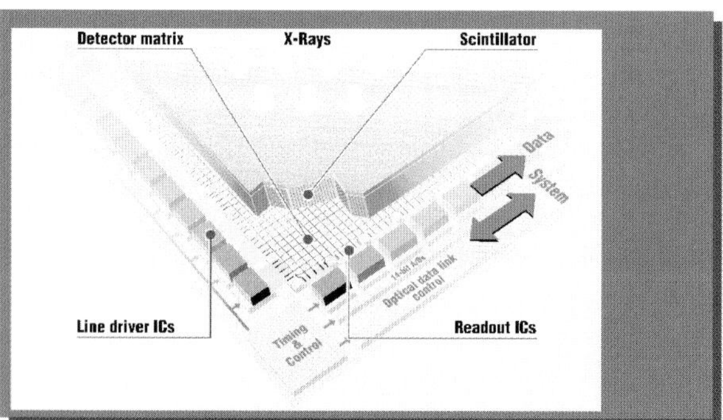

Fig. 2. Principle of a flat detector based on cesium iodide and amorphous silicon

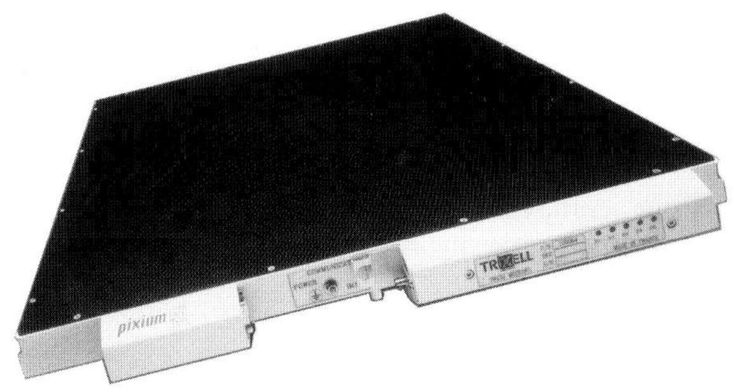

Fig. 3. Flat detector

1. "The amorphous silicon based system with a simulated speed of 400 provided images equivalent to screen-film-radiographs. For clinical tasks such as routine follow-up-studies, assessment of instability or orthopaedic measurements a radiation dose reduction of up to 75% may be possible" [9].
   (Dr. Strotzer et al., University of Regensburg, Germany)
2. "Subjective visibility of normal anatomy of the hands and feet using selenium-based digital radiography was similar to that achieved using conventional film-screen-radiography (100 speed!) [10].
   (Dr. Piraino et al., Cleveland Clinic Foundation, USA)
3. "In a first clinical comparative study, the flat detector exposures were assessed as being significantly better than those of conventional screen-film-combinations, particularly with respect to image latitude and the soft-issue rendition."
   (Dr. Hamers et al., Department of Radiology Zentralkrankenhaus Bremen, Germany) [11].

These very promising judgements from radiologists at an early stage show the potential of the oncoming method in terms of diagnostic accuracy and possibilities of dose reduction [15–17].

System components

Flat detectors basically represent the heart of a newly designed solution but there a many other system components which have to be optimized in order to create good usability for the needs of chest or skeletal radiography. The goal for a development must be an approach that takes advantage of the new technology with benefits like immediate imaging and large detecting area and, on the other hand, also optimizes the design of the other components like user interface, generator handling, table, 3D-overhead crane etc.

A simple example is the anti scatter grid. The new FD has very short exposure times. Oscillating grids are not working properly in this context and produce grid line artifacts that limit the image quality. A newly developed stationary grid with 80 lines/cm does not show this problem [18].

If the detector allows quick imaging the system should facilitate that, too. The user interface is going to be one of the tools to minimize the patient examination time. Ideally it supports the speed of the detector by minimizing the handling of patient and generator data. This is achieved through implementation of an efficient patient worklist and organ programming concept as well as through integration of the generator console into one user interface. The

Benefits of a procedure using a flat detector solution compared to conventional film screen technology

Film-screen	FD
A large variety of film sizes and cassette sizes have to be provided for specific exams	One FD for all examinations; the organ program automatically defines readout aperture
Different film-screen-systems have to be provided for specific exams	FD is programmable on the film-screen-equivalence
Selection of wrong exposure data leads to retakes	Initial wrong processing algorithm can be corrected via postprocessing, less retakes
More than one exam leads to handling and transporting cassettes	FD covers nearly every exam, no physical work is to be done
Identification after the exposure needs flash card devices or other manual actions	Patient data is entered via worklist or bar code or keyboard once and is then part of the digital data
Time-consuming readout of film-screen cassette before the patient is released from the table	Image appears on the monitor for review after a few seconds
Darkroom is needed	The darkroom can be eliminated
Transportation of the film to a radiologist for reading is time consuming	Transport of the image can be done electronically and preprogrammable
Film storage needs central or local archive with lots of space	Digital images can be stored on room saving devices
Film storage requires intensive labor to deliver and store films to the radiologists and back to the archive, images are often lost	Digital images allow fast and convenient access via Workstation, lost images are no longer a problem
For teleradiology you need to digitize the film	A second opinion on an exam is no problem
Film has to be transported to OR or consulting doctors	Images can be sent electronically in multiple viewing destinations

higher the integration level of such an approach the less working steps are necessary and the quicker the whole system works. This results in an optimized workflow with the benefit of no cassette handling and reduced generator setup time, less patient waiting time on the table or in front of the wall stand, immediate image distribution on a monitor combined with the possibilities of digital data in terms of networking and archiving. The overall performance of such a system will be superior to any existing conventional unit.

The optimized process for a routine patient X-ray examination can be described as follows:

Patient examination process
Request chest p.a./lateral

Patient demographics have been transferred via worklist, examination type has been defined

⇓

Technologist chooses patient name and organ program for chest p.a. automatically

⇓

Patient is positioned and exposure is done

⇓

Image shows up on the monitor to control positioning and quality of exposure

⇓

System loads organ program for chest lateral automatically

⇓

Patient is positioned and exposure is done

⇓

Image shows up on the monitor to control positioning and quality of exposure

⇓

Patient examination is complete

This very fast process – the first FD systems complete the above described procedure in approximately one minute – leads to the logical conclusion that with the use of FD systems in the future patient throughput is no longer dependent on the performance of a system but on the intelligent way to organize patient transport.

However, this is not the only impact, FD-imaging will have in the field of chest and skeletal radiography.

FD system design

Size and Weight of the flat panel device (see technical data) indicate limitations to the use of the detector [8]. Newer developments allow the device being used in the intensive care environment as an add on to a mobile X-ray device (Fig. 5), but the detector has an attached cable that limits the use and the patient weight should not exceed 300 pounds. Still, intensive care units will welcome this oppor-

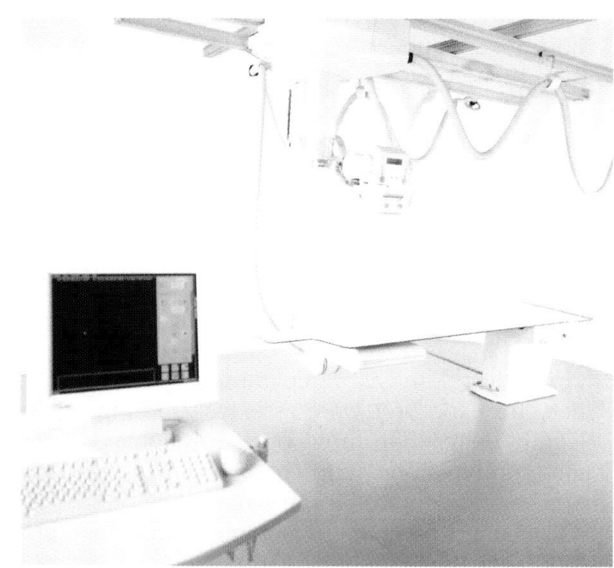

Fig. 4. One detector solution for chest and skeletal radiography

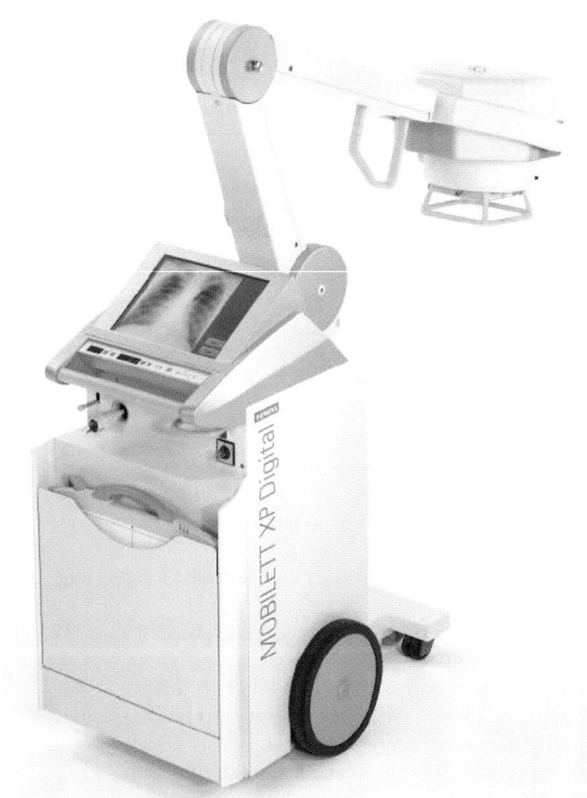

Fig. 5. Mobile unit with FD detector

tunity for they will be awarded with an quasi instant image (5s) after the exposure. In most cases the detector replaces the bucky tray either in a X-ray table or a bucky wall stand. The industry offers various solutions to be used in general radiography. In most cases an integrated solution is offered with two detectors, one for the bucky wall stand and one for the table, but you also find solutions that use only on mobile detector being carried around between wall stand and X-ray table. Even retrofit detectors to elder installed system are offered as of today.

The newest solution integrates one detector in a flexible 3D-crane with the X-ray tube mounted on a second crane (Fig. 4). Both are electronically coupled and can move simultaneous, so that by pressing an organ program on the generator the whole system can pre-position itself automatically. The design allows the use on one integrated detector to basically cover all angulations required, the only limit is the size of the device.

Digital mammography

A dedicated use for flat panel detectors is within digital mammography. The detector used to cover these examinations is based on amorphous selenium with a photoconductor to absorb the X-rays and directly generate an electrical signal without any intermediate steps. Latest developments allow a spatial resolution with >7 lp/mm and measurements show a superior DQE for better detection of small and low contrast objects compared to using indirect technologies.

Networking

More and more hospitals want to digitize all their imaging and share the benefits of communicating digital data throughout the radiological department [19]. Using multiple viewing destinations within the facility or via teleradiology to a second source. Flat panel detector systems allow chest and skeletal radiography to close the digital gap and participate in a procedure which other modalities like CT or MR include form their very beginning.

It has to be pointed out that the amount of data being acquired with flat detector systems will be huge and has to be thoroughly investigated before the systems are hooked up to a network. Hospitals with an existing PACS system or those who are investigating to enter into digital reading have to be aware of the fact that images acquired with the detector will have an impact on network and storage design. A fully acquired image with

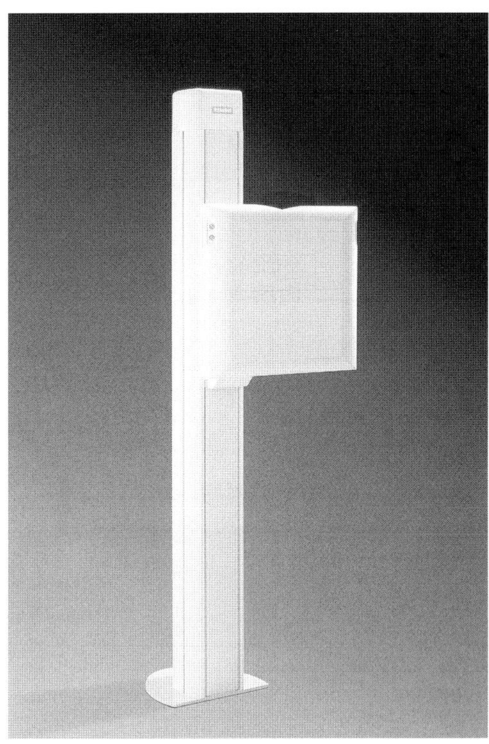

Fig. 6. Automatic chest stand based on flat detector technology

43 cm × 43 cm active area, 3K × 3K resolution and 12bit processing sums up to an amount of 18 Mbyte of data! The smaller the object the less the amount of digital data, logically.

The digital imaging concept as part of the new flat detector systems should therefore provide the necessary solutions to network the images in a proper way. This solution includes the possibility to accept a patient worklist out of an existing radiological information system (RIS) as well as the capability of DICOM-SEND CR-Objects and DICOM BASIC PRINT for those who want to continue working with hardcopy functionality.

Every flat detector system with the above described versatility can be easily hooked up to DICOM-capable network.

Integrated FD solutions provide additional benefits when used inside a network. Many devices are following a DICOM MPPS protocol (Modality Perform Procedure Step) which can be used within a PACS system for patient and system tracking.

When looking into the opportunities of a PACS system one can easily imagine that reading of MR/CT/CR/DR and other technologies in a combined fashion wherever and whenever is going to provide a major productivity step for every department.

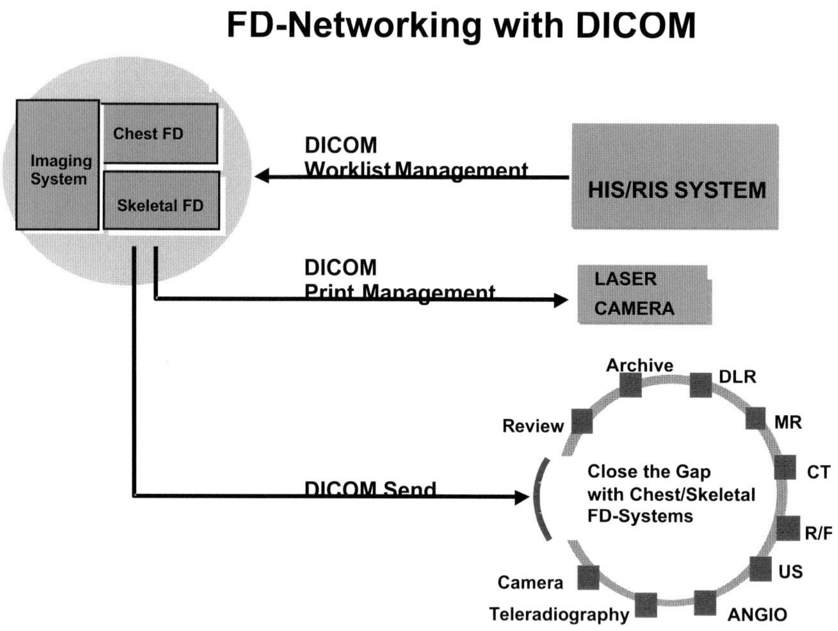

FD-Networking with DICOM

Imaging System
Chest FD
Skeletal FD
DICOM Worklist Management
HIS/RIS SYSTEM
DICOM Print Management
LASER CAMERA
DICOM Send
Archive
DLR
MR
CT
R/F
US
ANGIO
Teleradiography
Camera
Review
Close the Gap with Chest/Skeletal FD-Systems

Fig. 7. Networking capability of a flat detector system

Limitations

As briefly discussed flat detectors are widely used in various application within the enterprise. Limitations as of today are mainly due to size and weight of the device, it is not possible to reproduce certain exams where the detecting device needs to be positioned closely to the patient.

The biggest limitation for the overall use is the cost for these devices to be widely accepted. Manufacturing of the detector has been difficult and although the quality has improved over the last years the investment for such a system is still substantial and indirect technologies therefore are still the choice in most of the cases.

Fluoroscopy and angiography

As pointed out in the beginning of this article the combination of a cesium-iodide-scintillator and an amorphous silicon read-out-matrix has the potential to also being used in fluoroscopy, angiography and cardiology [20]. The substitution of these procedures was not as urgent as for skeletal and chest examination for current technologies using large image intensifiers combined with integrated digital readout systems were providing the digital images already in good quality and immediately.

First studies to use FD detectors for fluoroscopic as well as angiographic procedures have been performed in 1995 by the University of Freiburg and others on a technological prototype with a matrix of 1k × 1k and pixel size of 200 ym. The detector was adjusted to a cardiology C-arm worked with 12.5 and 25 frames per second and with half of the geometrical resolution.

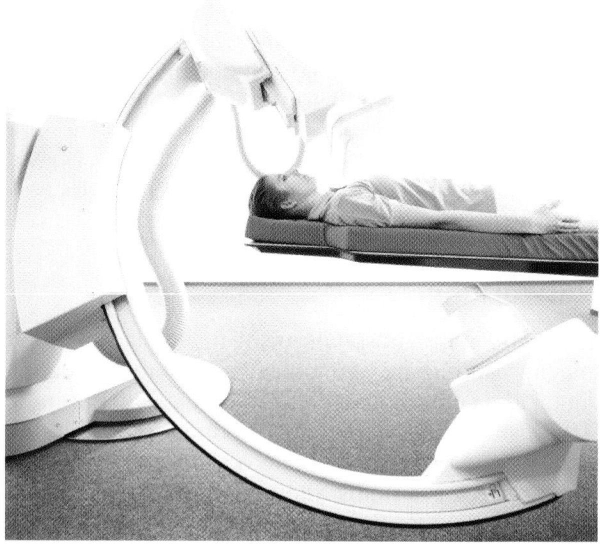

Fig. 8. FD cardiology solution

The initial tests demonstrated the principal capabilites of the new technology and over the last years many systems have been built and are used that work with flat detector technology in basic fluroscopy, angiography and even cardiology mono- as well as biplane.

The detectors used measure 20 × 20 cm (pixel size 184 ym) to 30 × 40 cm (pixel size 154 ym) and work with up to 30 frames/sec real-time image acquisition in 1025 matrix and 14-bit digitization depth.

The excellent spatial and contract resolution of the detector has lead to an overall improvement of image quality, the smaller size of the device allows the detecting system being smaller compared to image intensifiers and shows advantages in positioning at the patient.

Large 35 × 43 detectors in the future will allow fluoroscopy and general radigraphy being performed with one device.

Conclusions

FD-systems for chest and skeletal radiography are a revolutionary step to optimize the work for the majority of chest and skeletal examinations. The biggest benefit of flat detector systems is the optimization of the patient examination process to an extent, that FD-systems will no longer limit the patient workflow. Networking with DICOM-capable systems will be possible and will allow general radiography being part of an enterprise wide PACS solution with all benefits like distribution of images, interfacing with other clinical results and so on.

Earlier limitations to use flat detector systems in general for chest and skeletal work have been overcome with new solutions being provided by the industry, the investment into a digital device remains substantial. It remains to be seen if over time the total cost of ownership using flat detector systems in a networking environment will be in favor compared to indirect systems.

References

[1] Busch HP (1997) Digital radiology for clinical applications. European Radiology (3) [Suppl]: 566–572

[2] Zhao W, Rowlands JA (1995) X-ray imaging using amorphous selenium: feasibility of a flat panel self-scanned detector for digital radiology. Med Phys 22: 1595

[3] Antonuk LE, Boundry J, Huang W, et al (1992) Demonstration of megavoltage and diagnostic X-ray imaging with hydrogenated amorphous silicon arrays. Med Phys 19: 1455–1466

[4] Antonuk LE, Yorkston J, Huang W, et al (1995) A real-time, flat panel amorphous silicon, digital X-ray imager. Radiographics 15: 993–1000

[5] Chabbal J, Chaussat C, Ducourant T, et al (1996) Amorphous silicon X-ray image sensor. Medical Imaging. 1996: Physics of Medical Imaging. Prod SPIE 2708: 499–510

[6] Chaussat C, Chabbal J, Ducourant T, et al (1998) New superior CsI/a-Si 43 cm × 43 cm X-ray flat panel detector for general radiography provides immediate direct digital output and easy interfacing to digital radiography systems. In: Lemke HU (ed) Proceedings of the 12th International Symposium on Computer Assisted Radiology and Surgery CAR'98. Elsevier, Amsterdam 3–8

[7] Antonuk LE, El-Mohri Y, Siewerdsen JH, et al (1997) Empirical investigation of the signal performance of a high-resolution, indirect detection, active matrix flat-panel imager (AMFPI) for fluoroscopic and radiographic operation. Med Phys 24 (1): 51–70

[8] Neitzel U (1997) Integrated digital radiography with a flat electronic detector. Medicamundi

[9] Strotzer M, et al (1998) Clinical application of a flat-panel x-ray detector based on amorphous silicon technology: image quality and potential for radiation dose reduction in skeletal radiography. AJR 171: 23–27, 0361-803X/98/1711–23 © American Roentgen Ray Society

[10] Piraino DW, et al (1999) Selenium-based digital radiography versus conventional film-screen radiography of the hands and feet: a subjective comparison. AJR 172: 177–184, © American Roentgen Ray Society; AJR:172, January 1999

[11] Hamers S, Freyschmidt J (1998) Digital radiography with an electronic flat-panel detector: first clinical experience in skeletal diagnostics. Medicamundi 42 (3)

[12] Shaber GS, Lee DL, Bell J, et al (1998) Clinical evaluation of a full field digital projection radiography detector. SPIE 336: 463–469

[13] Yamazaki T, Morishita M, Kaifu N, et al (1998) Development of digital radiography system, Proceedings of the 12th International Symposium and Exhibition CAR'98, pp 536–541

[14] Hintze A, Maack I, Neitzel U (1998) Digital projection radiography with a full size flat panel detector bucky system, Proceedings of the 12th International Symposium and Exhibition CAR'98, pp 9–14

[15] Völk M, Strotzer M, Gmeinwieser J, et al (1997) Flatpanel X-ray detector using amorphous silicon technology: reduced radiation dose for the detection of foreign bodies. Invest Radiol 32: 373–377

[16] Strotzer M, Gmeinwieser J, Völk M, et al (1998) Clinical application of flat-panel x-ray detector based on amorphous silicon technology: image quality and potential for radiation dose reduction in skeletal radiography. Am J Roentgenol 171: 23–27

[17] Strotzer M, Völk M, Spahn M, Fründ R, Seitz J, Spies V, Gmeinwieser J, Alexander J, Feuerbach S (1997) Amorphous silicon (a-Si), flat-panel, X-ray detector versus screen-film radiography (SFR): Effect of dose reduction

on the detectability of cortical bone lesions and fractures. ECR'97 – 10th European Congress of Radiology: Scientific Programme and Abstracts 205, Springer

[18] Aichinger H, Staudt F, Kuhn H (1992) Multiline grids for imaging in diagnostic radiology – a physical and clinical assessment. Electromedica 60 (3): 74

[19] Siegel E, Flagle C, Reiner B, et al (1998) Cost benefit analysis of filmless operation. Presented at annual meeting of American Roentgen Ray Society, San Francisco, June

[20] Schiebel U, Conrads N, Jung N, et al (1994) Fluoroscopic X-ray imaging with amorphous silicon thin-film arrays. Medical Imaging 1994: Physics of Medical Imaging 1994: Physics of Medical Imaging. Proc SPIE 2163: 129–140

[21] Chabbal J, Chaussat C, Ducourant T, Fritsch L, Michailos J, Spinnler V, Vieux G, Arques M, Hahm G, Hoheisel M, Horbaschek H, Schulz R, Spahn M (1996) Amorphous silicon x-ray image sensor. SPIE 2708: 499

Digital radiology and its cost-effectiveness? – Experiences and recommendations from Vienna's Donauspital (Danube hospital)

W. Reinagl

SMZO Donauspital, Vienna, Austria

The Donauspital is Vienna's most recently built new hospital [1]. It is a hospital centre with 953 beds, which has three wards for internal medicine as well as bed wards in neurology, intensive care, general surgery, trauma care, neurosurgery, ortheopaedics, ophthalmology, otorhinolaryngology, urology, dermatology, nuclear medicine, obstetrics and gynaecology, paediatrics, paediatric surgery, oromaxillofacial surgery, and psychiatry. The hospital also offers outpatient departments in all specialties and institutes (radiology diagnostics, radio-oncology, physical medicine, laboratory medicine, pathology/bacteriology) [2].

Table 1. Performance data of Vienna's Donauspital, 2003

50,472	Inpatients
341,056	Care days
6.8	Average duration of patients' stay
85.6%	Use
1,993	Births
19,334	Surgical procedures

The Donauspital is part of the "Sozialmedizinisches Zentrum Ost der Stadt Wien" (Socio-Medical Center East, SMZO) of the City of Vienna. In addition to the hospital, the centre encompasses the geriatrics centre Donaustadt with 405 beds, a day care centre for elderly people, a school for general healthcare and nursing, and 500 staff flats. The centre is designed to be a centre of competence, providing medical and social care for the population in the part of Vienna that is situated on the other side of the Danube river (21. and 22. district, population about 280,000 [3]). It is at the heart of a network, the "Regionalverbund Donaustadt" (Regional Alliance Donaustadt, Health Care Network).

Planning for the Donauspital started in 1979, and building works started in November 1985, after a two-year gap in planning. The first of three developmental stages was taken into service in 1992. Building was finished in 1996 with the third stage, which included the psychiatric ward, magnetic resonance tomography, and the institute for radio-oncology with a linear accelerator and brachytherapy. In 2004, the orthopaedic ward was expanded by 20 beds (to a total of 52 beds) and a positron emission tomograph was installed in the department for nuclear medicine, diagnostics and therapy.

In 1989 the decision was made to build a digital radiology ward; the main aim was to be able to transmit imaging data not only within the hospital but also to other hospitals and to doctors with their own practices in the Regional Alliance Donaustadt. A strategic aim from the start was the capacity to incorporate the possibilities of tele-consulting. The qualitative advantage for patients was a main consideration, but so was the economic (hence financial) benefit:

- Avoiding duplication of examinations by electronic exchange of imaging data
- The opportunity to consult several experts on one image, and
- Tele-consulting

The decision to acquire the new facilities for radiodiagnosis (including ultrasonography) not in an analogue but in a digital format – in as far as the current industrial standards existed to make these available – was made at a time when the municipal council of the City of Vienna had agreed the entire cost for all facilities in the new hospital. The cost for the digital equipment, which was notably higher than that of conventional equipment, was covered by savings made in building the hospital so that the overall cost was the same. The City of Vienna as the funding body of the hospital was reassured that the running costs for the digital equipment with its quality advantages were not going to exceed those of analogue equipment. The

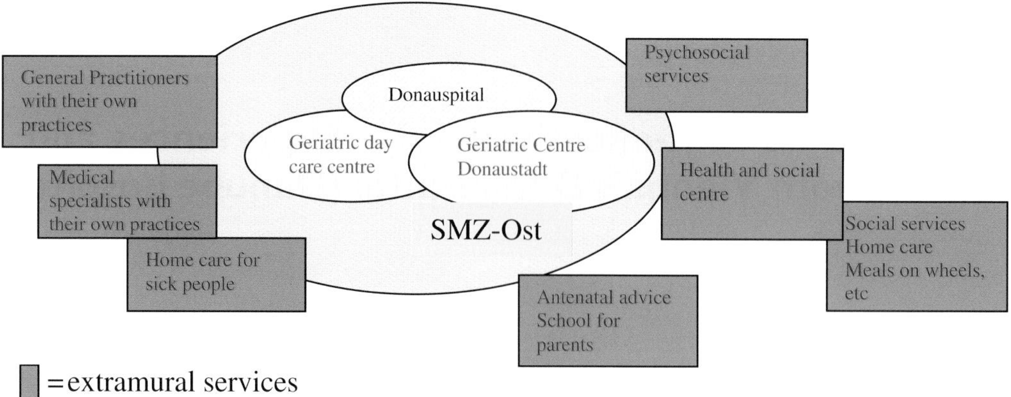

Fig. 1. Plan of the Regional Alliance Donaustadt

cost comparison was relatively easy. Comparing the cost of film and chemicals, savings on storage space [4], savings on staff working in the archives [5] with the statutory useful economic life of the PACS [picture archiving and communications systems] components showed no extra expense and convinced the funding body of the economic utility of the digital facilities (see Table 4). A cost-benefit analysis finally swayed those in positions of responsibility for planning to vote in favour of digital technology. The qualitative enhacements – very broadly speaking – even convinced most of the critics of the decision [6].

- A reduced radiation dose (especially important with regard to paediatric wards)
- Opportunities for further work on an image, improvement of image quality
- Clear improvement of the image communication within the hospital
- No more X-ray chemicals (disposing of used chemicals is an environmental hazard)
- Safe archiving, with great savings in terms of space and personnel

The Austrian Institute for Technology Assessment conducted a study into the "digital hospital" in 1996 at the request of the Federal Ministry for Education, Science, and Culture. The result with respect to the Donauspital's digital radiology was found to be as follows [7]:

The radiological institute at the Donauspital as digital equipment and has shown enormous productivity during its first year in operation. This is true for the numbers of patients per staff and the expense per staff. Substantial savings potential is in avoiding the cost of films and the associated costs for development and disposal. Cost savings have also been made in terms of space, although these will not reach zero. The desirability of and demand for radiodiagnosis are increasing; there is no proof that fewer radiographs are taken when digital technology is used than are in institutions that work with conventional technology. Therefore the reduced number of repeat images has to be compared with an increased number of control images and complementary images. The development of an efficient control system with targets and responsibility for the budget may develop a stronger cost consciousness in the clinicians. The demand for internal costs within the hospital may be influenced in this way (optimised, not minimised). Enticements (responsibility for the budget) on the one hand and interdisciplinary further training of clinicians and radiologists on the other hand seem promising, as does giving radiologists more of a vote in deciding the methods to be applied.

The recommendation made in the study, to control the demand for services using imaging for diagnostic purposes by integrating these internal services and costs into the departmental budgets, has now been put into practice in the Donauspital.

Cost-effectiveness

Acting cost-effectively means using the available means to meet as much of the demand as possible, i.e. to meet a high demand with as little expense as possible. When using this general definition of the principle of cost-effectiveness as a basis to take a closer look at the instruments of cost calculations, one comes to calculatory cost-effectiveness, which describes the relation of revenue from services over a budgeted period to expenditure over the same period. Since the reimbursements from the hospital insurance bodies do not cover the costs of the hospital's services, the deficit has to be covered by the funding bodies. The relevant reference value in this context is the extent of cost coverage that individual hospitals manage to achieve [8].

Table 2. Cost data from Vienna's municipal hospital centres

2003	Number of Beds	Number of Inpatients	Outpatient Frequency	Duration of Stay	Expenditure (in €)	Expenditure/ Inpatients (in €)
KFJ	745	29,235	220,194	7.7	119,104,279	4,074
Lainz	1,044	50,922	292,231	6.7	213,431,000	4,191
Rudolfstiftung	854	48,346	353,488	6.0	154,641,548	3,199
Wilhelminen	1,116	47,479	394,483	7.7	196,448,175	4,138
Donauspital	933	50,472	438,766	6.8	193,453,175	3,833

Beds: Number of beds; Outpatient frequency: Number of visits from outpatients to a main cost centre without beds; Duration of stay: The length of time, in care days, that an inpatient stays in hospital; Expenditure/inpatients: Total costs including those for outpatients, divided by the number of inpatients

Vienna's alliance of hospitals is one of the largest municipal hospital networks and allows comparisons between hospital centres within the alliance that still have with analogue technologies in place. Table 2 shows the degree of cost-effectiveness of the five hospital centres in the alliance. The Donauspital's cost-effectiveness is comparatively high. It can therefore be concluded that the running costs for digital radiology do not negatively affect the overall cost structure.

What follows is a business comparison for the radiology institutes of Vienna's five municipal hospital centres for 2003

The cost breakdown data are summarised every year by Austria's Federal Ministry for Health and Women on the basis of, firstly, cost data compiled in accordance with Paragraph 33 of the "Kostenrechnungsverordnung for Fondskrankenanstalten, BGBl. No 784/96" (the cost accounting regulation for Austrian hospitals financed by provincial funds), and, secondly, the statistical data compiled in accordance with paragraph 3 of the Statistikverordnung für Fondskrankenanstalten, BGBl. No 785/96 (the regulation for statistics relating to Austrian hospitals financed by provincial funds), and made available to the hospitals.

The comparison of costs per service unit ("total costs per frequency") shows clearly that the costs incurred by the Donauspital are favourable.

The data shown in Table 3 for the Donauspital [5] show a clear discrepancy to those from the compared hospitals. This discrepancy is almost entirely due to the data from the A&E surgery department, which does not exist in other KAV hospitals to the same extent as in the Donauspital. About half of all treatment and frequency data in the Donauspital are from the A&E department.

"Treatment" in the sense of the cost calculation means the "X-ray service." This does not mean the same in all the hospitals, so that a comparison is problematic. The term "frequency", however, is used unambiguously and unanimously and means one visit/day/cost centre.

Table 3. Reference points for central radiological institutes excluding magnetic resonance imaging and computed tomography (from baseline data evaluations 2003 from the Federal Ministry for Work, Health, and Social Affairs)

2003	Treatment Total	Costs for Treatment (in €)	Frequency and Total	Costs/ Frequency (in €)
Donauspital[1)]	150,198	92	114,412	121
Kaiser-Franz-Josef-Spital	87,666	118	71,461	145
Krankenhaus Lainz[2)]	32,842	127	26,780	156
Wilhelminenspital	76,466	132	65,840	153
Krankenanstalt Rudolfst.	72,895	114	60,355	138

[1]Including accident and emergency radiography. [2]Only central radiography, without decentralised modalities.

A comparison of costs and frequencies shows that the costs of the Donauspital with its digital technology are favourable compared with the other hospitals, which have only rudimentary digital technologies.

This comparison, together with the comparison in Table 2, shows that in spite of substantial qualitative advantages of digital radiology its running costs are no higher than those of analogue radiology.

The comparison of costs for a radiology institute of the size of the Donauspital (including A&E) as in Table 4, for analogue and digital facilities, confirms that digital technology is no more costly than analogue technology.

Experiences since 1992 and recommendations

The introduction of digital radiology is undoubtedly associated with high investment costs. The experience

Table 4

All in 1000 Austrian shillings	Analogue system (not required for digital system) per year	Over 7 years	Digital system (additionally required for digital system) per year[1]	Over 7 years[1]
PACS[2]				120,000
Servicing and maintenance	3,000	21,000	15,000	105,000
12 development machines		5,068		
2 laser imaging machines		3,200		
4 film copiers		240		
10 instruments to enable doctors to write on radiographs		60		
40 X-ray viewboxes		684		
6 alternators		1,800		
2 film viewers		200		
Archive of 1300 m^3 at ATS 5500,00; ATS 7,150,000, duration of use 70 years		715		
7 archive sta (24/7)	2,450	17,150		
X ray films	26,000	182,000		
Film chemicals including disposal	800	5,600		
Film bags	100	700		
Optical storage discs			600	4,200
Imaging plates				6,000
Expenditure over 7 years[1]		238,417		235,200

[1] Duration of use according to cost accounting regulation (Kostenrechnungsverordnung, KRV).
[2] Includes all costs of hardware and software; does not include the costs of X-ray equipment.

of the Donauspital shows that a total switch to digital technologies is highly recommended and one should not worked mixed digital/analogue. In the history of the technological development of digital radiology in the Donauspital this was initially necessary (in 1992 radiodiagnostics in the A&E department was performed on analogue equipment). The prevailing doubts about the usefulness/applicability of digital technology in the A&E ward resulted in rapid innovation in the industry, so that in 1998 the A&E department could be switched to digital radiodiagnostics.

Digital radiology has to be envisaged in connection with electronic image transfer and archiving, but also with the radiology information system. This system therefore has to be embedded in the hospital's own information system (KIS).

The decision about whether electronic images should be used in all wards and outpatient clinics of the hospital will have to be made individually by each hospital, on the basis of need but also potential restrictions. Surgical and intensive care wards, orthopaedics, and neurosurgery needed to be networked as a matter of course; these have to be furnished with viewing equipment with quality of primary medical findings.

In addition to the high initial financial outlay, substantial expenditure is incurred by running and servicing digital equipment.

The higher costs for these can be offset by remembering that digital radiology does not use the following, so costs incurred by analogue technologies will not be incurred:

- A gain in working time (maybe savings due to fewer necessary staff)
- No X-ray films
- No X-ray chemicals (economically as well as environmentally important)
- No archiving space required

The currently used multi-use phosphor imaging plates are over time replaced with tapes with an amorphous selenium flat panel detector. These tapes remain in the X-ray equipment, from which the image data enter directly into the X-ray system. By further simplifying the workflow, productivity and speed are enhanced. An additional saving is made in terms of working time, since the storage films do not need to be transported manually from the image capturing device to the selection device.

From today's perspective (2004), the question is not whether analogue or digital technology should be used, as digital radiology has unanimously won first place. Digital systems will pay for themselves after three to five years, depending on the mass structure, according to the managing director of Imaging Service

GmbH (ISG), Matthias Matzko [9]. The potential utility of digital radiology has by no means been exhausted. Economists urge to gauge the (hidden) synergy effects, which also mean clear quality improvements, reduction of the radiation load, automatic patient related dosage documentation, optimisation of the workflow, and the consequences of all these for the length of the patient's stay in the hospital, conditions for image fusion, further processing, etc.

Particular weight, however, is due to the qualitative and economic advantages in telemedicine projects. The creation of teleportal hospitals in regional alliances (networks health regions or regional healthcare partnerships [10]) will clarify the economic advantages only later on. Teleportal hospitals capture patient data on site, aided by modern diagnostic equipment. The data are then evaluated centrally in competency centres. The place for treatment is decided on the basis of available space. The Rhön-Klinikum AG is expecting the first teleportal hospitals to come into the network in 2005. The company is expecting optimised care and reduced total treatment costs by about 20% thanks to a division of labour in the organisation of work processes [11].

The administrative director assessed the first 12 years of using digital radiology in the Donauspital as follows:

1) The **costs of servicing** the modalities as well as the PACS are clearly higher than assumed originally. The equally clearly higher productivity results in a favourable relation between cost and service. The administrative director cannot, however, answer the question whether the higher output of digital equipment compared with conventional radiology is of diagnostic importance.

2) **Archiving:** New methods in diagnostic imaging are resulting in continuous increases in the amount of imaging data and make the implementation of economical archiving solutions into an ongoing task for the service providers in medical imaging diagnostics [12]. The storage amounts especially for long-term storage will have to be limited: the preselection of the data that are to be archived should be taken into consideration (from a legal point of view too), as should their compression. In Vienna's hospital alliance, a pertinent decision has been made.

Following the recommendations of Austria's Radiology Society, radiological images may be compressed for the purpose of archiving in a PACS with the lossy compression procedures that will in future be based on the DICOM [Digital Imaging and Communications in Medicine] standard (JPEG-LS or JPEG-2000) by a suitable factor (1:10 for images of the thorax, 1:20 for CT scans and magnetic resonance images.).

This image compression, which according to radiologists does not result in a notable loss in quality, can – in order to administer the storage space in the archiving systems in an economical manner – in future be applied also to the images transferred into a PACS archive.

This image compressions, which according to radiologists does not result in a loss of quality in the image can be used in future be applied to all images imported into the PACS archive – so as to administer the storage space in the archiving systems as economically as possible.

The lossy compression processes that are defined in the DICOM standard should therefore be implemented into existing "systems" in the framework/context of the technological and economical opportunities. When purchasing new equipment the implementation of such compression methods has to be taken into consideration during the purchasing process [13].

3) **Transparency with respect to radiation dosage:** Digital radiology enables the automatic inclusion of exposure data of imaging modalities into the electronic patient file within a digital, film-less hospital [14]. The assumed cost-effectiveness of online dosage documentation needs to be examined separately.

4) **Flat panel detectors:** As mentioned above, this technology should be inforced because the resulting simplification of the workflow saves waiting times for patients as well as working hours for staff. Additionally, direct readiographical systems based on flat detectors are physically superior to digital luminescence radiography (DLR): In experiments, the dose needed to achieve the same sharpness of contrast for visibility of detail is significantly higher when a digital storage film is used than when a flat detector is used.

The example of a thorax imaging workstation illustrates a clear advantage in terms of cost:

THORAMAT (four storage films, X-ray tube on a ceiling stand, additionally wall-mounted tripod): purchasing and running costs over 10 years €673,000.00

Thorax FD (thorax imaging workstation with flat panel detector): purchasing and running costs over 10 years €530,000.00.

5) **Image fusion:** Digital radiology, combined with other digital imaging procedures, enables "imaging postprocessing office" (clinical image fusion). This is a procedure in which the image series of diverse imaging modalities are combined in a new series so as to link the respective advantages of the modalities. The fused image normally contains as background information the information of a modality with high anatomical precision, such as images obtained by computed tomography or magnetic resonance

imaging. In the foreground of the image, the series is inserted, colour-coded and containing functional information, such as images obtained by positron emission tomography (PET), single photon emission tomography (SPECT), or magnetic resonance imaging [15].

Economists perceive this as an exemplary use of synergistic effects. The enormously expensive modalities are being integrated for the first time, i.e. used in synergy.

6) **Tele-portal hospitals:** see above.

7) **Networks:** In order to be able to use the advantages of electronic image communications without disturbances, the communications networks should enable the safe transfer of large amounts of data and should be oriented towards future developments.

As physical transfer media, fibreoptic cables and modern copper cables (level 5) should be used. Ideally, both these materials should be combined so that the fibreoptic cable is used as a "backbone" until the desired hospital floor is reached, and the copper cable is used on that floor itself [15].

In Donauspital (DSP) a completely new electronic data processing network will be built from 2004 onwards. The project manager is Peter Grünstäudl (peter.grünstäudl@wienkav.at), of the electronic data processing management and the management centre of the "Wiener Krankenanstaltenverbund" (Vienna hospital alliance) (http://www.wienkav.at/kav/tu3/emb/).

The network that is currently still in use consists of two networks: a base network (the so-called backbone) in the form of the optical fibre network and for the terminal equipment a coaxial cable network (copper) with a maximum bandwidth of 10 megabits per second and a separate X-ray network (FDDI ring).

The technology of the base network has the advantage that additional end user equipment can be connected to the network speedily and without great expenditure in terms of time and money. The disadvantage is that the network's power (10 megabits/second) is distributed among all end users that are linked to the network, which results in a longer response time especially during peak working hours and when additional equipment is connected to the network. This means that the transfer rate of 10 MBits/sec cannot be achieved.

Since the number of end user equipment has risen drastically over the years and the amount of data that needed transferring has increased substantially, the network is now not able to meet the requirements of the Donauspital any more and cannot be optimised any further.

In order to meet requirements now and in the future, a complete reorganisation (in a physical and logical sense) has become a matter of urgency. The X-ray network will also be affected by the new network. The entire network will be logically subdivided into segments.

The project network reorganisation DSP is therefore aiming to create the basis for transmitting all required data in electronic format so any user can call these at any place in the hospital, and at an acceptable and guaranteed speed (100 megabits/sec up to more than 1 gigabit/sec).

The physical reorganisation of the entire network is going to entail the base network as well as the end user network.

The old base network will be replaced by an optical fibre network of a newer and more powerful generation. Redundancies will be built in. This means that all network components in all cable spreading rooms will now be fed into in two different routes.

For end user equipment, twisted pair cables (copper) will be laid as a point-to-point connection. This will enable transmission on a bandwidth of 100 megabits per second. The transmission rate can effortlessly be increased to 1 gigabit/second – more than 100 times the speed achieved today.

A particularly innovation used in this project is that in the end user equipment a special cable will be used for the first time., which was developed especially for the Donauspital. This is a doubled and twisted pair cable, which has an empty tube, into which optical glass fibres can be inserted at a later stage without any major problems – i.e. without have to renew the cabling (see illustration). This will be crucial once market developments make the use of fibre optic cables for end user equipment economically viable in terms of cost or in individual cases as a matter of strategy. This would increase the transfer rate exponentially.

As each end user will need a network socket in their room as well as a free network socket in the relevant distribution box, each additional end user socket or connection point that needs to added in the future would necessitate re-cabling. This would

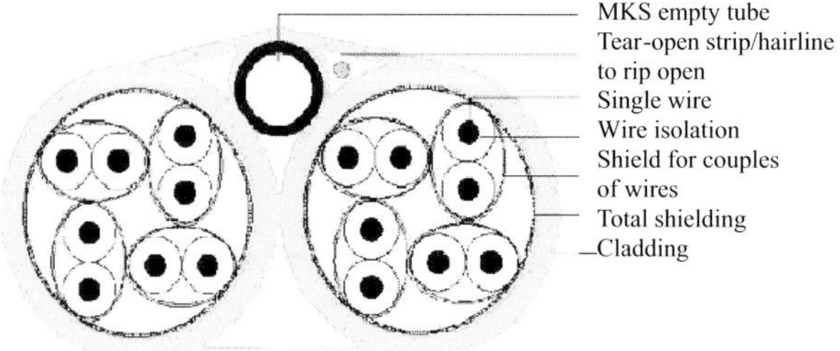

mean building measures, which are associated with substantial financial and organisational expenditure. For this reason the number of connections/extensions has been laid out in such a way that even potentially maximum requirements on capacity should be met [16].

Summary

After 12 years of using a digital radiology system, people's expectations during the planning phase have been confirmed. Its use rationalises processes in imaging diagnostics and contributes substantially to increasing quality and productivity in the core business of the hospital.

However, the manifold improvements and advantages of digital radiology, its ease of use, and the fascinating innovation itself lead to an increase in expectations and demand. Rapidly increasing numbers of referrals and service demands from the clinical sector may soon annihilate any financial gains achieved through digital systems. The implementation of digital systems therefore should be accompanied by controlling referrals (medical controls, diagnostic standards, etc).

References

[1] Construction time 1985–1992 (1st stage), 1994 (2nd stage), 1996 (3rd stage)
[2] s. http://www.wienkav.at/kav/dsp
[3] s. http://www.wien.gv.at/ma66/aktuell
[4] According to the Viennese Hospital Law, radiographs have to be kept for a total of ten years.
[5] The accident and emergency department and the paediatrics department require access to the archive 24/7.
[6] s.a. Sabina Schober, Digitale Radiologie im Donauspital [Digital radiology in the Donauspital] (diploma dissertation, School for Economics, Vienna, October, 1995).
[7] "The digital hospital. Technology assessment of modern telecommunications technologies in hospitals as exempluified by the Donauspital/Socio-Medical Center East." Final report on the study conducted by Austria's Academy of Sciences, Institute for Technology Assessment, Vienna, January 1997.
[8] Final report on the study conducted by Austria's Academy of Sciences, page 66
[9] ISG a company that has been separated out from the Institute for Clinical Radiology Großhadern, which is implementing a telemedicine project between the university hospital Großhadern in Munich and the Amper-Hospital in Dachau (see *Klinik Management Aktuell*, No 95-05/2004).
[10] s. model of the Working Group of Austria's Health Insurance Organisations (ARGE KV)", in *„Solidarität"*, September 2004, monthly magazine of Austria's Federation of Trade Unions.
[11] s. *Klinik Management Aktuell* [Hospital Management Today], Nr. 95-05/2004, S. 66.
[12] Presentation by W. Hruby at the 7th conference on medical law, Johann Kepler University Linz (December 2002)
[13] Instruction of the Viennese Hospital Group, dated 17 July 2002 (GED-150/02/TIM)
[14] s. *Wiener klinische Wochenschrift* 3a/2002, S. 10.
[15] s. Hospital for Radiology, Charitè Campus Virchow-Hospitals, Working Group Digital Radiology (http://www.charite.de/rv/str/forschung/digrad/charite/aufbau/index.php)
[16] The text on the Donauspital's network overhaul and modernisation is by Peter Grünstäudl; intranet of the DSP (2004).

Investing in PACS using real option theory

W. Rueger

Siemens Medical Systems, USA

Abstract

Frequently, traditional cost effectiveness models based on film savings and other productivity improvements indicate that an investment in PACS is difficult to justify. This paper offers a new evaluation perspective based on Real Option Theory that has been applied successfully in other industries. Other than the traditional savings centric model, it allows to account for managerial flexibility, risk, expansion opportunities, increased market share and other "intangible" key metrics.

It is based on the consideration that an initial investment may create opportunities for future investments, e.g. by way of expansion. The additional value associated with such real options uncovers the embedded value of the initial investment and may often favor an investment scenario where the traditional savings based approach falls short.

In the following, the valuation of a real option and its application to various PACS investment scenarios (option to wait, option to expand, option to learn) are discussed.

What is an option?

An option is a contract that confers upon its holder the right, *without the obligation*, to acquire or dispose of a risky asset at a set strike price within a given period of time. The holder may exercise the option by buying or selling the underlying asset before or on its expiration date if the net payoff from the transaction is positive. If the holder does not exercise the option by or on the expiration date, the option expires worthless. The value of the option is the value one would pay to buy the contract if it were traded in the capital markets. An option that gives the right to acquire an asset is called a *call option*; an option that gives the right to dispose of an asset is called a *put option*.

Options may have different types of underlying assets. A financial option's underlying asset is a security. The most familiar example is the stock option whose underlying security is the common stock of a publicly traded company. When the underlying asset is a real asset, such as the future cash flows of a risky investment, the option is called a real option. These are precisely the kinds of options that arise in capital budgeting projects. The right to delay an investment outlay, to abandon a project midstream, and to expand or contract operations, as well as future growth opportunities cast as follow-on projects are all examples of real options. A project or investment activity is said to *embed* a real option it the decision to undertake the project implicitly buys that option. Software projects and IT investments in general embed many types of real options.

The value of an option is intricately linked to its asymmetric nature: the holder has the right, but not the obligation to exercise an option, and therefore, does so only if and when it is beneficial. This asymmetry limits the downside potential for the holder, but leaves the upside potential unlimited.

The first real option transaction [4]

The first account of a real option is found in the writings of Aristotle. He tells of how Thales the Melesian, a sophist philosopher, divined from some tea leaves that there would be a bountiful olive harvest in six months' time. Having a little money, he approached the owners of some olive presses and bought the right to rent their presses at the usual rate. When a record harvest duly arrived and the growers were clamoring for pressing capacity, he rented the presses to them at above the market rate, paid the normal rate to their owners, and kept the difference for himself, proving for all time that sophism is not only an honorable profession, but a profitable one too. What is the real option in this story? First of all, Thales purchased the right, but not the obligation, to rent the presses. (He purchased a call option, the right to buy or rent. The opposite is a put option, the right to sell.) Had the harvest been poor, he would have chosen not to rent, and lost only his original small investment, the price of the option. Thales contracted for a predetermined rental price that in option pricing terminology is called the exercise or strike price. If the market price is higher than the exercise price, the call option is said to be "in the money" and Thales would exercise it. If the market price is lower than the exercise price, then the call is "out of the money" and would not be exercised. The underlying source of uncertainty in the story was the size of the olive harvest, which affected the market rental value of the presses. As the *value of the underlying variable* increases, so does the value of the option. In other words, the greater the harvest of olives to be pressed, the more valuable Thales' option to rent the presses will be. The value of the option also increases with the *level of uncertainty* of the underlying variable. The logic is straightforward. If there is no uncertainty over the size of the olive harvest, which is known to be normal, then the market rental value of the presses will also be normal, and Thales' option will be worthless. But if the size of the harvest is uncertain, there is a chance that his option will finish in the money. The greater the uncertainty, the higher the probability that the option will finish in the money, and the more valuable the option. So far we have mentioned three of the five variables that affect the value of the option. It increases with the *value of the underlying variable* and with its *uncertainty,* and it decreases as the *exercise price* goes up. The fourth variable is the *time to maturity* of the option. Thales purchased his option six months before the harvest, but it would have been even more valuable two months earlier, because uncertainty increases with time. To see why, suppose that Thales has agreed to pay 10 drachmas per hour to rent the presses, and the market rental price is also 10 drachmas. With only one second to go before his option expires, it has no value. But with a month to go, there is a good chance that the market value will rise above 10 drachmas and the option will finish in the money. Therefore, the longer the time to maturity, the more valuable an option is. Finally, the value of the option increases with the *time value of money,* the risk-free rate of interest. This is because the present value of the exercise cost falls as interest rates rise.

Option pricing model

The price of a financial call option is typically estimated by the application of the Black-Scholes formula with a modification from Merton (8, p. 263):

$$\text{Call Option} = Se^{-\delta t}N(d_1) - Xe^{-rt} * N(d_2),$$

$$\text{where } d_{1/2} = \frac{\ln(S/X) + (r - \delta \pm \sigma^2/2)t}{\sigma\sqrt{t}}$$

and where S = stock price, X = exercise price, δ = dividends, r = risk-free rate, σ = uncertainty, t = time to expiry, and N(d) = cumulative normal distribution function.

It should be noted that Myron Scholes and Robert Merton were awarded the 1997 Nobel Prize for economics for their financial options valuation model. Fischer Black, who died in 1995, was mentioned in the award.

The **stock price** (S) is the value of the underlying stock or asset on which an option is purchased. As such, it is simply the market's estimate of the present value of all future cash flows – dividends, capital gains, and so on – associated with that stock/asset. Its equivalent in a real option is, therefore, the present value of cash flows expected from the investment opportunity on which the option is purchased. It is also referred as the source of the uncertainty, as the value of S is assumed to fluctuate more with higher degree of uncertainty/risk associated with the project.

The **strike or exercise price** (X) is the predetermined price at which the option can be exercised. Its real-market equivalent is the present value of all the fixed costs (investment) expected over the lifetime of the investment opportunity.

Uncertainty or Volatility (σ) is a measure of the unpredictability of future stock price movements: more precisely, the standard deviation of the growth rate of the value of future cash inflows associated with the stock. The real-market equivalent is the same, but in relation to the cash flows associated with the asset. Typical values for σ can be placed in the context of equity volatilities of around 15%–20% for mature financial sector firms, 20%–30% for industrials or resources companies and 40%–65% for exploration concerns, information technology projects and R&D projects [12].

Time to expiry (t) is the period during which the option can be exercised. Its real-market equivalent is the period for which the investment opportunity is valid. This will depend on technology (a product's life cycle), competitive advantage (intensity of competition), and contracts (patents, leases, licences).

Dividends (δ) are sums paid regularly to stockholders. In real-market terms, dividend expense is represented by the value that drains away over the duration of the option. This could be the cost incurred to preserve the option (by staving of competition or keeping the opportunity alive), or the cash flows lost to competitors that go ahead and invest in an opportunity, depriving later entrants of cash flows. Or it represents the savings and revenue foregone when not investing.

The **risk-free interest rate** (r) is the yield of a riskless security with the same maturity as the duration of the option, whether with regard to financial options or real options.

Increases in stock price, uncertainty, time to expiry, and risk-free interest rate raise the option value. Increases in exercise price and dividends reduce it [9].

Traditional project evaluation

Lets look at the traditional approach called Discounted Cash Flow (DCF) analysis or Net Present Value (NPV) technique:

A hospital is considering a PACS investment decision. The initial investment is $I_0 = \$1M$. The cost of capital is estimated at $d_r = 8\%$, the discount rate. Cash flow per year generated by the project is estimated at $CFPY = 250,000$. The time horizon is 5 years. Other cost is ignored for simplicity.

First, all future cash flow is discounted back to the present – money in the future is less worth than money in the present – resulting in a Present Value

$$PV = \sum_{i=1}^{5} \frac{CFPY_i}{(1+d_c)^i} = \frac{\$250,000}{(1+8\%)^1} + \frac{\$250,000}{(1+8\%)^2} + \frac{\$250,000}{(1+8\%)^3} + \frac{\$250,000}{(1+8\%)^4} + \frac{\$250,000}{(1+8\%)^5} = \$998,178$$

Thus, the Net Present Value of the project results in

$$NPV_{hospital} = PV - I_0 = \$998,178 - \$1,000,000 = -\$1,822,$$

almost at break even.

The DCF method is simple: projects with positive NPV are believed to create value and are to be accepted; negative NPV projects are thrown out. Thus, the above project should be not be implemented – at least not from a DCF perspective. The time horizon impacts NPV considerably. Its choice should reflect the realistic useful life of the project. For PACS, 5 years are assumed to be appropriate.

Impact of real options on project valuation

In expanding on the example of the prior section, we will assume the hospital has the opportunity to acquire the imaging center across the street that creates the option of extending PACS to the imaging center. The size of the project is half of the hospital PACS project. The present value of the cost of the follow-on investment is estimated at $I_3 = \$500,000$, savings per year are \$125,000. Time horizon is 5 years; the cash flow is again discounted at 8%. Thus, the

$$NPV_{imaging\ center} = NPV_{hospital}/2 = -\$911,$$

half the net present value of the hospital PACS project. Similarly, the PV of the cash flow for the imaging center is half of the hospital's cash flow, equating to \$499,089. The combined NPV of both projects is –\$1,822 –\$911= –\$ 2,734 which is to be expected.

What is the value of the expansion option? Assuming the window of opportunity (to acquire the imaging center and implement PACS) is open for 3 years, the option is valued as follows:

$$\begin{aligned} S &= \text{Source of uncertainty} = \text{PV of cashflow} \\ &\quad \text{generated by project} = \$499,089 \\ X &= \text{Strike price} = \text{PV of investment} = \$500,000 \\ t &= \text{time to expiry} = 3 \text{ years} \\ \delta &= \text{Dividends} = 0 \\ \sigma &= \text{Volatility} = 40\% \text{ per year} \\ r &= \text{risk-free interest rate} = 5\% \text{ per year} \end{aligned}$$

$$\begin{aligned} \text{Option} &= \$499,089 \cdot e^{-0 \cdot 3} \cdot N(0.560) \\ &\quad - \$500,000 \cdot e^{-.05 \cdot 3} \cdot N(-0.133) \\ &= \$499,089 \cdot 1 \cdot 0.712 \\ &\quad - \$500,000 \cdot 0.861 \cdot 0.447 \\ &= \$163,041 \end{aligned}$$

The value of the option results in an expanded or strategic net present value:

$$\text{Expanded NPV} = \text{NPV} + \text{Option},$$

with

$$\text{NPV} = \text{Present Value of cashflows} - \text{Investment} = PV - I$$

Considering the option, the adjusted NPV for the hospital PACS results in

$$\begin{aligned} &NPV_{hospital\ with\ option\ to\ expand} \\ &= NPV_{hospital} + \text{Option} \\ &= -\$1,822 + \$163,041 \\ &= \$161,218 \end{aligned}$$

rendering the decision to proceed with the project in a much more favorable light.

Where is the additional value coming from? Is it tangible, is it realistic? What projects benefit?

The real option model adds an important fact: It uncovers the hidden strategic value of the first investment IF a sensible follow-on investment is possible. Thus, the initial investment creates more value than indicated by traditional DCF. However, without the existence of the expansion opportunity, the value of the option equaled \$0.

The value of real option is in every way real and tangible. It accounts for – what is also supported by common sense – the lower risk introduced by staging the investment and allowing for flexibility to decide for the follow-on investment at a later point. Risk can be multifacetted, such as staff acceptance of the project, cost of capital and/or technology in the future, certainty or uncertainty of projected cash flows, or committing only a fraction of the total investment initially [12].

Of course, there are limitations to the sensible use of real options. They are most important in situations of uncertainty where management can respond flexibly to new information, and where the projects value without flexibility is near breakeven. If the NPV is very high, the project will go full steam ahead, and flexibility is unlikely to be exercised. And if the NPV is strongly negative, no amount of flexibility will help. Optionality is of greatest value for the difficult decisions – the close calls where the traditional NPV is close or below zero [4].

Examining the probability distributions or risk profiles of the expected value of a project shows the difference between a traditional and a dynamic valuation approach.

A traditional net present value analysis generates a range of probable expected values by random variation of the project parameters with the most likely value in the center of a symmetric normal probability distribution as shown in Fig. 1. An adjusted present value analysis, including the value of the real options, incorporates into the analysis process management's flexibility to improve a project's upside potential while limiting the impact of the project's downside losses – when not exercising the option should the future investment climate be unfavorable. This results in a project with a higher net present value NPV_{p+o} and causes the distribution to be skewed to the right [6].

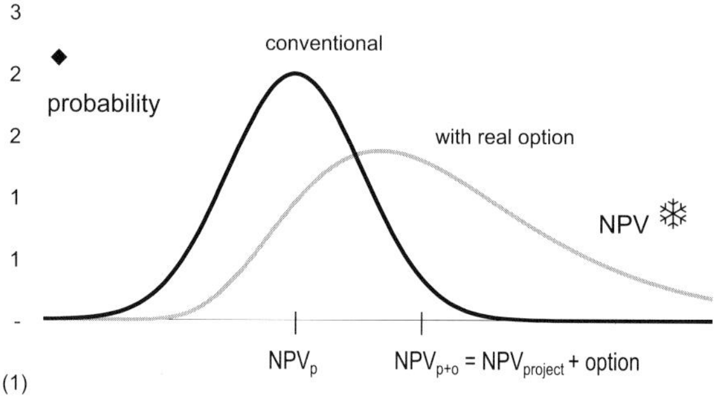

Fig. 1. Impact of Real Options on Net Present Value risk profile. The real option takes advantage of positive NPV changes due to environment changes and mitigates downside risk

Taxonomy of real options

Previous work in real options has generated a taxonomy that has broken down real options into several categories based upon the type of flexibility provided [1,11]. It is also possible for a project to have more than one category of real options be applicable that leads to multiple interacting real options.

Waiting-to-invest option: By investing in a project, revenues or productivity can be increased. However, immediate investing means assuming immediate risk. The losses of waiting are balanced again the risk of earning future profits.

Learning option: The risk of investing in new technologies can be mitigated by starting with seed investments – prototyping – and observing the results.

Expansion (staging) options: When benefits are uncertain, commit investments in smaller stages, even if the first stage may not be profitable by itself.

Thus, retaining the option to abandon at different stages while retaining the ability to grow.

Exit options: Exit when opportunities do not present themselves as planned. By keeping the option to exit or to abandon open, the NPV of a project may increase and favor an initial investment.

Insurance option: Protects the investor from a future upside or downside at the expense of the option premium that is typically a fraction of the value to be protected.

Cost modeling in PACS

PACS allows improving productivity as well as increasing revenue. Productivity improvements fall in two classes:

- Film related savings (film material, handling, processing, re-takes, archiving, increased throughput at modalities, less space requirements, no more film loss)
- Physician (radiologist and referring physician) time saved [10]. Only of relevance when physicians are employed by the PACS investor.

Table 1. Discounted Cash Flow analysis of the full PACS solution for a hospital with "1" procedure per year, project "One Shot". In year 1, savings are only counted from months 7–12 (1/2 of total) to account for implementation time. NPV scaled to I = 1.7%

Year	0	1	2	3	4	5	Comment
Investment I	−$40.00						for "1" procedure
Support			−$4.00	−$4.00	−$4.00	−$4.00	10% of investment
Savings		$7.50	$15.00	$15.00	$15.00	$15.00	$15 per procedure
Cash flow		$7.50	$11.00	$11.00	$11.00	$11.00	
Discounted Cashflow		$6.94	$9.43	$8.73	$8.09	$7.49	8% discount rate
Present Value of Cashflow		$6.94	$16.38	$25.11	$33.19	$40.68	
Net Present Value		−$33.06	−$23.62	−$14.89	−$6.81	$0.68	NPV = PV − I

Typical cost for film related savings vary between $10 [13] and $18 [2] per procedure for the average mix. They tend to be higher for teaching institutions.

The cost for investing in PACS can be estimated at $40 per procedure for a high-end turnkey solution, including computed radiography, interfaces and network. Thus, for a hospital with 100,000 procedures per year, the investment is $4 Million.

Support including equipment service is estimated at 10% of the initial investment, starting in year 2.

Increasing revenue is quite a realistic possibility due to attractiveness of vastly improved turnaround time and instantaneous electronic distribution capabilities of a PACS to the referring physicians.

The examples in the application section use the DCF model in Table 1. Note the cost of support start in year 2, savings from i.e. film related operations amount to 50% of the full amount in year 1, taking implementation time into account.

Applications of real options in PACS

Waiting-to-invest option

There is a cost to delaying taking a project, once the net present value turns positive. Each year of delay translates into one less year of value-creating cash flows offsetting the investment in PACS, increasing the cost of the delayed opportunity. However, waiting also reduces the uncertainty associated with investing [3,5].

Figure 2 shows two scenarios for the option values as a function of the savings. The model is based on the DCF analysis in Table 1. The potential savings or foregone earnings *before* the PACS implementation are described by δ. For instance, δ = 20% correspond for a $40 investment (for the "1" procedure hospital) with $10 savings per procedure and year. The option values are plotted against the savings per year *after* PACS has been implemented, already considering the 10% cost of support.

Conventional DCF analysis commands, take the project when NPV turns positive. However, when considering the option, it says there is actually value in waiting. Thus, NPV must meet or exceed the option value, indicated by the crossovers marked in Fig. 2. At the crossovers, the "value to wait" indicated by the arrow turns zero. With higher expected savings equivalent to higher savings foregone before PACS, waiting times are shorter and the value to wait is less. Projects with option values below the NPV graph should be implemented immediately.

Waiting times result from the consideration that investing later is more affordable due to the discounting of future values. Moreover, waiting times increase with increasing uncertainty σ that inflates the option value. Balancing the discounted investment against the present value of cash flows minus the option value

$$\frac{I}{(1 + d_r)^t} = PV_{cashflow} - Option$$

allows resolving for the waiting time t.

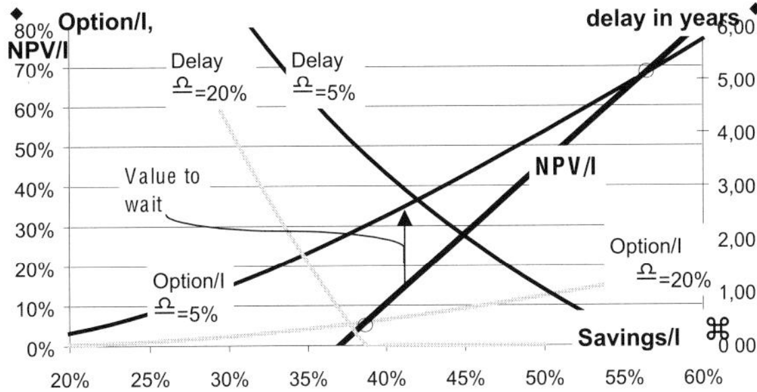

Fig. 2. Waiting-to-invest Option. Option parameters are scaled: S = Savings/I, X = 1, r = 5%, δ = either 5% or 20% of I, δ = 40%, time to expiry 5 years. Savings = Savings (present value) per procedure generated by project per year, I = Investment. Waiting times are optimal when Option/I values cross NPV/I line, setting the "Value to wait" as indicated by the arrow to 0. Other parameters from Table 1

For practical considerations, most PACS projects with positive NPV command waiting times of 1 year or less which is easily consumed by the budgeting and vendor selection process.

Expansion option

We are considering two cases:

- "Partial PACS first": Starting with a partial PACS, a Critical Care Image Distribution application, and completing the installation in phase 2. Film related savings are equivalent to $3 per procedure in phase 1.
- "Complete Archive first": Installing the complete archive first and adding all other modules in phase 2. In phase 1, there are no film related savings.

For modeling, both cases are based on the project in Table 1, from now on referred to as "One Shot", split in 2 phases, with phase 1 requiring 25% of the investment in the original project. Phase 2 is assumed to begin in year 3. Numbers are shown in Table 2.

Both phases combined will last through year 7, making a "re-investment" for the phase 1 part in year 5 necessary.

Comparing the traditional NPVs favors obviously the "Partial PACS first" over the "Complete Archive first", as common sense would tell. It is interesting to note that the total NPV for "Partial PACS first" is slightly less than for "One Shot", caused by the comparatively lower savings achievable with Critical Care Image Distribution during the first 2 years.

However, traditional DCF analysis is not in favor breaking "One Shot" either way, as the resulting NPVs are negative.

Including the value of the real option in the analysis leads to a drastically changed evaluation:

- Breaking the project into phases is by far superior as indicated by the expanded NPV, accounting for the reduced overall risk while delaying part of the implementation. The real option approach allows valuing such a strategic measure in financial terms.
- "Partial PACS first" is still superior over "Complete Archive first", as positive cash flow due to film related savings is generated sooner.
- "Complete Archive first" becomes a financially sensible alternative. It is more convenient for the radiologists who will have the exams for the recent 2 years readily available on the workstation when beginning with softcopy reading in phase 2.

However, other circumstances may prohibit phasing, e.g. when equipment needs to be selected for a new hospital [7] and switching between technologies inflates the overall investment. Such cases can be analyzed with the option "to switch" [1,11].

Table 2. Impact of expansion option on staging PACS implementation for 2 different approaches "Partial PACS first" and "Complete Archive first". Both approaches become viable after considering the value of the expansion option. Risk-less rate r = 5%, other parameters as in Table 1

Scenarios	One Shot	Partial PACS first			Complete archive first		
Phases	Total	1	2	Total	1	2	Total
Investment in year 1	$40	$10			$10		
Investment in year 3			$30			$30	
PV Re-investment year 5		$2.7			$2.7		
PV Savings/year	$15	$3	$12	$15	$0	$15	$15
Start of investment (year)	1	1	3	–	1	3	–
Duration (years)	5	7	5	7	7	5	7
PV (present value) investment	$40.00	$12.72	$25.72	$38.44	$12.72	$25.72	$38.44
PV (present value) project	$40.68	$9.95	$28.43	$38.38	−$4.28	$37.51	$33.22
NPV w/o option	$0.68	−$2.77	$2.71	−$0.07	−$17.00	$11.78	−$5.22
Option Value	n/a	$15.10	$0.00	$15.10	$10.95	$0.00	$10.95
NPV including real option	n/a	$12.32	$2.71	$15.03	−$6.06	$11.78	$5.73
Option parameters							
S = PV project for years 3 thru 7		$38.38			$33.22		
X = PV investment for years 3+		$28.44			$28.44		
Dividend Ω		0%			0%		
Volatility ◆		40%			40%		
Time to expiry (years)		2			2		

Some comments on computing the option parameters: For S, the underlying asset, the present value of the total cash flow of the project between years 3 and 7 is used, not just the values of phase 2. The equivalent applies for the exercise price X. Other than for the "waiting-to-invest option", the dividend $\delta = 0\%$. For the expansion option, it is relevant to consider "leakages of the asset" [1] during and not before the term of the option. Leakage is e.g. a dividend payment for a stock, which lowers the stock value accordingly. And such leakages are not present in PACS projects.

Insurance option

Options can also be used protecting an investor from up- or downside risk. As an example, let us consider the PACS investor who needs to re-invest in upgrades or system expansions or re-negotiate equipment service contracts. For simplicity, we assume a complete re-investment may be necessary after 5 years of operating PACS.

Will the investor be able to buy at the same or a lower price as he did initially? It is common knowledge that the cost of PACS is subject to price change (erosion), much as other IT solutions are. On the other hand, functionality of a future PACS will be richer at a possibly richer price, and who would not want to take advantage of more features? It may be beneficial, both for seller and buyer, to evaluate the cost of an option that offers a price cap to the investor, simplifying long-term budgeting.

We are considering the example of pricing an option for an organization that buys a full featured PACS today and wants to lock in an upper limit of the price for a yet again a full featured system in 5 years from now, not knowing what the future features might be. Buyer and Seller agree on average price chance of −9% per year for the 5 year term, translating the initial system price of $1 Million in $624k present value dollars for the estimated market price of the future system. With the parameters in Fig. 3, the option to lock in an upper limit of −9% annual price change equivalent to a $624k price cap is valued at $268k which is 5.4% annually of the initial investment of $1M.

The seller assumes the risk of less price erosion and is thus compensated with an insurance premium, the option value.

Since the buyer has to pay the option premium, his effective price cap is inflated by the option value, putting it at an price erosion level of only 2.3% (−2.3% avg. price change) per year. Should the future market price be higher than that, then it is the buyers gain and the seller's loss. On the other hand, the seller benefits from higher price erosion levels exceeding 9%.

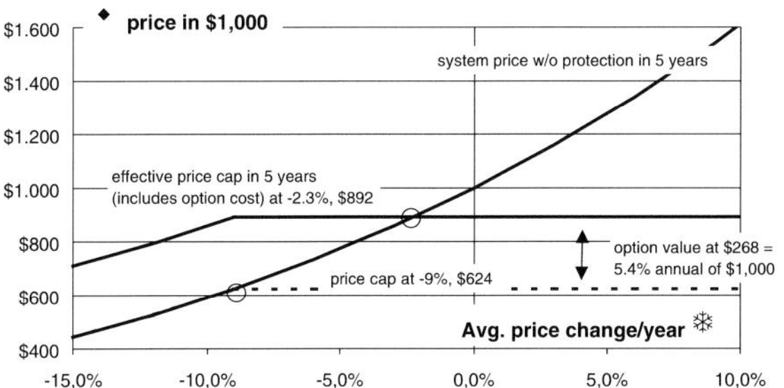

Fig. 3. Insurance option for protecting the cost of a future system replacement against price change. Option parameters: S = $624k, X = $624 k, $r = 5\%$, $\delta = 0\%$, $\sigma = 40\%$, $t = 5$ years. Graphs show situation in 5 years from today, when the option is about to be exercised

Other scenarios for applying real options that include a transfer of risk from the buyer to the seller at the expense of option premium might be obsolescence protection, for HW and/or SW.

Growth option

The 100,000 procedure/year hospital that implemented project "One Shot" is considering an aggressive marketing campaign to increase its procedure volume. Convinced of the attractiveness of its superior electronic imaging infrastructure, it plans to offer 100 selected referring physicians a free PC with a high speed DSL link to the hospitals web-server, allowing instantaneous access to images and reports.

The investment for PCs, webserver, software and network access cost for 5 years are estimated at $1.5 Million or $300k equivalent to $3 per procedure and year. Maintenance is estimated at 10% per year. For the procedure volume, moderate single digit percentage increases are expected each year that can be handled with the existing imaging equipment. Thus, the profit of incremental procedures is estimated at $60 per exam.

For instance, 1% annual growth puts the project's present value at $3.5M for the five year term. The results in Fig. 4 show NPV relative to total investment of the initial PACS at $40 per exam plus the $3 per exam for the distribution system. Compared to the NPV/I = 1.7% of "One Shot", even modest revenue increases turn out to be highly significant.

Obviously, the NPV including the real option exceeds the conventional NPV. In this case however, the conventional NPV by itself is significant enough to support a positive investment decision.

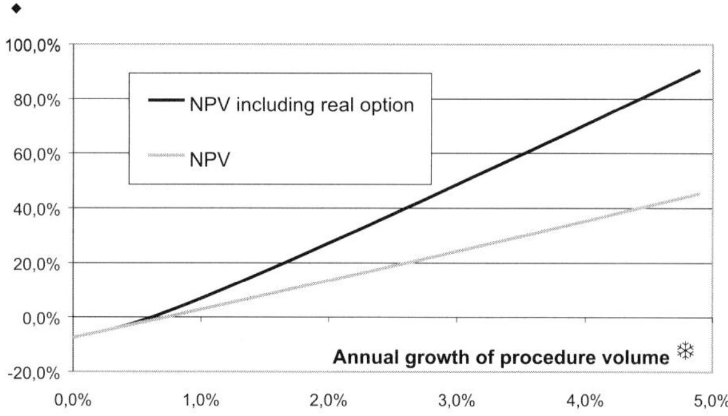

Fig. 4. Effect of annual single digit percentage growth of procedure volume. NPV is scaled to the combined investment for full PACS and the distribution system of I = \$43 per exam. Option parameters: S = \$3.5 per exam for 1% growth, X = \$3 per exam, r = 5%, δ = 0%, σ = 40%, t = 5 year.

Summary

Real options allow to put a value on crucial factors for investment success such as managerial flexibility, strategic or "intangible" values as well as uncertainty. As a tool, they can be used to expand conventional discount cash flow analysis to gain better numerical insight in investment opportunities. As decision support, they can be used to translate the strategic and operational value of a PACS into dollars and cents and make it thus transparent for financially oriented decision-makers. They prove beneficial for PACS investments, especially for organizations that are limited to rely on productivity improvements for cost justification.

References

[1] Amram M, Kulatilika K (1999) Real options. Boston: Harvard Business School Press. www.real-options.com

[2] Arenson, et al (1989) Proceedings SPIE. 1093: 50–58

[3] Brennan M, Trigeorgis L (2000) Project flexibility, agency, and competition. Oxford University Press, New York

[4] Copeland T, Keenan P (1998) How much is flexibility worth. The McKinsey Quarterly 2: 38–49 www.mc-kinsey.com

[5] Damodaran A (1999) The promise and peril of real options. working paper www.stern.nyu.edu/~adamodar

[6] Flatto J (1996) Using real options in project evaluation, The Magazine for Life Insurance Management Resource. www.puc-rio.br/marco.ind/LOMA96.html

[7] Hruby W, Mosser H, Urban M, Rueger W (1992) The Vienna SMZO project: the totally digital hospital. Eur J Radiol 16: 66–68

[8] Hull J (1997) Options, futures and other derivatives. Prentice Hall, Upper Saddle River, NJ, USA

[9] Leslie K, Michaels M (1997) The real power of real options. The McKinsey Quarterly 3: 4–22 www.mckinsey.com

[10] Straub WH, Gur D (1990) The hidden costs of delayed access to diagnostic imaging information: impact on PACS implementation. AJR 155: 613–616

[11] Trigeorgis L (1995) Real options in capital investments. Praeger, Westport USA

[12] Veritas (1999) Real options – An analytical approach to aligning risk management and corporate strategy. Boston: Corporate Finance Review. www.categoricalsolutions.com.au

[13] Young J (1997) Decisions in imaging economics. Supplement May/June 1997 www.imagingeconomics.com

Process benchmarking in radiology

D. Weseloh and U. Viethen

Siemens AG, Medical Solutions, Erlangen, Germany

Introduction

The availability of people, information and materials, at a certain time and place, characterize modern industrial production, which has influenced many branches since the middle of the 20th century. The attributes of this philosophy, summarized under the term "lean production", are large-scale production at low cost, high quality and the flexibility to customize goods [1].

When comparing the clinical workflows of healthcare facilities with industrial manufacturing processes, one might get the impression that there is a backlog demand for the healthcare facilities. Apparently, there are differences in the quality of processes: missing data results in additional communication effort, personnel is not available or is insufficiently skilled, imaging modalities are working at low capacity, to mention only a few examples.

When analyzing the transferability of industrial process implementations with regards to healthcare, one is instantly struck by a significant difference. While in industry all produced goods are the same (still with customization), the patient is always different. It makes good sense to define standardized treatment for disease patterns, but a hundred per cent standardization is not possible. Neglecting this fact not only makes it impossible to improve processes, but is also in essential contradiction to the Hippocratic oath, which emphasizes the individuality of treatment. This individuality can never be replaced by predefined procedures [2]. However, if sufficient freedom is ensured to fulfill this commitment, the introduction of standardization and other manufacturing principles such as just-in-time, failure control by autonomation, and reduction of process fluctuations, seems feasible and promising.

Advanced steps are now being taken, e.g. by introduction of quality control systems, disease-oriented standardization of processes, or development of integrated IT networks. Further improvements are necessary in the near future, to cope with aging society and growing cost. Pressure is also coming from new developments in science. The human genetic code is being revealed and its interaction with diseases. This technology can release its enormous potential for prevention and therapy only if embedded in well established and refined clinical processes [3].

How can we speed up this development? In this stage of relatively poor process implementations, a possible method is to observe existing clinical processes and measure efficiency-related parameters such as process cost and time or satisfaction values. Based on this comparison, measures for improvements in technology and organization can be developed. This article describes the selected results of a benchmarking project that focused on radiological processes and was conducted by Siemens together with 15 radiology institutes in Germany.

Key parameters of radiological processes

The comparison of processes generally begins with the definition of parameters by which the quality of the processes is assessed. In the case of a radiology institute, one can start with the picture of a facility generating *high quality reports*, which has *inexpensive and short processes*, and an excellent *perception as a service provider* by the referring physicians as well as the patients. These parameters are determined by the general organizational and technological framework (see Fig. 1).

The *quality of reports* covers the quality of diagnostic images as well as the written report. It is the essential service of the radiologist, and influences significantly the radiologist's perception as a service provider. However, the satisfaction of referring physicians cannot be the only criteria for report quality.

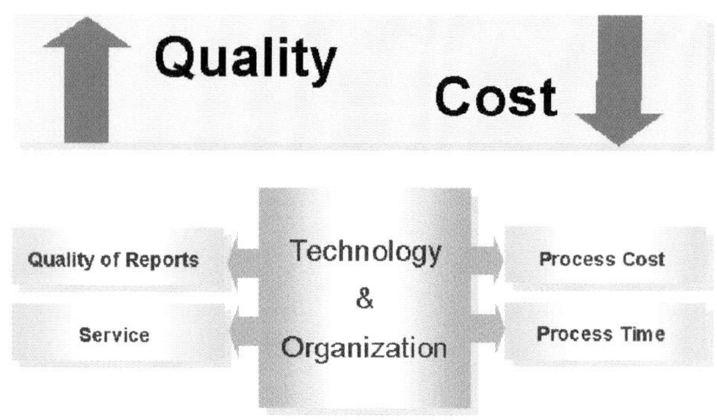

Fig. 1. Process optimization in radiology

The perception as a *service* provider is influenced by turnaround time, report quality, communication skills of the staff interfacing with referrals and patients, to name only a few examples.

Process cost in radiology, is composed of staff cost including overhead, IT and modality depreciation, costs for consumable supplies, lease rental charges, etc. Staff cost normally makes up the largest part.

Process time is the duration of one ore more process steps. Shortening process steps can lead to cost reduction, if not compensated by additional staff or other cost-sensitive measures. Short process time is a precondition for high patient throughput.

It is clear that to *succeed economically*, mature processes are a precondition, but are not the only requirement. Especially for practices, the share of patients with rewarding insurance contracts, or the integration of the facility into a network of referring physicians, ensuring a constant flow of patients, influence business success considerably.

Methodology

The participants of the benchmarking project were radiology institutes from university hospitals, community hospitals, practices, or practices associated to community hospitals. All of them were working with a RIS/PACS system[1]. Table 1 shows the technological profiles of the consortium.

The analysis was conducted in cooperation with a consulting firm, which is normally not active in the area of healthcare processes, but well experienced and acknowledged in the field of industrial process optimization. The combination of deep product and clinical workflow know-how, provided by the project participants and Siemens, together with long lasting experience with tools and methodologies for process analysis and optimization, turned out to be an effective way to identify process shortcomings and best practice elements.

The analysis was conducted on predefined reference workflows to allow subsequent comparison. Six radiological cases, which were performed on a regular basis in the participating institutes, were defined:

1. Standard X-ray of wrist or ankle in two planes, mobile patient
2. Standard X-ray of abdomen in two planes, with contrast medium, immobile patient
3. Chest X-ray examination in bed, on ward
4. CT examination of head, with contrast medium, mobile patient
5. MR examination of head (oncology), with contrast medium, mobile patient
6. Fluoroscopy: esophagus or phlebography, mobile patient

The primary focus of our investigations was on process time and staff cost (without overhead). For each of the six reference workflows, these parameters were assessed for all process steps with involvement of the patient, the patient's image or text data, or material required for the examination. The timeframe was from the request for examination, to the delivery of report. The time values were assessed in interviews with the personnel usually involved in the corresponding process step, i.e. radiologists, technicians, typists and registration staff. 3–5 people were asked to estimate the length of each process step, based on their daily experience.

The corresponding staff costs were calculated from the individual salary of the people involved, and the length of the process step.

In addition, satisfaction values from referring physicians and patients were obtained in interviews, to assess report quality and the perception of the department as a service provider. However, due to the limited number of the interviews, significant propositions on these quality-related parameters could not be derived.

For selected workflows, we investigated the costs for consumable supplies and depreciation of technical equipment, too.

Results

Composition of process cost

An analysis of the composition of process costs was conducted for the radiological workflows of a MR head and a standard X-ray examination (reference

[1]Exception is participant no. 6, who didn't use its RIS system.

Table 1. Technological profiles of project participants (E.I.D. = Electronic Image Distribution)

Type	No.	PACS	RIS	HIS	E.I.D.	Org. Specifics	Techn. Specifics
University Hospitals	1	Siemens	GAP	SAP/ISH	yes	decentral, one unit assessed	electronic dictation, teleradiology
	2	Siemens	Medos	SAP/ISH	yes		teleradiology
	3	Siemens	Innomed	SAP/ISH	no	decentral	teleradiology
	4	AGFA	locally dev.	SAP/HR3	yes	decentral, one unit assessed	
Community Hospitals	5	Siemens	WRAD	Clinicom	no		
	6	Siemens	–	GWI	yes		
	7	Siemens	Medos	Medico	yes		teleradiology
	8	Siemens	ITB	SAP/ISH	yes		
	9	Siemens	Medos	GWI	yes		teleradiology
	10	Siemens	GAP	GWI	yes		
Associated Practices	11	Siemens	GAP	Micom	yes		speech recognition, electronic request, teleradiology
	12	Siemens	MacDoc	Medico	yes	decentral, one unit assessed	teleradiology
Practices	13	Siemens	GAP	–	yes		teleradiology
	14	Siemens	GAP	–	no		speech recognition
	15	AGFA	GAP	–	no		speech recognition

workflows 5 and 1). For this analysis, we only considered participants 5 to 12 (community hospitals and associated practices), because the inclusion of university hospitals and practices with their strongly different organizational structure and composition of cases would not allow a direct comparison.

Table 2 shows the variations in staff cost. In all cases, the nominal working time according to German labor agreements was assumed. Overtime was not considered.

Figure 2 provides an overview on the cost composition along the process chain for the MR reference workflow. The average cost for staff as well as the average depreciation cost for technology and the cost for consumable supplies are indicated with their individual shares. Reporting was done on the monitor, except department no. 5, which was in the transition process to softcopy reading. The corresponding film and printing costs were not considered in the diagram.

Staff cost was derived from the individual salaries (see Table 2), which were averaged over the accounted departments. Overhead costs or other assignable costs for room lease, electricity, etc., were not considered.

For the estimation of technology cost, we calculated the yearly depreciation for the imaging system and the RIS/PACS system (which was considered as one unit). Service costs were included, while energy, imputed interest, and room cost were neglected. Divided by the availability time per year of the systems (i.e., the number of minutes per year, where the system is available for usage), we obtained the cost for usage per minute[2].

Cost for consumable supplies mainly consisted of contrast medium, canula, and infusion tube (37.24 €).

Figure 3 shows how the overall process cost of 110.83 € distributes to the different cost types.

Figures 4 and 5 illustrate the corresponding results for the standardized X-ray examination. Again, only the community hospitals and associated practices (5–12) were considered. For the overall process cost, we obtained 18.66 €.

[2]Depreciation spans of seven years for the modality and five years for RIS/PACS were assumed. For the RIS/PACS system, the usage cost per minute was corrected by a factor, which allowed for the parallel usage of a RIS/PACS system. Unlike an imaging modality, the RIS/PACS can be used by several parties at a time. We calculated the average permanent usage of the system by physicians, technicians, and registration sta, and could thereby correct the cost per minute for a particular process. Usage by the clinicians was not considered, nor – consequently – the investment in image/report distribution technology.

Table 2. Range of staff cost in radiology

Job Type	Staff Cost per Year	Work Time per Year	Cost per Minute
Radiologist	58000...92000 €	93420 Min.	0,62...0,99 €
Technician	24000...45000 €	93420 Min.	0,26...0,48 €
Typist / Registration	21000...45000 €	93420 Min.	0,23...0,48 €

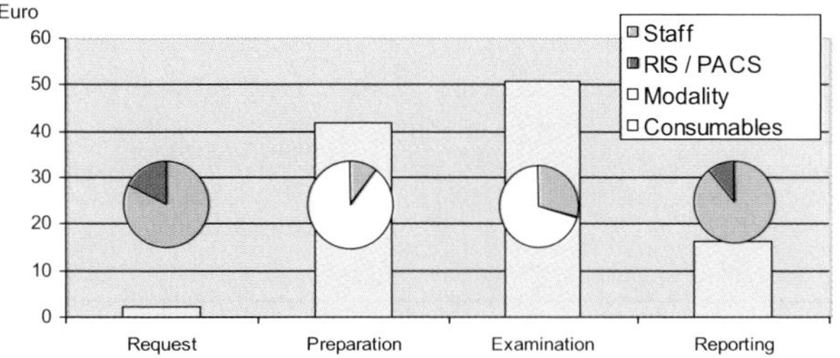

Fig. 2. Cost composition for radiological process chain (MR Head Examination)

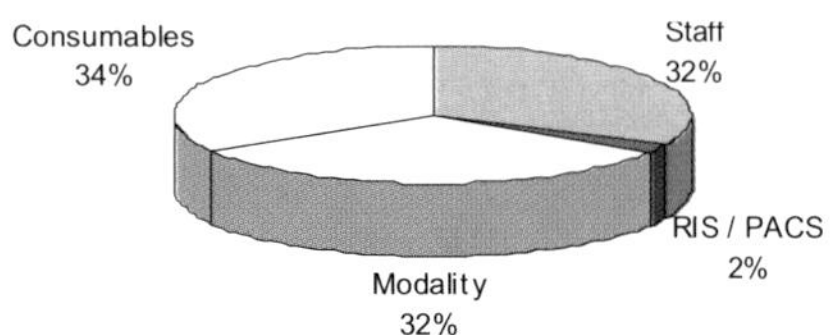

Fig. 3. Cost composition for MR head examination

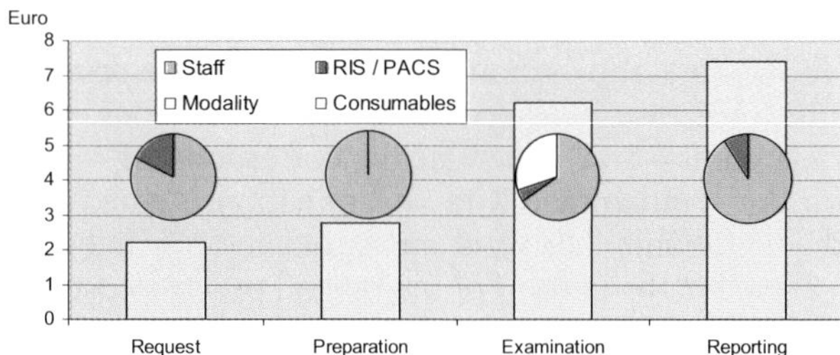

Fig. 4. Cost composition for radiological process chain (X-ray Examination)

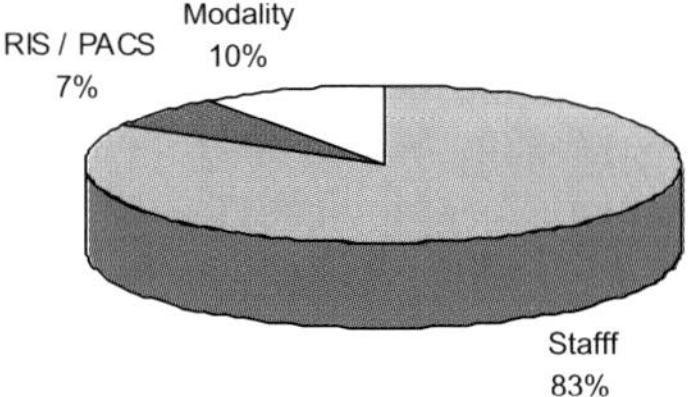

Fig. 5. Cost Composition for X-ray examination

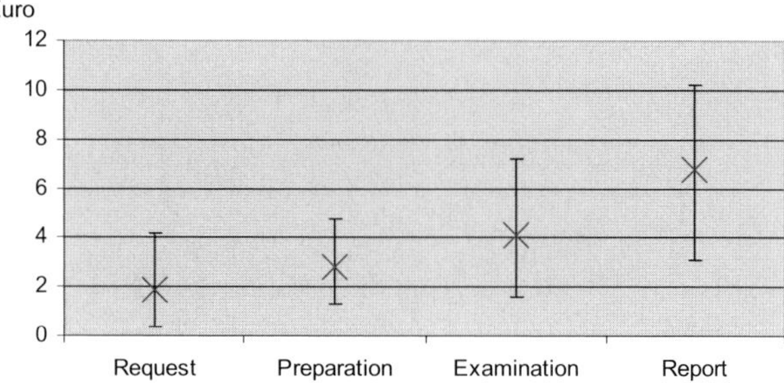

Fig. 6. Variation of staff cost for X-ray examination

When comparing the cost structures of these two cases, one finds the high share of staff cost of 83% for the X-ray examination, compared with 32% for the MR examination (due to high costs for consumables and depreciation of the MR system).

X-ray examinations normally make up the largest part of the yearly number of procedures (72–83% in the observed group), compared to few MR examinations (2–12%). On the other hand, MR examinations are more expensive; the comparison of the two examples above results in a factor 6, but should be lower when considering also X-ray examinations with use of consumables, like contrast agents.

The variations in staff cost for the X-ray examination within the observed group are displayed in Fig. 6.

While the average values sum up to 15.48 €, the lowest values result in 6.33 €, and the maximum total along the process chain is 26.34 €. The difference between these two cases is 20 €, which multiplies to 600,000 € per year, assuming 30,000 procedures.

According to Figs. 3 and 5, the reduction of staff cost is the most effective lever for process cost reduction in radiology. Organizational and technological measures can be taken to reduce process cost (see Fig. 1). The following section provides an example of improvement, based on intelligent use of RIS/PACS technology.

Differences in the request process

We investigated the duration of the examination request process. Personnel from the wards, from

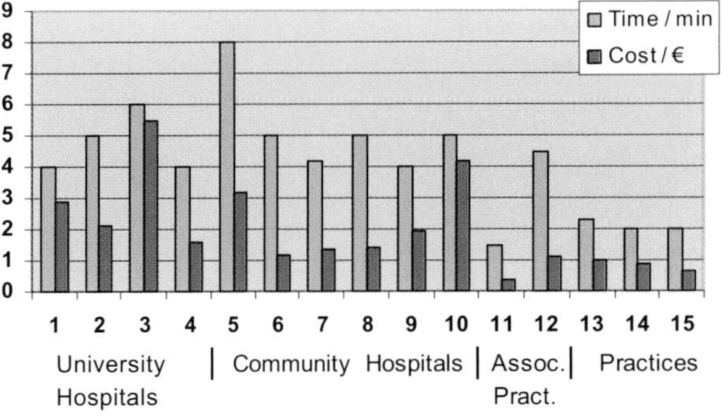

Fig. 7. Process time and cost for the request process

referring physicians, the radiology's registration desk, but sometimes also technicians and physicians are involved in this process step. Differences are usually small and in the range of few minutes, but the yearly number of procedures multiplies the differences to considerable amounts.

Figure 7 provides an overview on process time and cost. Ambulatory and stationary cases, as well as the different examination types, were considered with respect to their individual weight. The working time and associated cost of all radiology employees involved in this step were added together.

Radiology departments in hospitals obviously have higher time and cost values compared to practices. This seems feasible due to the higher complexity level of stationary cases, requiring more communication for the scheduling process. Another factor could be the heterogeneous communication structure in hospitals: in all observed hospitals, the wards were communicating not only with a central registration desk but also with the modality technicians and (partly) the physicians, mostly for CT and MR examination planning. This involvement of relatively expensive personnel could especially be observed in departments 3 and 10, leading to a high cost per time ratio. In the practices, on the other hand, the communication for scheduling was nearly completely covered by the central registration desk.

The best practice representative is department 11 with an average process time of 1.5 minutes and associated costs of 0.35 €. The main reason for this was the reduced communication effort for the scheduling of the stationary patients (share 35%), caused by electronic scheduling software as part of the RIS. Participant 11 was the only one in the consortium who used such technology. The module, available on the hospital ward's PC terminals, obliged the referring physicians to enter necessary information into mandatory fields, reducing telephone conversations effectively.

Room for improvements could be observed especially in departments 3 and 5. Communication due to illegible referral slips, missing laboratory data, or inconsistencies in the request made up the additional time. In hospital 5, the scheduling of 35% of the CT/MR procedures required a 5 minutes clarification on telephone between the referring physician and a radiologist.

When comparing good with poor process implementations within the group of community hospitals and associated practices, one obtains a cost difference of 2.81 € (hospital 5 versus 11). Considering 50,000 examinations per year, this amount multiplies to 140,000 €.

Improvements seem to be feasible by software for electronic request. But also organizational measures like guidelines for fast and accurate communication are helpful. The question whether hospitals could implement a central examination planning, like practices, remains open and requires further discussion. Especially a network based electronic scheduler in radiology, high skill level of the registration staff, and the strict adherence to defined communication paths, seem critical.

Reporting time span

We investigated the time span from the completion of the radiological examination to the clearance of the report (see Fig. 8). The reduction of this time span is essential for an early diagnosis and beginning of therapy, as well as reduction of hospital days, and influences seriously the image of the department as a service provider. For this analysis, only the community hospitals and associated practices were considered, due to their comparable organizational structure.

A short time span can be expected when the capacity boundary of the affected processes allows handling the natural fluctuations in the daily number of procedures. This boundary depends on the average workload of typists and reporting physicians, but also on the technological equipment supporting the reporting process.

The manning levels and procedures per FTE (Full Time Equivalentone full-time employee) are indicated in Fig. 9.

We observed the shortest process times at the associated practice no.11. All reports were finished on the same or at latest on the next day. On the other hand, hospital department no. 7 had process times of 2–5 days.

The comparison of the procedures per FTE (Fig. 9) did not reveal any anomalies for department no. 7., but the analysis of additional workload gave a high

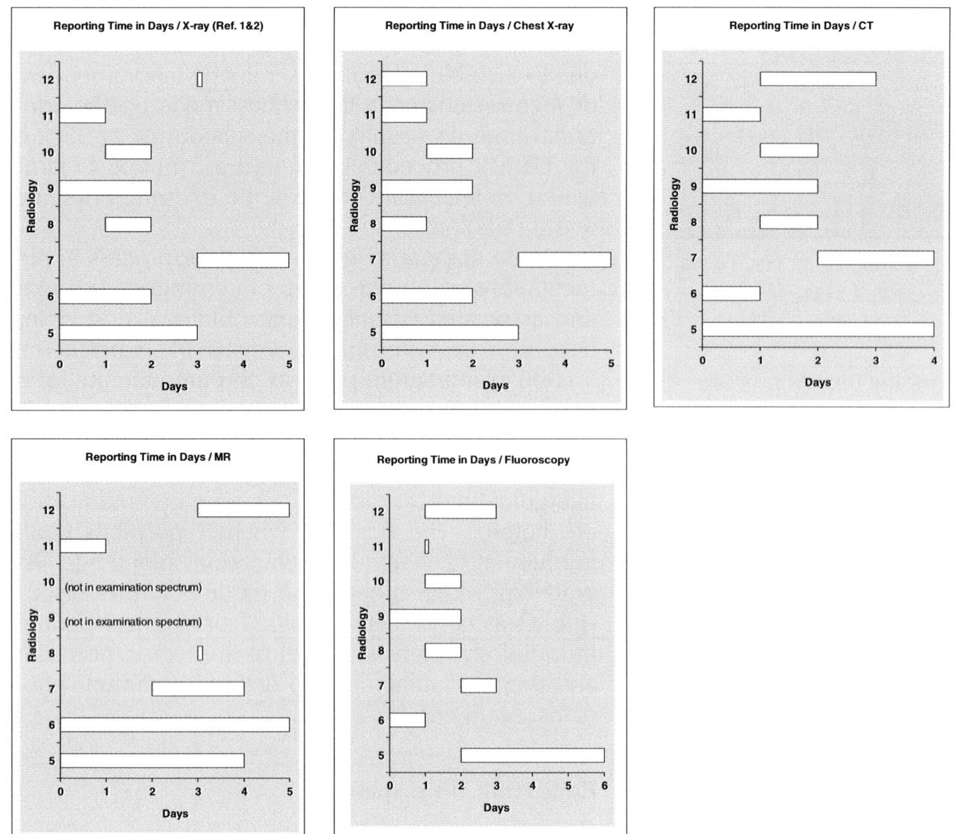

Fig. 8. Reporting Time Spans for Reference Workflows. The indicated bars cover 90% of the cases. Departments 5–10: community hospitals. Departments 11, 12: associated practices

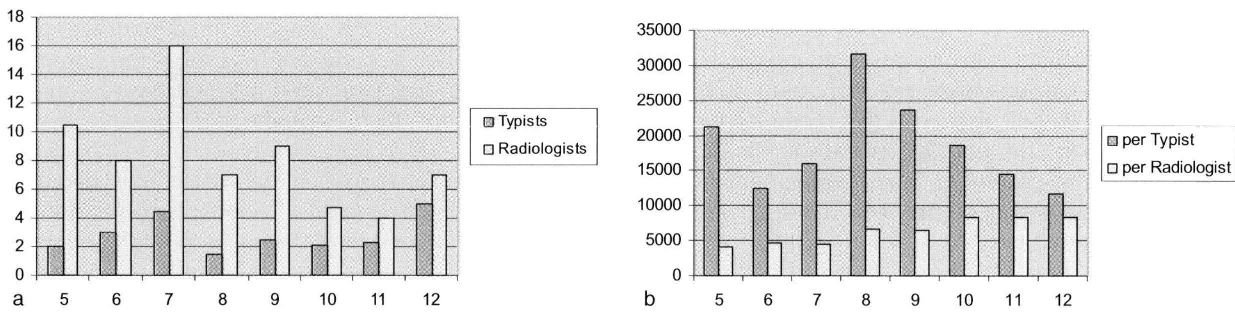

Fig. 9. Manning Levels (**a**) and Procedures per FTE (**b**). Departments 5–10: community hospitals. Departments 11, 12: associated practices

number of clinical demos (Fig. 10), which tied up radiologists for 15–30 minutes, each.

An important factor for the short process time in department no. 11 was the use of speech recognition software as part of the RIS. No.11 was the only participant of the group using this technology. In 30% of all radiological cases, the physicians corrected the reports right after the dictation, making correction cycles with the typists obsolete. The remaining 70% were processed through background speech recognition.

A further reason might be the high share of ambulant cases (65%) for no.11 compared to no. 7 (45%), with their relatively low complexity level, reducing the process time for reporting.

The waiting queue in department no. 7 can be seen as a typical evidence for a process bottleneck. The reasons for the occurrence of bottlenecks in

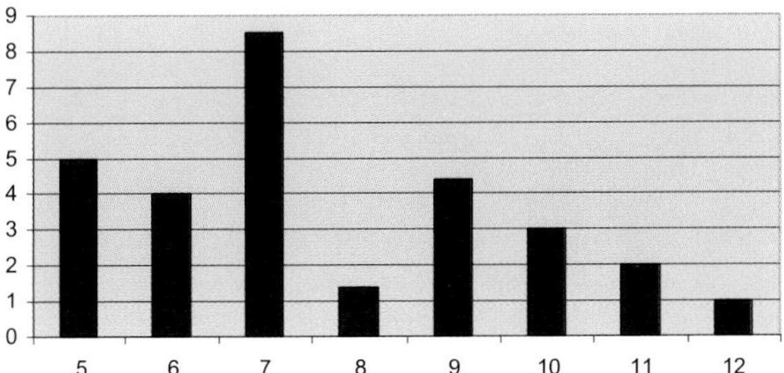

Fig. 10. Number of Clinical Demos per Day. Departments 5–10: community hospitals. Departments 11, 12: associated practices

process chains (in industry or anywhere else) are fluctuations and insufficient capacity buffers [1]. Fluctuations in radiology are caused by the natural variations in the number of cases. It remains to be discussed whether and how these fluctuations can be reduced by, e.g., flexible and short-term scheduling, without loosing the capability for instant processing of emergency cases [4]. Insufficient capacity buffers on the other hand are mostly caused by overloading personnel with work, taking away their ability to process peaks in the number of requests.

Conclusion

Cost pressure is one of the main drivers for the organizational and technological changes in healthcare. The self-conception of hospital radiology in Europe will change from the image of a functional unit towards the image of a service provider for patients and referring physicians. University hospitals with their specific sourcing structure might be less affected by this development than privately owned facilities. Private practices on the other side have been in a competitive situation since years.

Process optimization is necessary to transform a radiology department into a high-performance and cost-efficient organization. The examples provided above show the performance differences existing today. The intense exchange of ideas between organizations, accompanied by continuous measurement and comparison of performance parameters, can lead to the creation of a knowledge base for radiological processes. This is essential for the further development of clinical care plans, and in addition provides the industry with valuable input for future products.

References

[1] Ohno T (1978) Toyota Production System, Tokio 1978 (English: Portland 1988)

[2] Hoppe JD (2002) Gesundheitspolitische Positionen der deutschen Ärzteschaft, Position Paper of the German Medical Fraternity, 29.8.2002

[3] Bayat A (2002) Bioinformatics. BMJ 324: 1018–22

[4] Pfaffenberger P (1999) Moderne Patientendurchlauf-Organisation. In: Braun GE (ed) Handbuch Krankenhausmanagement, Stuttgart

[5] Shieh YY, Roberson GH (1999) Integrated radiology information system, picture archiving and communications system, and teleradiology – workflow-driven and future-proof. J Digit Imaging 12 [2 Suppl 1]: 199–200

[6] Saini S, et al (2000) Technical cost of radiologic examinations: Analysis across Imaging Modalities. Radiology 216: 269–272

[7] Saini S, et al (2000) Cost of hospital-based radiological examinations: an update. Eur Radiol 10 [Suppl 3]: 368–369

Mobile IT adoption in the enterprise: 2004 update*

C. Zetie

Giga position

Most informal and formal signs point to renewed growth in enterprise interest in exploiting the possibilities of mobile technology. Among Giga clients, the demand from major companies in particular for advice on a strategic approach to enterprise mobility is noticeably higher. This renewed interest confirms that mobile IT is once again seen as a catalyst for strategic change rather than a tactical technology initiative; for example, in the form of mobile e-mail for a handful of "VIP" users.

Among the strongest technology drivers of adoption are improved levels of wireless coverage for both wide area network (WAN) and local-area network (LAN), increasingly powerful mobile devices, and lower costs in all aspects of the technology. During 2004, the growth of radio frequency identification (RFID) will create additional demand, as companies that may not otherwise consider deploying mobile applications are forced to come to terms with the realities of highly distributed architectures for both data and function. Among the greatest technical barriers to adoption is increased concern about all aspects of security and confidentiality, as well as management complexity. The latter is fueled in part by a frustratingly rapid turnover in platform technology.

The biggest business driver of all is clearly the improving US economy, which is likely to disproportionately benefit mobile technologies. Some economists predict that companies will treat the early stages of recovery with caution and emphasize the need to address increased demand at least initially through improved productivity and better utilization of existing assets – a so-called "jobless recovery." If so, mobile technology will be one of the more significant IT investments as an enabler of that strategy. Consequently, mobile technology is likely to see more than its fair share of growth in any economic recovery that continues into 2004.

Recommendations

- Include mobile IT in architecture, infrastructure, channel, technology or vendor selection planning. Although mobile IT has not quite reached the point where a majority of companies have production deployments, it is likely to surpass that milestone in 2004. Mobile IT planning should be incorporated into strategy rather than left to tactical projects. Correspondingly, strategy and planning for back-end platforms should take into account potential future requirements for mobile IT.
- Select vendors with more confidence, even smaller players. Vendors that made it this far are, for the most part, by definition the strongest of the species. Vendors that have a referenceable client list, a decent cash position, and a respectable product roadmap that will keep them from being overtaken by the infrastructure majors should do disproportionately well in the upturn.
- Platform (device) choice chiefly remains a tactical, sometimes even project-level decision, rarely a strategic and exclusive one. Expect to find a demand for various kinds of devices, from smartphones to laptops, according to business needs. The more comprehensive the adoption of mobile technologies, the more true this will become.

- Understand how business process change can be catalyzed with mobile IT. This will deliver greater business impact than applications that merely improve productivity or accuracy of operations. Never forget that mobile IT is merely a technology, not a business solution in its own right.

Proof/notes

Overview: reasons to be cheerful

At end-user events targeted at senior IT executives, mobile IT is back on the agenda alongside such high-profile topics as on-demand computing and the impact of the Sarbanes-Oxley legislation. Despite casualties among small vendors, an economic climate inimical to all but the most conservative investments throughout much of 2002 and into 2003, and a backlash caused in part by disappointment with 2G network services, mobile IT deployment survived the downturn and remains robust. In fact, a renaissance appears to have been underway for at least the last half of 2003 – this time, without over-inflated expectations.

The past six months have seen a number of leading indicators that growth is back and that enterprises are increasingly willing to invest in mobile technology. Among informal signs of green shoots and strong enterprise interest for mobile IT:

- **Intel**'s recent Mobile Software Occasion was extremely well attended.
- A recent London roundtable on mobile IT hosted by Giga was oversubscribed, and was filled with FTSE100 user companies alongside major government users.
- Discussions with major user organizations are increasingly strategic (how mobile IT can help the business) rather than economic (how mobile IT can help lower costs and improve productivity) or tactical (which vendor or technology to consider).
- Levels of interest as indicated by Giga inquiry statistics have seen a distinct upsurge in the second half and particularly in the last quarter of 2003.

In another key indicator of improved expectations, the trade press has turned more positive. Numerous specialist daily and weekly e-mail newsletters report on the market, filling their pages with vendor announcements and press releases. Leading trade press publications such as *Computerworld* and *Information Week* have created special Web site sections and e-mail news roundups on the topic. There is even a new dedicated Web site from **CMP**, called *Mobilized Software* (www.mobilizedsoftware.com), which boldly enters a space that has been a graveyard for both print and online publications, with MobileCommerceNet being one of the most recent casualties (see www.mobile.commerce.net/story.php?story_id=3295&s=). The fact that CMP launched a specialized site in this area so soon after a previous site failed to garner adequate support is a significant vote of confidence in the ability of mobile IT to attract both readers and sponsors (the moribund online *M-Business Daily* does not appear to have been updated since March 2003 and its associated print version, *M-Business Magazine*, last published in March 2002).

This anecdotal evidence is supported by more objective Giga polls. For the past several years Giga has polled attendees at various events and conferences about their state of mobile IT adoption, and the aggregated results for 2002 and 2003 are shown below in Fig. 1. Since these audiences are self-selected by their attendance at the relevant events, these figures should not be extrapolated to the IT market as a whole. In particular, these figures are overwhelmingly drawn from US audiences, and other geographies may differ significantly. However it is reasonable to compare numbers from year to year as the respondent mix across a number of polls is reasonably comparable.

These numbers indicate that levels of adoption are once again rising, after stagnating or showing tepid growth at best for a year or more. Assuming that levels of activity in application development are a valid leading indicator of next year's deployment

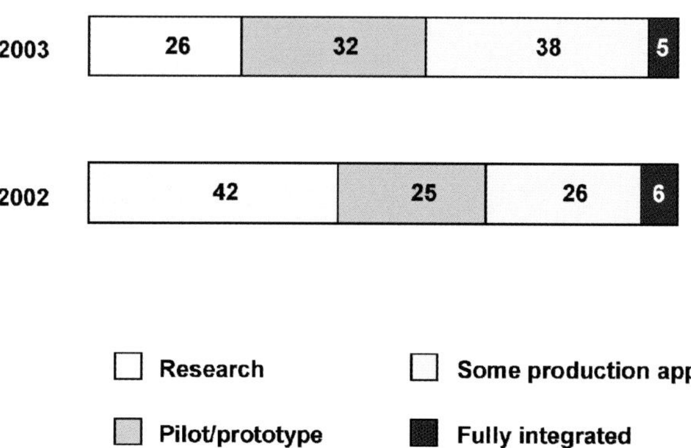

Fig. 1. The state of enterprise adoption (Source: Giga Research, a wholly owned subsidiary of Forrester Research, Inc.)

trends, we anticipate that growth will continue into 2004.

Life is also improving for the individual mobile professional. New integrated devices (such as the **palmOne** Treo 600, Symbian devices from **Nokia** and **Ericsson**, new models of **Research in Motion** (RIM) BlackBerry, and **Microsoft** Smartphone devices) are garnering positive reviews after a period of backlash against clunky, failed communicator designs. Meanwhile, new software releases from RIM, Microsoft and others provide an increasingly integrated personal information manager (PIM) e-mail experience. This confluence of factors will make the PIM e-mail environment considerably more effective and popular with mobile professionals. As professional adopters of mobile e-mail are often advocates for and harbingers of wider wireless adoption in the enterprise, their satisfaction levels will contribute to the general optimism.

It should also be noted that RFID is likely to drive further adoption of handhelds. Even in conventional supply chain and warehouse-type applications where fixed readers carry the bulk of the workload, there will be a need for exception handling (e.g. a case or pallet that fails to read at the door cannot be allowed to hold up unloading of the pallets behind it and must be moved aside, probably to be rescanned with a handheld reader). Outside of the supply chain there will be many uses for handheld RFID scanners, most likely based on a standard PDA platform, for example to identify tagged assets in the field or identify baggage at airports.

Vendor expectations

This general optimism is reinforced by key vendor revenue. Although many small vendors continue to struggle, and some will still fail before the end of 2004, the worst of the consolidation is over. Vendors both large and small that have ridden out the past two years of retrenchment and caution are well poised to reap the benefits of the emergent upturn (see Planning Assumption, Market Overview 2004: Mobile Application Development, Carl Zetie).

Many small vendors simply did not survive the lean years, and as a result, those left standing will claim a larger share of the recovering market. During the early hype-fueled market boom there were simply too many vendors – many of them opportunistic startups with little distinguishing intellectual property – it was impossible for all of them to do well, and selecting any small vendor was something of a lottery. By contrast, the chances of viability for vendors that made it this far in reasonable shape are dramatically improved, even for those that are not yet profitable. The distinguishing characteristics of well-positioned vendors include:

- *Referenceable customers*: At this stage in market development, there are a number of vendors with solid proof points for their capabilities. Correspondingly, there is little space for unproven products or brand-new companies that claim to deliver the same capabilities but without the same level of proof. Unless these companies have some truly unique, innovative, and valuable technology that an early adopter is willing to take a risk with, they should be avoided.
- *A strong cash position*: Even though prospects are improving, vendors still need to be able to ride out the longer evaluation cycles that have become common during the economic downturn. They also need to be able to fund expansion as prospects improve. Look for companies that can demonstrate a cash position that can sustain several quarters at their current burn rate.
- *Unique value-add*: Many smaller vendors in the last wave disappeared because they offered little value beyond what major infrastructure vendors were readily able to replicate. Smaller vendors that want to avoid the same fate this time around still need to offer rich capabilities that are not easily imitated by larger players.

In the realm of the larger vendors, the most notable trend is an increasing emphasis on solution selling. The positioning from vendors such as Microsoft and **IBM** increasingly emphasizes the completeness and integration of their offerings. **HP** has created an organization responsible for coordinating its products across multiple product and service groups. Even Nokia, best known as a handset and carrier equipment maker, has created a group focused on enterprise solutions. This kind of transition is one more indicator of a maturing market, a response by vendors to the user shift from tactical to strategic needs.

One useful quantitative measure of the market from the vendor side is to look at RIM. This company is a good predictor for the market as a whole because its product crosses all verticals and its channels include both enterprises and carriers. It can be a powerful leading indicator as enterprise e-mail deployment is often the first step into mobile IT for an organization. As shown by RIM's earnings statements (see Fig. 2), slow but steady increases in revenue

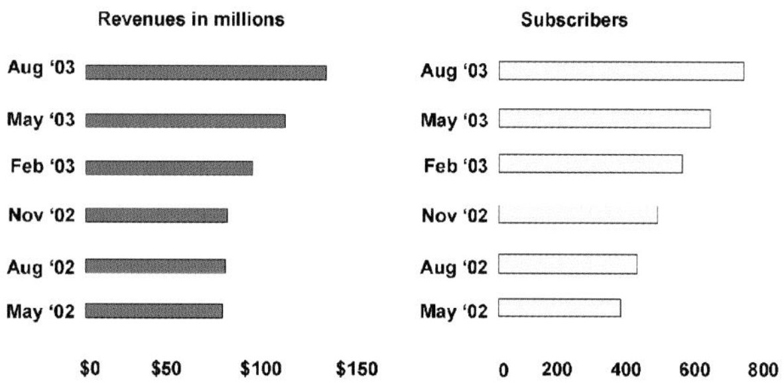

Fig. 2. RIM revenues and subscriber numbers (Source: Giga Research, a wholly owned subsidiary of Forrester Research, Inc.)

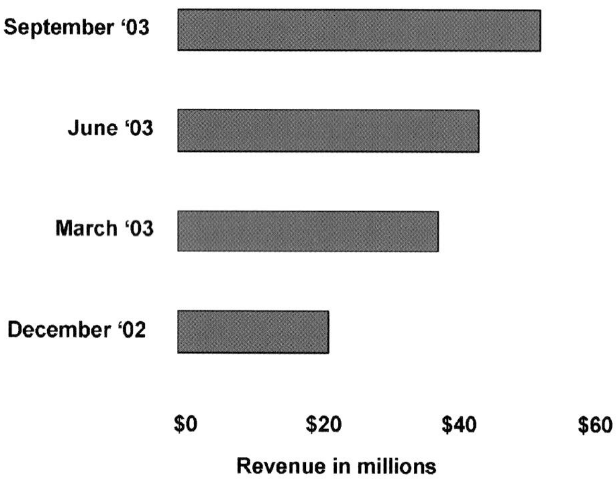

Fig. 3. Microsoft revenues attributed to mobile and embedded devices (Source: Giga Research, a wholly owned subsidiary of Forrester Research, Inc.)

through 2002 and into early 2003 accelerated rapidly later in 2003. (Note that RIM's fiscal year runs to the end of February.) This is good news for RIM, and a positive sign for mobile IT adoption as a whole.

Revenues attributed by Microsoft to mobile and embedded products show a similar direction of growth (see Fig. 3). Microsoft's revenues are less directly interpretable than RIM's in this regard, not least because Microsoft's revenue represents only a small fraction of the total revenue associated with the economy created around its mobile and embedded offerings. It is also misleading to look too far back into the historical record, as Pocket PC in particular was a late entrant compared to **Palm** and is catching up from a slow start. Nonetheless they provide additional confirmation of the direction of the market.

Another key vendor in this space that would normally be considered a barometer of adoption is Palm. However, during the past 12 months Palm has been in the process of splitting itself into two companies (palmOne and PalmSource), merging with a

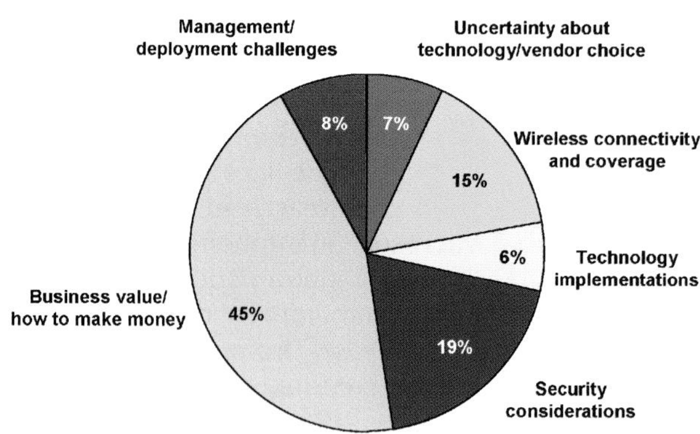

Fig. 4. What do you consider the biggest challenge facing your wireless strategy? (Source: Giga Research, a wholly owned subsidiary of Forrester Research, Inc.)

former rival (**Handspring**), and releasing a slew of new products that have affected revenue cycles. Palm revenue is also seasonally distributed, as many individuals purchase these units during the holiday season. Consequently it is hard to read too much into Palm's up-and-down year. However, it is worth noting that palmOne CEO Todd Bradley recently raised his revenue forecast for the second quarter (ending November 2003).

Economic reality counts more than ever

In the early stages of a tentative economic recovery it should be no surprise that business value remains top-of-mind for many potential adopters. However, security concerns are at a substantially higher level than ever before. This partly reflects a more security-conscious environment overall, but it also reflects growing awareness of the specific risks of PDAs, fueled by some high-profile press. PDAs have become not only repositories of large amounts of confidential data, but also potential points of access into corporate networks. For example, virtual private network (VPN) clients are sometimes hosted on the same device where passwords are handily recorded. A lost or stolen PDA, inadequately protected, becomes a risk not only to the data stored on the device, but also to the corporate networks that the device is capable of logging on to.

Also growing in importance is the challenge of systems management. As companies deal with larger deployments, longer-lived projects, the complexity of patching or upgrading devices in the field and replacing lost or broken units is beginning to register as a significant cost. This problem is exacerbated by the too-rapid turnover of platforms that enterprise see from device manufacturers, One consequence is that vendors must understand platform loyalty is, for most companies, relatively low (in contrast to individual adopters, whose loyalty is typically very high). Platform choice chiefly remains a tactical, even project-level decision, rarely a strategic one. Mixing or switching are common, and the need to support mixed environments is also commonplace.

A distinct change in tone is noticeable in Giga's interactions with clients. User organizations are now far less likely to ask whether there is business value in mobile IT – that case is substantially proven – but how much. Mobile IT can contribute to business goals at all levels (see Planning Assumption, Identifying Business Opportunities in Mobile IT, Carl Zetie). Based on projects we have seen during the past two years, Giga has observed a number of common characteristics that can be used to identify business opportunities with medium and high value. Identifying characteristics for medium-value business cases include:

- Rich customer interaction opportunities, such as sales force automation or healthcare administration.
- Data is generated at point of customer contact, where data can be more accurately collected and verified at the point of collection. Examples include car rental, equipment hire, regulatory inspections, and poll taking or surveying.
- A need for improved productivity and accuracy; for example, verifying inventory in the retail supply chain, field service, and delivery scheduling.

While situations such as these regularly generate viable business cases, there are other situations that offer compelling returns. In general, when mobile technology can be leveraged to improve downstream business processes, the value can be dramatic. Typical characteristics of high-value business cases include:

- Complex paperwork or regulatory compliance: Examples include finance, healthcare, flight maintenance, or government regulations. The costs of compliance can be high, but are minor compared to the potential costs of failing to comply.
- Dynamic, unpredictable, time-critical events: Business processes such as delivery, field service, and especially any situation involving service levels and high-value asset utilization can be dramatically impacted. With greater flexibility and responsiveness, for example, it may be possible to reduce inventory levels or standby staffing. Companies such as Cemex show the business value of being able to provide more predictable service to customers by absorbing unpredictability in their processes.
- Risk must be mitigated: Mobile technologies and associated applications can enable companies to reduce costs associated with guaranteeing service levels; for example, reducing the need to maintain excess or standby capacity and by increasing utilization and efficient scheduling of existing assets.

Note in particular the difference in value between regulatory *inspection* and regulatory *compliance*. For government bodies, mobile technology can improve the productivity, accuracy and completeness of many kinds of inspection activity. It can also improve the downstream dissemination and processing of inspection results, leading to more comprehensive followup and higher levels of compliance. As valuable as this is, it pales compared to the potential cost to a business of failing to comply (or even being unable to demonstrate compliance) with a regulatory regime.

One lesson that has been borne out again and again during the past 18 months of adoption is that business opportunities are identified not by technology but by business circumstances and processes specific to a particular opportunity. An illustration of this key principle can be found in mobile or wireless e-mail. This technology has the potential to add value (and succeed, in business terms) when:

- There is a need for employees to respond and react quickly to important messages.
- Downstream processes are highly reactive, and can consume e-mail decisions in real time, improving the responsiveness of the business process as a whole.
- It allows other important work to continue; for example, where continuing a process is blocked by incoming e-mail.
- It unshackles the user from the desk. The users can conduct other business, go to meetings, attend conferences, etc., rather than being trapped at the desk because of the need to respond to an urgent message.

Note that increased productivity does not figure highly on this list. Merely responding to more e-mail more quickly does not inherently have value (indeed, it may be detrimental to productivity), so the argument that users will be more productive merely because they can send and receive e-mail in what would otherwise be dead time is hard to prove. There are circumstances under which it can be argued that wireless e-mail has very low value at best, and is a distraction from being fully focused on the activity or meeting if front of the user, at worst. Such situations are typified by the following characteristics:

- User responses are essentially frequent but unimportant, usually conversational exchanges that have little business value or would be more effectively conducted as a brief phone call.
- Downstream processes are by batch or are slow to react, so the immediacy of the employee's response does not translate into more rapid business response.
- It enables the employee to fill idle minutes. While some employees may be able to contribute more in these otherwise lost minutes, the biggest danger is employees simply generate more e-mail noise by adding traffic to threads of discussion without adding much value – because they can.
- It shackles the employee to e-mail. This is the greatest challenge in managing the personal productivity impact of wireless e-mail. Almost everybody is aware of a colleague or business contact who is so constantly checking e-mail that they are distracted from other meetings or activities to which they should be devoting full attention.

Examples of mobile e-mail that delivers business value includes improving the responsiveness of customer service agents and sales account managers, improving communication between executives, and enabling rapid decision-making even while key participants are remote or traveling. When conference attendees are asked, "who here could not be at this conference today if wireless e-mail didn't allow them to stay in touch with vital decision-making back at the office?" the question invariably draws a large affirmative response. It is still common to find business processes other than straightforward e-mail communication delivered using e-mail as the transport and the client. Examples include simple approvals (such as a manager approving a travel or expense request, or a sales district director approving a discount that falls outside normal guidelines) to more transaction steps in a complex process such as mailing an order or a request for inventory replenishment using a structured form, or informing a service technician of a changed schedule. E-mail is frequently used for such purposes in place of custom clients because it is relatively easy to deploy and, providing that the client user interface requirements are not complex, avoids the need for multiple client applications. In other words, e-mail is the universal transport and the universal client for straightforward requirements.

Alternative view

Despite these optimistic indications that mobile IT is becoming increasingly accepted as a mainstream deployment channel, it is possible that the best is already past. The pessimistic view is that the majority of business uses for mobile IT have already been found – delivery, warehouse, etc. – and what remains is an uptick in personal/professional use and a few unexplored niches such as handheld RFID readers. One indication that the market is indeed heading for a long-term plateau would be a flattening of revenues of vendors other than RIM and its immediate competitors in the professional PIM e-mail space. This outcome would also require that the overarching trend toward increasing mobility of the workforce itself halt or even reverse, and therefore under current indications it does not yet seem likely.

References

Related Giga Research

Planning Assumptions

[1] Identifying Business Opportunities in Mobile IT, Carl Zetie
[2] Mobile Enterprise Summit 2002 Surveys: Mobile Application Momentum Grows, Lisa Pierce and Carl Zetie
[3] Mobile Enterprise Summit 2002 Surveys: Wireless Voice Walking, Not Running, and Wireless Data Still Crawling, Lisa Pierce and Carl Zetie
[4] Mobile Enterprise Summit 2002 Surveys: Pocket PC Leads Enterprise Mindshare, Carl Zetie
[5] Market Overview: The State of Mobile and Wireless Adoption, Carl Zetie

Epilogue

Virtual reality – symbiosis of science and art

R. Bulirsch and M. Hardt

Department of Mathematics (SCB), University of Technology, Munich, Germany

Dürer and the perspective

Non mi legga qui non è matematico, nelli mia principi ... In plain English: No one should read me, my writings who is not a mathematician. ... That was Leonardo da Vinci (Figs. 1 and 2) speaking about himself. Leonardo's works, his visionary insight, still today create a certain fascination. The other one, Raffaello Santi (il divino), Raffael (the divine), sees himself more as a disciple of geometry than a painter. In his "School of Athens", he celebrates geometry, shows us philosophers and mathematicians, and even poses with the group of mathematicians in the right of the picture.

In the Renaissance, the visual arts discovered geometry; mathematical dogmas of architectural perfection once thrown out were resurrected. The great architects of that time were convinced that the visible world, seen through a geometrically perfect church architecture, can be a door to the metaphysical world.

The Renaissance and the "New Vision" (Fig. 3). The Italian artists were careful to keep the knowledge about the newly discovered perspective as a big secret (Fig. 4). Albrecht Dürer (1506), friend of Raffael, wrote from Venice to Willibald Pirckheimer in Nuremberg ... *I ride to Bologna for the sake of a secret perspective in the arts that someone is willing to teach me. ... Afterwards I will come with the next messenger.*

Geometry was for Dürer the manifestation of the natural laws (Fig. 5). Someone who did not master algebra and geometry, and who similarly did not fully understand astronomy and the natural sciences, was for him not a complete painter. Dürer studied Johannes Müller, a reformer of mathematics from the Renaissance. Müller was known to the world as *Regiomontanus*. Columbus and Amerigo Vespucci supposedly sailed according to Regiomontanus' star maps. Dürer also read the writings of another great person with amazement and delight.

He was famous already in his own lifetime (Fig. 6), *Nikolaus von Kues, Cusanus, Cardinal Nikolaus from St. Peter in chains.* The Dominican Giordano Bruno, the great Italian and rebel, praised Cusanus ... *he was not an equal of Pythagoras, rather he was* greater .... In his writings *De mathematica perfectione*, he, Cusanus, the Cardinal of the catholic church, made the following comments ... *Mathematical insights lead us to ideas of an almost divine and eternal nature.* Cusanus occupied himself with curve and surface measurements and almost invented calculus 250 years before the great Leibniz and Newton.

In Nuremberg, Albrecht Dürer placed all his discoveries about the New Vision into his book, *Instructions for measurement with the compass and ruler* (Fig. 7)... Dürer's words to Pirckheimer: *Because this is really the foundation of all painting* (Fig. 8), *I have taken it upon myself ... to create a foundation such that the real truth may be recognized ... so easily are the arts lost, only difficult are they invented again.* Dürer had written his book with his whole heart; he prized it higher than his works of art.

The High Renaissance was a great time for mathematics in the Holy Roman Empire. In Augsburg, books appeared about mathematics; it was seen as an important science. Even the Fugger, the Augsburg noblemen, showed their interest in them through their support for publishing the works of Euclid. In the Benedictine Abbey of St. Ulrich and Afra, the scholarly monk Vitus wrote instructions for arithmetic. In his German text from the year 1500, there appeared for the first time the word *computus, computi* (*computing*).

We can see how perfect the great painters of the Renaissance mastered the geometrical laws of the perspective with the master work of Hans Holbein, the younger, *The Ambassadors* (Fig. 9) Holbein was from Augsburg, though later he went to London. In

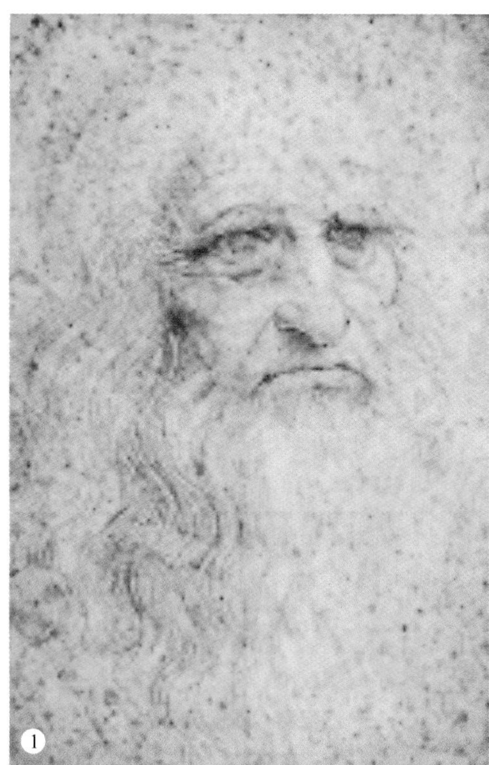

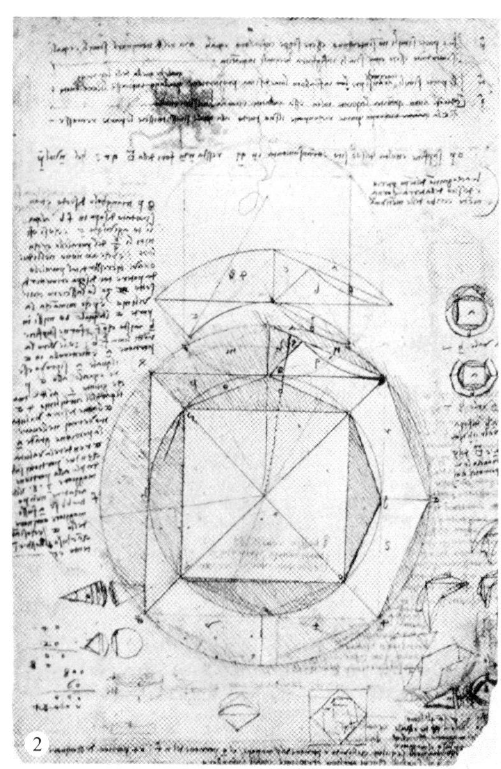

Figs. 1 and 2.

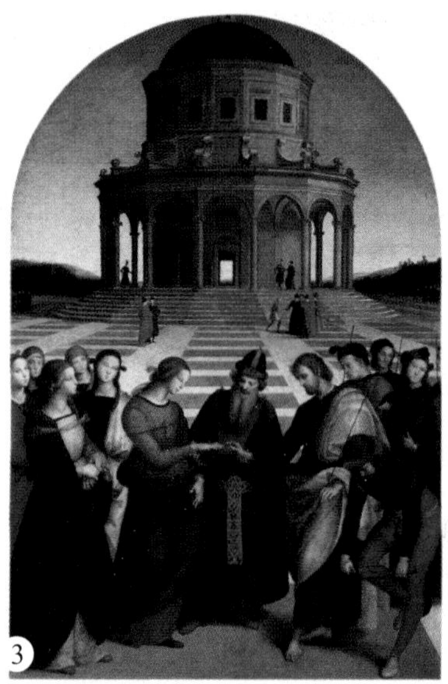

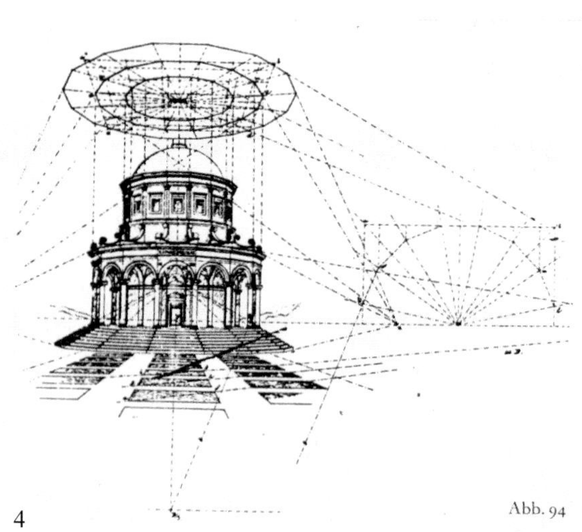

Figs. 3 and 4.

the painting, we can see pictured the French ambassador Jean de Dinteville and the Bishop of Lavour George de Selve. The elongated object, not appearing as anything in particular towards the bottom of the picture (Fig. 10), is in fact a skull distorted in perspective. By manipulation on a computer, it is possible to completely reverse the process of distortion (Fig. 11), thereby presenting us with a

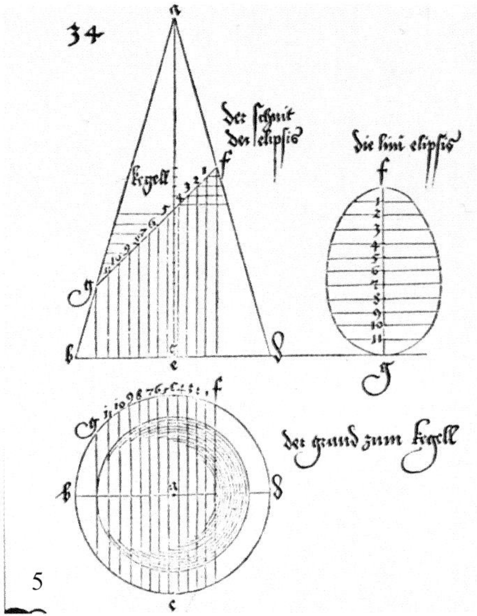

Fig. 5.

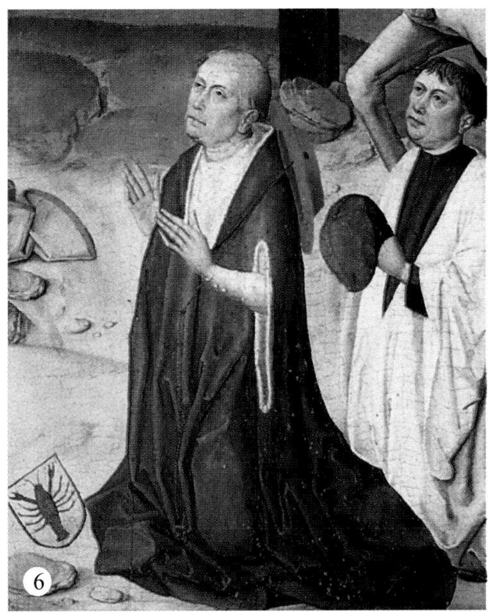

Fig. 6.

proportionally accurate depiction of a skull. Holbein's creation of the distorted skull is a masterpiece revealing how he mastered the geometrical laws of the perspective. (The following pictures display his mathematical instruments and textbooks, Figs. 12 and 13).

But what can Dürer mean to us today, us – who believe we are so smart, who live in an era of computers? What possibly could someone mean to us who has been dead for almost 500 years? Every computer goes about creating image perspectives just like Dürer, the machine can only do it quicker, much quicker. We see as the most natural thing the many discoveries of science, insights which were perhaps struggled with for hundreds of years. We see these as a triviality, unfortunately.

Mathematics and modern painting

Perspective vision in art is not everything today any more. Cézanne, Klimt, Monet, and van Gogh (Fig. 14) lead us into other art worlds, but also the

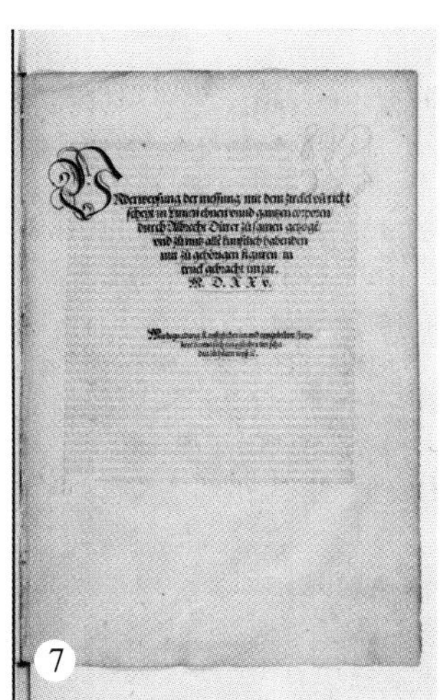

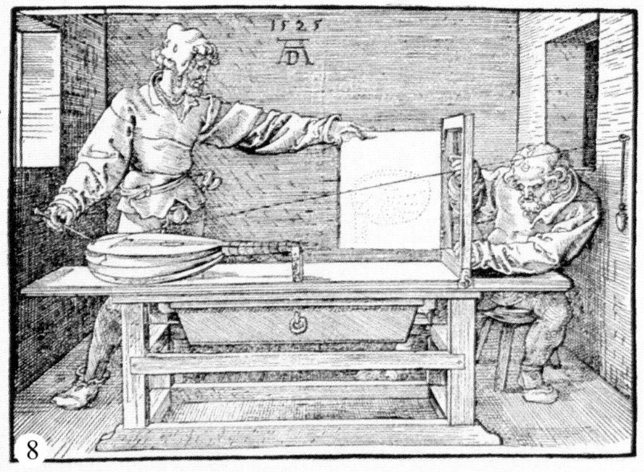

Figs. 7 and 8.

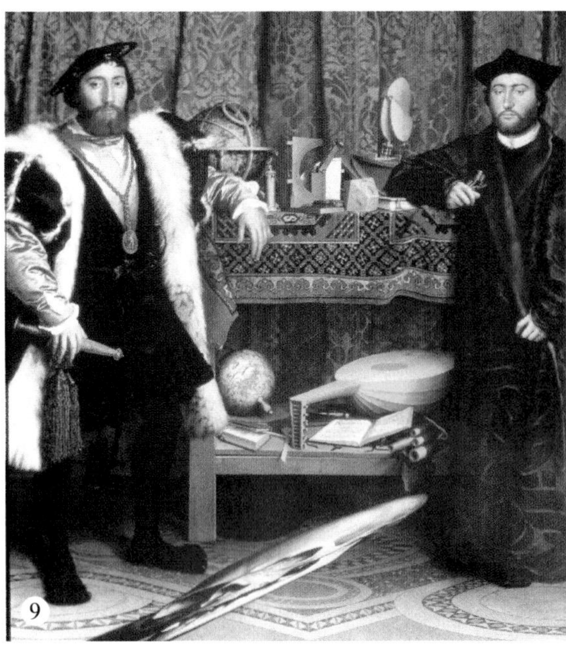

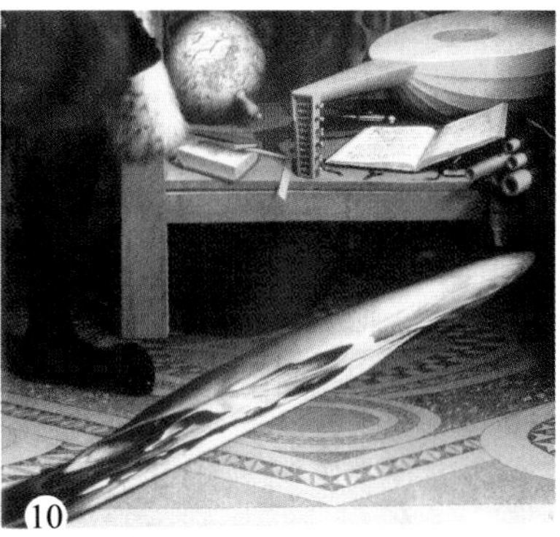

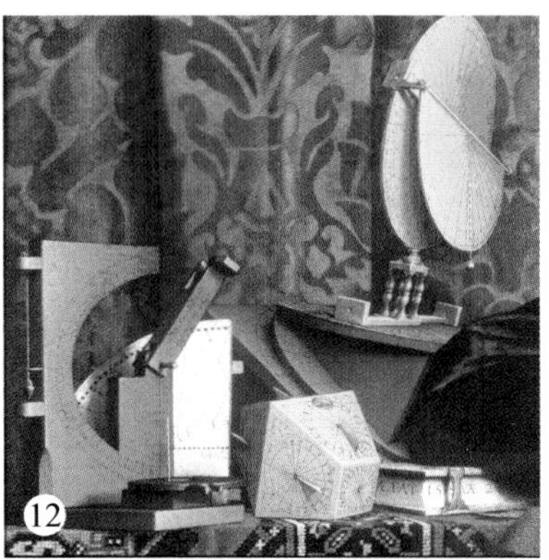

Figs. 9, 10 and 12.

experience of vision has changed and computers were partly responsible.

Great painters shared Dürer's enthusiasm for strict and rational sciences. Paul Klee was convinced that there was a mathematical foundation for all areas of existence. The *Cardinal-Progression* (Sequence 1,2,4,8,16,...) (Fig. 15) made a profound impression on him, and he placed it in his paintings.

The Russian painter Wassily Kandinsky (Fig. 16) once said: ... *Everything can be portrayed ... as a mathematical formula.*

From art as a mathematical structure said the Swiss Max Bill, where he was expressing how it was possible using a mathematical framework to develop art in far-reaching ways and to connect nature and art in mathematics.

Raffael made a profound impression on the Spanish painter Dalí. Dalí gave his own version of the School of Athens. Dalí was especially interested in geometry. One of his paintings, for example, carries the title *Search for the fourth dimension.*

In 1972, a book appeared written by the French mathematician René Thom, *Stability and Morphogenesis.* Thom investigated in his book the mathematical relationships which describe the sudden conversion of one state into another state, for instance, when water suddenly freezes to ice or when water evaporates. René Thom describes the conversion through mathematical equations that may be represented as surfaces. One he calls, for example, Swallowtail, and another Butterfly. Thom's book is filled with an abundance of interesting pictures. Thom, with his investigated state conversions, coined the term "catastrophe", catastrophe élementaire, etc. The phrase "Catastrophe Theory" from Thom's book circulated through the media like a released seismic wave. Thom was not very pleased about that since his "catastrophes" had little to do with our "everyday catastrophes".

Dalí loved Thom's book; again and again he had it read to him. (There is Dalí in the photograph with the Spanish poet García Lorca.) Dalí painted then only Thom's pictures (Fig. 17, Fig. 18). One of his last ones had the title *Topological Separation of*

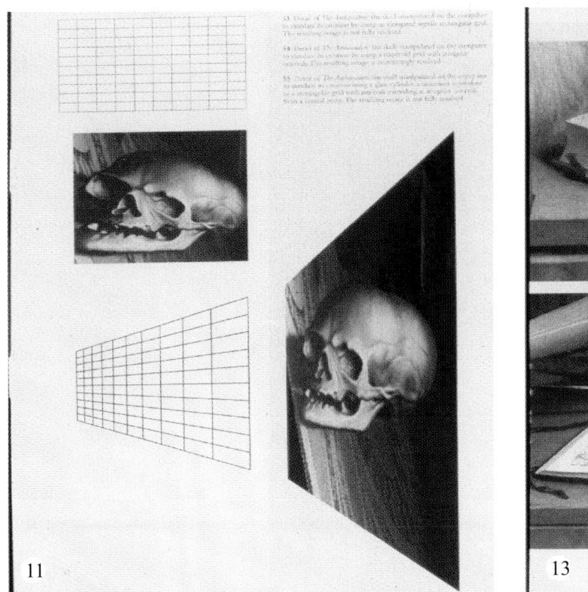
11

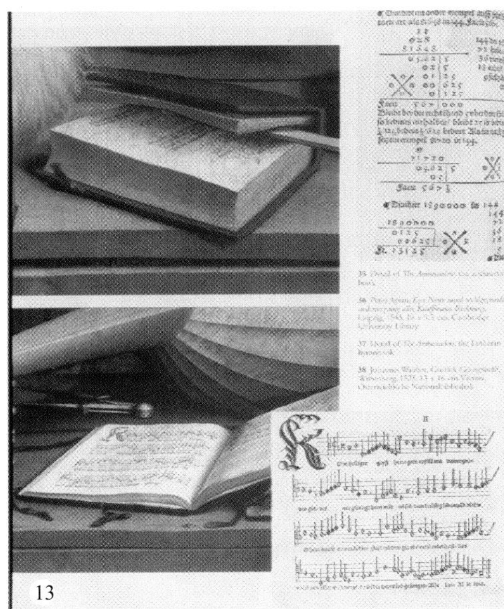
13

Figs. 11 and 13.

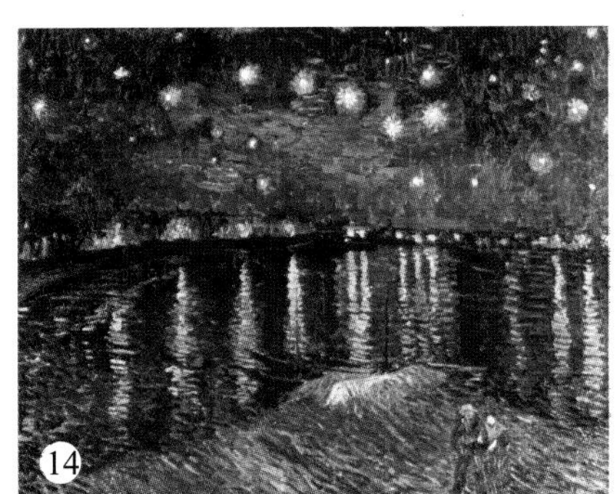
14

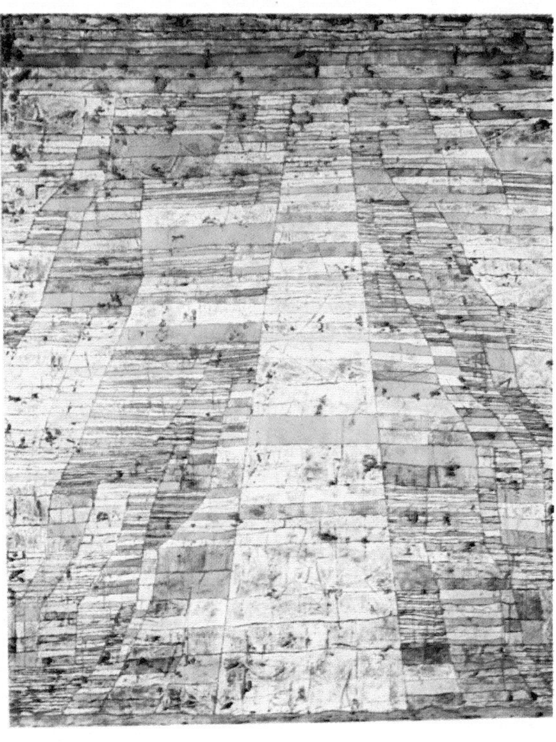
15

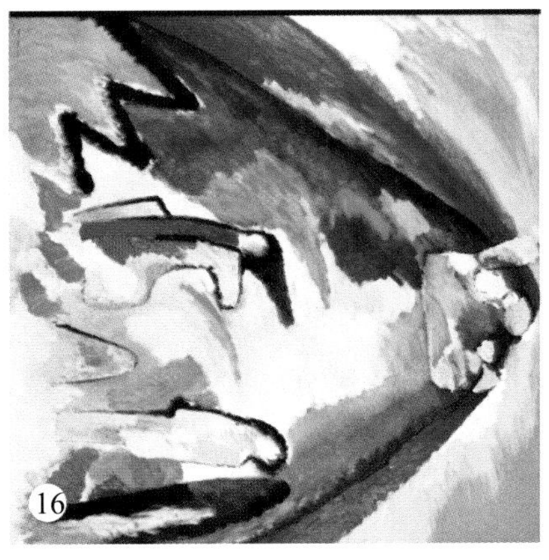
16

Figs. 14–16.

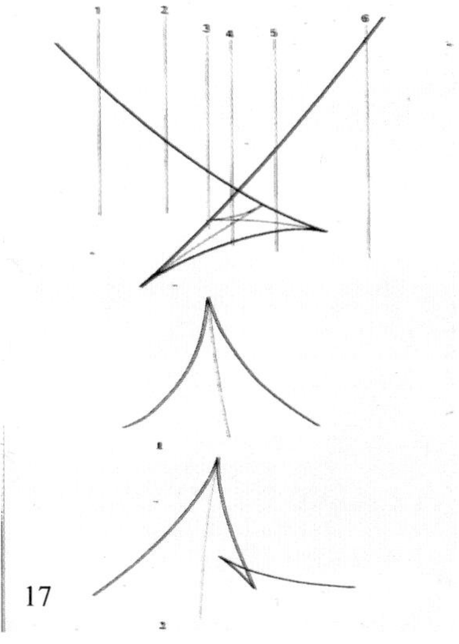
17

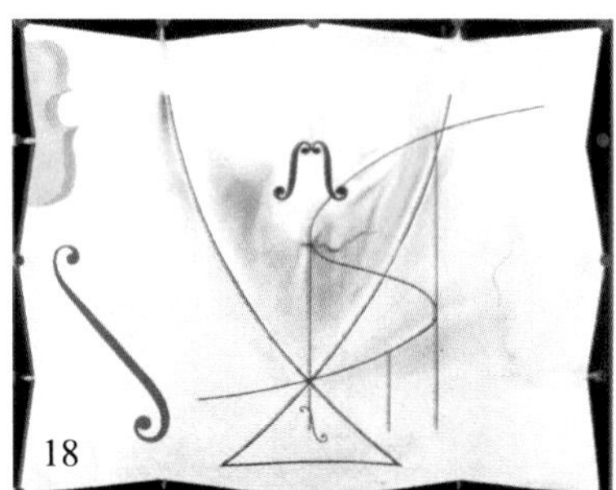
18

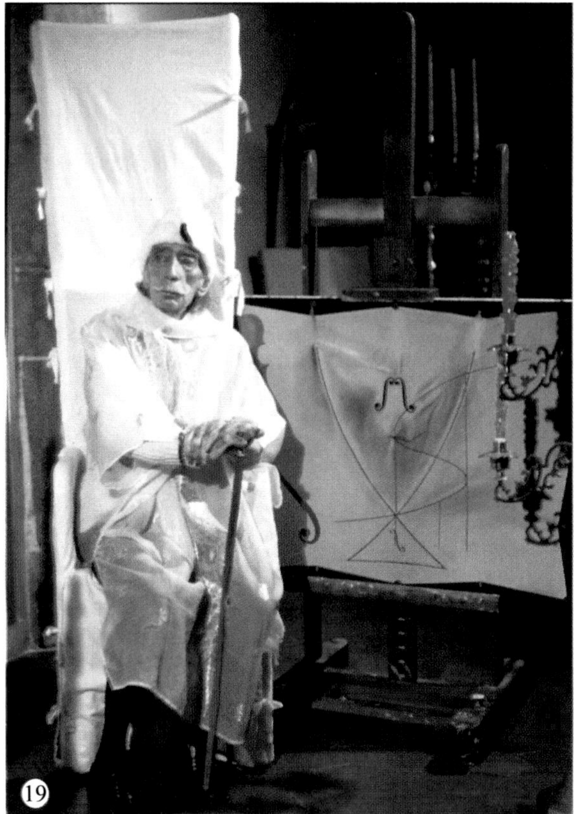
19

Figs. 17–19.

Europe, in homage to René Thom, where underneath are the mathematical formulas for the Swallowtail, mathematical abstractions in Dalí's artistic world [1] (Fig. 19).

Franck Kupka (Fig. 20) or François Kupka, actually Frantiek Kupka, was a great artist. The Czech from Prague, born still under the Austro-Hungarian monarchy, passed through Vienna on his way to Paris. He stayed in France until his death in 1957. Kupka attended lectures at the polytechnical college and at the department of medicine. It was his firm belief that every modern artist should have such an education, the same idea Dürer had 400 years earlier. He did not understand modern painters who did not at least make some use of a telescope or a microscope. Kupka painted first with objects (Fig. 21), but his view of things later changed; he started painting images that would affect you in a strange way. Kupka built his work upon irregular, invisible forms (Fig. 22) which would, in fact, exist in nature (Fig. 23). As a painter working apart from all fashionable trends, he brought much ridicule upon himself. And Kupka was forgotten – 80 years later one can see Kupka's images again, created by someone else other than Kupka, produced in a computer following strict mathematical laws (Fig. 24). Kupka's images: Snapshots of fractal sequences. Kupka knew nothing about fractal geometry, this mathematical discipline was not around at that time.

Goethe's fractal mountains

Kupka worshiped Goethe. In Goethe's undated writings we can read [2] ... *there is a universal law from which all tangible matter is formed, and this law*

[1] The mathematician Thom was possibly flattered, but he thought Dalí lacked the necessary mathematical understanding. We overlook this point.

[2] Probably originated around 1817. Goethe, Volume 11.2, page 550, Hanser München.

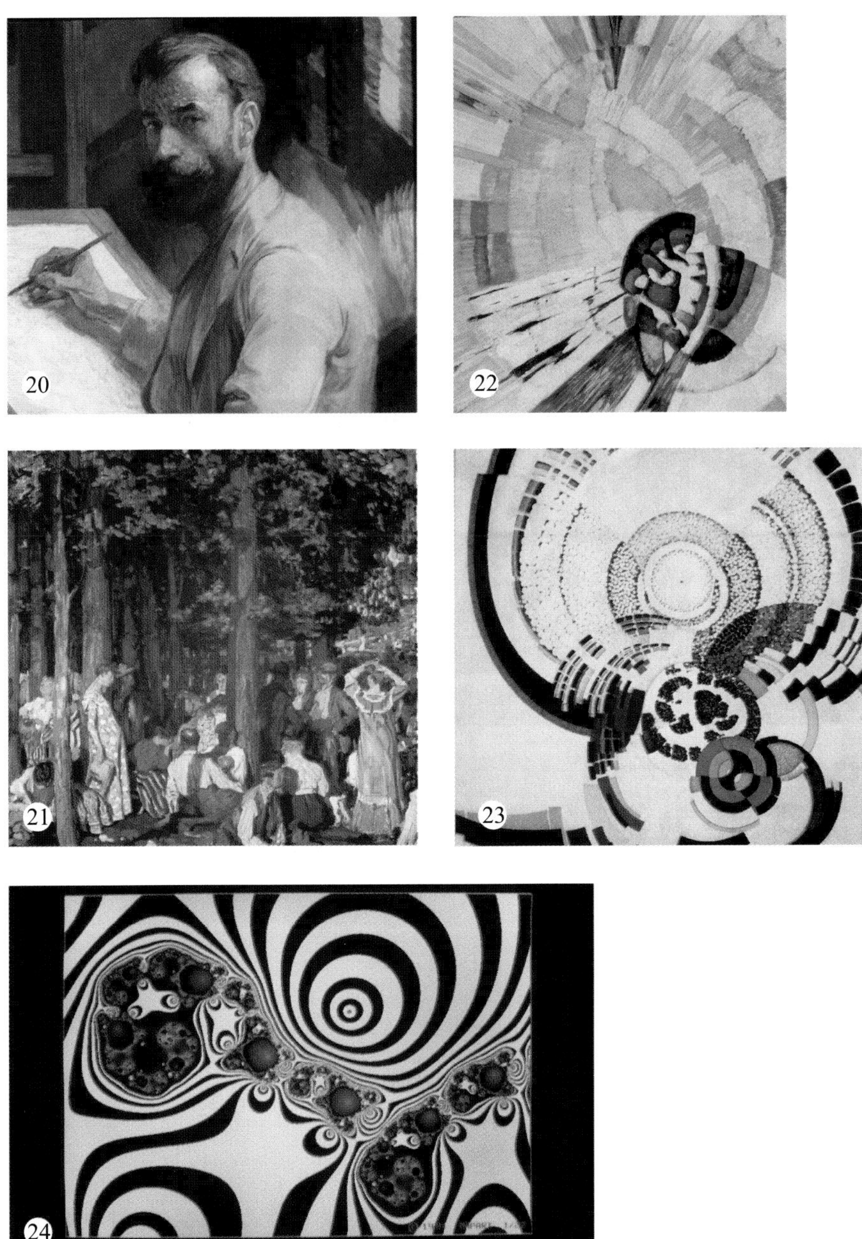

Figs. 20–24.

reveals to us the mountains. . . . The form of an object requires that it can, in some given manner, be separated into similar pieces. The inorganic is the geometrical foundation of the world.

Self-similar quantities. This is a familiar concept in the context of fractal geometry: if one subdivides collections of points (Fig. 25) following the laws of this field, and always subdividing more, thereby generating an infinite sequence of similar pieces (Fig. 26), one obtains amazing results (Fig. 27). Staying in two dimensions, there appear the outlines of continents (Fig. 28), coast lines (Fig. 29), surfaces like you might see in nature; if the output quantities are three-dimensional, one obtains, depending upon how the calculations were conducted, pictures of mountain formations (Fig. 30) and much, much more.

Mountain contours as the result of mathematical processes (Fig. 31) which are infinite sequences of self-similar parts. We cannot know what Goethe's

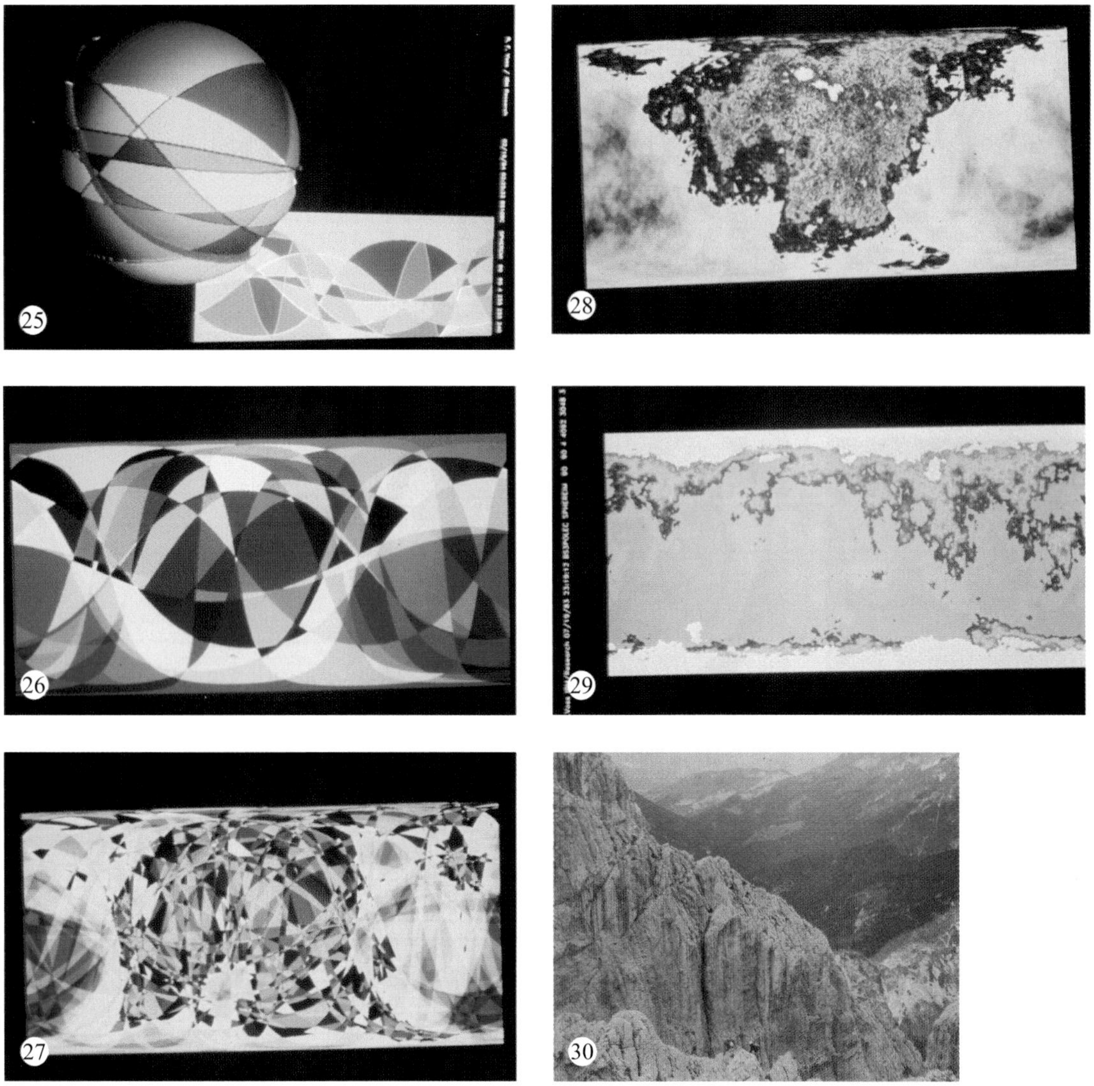

Figs. 25–30.

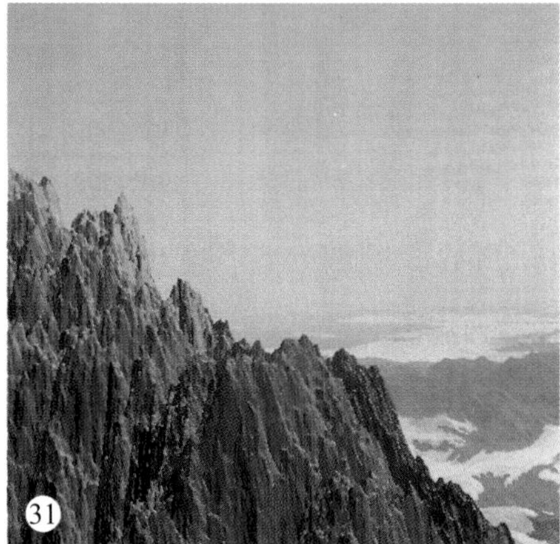

Fig. 31.

inner eye had seen, we can only look at pictures algorithmically produced according to mathematical laws on the computer. Goethe's sensual fantasies resulting in a connecting link between art and science. We are at least left with admiration for Goethe's insight and vision.

Image generation in computers

The *new archaeology, virtual trips into the past* is the title of a new book by Maurizio Forte and Alberto Siliotti. One can see the remains of ancient cultures (Fig. 32), familiar pictures, and right next to them reconstructions of these structures – generated in a computer. Let's have a look at some (Fig. 33).

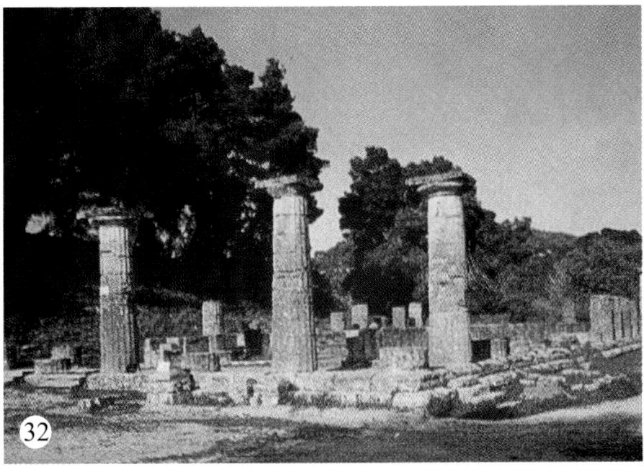

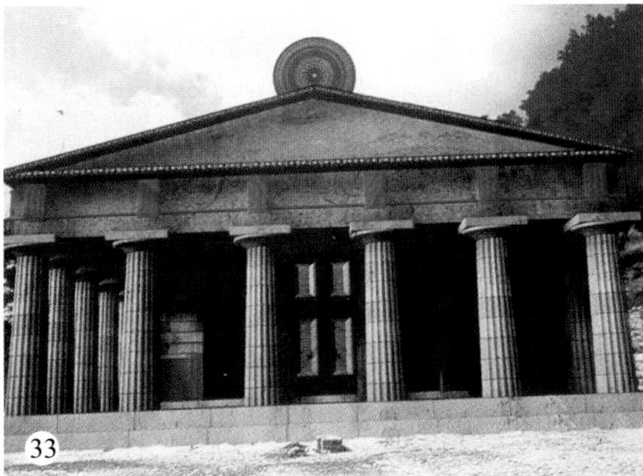

Figs. 32–33.

Virtual worlds. [3] The picture maker, picture generator is the computer, and with help from mathematics it's possible to calculate pictures of reality. That had been known for a long time; it didn't help much though, since mathematical structures could not be made visible. Today that is different. The powerful means available is the electronic computing machine. But how does the machine do it?

Cluny (Fig. 34), the large monastery in Burgundy with its enormous church the size of 5 ships, over 200 meters long and with seven towers, was destroyed in the French revolution. In the computer the church was built up again; Cramer and Koob documented it in their book. A wire model (Fig. 35) is created that takes forms (Fig. 36) down to regular basis elements (Fig. 37) of geometry and through unification and intersection establishes new forms. Individual components are bundled into component groups (Fig. 38), supports, arcades, halls, arches. Afterwards, they are "constructed together" again following the old, surviving plans (Fig. 39).

The necessary computational effort for the generation of the images is tremendous, especially when animated images need to be created. *Numerical Simulation,* the explicit solution of mathematical equations and its translation into images on computers following the laws of projective geometry, is of enormous significance for commercial applications. These include such key industries such as automotive and aerospace, space travel, and electronic and chemical industries. Progress in industrial production and research are no longer imaginable without numerical simulation.

[3] Virtual, from middle-latin "virtualis", existing with respect to forces but not in reality.

Faster computers through miniaturization

Higher performing computers were first made possible through the miniaturization of electrical components. Everything began in October 1957 as the Soviet Union shot its first satellite, the Sputnik, into orbit around the Earth. What a shock for the United States. A new space program was immediately established, and for this space program small computers were desperately needed. Luckily, the transistor was there, discovered in the Bell labs in 1947: two wires out of bronze phosphorous on a germanium crystal, and this made it possible to amplify weak electrical currents. Initially, there was no interest in transistors, but then in 1957, while in a sort of "emergency state," transistors started being built and being welded into circuits. They were, however, expensive to produce. Then came the idea to put everything together on a silicon plate using thin metal conduits for connectors. They called it a chip, a microchip. This microchip was built into NASA's Gemini rockets, and it continued to be used in every space program up until the Apollo program. In 1968, they could already place 64,000 tiny circuits on a chip.

Interestingly enough, space travel was responsible for pushing forward computer development through miniaturization.

High computing speeds and large memories

On a memory chip, a 4 Megabit chip, there are 4 million transistors packed tightly together. A 16 Megabit chip (Fig. 40) contains around 16 million

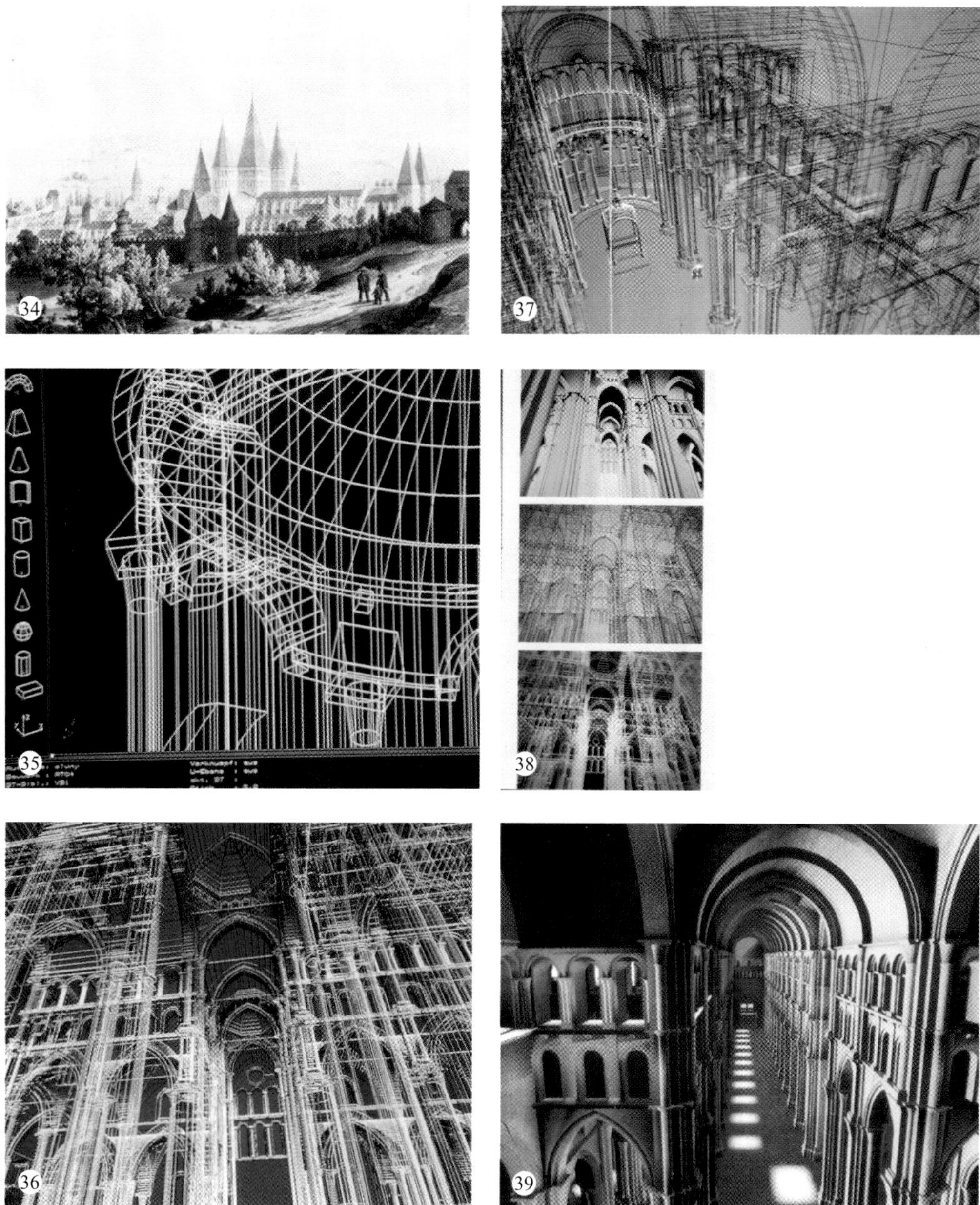

Figs. 34–39.

transistors inside the area of one penny. The whole Bible, Old and New Testaments together, can easily be saved on two of them. Of course, without any beautiful pictures, like for example those of Doré. Maybe twenty of those pictures would fit on a chip.

One of the newer ones is the 256 Megabit chip (Fig. 41) it is currently being marketed. You can store several seconds of a 35 mm color feature film on it. This new chip could also store all 80 of the new Bible pictures from the famous Viennese painter Ernst Fuchs on it.

Robots and automobile construction, the Moose test

Cars may be put together by robots, but they are designed on a computer. Chassis simulations for an automobile work like this. An automobile is

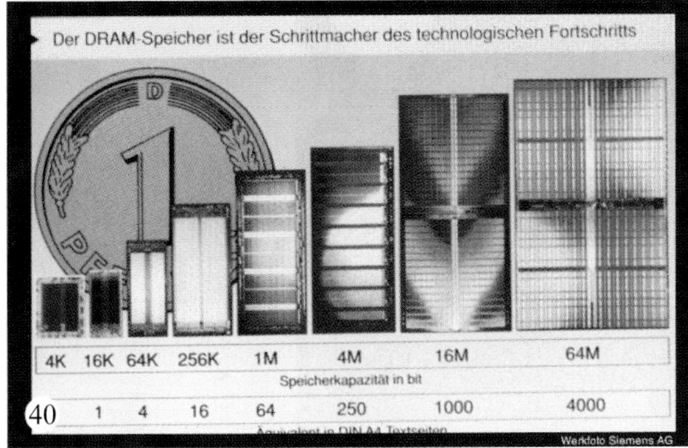

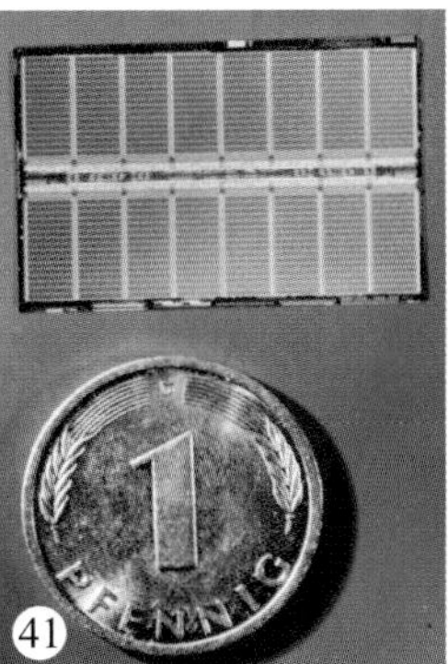

Figs. 40–41.

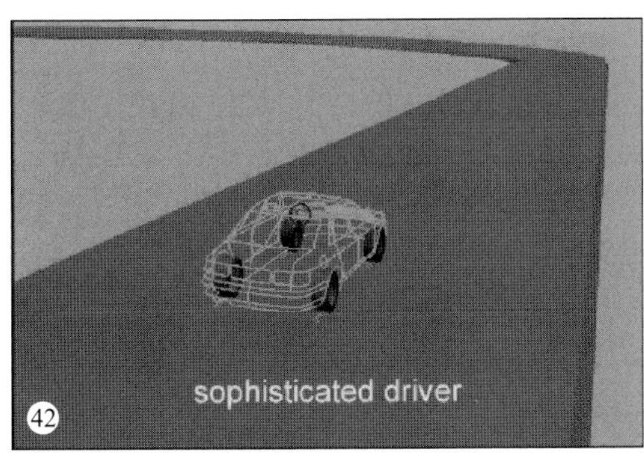

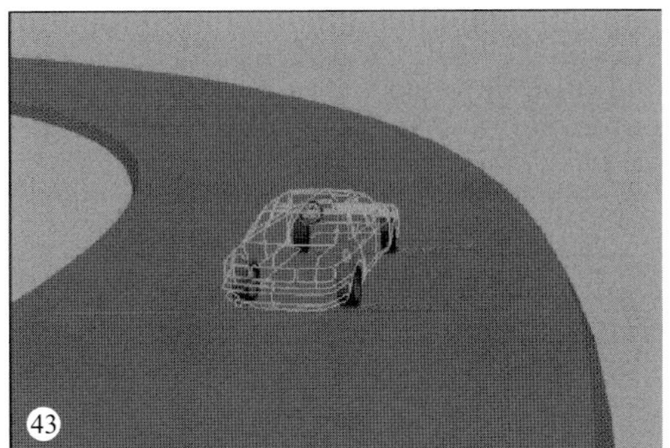

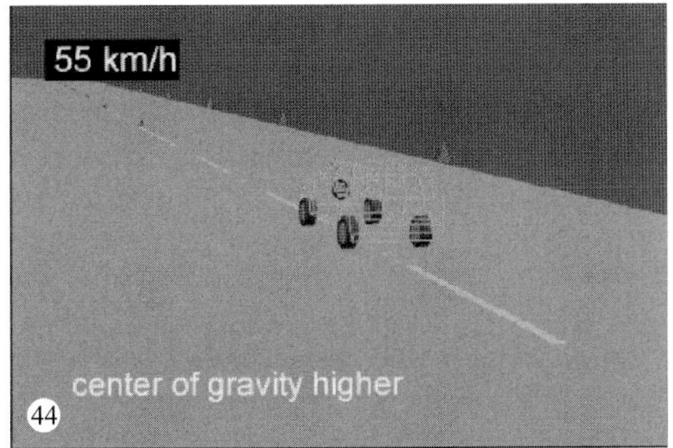

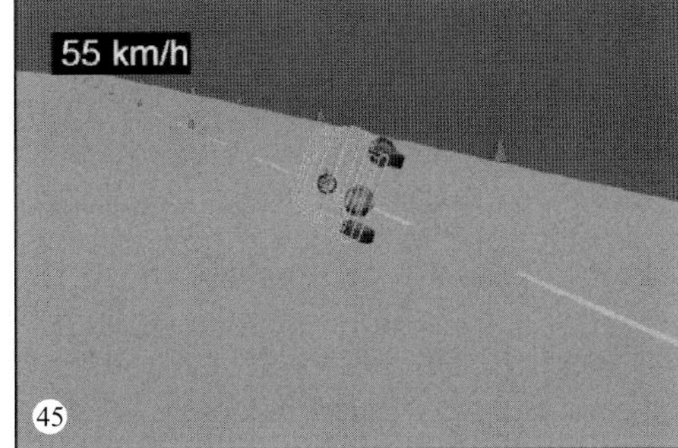

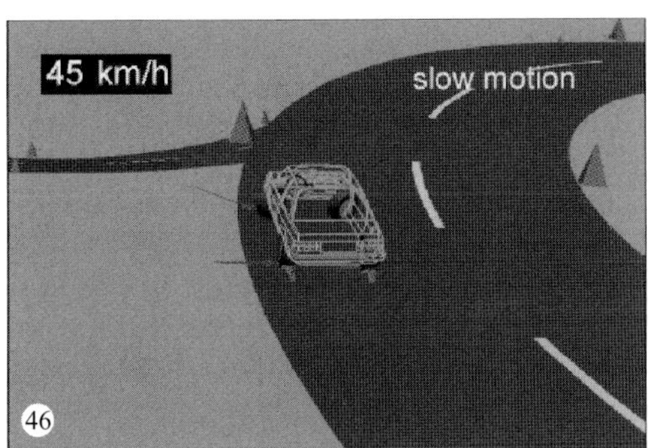

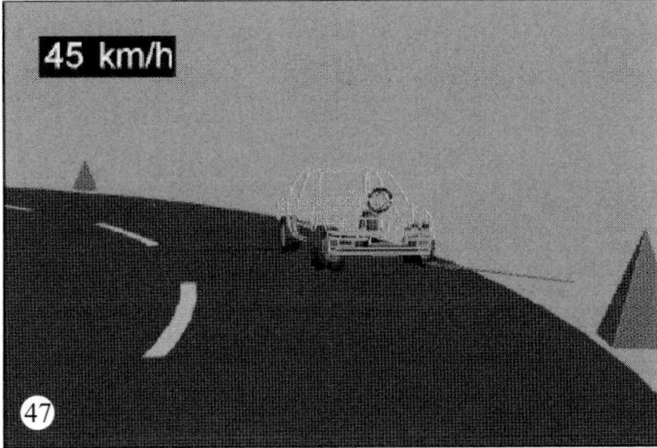

Figs. 42–47.

48

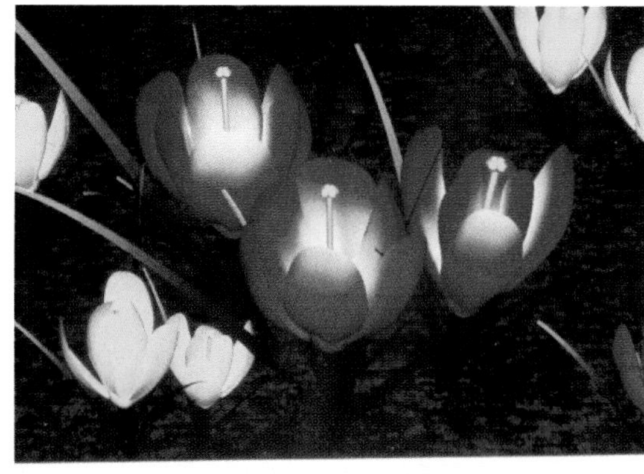

```
#define T_A 7                    /* developmental switch time */
#define T_L 9                    /* leaf growth limit */
#define T_K 5                    /* flower growth limit */
#include L(0),L(1),...,L(T_L)  /* leaf shapes */
#include K(0),K(1),...,K(T_K)  /* flower shapes */

ω  : a(1)
p1 : a(t)  : t<T_A  → F(1)[&(30)~L(0)]/(137.5)a(t+1)
p2 : a(t)  : t=T_A  → F(20)A
p3 : A     : *      → ~K(0)
p4 : L(t)  : t<T_L  → L(t+1)
p5 : K(t)  : t<T_K  → K(t+1)
```

49

Figs. 48 and 49.

designed with 56 variables in a mathematical coordinate grid. The movements of the front and rear axle, the tires, the motor block, the center of gravity, etc.: for every one of these movements there exists a variable as a function of time. 56 time-varying quantities for the car connected through the laws of mechanics by (differential) relationships. With fewer variables it doesn't work, more would be better. Icy conditions, ground unevenness, spring strength, steering inaccuracy, tire quality, and motor power to name only a few are given as parameters. The virtual car is sent onto a test track. A virtual driver uses a steering wheel, gas pedal, brakes and tries as quickly as possible to complete the test circuit. You can see the moving car on the screen, but this car is only the visual image of the solution of a system of 56 differential equations in a 56 dimensional solution space. On an ice sheet, this virtual car starts slipping, and by incorrect braking it loses control and flies out of the curve. The car on the screen behaves as truly as a real car on a test track (Figs. 42–47).

If the car (in the computer) is loaded poorly with additional weight with the center of gravity shifted upward, a disaster occurs. By forced slalom driving, the virtual car turns over like in reality. The mathematical solution predicts the accident even before the automobile is built.

Metamorphosis of plants in the computer

On the side of triangle we place a smaller triangle, and on its side an even smaller one, and so on infinitely often. Snowflakes (almost) look like that (Fig. 48). Another example: In a square we place a smaller square, and in this a smaller one, and keep doing this forever. Result? A curve which fills an entire square!

The laws by which both of these curves are created can be written according to a strict set of rules in the form of an algorithm. A computing machine can, in connection with a screen, make the thereby created curves visible.

The simple calculational rules may be altered in such a way that we move from a sheet of paper, the plane, into a 3-dimensional space. With each successive iteration, another spiral twist of the short sections of the curve may be undertaken. It is not required that the curve sections be of the same length: one can be made shorter, the other longer, leaving things up to chance. All of these things can be represented by a set of computer instructions, a so-called "string" (Fig. 49). The computing machine processes the algorithm. The result appears on the screen: It has a strong resemblance with a plant. We can make the rules more complicated, coloring the resulting image

```
#define S          /* seed shape */
#define R          /* ray floret shape */
#include M N O P   /* petal shapes */

ω  : A(0)
p1 : A(n) :  * → +(137.5)[f(n^0.5)C(n)]A(n+1)
p2 : C(n) :  n <= 440              → ~S
p3 : C(n) :  440 < n & n <= 565    → ~R
p4 : C(n) :  565 < n & n <= 580    → ~M
p5 : C(n) :  580 < n & n <= 595    → ~N
p6 : C(n) :  595 < n & n <= 610    → ~O
p7 : C(n) :  610 < n               → ~P
```

50

Figs. 50 and 51.

and thereby obtaining strange pictures which look extremely similar to plants. It depends sometimes only upon the insufficient resources at our disposal that they do not completely look like plants.

Goethe's metamorphosis of plants, the derivation of all plants from one primordial plant, follows the laws of contraction and stretching, with possibly a spiral twist, which all takes place in a vertical system. [4] In this way Goethe viewed the plant kingdom, and for that he earned the ridicule of his contemporaries and their followers. It affected Goethe deeply, but during all his life he clung confidently to this idea: *... like I was absorbed and driven by a passion, with which I must occupy myself through my entire remaining life. ...* Already in 1787, he wrote enthusiastically from Rome to Frau von Stein: *The primordial plant will be the most incredible creation in the world. ...* With ... *the key for it one can ... invent plants into infinity, ... which even though they might not exist ... will have an inner truth and consequence.*

Mathematical sciences deliver the key. The key: computer programs [5] in which "shrinking", "stretching", "rotation", "spiral twist" and other effects can be created algorithmically through geometrical transformations with the highest speed and in a large diversity. By the fixing of input parameters (Fig. 50), insertion of number combinations, the program creates images which look like natural plants. By changing the input parameters, one may obtain new plants. Also, by varying these parameters, a noticeable abundance of botanical objects can be created. Plant shapes, a virtual, artistic world out of the computer, a "materialized" idea from a primordial plant (Fig. 51).

Space travel

Modern mathematics and computer science can find important applications in space sciences. According to Ambros Speiser, the great engineer from ETH Zürich, it is called the *kings discipline of the engineers*. Within this field one may find problems such as the calculation of optimal flight paths to the planets and the transmission of images from space probes to Earth.

Life of the sun

Stars are born just like us. In the Orion nebula (Fig. 53) we can look into one of the cradles of creation; there we can see new stars, new suns which are

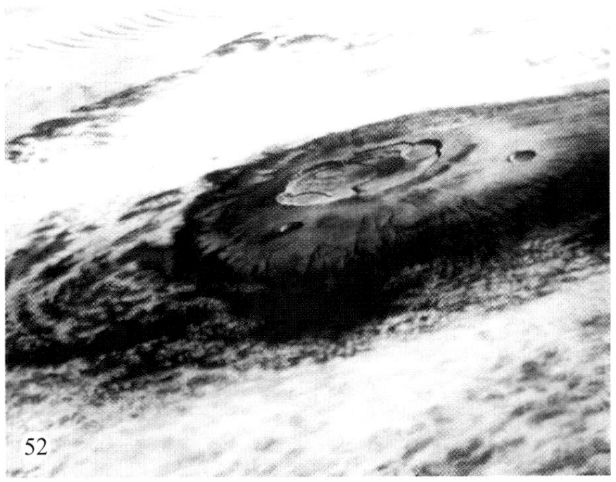

Fig. 52.

[4] For Schiller an "idea".

[5] See for example the plant modeling program of B. Lintermann and O. Deussen, xfrog (http://www.greenworks.de).

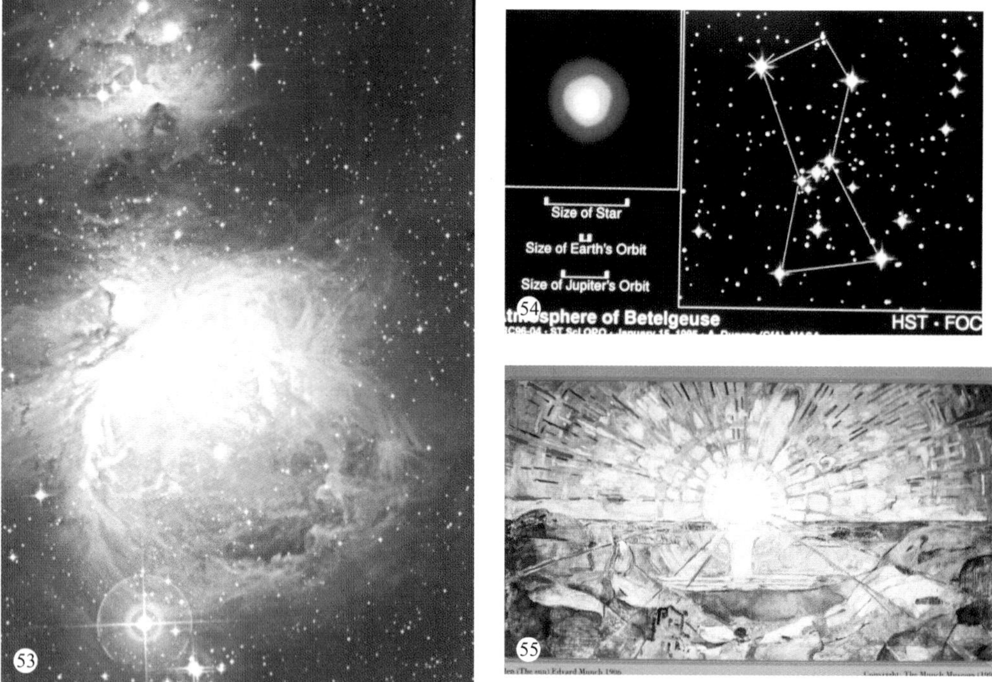

Figs. 53–55.

just being created. Stars, however, are also mortal – just like us. Large stars explode at the end of their lifetimes with an unimaginable power into a glowing ball of light. The shock waves emanating from the center of explosion rush then for millennia through the universe, compressing there any previously existing matter and giving birth to new stars. Our solar system was created, with high probability, as a consequence of the explosion of a giant star which would have happened an endless amount of time ago.

In the constellation of Orion, we can see a dying star (Fig. 54) a dying sun, the Betelgeuse (Alpha Orionis).

No star is for us so important as the sun (Fig. 55). Faust in Goethe's play watching the setting sun:
It sinks and fades away; the day is spent,
The sun moves on to nourish other life.
Sie rückt und weicht, der Tag ist überlebt
Dort eilt sie hin und fördert neues Leben.

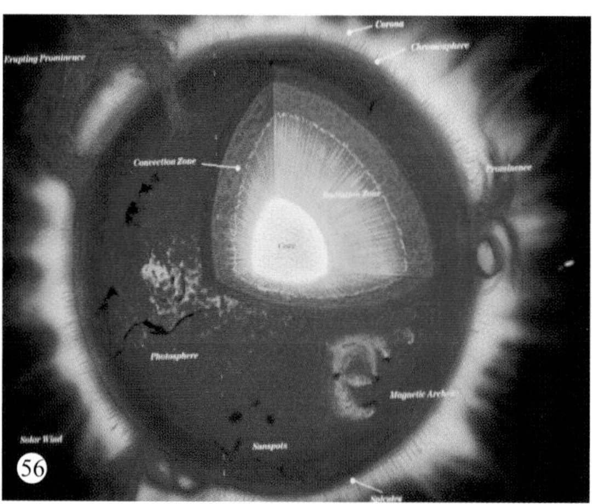

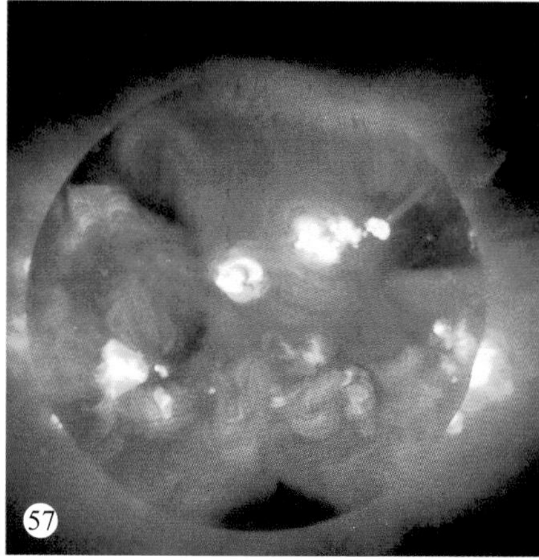

Figs. 56 and 57.

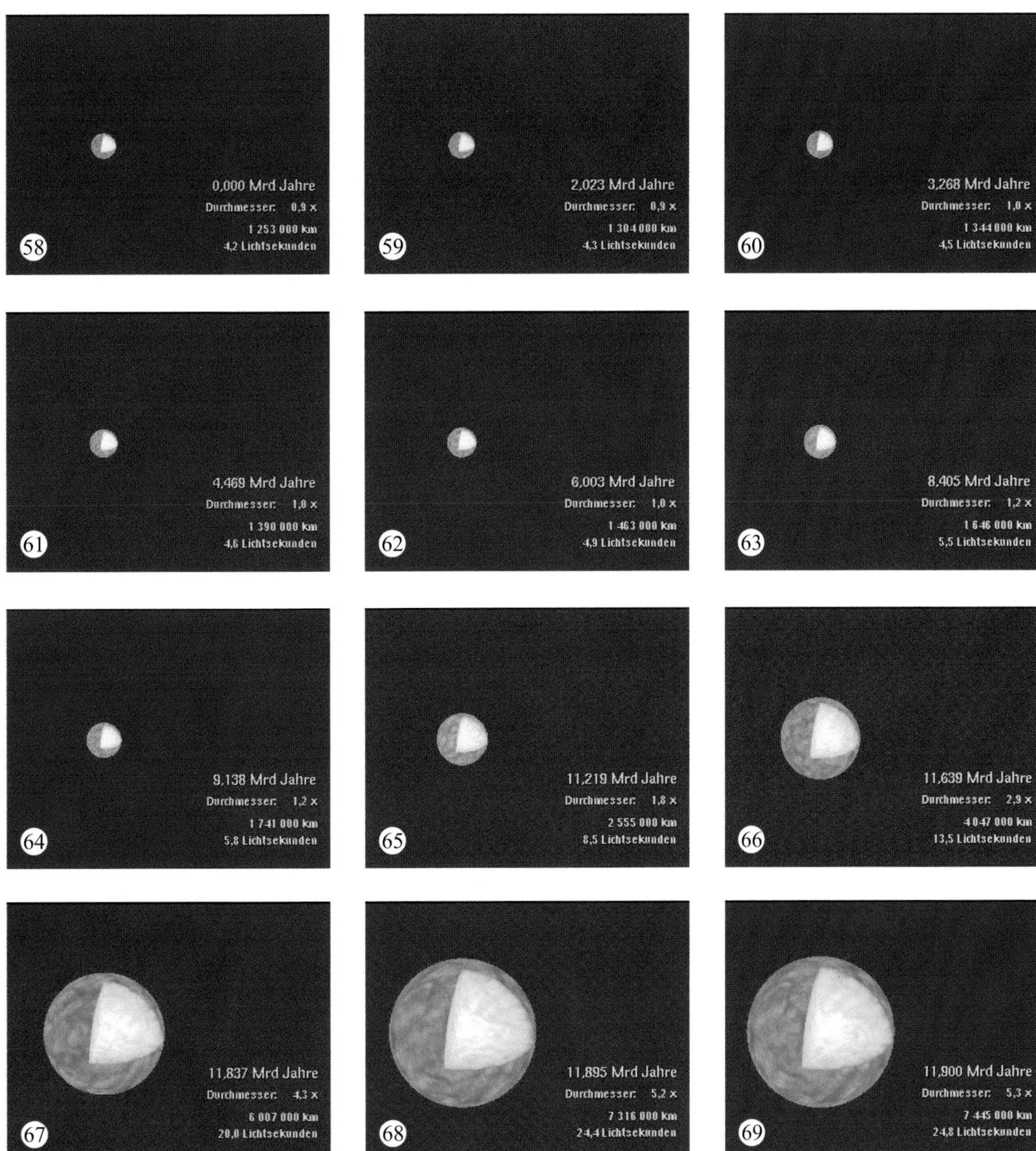

Figs. 58–69.

In the same play the archangel Raphael is praising the sun: [6]

Its vision gives the angels strength.

Ihr Anblick gibt den Engeln Stärke.

Deep in the sun's interior, hydrogen is converted by fusion into helium, and energy is thereby given off in the form of intense X-ray radiation. On the million-year long way to the sun's surface (Fig. 56) it will be converted into light and heat. In every second, 4 million tons of mass are transformed into radiation, and in every second the sun becomes 4 million tons lighter. But the sun is so huge that even after billions of years the loss is only very small. The gas pressure pushing outward and the gravitational force pulling inward keep the sun in a stable equilibrium.

The sun (Fig. 57): a ball made out of ionized hydrogen and helium floating freely in space; a

[6] Faust: Version 247.

self-regulating, gigantic nuclear reactor held together by its own gravity.

The life of a star can be described by a system of partial differential equations, whose calculated solutions for pressure, temperature, brightness, mass, chemical frequencies, etc. as given functions of state and time, describe the life of the sun. We solve the respective differential equations for the sun, a highly nonlinear system of partial differential equations of parabolic type. They will fill several pages if completely written out. It is a free boundary value problem with 3 free (moving) boundaries. The life of the sun: a story beginning with the ignition of nuclear fusion about four and a half billion years ago until its end in about seven and a half billion years from now, all to be seen in a computer. The earth will be able to support life for another one and a half billion years, an endlessly long time, then it will get so hot that the oceans evaporate. The sun will then shine for yet another 6 billion years, and before its end it will stretch out into a red shining giant star, which when viewed from Earth will take up almost half the sky and be so large that it extends past Mercury's orbit. The sun will then in quick succession eject gas clouds, pull itself together, stretch out again, eject new gas clouds. ... A planetary gas nebula is formed which will soon disappear into space, and a tiny but very heavy and slowly dying dwarf star is left behind. A cubic centimeter of mass from it would weigh about 12 tons.

Here we have the life of the sun on film [7] (Figs. 58–69). The film compresses the 12 billion years of life of the sun into a few minutes. On the same scale, the life of a hundred-year old person takes exactly 1 millionth of a second.

In order to get a better feeling for this large expanse of time, let us characterize a billion years as one kilometer, then the life of the sun will be 12 kilometers long, perhaps the distance to cross the city of Vienna. At the beginning of this 12-kilometer stretch corresponds the birth of the sun. If we start walking, after four and a half kilometers we will have reached the point in time of our own existence. In our last step, we would have passed over the one-half centimeter distance corresponding to all recorded history of the human race. The origin of the human species would lie only 4 meters away, and the lifespan of a 100-year old person would not be much thicker than that of a sheet of paper. Continuing our walk, we would have to be very optimistic if the human race will continue to exist for another meter, that is a million years. Life on Earth, in general, should continue for at least another kilometer after which the sun will continue to radiate energy for the last 6 km. Then at the milestone 12.3 km, our walk will end.

If the sun were only a little bit larger, the solutions of the mathematical equations show us that it would burn so fast that no life could develop on its planets. With only a 20% larger diameter, not even that much, after 1 billion years everything would be over for the sun. What if the sun had ten times as much mass? Already after a couple of million years – million, not billion – all the sun's fuel would be exhausted. If the sun were smaller, it would be better, but then it would not be hot enough and the planets would have to circle closer around it. They would be subjected to intensive X-ray radiation and powerful tides would rampage, all naturally extremely dangerous for life; life could never have developed.

Who could have built the sun better?

[7] In teamwork with the Max-Planck-Institute for Astrophysics, München.

Internet activism – Beyond Microsoft's walls

P. Weibel

In *How to Do Things With Words* (1962), linguist John L. Austin described the "performative" as a spoken expression that not only describes the world but changes it and creates new facts. The effectiveness of verbal action is tied to certain conditions. The most important of these aspects is context – the history, culture and legal system – to which it relates and from which the quote is derived. The performative derives its authority from all these aspects. The internet has established itself as a text medium and only secondarily as an image medium. Speech as text is its predominant form of action.

The text – which is entered via computers, then stored, processed and distributed – has a different relation to space and time to printed text: it can be accelerated, and displaced. The internet is a communications medium, not an archive; at the most it is an intermediate storage medium. Any document can be made available worldwide via a server within seconds and can be edited or read from anywhere in the world. It is normally not of any importance in which country the server is based. The time interval between production and publication of the text is reduced; the potential readership is not defined by its location but by its access to the infrastructure of information and communications' technology; its financial, educational and ideas background. This infrastructure, which enables rapid and dislocated communication, is not the a priori of the current political and economic distribution of power. It has, however, proved itself as the technical "dispositive" of the present, which is suspected of stabilising or radicalising the dominant condition, in the sense of an increased concentration of capital and power. The technical dispositive structures the actions of states, corporations and non-governmental organisations (NGOs), activists and groups of artists.

A new generation of artists is moving about in the data landscapes of networked computers and delivers critical insights into the results of the globally distributed processes that our society is built on. The global information space of our network, and not the framed blackboard image, is the new frame of reference, the arena of action. Artists' field of action has moved from the closed object of modern art to the open action arenas of the postmodern age. Through global information technology, new communities are formed that may have similar social structures in some sense but are not defined by their location. Art, which in the mid-20th century expanded its field of action from the picture to include physical space, now uses the data space too. Locally defined methods of production and perception of the classical arts have become non-local, telematic communication and action spaces. The aesthetics of processing and networking aim at re-civilising certain areas of the military and commercial complex of our information society. Artists in the net-world act as hackers and software experts in much the same way as guerrillas. They do not only bring the standards of civil society to the forefront but they implement these in the practical application of their software art.

Network-based artistic works represent the current form of art in which political hopes have been expressed most clearly in recent years. The socio-revolutionary utopias of historical avantgarde movements and enlightenment movements are supposed to become reality with the help of the new internet technology – which, like the telegraph, the railway, the telephone, etc stirred into life social visions of emancipation and justice [1]. Network-based art is currently the clearest form of action, which transforms the closed system of the aesthetic object of the modern age radically into the open system of the arenas of action of the postmodern age. Art that sees itself as a form of action with a social dimension will give its attention to forces that structure society, and thus to those technologies that it discovers for itself and that in turn transform it. The already noticeable and future changes brought about by the information and communications' technologies were the subject of my ZKM-exhibition *net_condition* as early as 1999. Here, works of art based on networking technologies were presented that reflected the new conditions at an aesthetic, economic and social level.

Artists react to the fundamental effects of information technology, which cannot be separated from the global economy. The ascent of neo-liberalism is also based on the global expansion of information technology. It produces a fourth world, as Manuel Castells called it [2], which is excluded from the global information flow and which may be encountered on a selective basis even in the current first, second and third worlds. The mega-fusions of large telecommunications and information technology companies, of print and electronic media, of content providers and distribution companies aim at controlling the technology as well as determining the hierarchy of the contents for which it is the vehicle. The artists and activists of the internet culture see the use of the internet as a historic opportunity to make communications' technology available to the emancipated citizen, i.e. the individual who has rights, and thereby to free the technology from the dictates of money, commerce and the military. Net-based art is trying to contribute to re-civilising global media technology by criticising the economic, social and technical conditions and limitations of the internet, analysing software, and attacking the global monopoly of software and hardware and the adoption of the new media by corporations. Internet-based activism acts at the level of the technical dispositive itself, i.e. in the network, via distributing network-based documents and software and by attacking hardware, but it also uses the digital action space to organise criticism and protest in real space in a new way and to speed it up. Beyond sensitising or alerting and educating users, network activism uses digital blockade or sabotage as well as innovative forms of political mobilisation.

Enlightenment and informing

The attacks by artists' groups are directed, for example, against the norms of technology itself but also against the monopolists implementing these norms. Their resistance in its most basic form is directed against the browser, the programme that enables graphic representation of the information that is accessible via the worldwide web, but which also determines how the signs are represented, and therefore interprets them and determines their effect. The formal commitment to the commercial browsers of Netscape and Microsoft, which are used by more than 90% of users, is interrupted by artists' re-programmed browsers. Although media artists are subject to the development and sales strategies of software manufacturers to a much greater extent than any other user (media art always justifies its existence with its technological advances, among others), media art aims at emancipation in acquiring and customising products, especially software, to an individual's own aesthetic and functional ideas. The explicit aim of avantgarde artists and internet activists is to leave the role of the consumer by descending to the source code of the purchased product or even to produce the source code. Art is to be seen not only as the consumption of ready-bought products but as a productive, selective force. The browser as the interpreter of the information on the net was at the centre stage of artistic interest even before the "browser war" between Netscape and Microsoft in 1997. In 1997, I/O/D presented their art project "web stalker"[3], which linked seamlessly to the events in the browser war. It was offered for downloading free of charge and could, at least in theory, be used as an alternative to the commercial products. Instead of showing the familiar HTML interpretation of a web page, however, it showed the structure of the internal and external links of a selected web page.

The user was encouraged to leave the closed surface of the normal product. While Netscape and Microsoft adapted their browsers to the reading habits of their users, to enable them to switch to the internet from traditional media more easily, the web stalker depicts graphically the characteristics of the worldwide web.

Another example is the "netomat" [4], conceived by artist and programmer Mciej Wisniewski as a work of art. This also tries to overcome the limitations of standard web browsers and shows new ways of using information. It detaches images, texts and sounds from the existing web pages and connects them to a flowing net that changes constantly when new search terms are used. "Netomat" is open-source software and can be modified by anyone. Its creators put their main emphasis on the fact that uncountable interfaces and functions can be developed by the worldwide community of users.

Jodi, the pseudonym used by artists Joan Heemskerk and Dirk Paesmans, subverts the normed user surface with desktop, trash bin, and pull-down menus by programming non-semantic events, gestures of destruction, which make interacting in the sense of a targeted instruction with a processor impossible. The programme has to be read as a dysfunction of the computer. The unfathomability and the abstraction of information processing become visible. The artists, who have been working on the worldwide web since 1995, force web users, for example, with "7061.jodi.org", to explore their machines virtually, to leave the user surface and therefore step out of their self-inflicted immaturity. Examining the specific material conditions of the web serves as a confrontation with the socio-economic forces that force particular hardware and software upon us. The aesthetic intervention aims at the structure of everyday life by software as a technical given that cannot be selected freely.

The emancipatory attitude inherent in disrupting the consumer perspective essentially depends on artists' technical know-how and ability to write programmes. These determine the scope and decide whether the artist remains at the level of the consumer. Protest is formulated in explicitly artistic ways of acting and programming strategies, as seen for example in Jodi's work, whereas the group "etoy" (www.etoy.com) or members of the group RTMark [5] act in an overtly political way. The objective is an emancipated society, whose means of cultural production does not depend on the monopoly of corporations. The internet is the ideal place to express resistance as access is principally open. Organisations that are independent of governments (NGOs or artists) can encounter corporations in a space that is, at least in theory, not subject to hierarchical structures. The resistance movement uses the same media as those that it criticises. Groups such as "etoy" or RTMark choose the appearance of their opponents in order to criticise these. Copyright, trademarks, concepts of the market economy are elements that are being used subversively against the keepers of these rights, marks, or concepts.

Since 1994, the website of the net group "etoy" has copied the appearance of a real e-commerce enterprise, "etoy.corporation." Users can find out about product offers and fluctuations in the share value of the company and invest in it. Predecessors in terms of copying political structures or artists organising themselves in fictitious enterprises date back to as early as the beginning of the 20th century – for example, the fictitious companies of the Dadaists, who made their companies "real" with business cards and newspaper advertisements. "etoy" mimics and thereby analyses in a playful manner the mechanisms of the New Economy. Its criticism is directed at the shareholder value, which became obvious in the "Toywar" between the toy manufacturer "eToys" and the artists' group "etoy".

"etoy" also contributed to the browser war. For the project "Digital-Hijack," the most popular word combinations used in search engines were analysed. "etoy" offered search engines sites on its server to help users to do so. Users clicked on a result found by the search engine and, reached instead of, for example, a pornography site, an "etoy" server. The message displayed was "Don't fucking move. This is a digital hi-jack." The return button was invalidated. "etoy" intended this action to point at inattentive users who are not aware that they are being manipulated by the big software manufacturers, but mainly by search engine companies. A few big corporations – Yahoo and Altavista among the search engines, Netscape among the browsers, and Microsoft among the operating system manufacturers – have had control over their users for quite some time. The artists' criticism is, however, also directed against the users themselves, against their uncritical and passive use of the new medium. "etoy" makes transparent the functional particularities of the internet, especially its search engines, which promise access to a non-hierarchically defined medium but in reality enforce directed search results.

RTMark act on the internet as a platform for the most diverse forms of cultural sabotage. The appearance of the group in the worldwide web since 1997 is similar to the unspectacular appearance of any enterprise. RTMark emphasises that it is not possible any more to position oneself into the great tradition of resistance as has evolved historically against political power. The power of the corporations under criticism is fundamentally different in that their position cannot be seen clearly, and they cannot be attacked as opponents. Since RTMark operates as a commercial company, its members benefit from its limited liability, which is a legal requirement in the USA. A project from the environment of RTMark was targeting the influence of Microsoft on the education system. Andy Mingo, a student in English and comparative literature at San Diego University, developed as a term project a website entitled www.microsoftecu.com (RTMark project SOFT). Microsoft challenged him to remove the site immediately as it infringed the company's copyright. Mingo declared his project an attempt at exploring the postmodern age through the appropriation of literature, in which he had decided to appropriate Microsoft in a satirical manner. Microsoft did not pursue its challenge. "I've been waiting a long time to prove that Microsoft is committed to technological diversity in our universities and diversity in general," Andy Mingo writes with irony on his website.

"Microsoft isn't only a supporter of diversity, they're concerned with protecting the environment and upholding the freedom of speech, which contains within its walls postmodern theory and narrative appropriation–artistic practice is a mode of production." [7]

Josh on and the FutureFarmers (USA) show with "They Rule"[8] how, by visualising databases, the relations between the most influential economic forces can be laid open. Users can browse through a selection of cards that depict the links between corporations and their management. Board members are shown with small icons depicting briefcases, which contain information about themselves and their companies – for example, about donations to politicians. "They Rule" uses the attributes of network technology, such as dynamic mapping and hyperlinks, and thus creates a sub-network of the power system. "They Rule" shows the network of those who rule. Microsoft, for example, is placed within this network of power, linked to the corporations Merck, Hewlett-Packard, Boeing, etc. "They Rule" attempts to transgress the internet as a mere marketing tool and reminds us of the medium's original promise to be a democratising medium. The internet is being used as a weapon of Enlightenment or informing against the network of power.

Artistic projects of network activism create new documents, software and user interfaces that visualise the technical conditions of computer-based communications on the one hand, and those that show the power structures and inextricable intertwining with technology – for example, in the area of search engines, through which an infinite amount of information is indexed. Hence the insight of Philip Quéau, who demanded that technologies that have as great an influence on life as laws should undergo an examination and create tools for a new Enlightenment [9].

Digital attacks

Network activism can transcend enlightenment in the sense of instruction and conveying of insights, to pushing through demands, as has been proved by "Etoy's" "toywar". The US toy manufacturer "Etoys" withdrew its lawsuit against the artists' group "etoy" after it had effected a preliminary court decision in November 1999 to prohibit "etoy" from using its domain name "www.etoy.com". "eToys", an US online shop for children's toys, which offers its services at the URL "www.etoys.com", had felt that the similarity of its own name to the name of the internet artists had affected the company's business. What followed in the months after is an example for the possibility of virtual resistance. The existing international web community was informed via mailing lists about all ideas and action plans and reacted on a massive scale. In the first night, the access screens of "eToys" website were bombarded with protest messages. Shortly afterwards, RTMark started its "professional revolt". The resistance culminated in the "toywar platform" at the end of that year, through which actions against the toyshop were coordinated and to which about 1800 "soldiers" from all over the world subscribed during the "war", to demonstrate the scale of the protest. The website also contained messages to participate in investor forums. Investors were encouraged to sell "eToys" stocks and shares and potential investors not to buy them. On the website "Quit eToys!", RTMark made available the email addresses of "eToys"'s employees, who were to be motivated to quit their jobs. In addition, a list of alternative online toyshops was offered.

In addition to these well-known patterns of protest and informing, readers were asked to support acts of digital sabotage: Through virtual "sit-ins". The website of "eToys" was blocked and therefore made inaccessible to others. To achieve this, as many activists as possible had to log on simultaneously to a particular internet site at a certain time. Such sit-ins were limited to 15 minutes but served more as a warning strike than a total blockade. In addition the script "killertoy.html" was made available, which can be installed on any server or personal computer and helps to keep filling the "eToy" shopping basket without ever confirming the purchase. This forced the webserver of "eToys" to calculate ever-growing lists and reduced its power. Announced and time-limited "distributed denial of service attacks" (DdoSA) are among the methods of network activists that may cause great potential harm to enterprises, no matter whether the inquiries blocking the server stem from programmes or individuals. "Electronic blockage can cause financial stress that physical blockage cannot"[10], according to the Critical Art Ensemble, which in 1999 coined the term ECD (electronic civil disobedience). Beyond the artistic context, electronic blockade has become an established "weapon" that was used to protest against German airline Lufthansa for its cooperation in turning away asylum seekers as well as against the World Trade Organisation (WTO). The power of international organisations and corporations is dispersed, strategic resistance is adapting, decentralised power is being fought with decentralised means [11].

Artistic and political action become intertwined. An example for this is the global internet activism of Mexico's Zapatistas and their followers. Since their revolt in 1994, Zapatistas have been using the internet to distribute emails from the leader, Subcommander Marcus, about the living conditions in Chiapas. Supporters of the Zapatistas have put up internet websites and discussion groups with reports on the situation vis-à-vis human rights in Chiapas, which are updated on a daily basis. Two of these activists, Stefan Wray and Ricardo Dominguez, are members of the group Electronic Disturbance Theater (EDT), which has become known for its software FloodNet. Since 1998, EDT has, among others, attacked the Mexican government website for the continued, covert war against Zapatistas in Mexico's south, with its Flood Net software. FloodNet relies on mass participation and automatically calls up the website that is to be attacked. If enough people participate in a FloodNet attack, the server is overwhelmed by inquiries and cannot cope with the volume. The website is consequently inaccessible. The attack was directed against the site of Mexico's government but also against the Pentagon, as the US Ministry of Defense had sold helicopters to Mexico's army that had been used in Chiapas. The real political effectiveness of the action is not in taking a website out of action temporarily but in attracting the attention of the media. As Ricardo Dominguez said:

"We began to notice that 1980s activist tactics were getting less media attention. Power had shifted from the streets to the information highway, so we started thinking about how to create political gestures on the web equivalent to lying down in the street and refusing to move." [12].

Network activism covers a wide spectrum, from the temporary and relatively harmless attack that becomes effective only via television, radio and newspapers, to something approaching information warfare, which can cause substantial financial harm to enterprises.

Protest >real space

The internet has created communities as well as new forms of enlightenment and informing and demonstration of resistance, which are expressed in digital attacks on the internet's infrastructure. It has also invisibly transformed traditional forms of protest taking to the streets, via global mobilisation of interest groups. With the help of the convergence of the internet and the mobile phone, a hitherto unknown degree of resistance against free trade was initiated on the occasion of the third conference of the WTO in Seattle in late 1999. The demonstrators had organised themselves online. Groups could form and disperse quickly and through networking could keep a clear overview of the situation. In Seattle, the first of now 30 independent media centres was founded, whose freelance writers, armed with laptop and mobile phone, reported speedily and independently about the protest.

Howard Rheingold called the groups that form when computer and communications' technologies that strengthen human beings' capacity for communication, "smart mobs". These can be used to support democracy but also to attack it [13]. The increasing integration of mobile telephones, computers and cameras into small, portable devices has the potential to transform the process of demonstrating as well as reporting such events, since they can subvert the regime of the mass media.

"Flashmobs" are a current example for the changed scope of action in public spaces. The term describes brief, seemingly spontaneously occurring groupings of people in public and semi-public places. They are organised through weblogs, newsgroups and email chain letters. They do decidedly not represent political ideas. Howard Rheingold's vision of the next social revolution, which can be initiated technologically, therefore seems remote. Participants follow an internet message and meet in a place where they receive further instructions as to the actual place of action and the proceedings. Typical of flashmobs are the sudden formation of a crowd from nothing, identical actions (for example, applauding, making telephone calls by using the same script, etc), and the sudden dispersal after a few minutes. In Juli, 200 people suddenly congregated in the mezzanine of the New York Hyatt Hotel, applauded for 15 seconds, and then disappeared [14].

Authority without force

The fascination of the electronic bourgeois resistance lies in the hope that the principle of "mystical foundation of authority" (Derrida) [15] and the law, the principle of force can be broken. The internet as a medium contains the utopian idea that reality can be changed through textual and visual performances without having to extract authority from an institution or legal framework that was originally formed by force. The idea is that spontaneous appointments between individuals who communicate via the internet can create new agreements that abolish the traditional ones without using force and without merely concealing the force used in their formation, as has happened in democratic state systems.

Derrida, in "Force of Law: 'The Mystical Foundation of Authority" pointed out that even the expression "to enforce the law" shows that force is inherent in justice as a right. It is therefore the foundation of any act of political performance. No law exists without applicability and therefore force. Derrida asks what the distinction is between the "force of the law" as a legitimate force and the "original act of force" that has installed this power without being able to resort to existing law and therefore can be neither legal nor illegal. His question is targeting the foundation of any law. Derrida quotes Pascal in that if one follows reason, nothing is "just" in and by itself [16]. Someone who follows back justice to its principles destroys it. Citing Montaigne, Derrida concludes: "Laws have authority because they are laws. This is the mystical foundation of authority and there is no other. As laws, laws are just. People follow them, however, not because they are just but because they possess authority. Montaigne speaks of "legitimate fictions" that the law contains; these are what the truth of justice/the legislative is based on. The origin of authority, the setting of the law is "an "un-"founded act of violence", [17] which is neither legal nor illegal. Even if performative acts that found the law (foundation of state) succeed and thus assume existing agreements (for example, in the international sphere), the "mystical" borderline is visible where these conditions originate. The structure is a structure in which the law can be deconstructed in its essence, because its final foundation is by definition un-founded. "That the law can be deconstructed is not a disaster," according to Derrida, but a political opportunity [18]. Through the internet and the convergence of computers and mobile communications, opportunities present themselves to negotiate agreements and make decisions. At a technical level, for the development of new standards for information and communications' technology, this has been practised for a long time, and the standards have been successfully defended against monopolists. In the political and social arena, a new negotiation space is coming into view, beyond authority that is based on force.

References

[1] Vgl. Armand Mattelard, "Une éternelle promesse: les paradis de la communication", in: Le Monde diplomatique 1995/1, Paris 1995

[2] Castells, Manuel, End of Millennium, Oxford: Blackwell Publishers 1998, S. 165

[3] (http://www.backspace.org/iod/),

[4] http://www.netomat.net/began.html

[5] http://www.rtmark.com/

[6] vgl. Reinhald Grether, "How the etoy Campaign was Won. An Agent's Report", in: Peter Weibel, Timothy Druckrey (Hg.), net_condition, MIT-Press, Cambridge/ Mass. 2001

[7] http://www.microsoftedu.com/FAQ.html

[8] http://www.theyrule.net

[9] Quéau, Phillipe, "Das globale Gemeinwohl", in: Florian Rötzer, Megamaschine Wissen: Vision: Überleben im Netz, Frankfurt/New York 1999, S. 218 f.

[10] Critical Art Ensemble, Electronic Civil Disobedience and other Unpopular Ideas. New York 1996, S. 18

[11] Critical Art Ensemble, Electronic Civil Disobedience and other Unpopular Ideas. New York 1996, S. 23

[12] Ricardo Dominguez. In: Jeanne Carstensen, 'Hey, Ho, We Won't Go – Civil Disobedience Comes to the Web', in: Nettime <http://www.nettime.org/>

[13] Howard Rheingold, Smart mobs: the next social revolution, Cambridge: Perseus 2003

[14] Maureen Ryan, "All in a flash: Meet, mob and move on," in: Chicago Tribune, 11. Juli 2003

[15] Jacques Derrida, Der "mystische Grund der Autorität", Frankfurt am Main: Suhrkamp 1991

[16] Jacques Derrida, Der "mystische Grund der Autorität", Frankfurt am Main: Suhrkamp 1991, S. 24 ff.

[17] Jacques Derrida, Der "mystische Grund der Autorität", Frankfurt am Main: Suhrkamp 1991, S. 29

[18] Jacques Derrida, Der "mystische Grund der Autorität", Frankfurt am Main: Suhrkamp 1991, S. 29

Subject Index

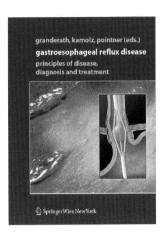

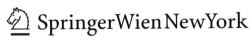

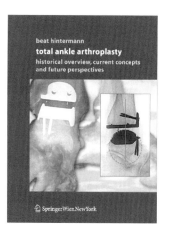

Springer-Verlag and the Environment

We at Springer-Verlag firmly believe that an international science publisher has a special obligation to the environment, and our corporate policies consistently reflect this conviction.

We also expect our business partners – printers, paper mills, packaging manufacturers, etc. – to commit themselves to using environmentally friendly materials and production processes.

The paper in this book is made from no-chlorine pulp and is acid free, in conformance with international standards for paper permanency.